Realities of Canadian Nursing

PROFESSIONAL, PRACTICE, AND POWER ISSUES

Realities of Canadian Nursing

PROFESSIONAL, PRACTICE, AND POWER ISSUES

Marjorie McIntyre, RN, PhD
Professor
University of Victoria
Victoria, British Columbia

Carol McDonald, RN, PhD
Associate Professor
University of Victoria
Victoria, British Columbia

Edition
4

Wolters Kluwer | Lippincott Williams & Wilkins
Health

Philadelphia · Baltimore · New York · London
Buenos Aires · Hong Kong · Sydney · Tokyo

Acquisitions Editor: Christina C. Burns
Product Manager: Annette Ferran
Editorial Assistant: Zack Shapiro/Dan Reilly
Production Manager: Priscilla Crater
Design Coordinator: Holly Reid McLaughlin
Illustration Coordinator: Brett McNaughton
Manufacturing Coordinator: Karin Duffield
Production Services/Compositor: Aptara, Inc.

4th Edition

9 8 7 6 5 4 3 2 1

Printed in China

Library of Congress Cataloging-in-Publication Data
Realities of Canadian nursing : professional, practice, and power issues / [edited by]
Marjorie McIntyre, Carol McDonald. – 4th ed.
    p. ; cm.
  Includes bibliographical references.
  ISBN 978-1-60913-687-1
  I. McIntyre, Marjorie, RN, Ph. D. II. McDonald, Carol.
  [DNLM: 1. Nursing–Canada. 2. Nurses–Canada. WY 16 DC2]
  LC classification not assigned
  610.730971–dc23

                                        2012036191

RRS1211

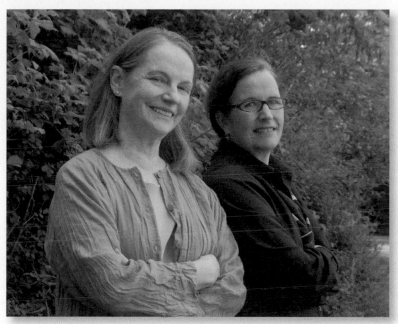

Authors Marjorie McIntyre (left) and Carol McDonald (right).

Marjorie McIntyre, RN, PhD, attended the Royal Alexander School of Nursing in Edmonton and practised in both acute care and community settings. She earned a BN at the University of Victoria, an MN at the University of British Columbia, and a PhD at the University of Colorado in Denver. She is currently a Professor at the University of Victoria in the School of Nursing, where her interests include issues in health and healthcare, leadership in nursing education, and curriculum design.

Carol McDonald, RN, PhD, is currently an Associate Professor at the University of Victoria School of Nursing. Following a 20 year practice career in mental health nursing, Carol earned a PhD in nursing from the University of Calgary. Among her current interests are nursing education, philosophical hermeneutics, and issues for nonheterosexual people in the healthcare system.

Contributors

Pat Armstrong, PhD
Distinguished Research Professor of Sociology
York University
Toronto, Ontario
Chapter 9

Anne Bruce, RN, PhD
Associate Professor
University of Victoria, School of Nursing
Victoria, British Columbia
Chapter 20

Laurel Brunke, RN, MSN, BScN
Registrar/Chief Executive Officer
College of Registered Nurses of British Columbia
Vancouver, British Columbia
Chapter 8

W. Dean Care, RN, MEd, EdD
Professor and Dean
Brandon University
Brandon, Manitoba
Chapter 13

Wanda M. Chernomas, RN, PhD
Associate Professor
University of Manitoba
Winnipeg, Manitoba
Chapter 13

Susan Duncan, RN, MSN, PhD
Associate Professor
Thompson Rivers University
Victoria, British Columbia
Chapter 26

Noreen Frisch, BSN, MSN, MSW, PhD
Professor and Director
University of Victoria, School of Nursing
Victoria, British Columbia
Chapter 19

Angela Gillis, PhD, RN
Professor
St. Francis Xavier University
Antigonish, Nova Scotia
Chapters 12 and 24

Judith Skelton-Green, RN, MSN, PhD, FCCHSE
President
Transitions: HUD Consultants Inc.
Penetanguishene, Ontario
Chapter 6

David Michael Gregory, RN, PhD
Faculty of Nursing
University of Regina
Regina, Saskatchewan
Chapter 13

Karen MacKinnon, RN, MScN, PhD
Assistant Professor
University of Victoria, School of Nursing
Victoria, British Columbia
Chapter 18

Kathryn McPherson, PhD
Associate Professor
York University
Toronto, Ontario
Chapter 10

Gail Mitchell, RN, PhD
Professor of Nursing
York University
Toronto, Ontario
Chapter 5

Andrea Monteiro, RN, MN
PhD Student
University of Victoria, School of Nursing
Victoria, British Columbia
Chapter 24

Jacinthe Pépin, RN, PhD
Professor
Université de Montréal
Montreal, Quebec
Chapter 3

Olga Petrovskaya, RN, BScN
Doctoral Candidate
University of Victoria
Victoria, British Columbia
Chapter 14

Joy Richards, RN, PhD
Vice President of Professional Affairs,
    Chief Nurse Executive
University Health Network
Toronto, Ontario
Chapter 5

Margaret Scaia, RN, BScN, MN
Senior Instructor
University of Victoria, School of Nursing
Victoria, British Columbia
Chapter 10

Judith Shamian, RN, PhD, LLD (Hon),
DSc (Hon), FAAN
President and CEO
VON Canada
Ottawa, Ontario
Chapter 6

Linda Silas, RN, BSCN
President
Canadian Federation of Nurses Unions
Ottawa, Ontario
Chapter 9

Janet Storch, RN, BSCN, MHSA, PhD,
DSc (Hon), LLD (Hon)
Professor Emeritus
University of Victoria, School of Nursing
Victoria, British Columbia
Chapter 2

Sally Thorne, RN, PhD, FCAHS
Professor Emeritus
University of British Columbia, School of Nursing
Vancouver, British Columbia
Chapter 11

Colleen Varcoe, RN, BSN, MEd, MSN, PhD
Professor
University of British Columbia, School of Nursing
Vancouver, British Columbia
Chapter 25

Michael Villeneuve
Executive Lead, National Expert Commission
Canadian Nurses Association
Ottawa, Ontario
Chapter 6

Nancy Walton, RN, PhD
Associate Professor; Chair of Research Ethics
    Board
Ryerson University
Toronto, Ontario
Chapter 21

Fjola Hart Wasekeesikaw, RN, MN
Self-employed
Hart Consulting & Associates
Winnipeg, Manitoba
Chapter 4

Reviewers

Brenda Cameron, RN, PhD
Professor
University of Alberta
Edmonton, Alberta

Tracy Christianson, BSN, MSN, PhED
Instructor
Thompson Rivers University
Kamloops, British Columbia

Lynn Corcoran, BN, MN
Academic Coordinator
Athabasca University
Athabasca, Alberta

Genevieve Currie, RN, BN, MN
Associate Professor
Mount Royal University
Calgary, Alberta

Isolde Daiski, RN, BScN, EdD
Associate Professor
York University
Toronto, Ontario

Sally Dampier, RN, DNP
Professor
Confederation College
Thunder Bay, Ontario

Denise English, RN, BN, MN
Nurse Educator
Centre for Nursing Studies
St. John's, Newfoundland

Helene Ezer, RN, PhD
Associate Dean
McGill University
Montreal, Quebec

Vee Faria, MCE, BScN, RN
Nursing Faculty
Aurora College
Yellowknife, Northwest Territories

Linda Ferguson, RN, PhD
Professor
University of Saskatchewan
Saskatoon, Saskatchewan

Katherine Haight, MSN
Academic Assistant/Nursing Instructor
Faculty of Health Sciences
University of Lethbridge
Lethbridge, Alberta

Evelyn Kennedy, PhD, RN
Associate Dean/Associate Professor
Cape Breton University
Sydney, Nova Scotia

Kathleen Kennedy, RN, BA,
MPA (Health Specialization)
Professor
Laurentian University/St. Lawrence
    College
Kingston, Ontario

Ken Kustiak, RN, RPN, BScN, MN
Nursing Instructor
MacEwan University
Ponoka, Alberta

Daniel Nagel, RN, BScN, MSN
BSN Faculty
Douglas College
Coquitlam, British Columbia

Bernie Pauly, RN, PhD
Associate Professor
University of Victoria
Victoria, British Columbia

Dawn Prentice, RN, PhD
Associate Professor
Department of Nursing
Brock University
St. Catharines, Ontario

Derek Sellman, RN, PhD, MA, BSc (Hons)
Associate Professor
University of Alberta
Edmonton, Alberta

Debra Sheets, PhD, MSN, RN-BC, CNE
Associate Professor
University of Victoria
Victoria, British Columbia

Carla Tilley, RN, MN
PhD Student
Nursing Practice Consultant
Vancouver Island Health Authority
Duncan, British Columbia

Trish Whelan, RN, BScN, MHS, ENC©
Assistant Professor
Mount Royal University
Beaumont, Alberta

Preface

The vision for *Realities of Canadian Nursing* has been and continues to be an exploration of current issues for nurses from a uniquely Canadian perspective that will prepare and inspire students to participate in political action alongside the generations of nurses who have already taken the lead. *Realities of Canadian Nursing* will engage readers in such a way that they will be prepared to work with others in addressing the long-standing barriers to many of the issues that confront nurses and the people who seek nurses' services. We believe that, in addressing these issues, nurses who understand the barriers to resolving these issues are in the best position to make significant contributions to their resolution. We want to dispel the many myths that question the need for nurses to be political and put to rest the notion that others will act on our behalf.

With this, the fourth edition of *Realities of Canadian Nursing,* we have expanded the original intent with even more breadth and depth of relevant topics and national authors from distinct geographic locations, providing representation from across the country. In addition to the authors of individual chapters, we are particularly thrilled to include photographic images of the North. At a 2012 Nurse Educator Conference in Yellowknife, Northwest Territories, we were introduced to the words "Under One Sky," which for us speaks so clearly to the intent of this text. At that same conference, standing beneath the magnificent Aurora Borealis late at night, the idea for the cover photo was brought to life. This photograph of the northern lights by Melvin R. Genge of Yellowknife, as well as the chapter photographs taken at Aurora College by Anne-Mieke Cameron, exemplifies our appreciation for the diversity of Canadian nurses, educators, and students gathering to explore the possibilities for healthcare under one sky.

This edition includes three new chapters addressing current issues for nursing practice. Three topics from earlier editions have been rewritten from the exciting perspectives of new authors, and three topics have been revisioned and revised by the previous authors. All chapters and topics have been updated. We are excited to include a new Chapter 3, "Nursing Education and Healthcare in Quebec," an addition to the previous chapters on nursing education and the Canadian healthcare system. In this chapter by Jacinthe Pépin of Quebec, readers will encounter issues particular to Quebec as well as issues it shares with other provinces.

In response to book reviewers, a new and timely Chapter 22 by Angela Gillis of St. Francis Xavier University in Nova Scotia, "Issues in Healthcare for an Aging Population," brings an in-depth look at this topic. Angela, herself an established scholar in issues in Canadian healthcare, brings a wealth of knowledge and enthusiasm to this topic.

From the opposite coast of the country, a newly emerging scholar at the University of Victoria, Olga Petrovskaya, critically explores the expanding influence of interprofessional healthcare practice and education for Canadian nurses in Chapter 14, "Changing Picture." This chapter also questions the current trend in intraprofessional staff mix for the provision of nursing care.

The diverse regional representation in the text thus extends from coast to coast to coast not only in chapter contributors but also in topics of issues themselves. In addition to Pepin, Gillis, and Petrovskaya, we welcome the valued work of respected scholars and practitioners Gail Mitchell and Joy Richards as new contributors. Using complexity theory, and a vision for phases of leadership throughout professional nursing practice, Gail and Joy have brought new energy to the rewriting of Chapter 5 on "Issues in Contemporary Nursing Leadership." Similarly, Chapter 21, "Ethical and Legal Issues in Nursing," has been revisioned and rewritten by Nancy Walton, a recognized expert in the area of nursing and healthcare ethics. Finally, Susan Duncan, an accomplished nursing scholar and leader in British Columbia, brings a new perspective to the future of nursing in the 21st century and beyond in Chapter 26, "Looking Back, Moving Forward."

Chapters addressing issues for First Nation's Ppeople and nurses in rural healthcare settings, topics pivotal to the Canadian perspective, have been revisited by their original contributors and significantly updated. Similarly, a chapter on the gendered nature of nursing has been revised and in response to reviewer comments now explicitly addresses the topic of men in nursing. Emerging scholar Andrea Monteiro brings her voice to the growing topic of environmental issues for nurses. National figures and contributors Skelton-Green, Shamian, and Villeneuve have reshaped the policy chapter, bringing an understanding of the practical usefulness and application of policy to nurses at all levels of education and practice.

In addition to new content in the text, every chapter in this edition synchronizes with Lippincott's thePoint, providing online resources and additional text. Further, chapters and issues no longer included in the hard copy version of the text will continue to be available to readers through thePoint. As authors and educators, thePoint provides us with an expanded reference of excellent chapters on issues that remain relevant to nursing and healthcare.

As with the previous editions of the text, *Realities of Canadian Nursing* brings to readers more than information about relevant issues in nursing and healthcare; each chapter builds on the frame for analysis introduced in Chapter 1 of the text. This frame for analysis provides readers, students, and educators with an organized format through which to identify and analyze issues, and, most importantly, to recognize barriers and strategies to a resolution of the issues. New to this edition is an expanded category of critical analysis using a post-colonial position. Drawing on a post-colonial position and other forms of critical analysis such as feminist, our contributors offer strategic points of resistance to dominant discourses by attributing significance to that which is too often considered insignificant—the underlying experiences and unheard concerns of nurses. Thoughtful exploration of these issues calls us all, nurses and non-nurses, to reflect on the ways in which we disrupt and maintain complicity in dominant discourses and on how we can deliberately use our knowledge to break through barriers and act strategically to resolve issues.

Now more than ever the conditions of nurses' workplaces, the settings and contexts of nurses' work, and the realities of contemporary society challenge, on a daily basis, nursing practice and the availability of resources needed to support this practice. An explicit goal of the fourth edition of *Realities of Canadian Nursing* is to disrupt the notion that changes to nursing and healthcare will happen without informed political action on the part of nurses: We hope to instill in more nurses the obligation to use their regulatory power, collectively and individually, to influence decision making in professional associations, collective bargaining units, government, and workplaces.

Acknowledgments

This book could not have happened without the dedication and hard work of many individuals, among them the reviewers, contributors, photographers, and not least of all the staff at Wolters Kluwer Health | Lippincott, Williams & Wilkins. In particular, we want to acknowledge the support and encouragement of Christina Burns, Acquisitions Editor, and Annette Ferran, Supervising Product Manager. Project Manager Fred Burns has been an exemplary partner in this process; over many months we were in nearly daily email contact, exchanging revisions, queries, and reminders. We have so much appreciated not only his excellent editorial ability but also the consistently good humor he brings to the work. In addition, we wish to thank Olga Petrovskaya, a doctoral student at the University of Victoria, for her work as an editorial assistant early in the project.

Authors acknowledge the significant contribution of Christine Ceci, Heather Clarke, Laurie Hardingham, and Dorothy Pringle to this book through their authorship of earlier chapters. Michael Villeneuve wishes to acknowledge the contribution of Nancy Field to the revision of Chapter 7, "Canadian Nurses Association and the International Council of Nurses." The CNA section of the chapter could not have been completed without the personal communications of CNA's executive leaders, policy directors, and staff, and the extensive information contained in CNA's Web site (2008 and 2012). The ICN section of the chapter is based on research conducted by Barbara L. Brush, Joan E. Lynaugh, Geertje Boschma, Anne Marie Rafferty, Meryn Stuart, and Nancy J. Tomes for *Nurses of All Nations: A History of the International Council of Nurses, 1899–1999* (Philadelphia: Lippincott Williams & Wilkins, 1999), used in this chapter with permission from the publisher. A series of articles on the history of the ICN, published by the same authors, have also been used with permission.

Others who worked behind the scenes include peers who reviewed the text and provided valuable feedback and advice. Despite the apparent invisibility of the work of reviewers, those of us with the insider's view see and appreciate the significant contributions they have made to earlier editions as well as to this edition.

As we have discussed in the preface, the photographs chosen for this edition contribute to the diversity of Canadian nursing, "Under One Sky." We are indebted to the photographic work of Melvin R. Genge for the cover photo of the Aurora Borealis. A special thank you to Anne-Mieke Cameron for her generosity in sharing photographs from Aurora College, and to each of the contributors who selected a photograph to complement their written text. Speaking of the contributors: With each edition of the text, we have been faced with decisions to bring in new chapters addressing current issues, which inevitably means moving some chapters from the print copy of the text. We are indebted to each of the chapter authors, of this and previous editions, for your contributions to this book and to Canadian nursing education.

Our collegial relationships with faculty and with both graduate and undergraduate students have inspired and sustained this work. We appreciate the companionship and the challenges that enliven these relationships and bring new energy to ongoing work.

Finally, we wish to thank our family and friends for their fine company on the journey.

Contents

xvi Contents

Nurses, Nursing, and the Healthcare System

1

Nursing Issues: A Call to Political Action

Marjorie McIntyre and Carol McDonald

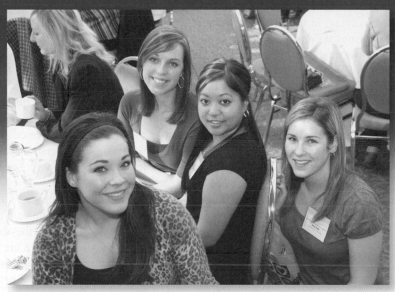

Undergraduate student nurses from the University of Victoria participate in the Western Region Canadian Association of Schools of Nursing. (Photography by Chris Marshall. Used with permission from University of Victoria.)

Critical Questions

As a way of engaging with the ideas in this chapter, consider the following:

1. What comes to mind when you think of political action?

2. Do you think of yourself as a social activist?

3. Would you consider nursing practice a political act?

Chapter Objectives

After completing this chapter, you will be able to:

1. Distinguish between problem solving and the process of issue articulation and resolution.

2. Use a framework for the articulation and analysis of an issue.

3. Describe strategies for addressing barriers and moving issues toward resolution.

Nurses across Canada are grappling with what seems at times to be irresolvable issues embedded in healthcare delivery, nursing practice, and education. Nurses struggle to solve recurring problems within a context of inadequate resources and insufficient support. Sometimes a short-term solution is what is called for; indeed, the everyday work of nurses frequently requires immediate problem solving. We, however, would like to emphasize the difference between a problem and an issue. In this text, we raise the questions of how we might understand problems that nurses encounter in day-to-day practice differently. How might we move beyond an approach to problem solving, in which problems are viewed as simplistic and isolated, toward an understanding of issues as complex and interrelated, with a breadth and scope not accounted for solving problems? How might we benefit from a new approach to issue articulation and issue resolution? The premise of this chapter and, in fact, of this entire book is that reconceptualizing seemingly irresolvable problems as issues situated in political, material, and social contexts opens us to the realities and possibilities previously obscured. It is important for nurses to question the ways in which issues are conceptualized, because how a nursing situation is understood by nurses and other decision makers will have implications for how it is likely to be addressed. The many issues affecting nurses, the profession, and the healthcare system can be understood and articulated as political issues in that they ultimately involve influencing others for the purpose of quality patient care.

Thoughtful exploration of these political questions calls us all, nurses and non-nurses, to reflect on that which constrains—and enables—the ways we can communicate and think about nursing. When nurses find themselves unable to nurse as they envision, as they believe they can or should, or when their interpretations of what is occurring in healthcare are excluded from policy discussions, a sense of being incorrect, in some essential sense, in their understanding of themselves and their work, comes into play. A profound dissonance emerges between what one believes one is called on to be and do and what the world, and one's relationship to it, allows. This distress deepens when it remains unheard, when what is of concern to nurses remains stubbornly invisible to others (Ceci & McIntyre, 2001). The ability to articulate issues is one of the means of preparing nurses for political action. Box 1.1 presents an example of a serious healthcare issue affecting a marginalized population that was identified and acted upon by community nurses. Although this exemplar originated in 2000, the issue of the need for tuberculosis (TB) screening among people without permanent accommodation continues to be relevant today.

BOX 1.1   **Healthcare Issue: Political Action Results in Screening Program**

Four community nurses working with homeless people suspected there was an increase in tuberculosis (TB) based on several cases of active TB and an increase in positive skin tests among their patients. However, when they approached the public health department, they were informed that the statistics did not indicate an increase. Although the nurses asked that TB screening be conducted in homeless shelters and drop-in centers, the health department refused.

The nurses believed that TB was increasing and, therefore, decided to press the health department to initiate a screening program. They proceeded with the following steps:

- Calling a meeting with other healthcare workers, shelter and drop-in staff, and homeless people
- Forming an action group
- Educating group members about TB
- Researching the experiences of other cities
- Making representations to health departments
- Offering to assist with screenings

These efforts resulted in a major screening program that demonstrated the increased numbers of people with TB. The group then expanded its focus to include other issues.

Source: From Canadian Nurses Association. (2000). *CNA Today, 10*(2), 11, with permission.

This chapter introduces the topic of nursing issues and provides an overview of issue articulation and its significance to nursing. Specifically, it provides a framework to explore, articulate, analyze, and generate possibilities for increased understanding and, when feasible, for resolution of nursing issues. Examples of barriers to issue resolution and specific strategies to generate possibilities for resolution are also discussed.

SIGNIFICANCE FOR NURSES

What is the significance of understanding problems in healthcare as complex and multilayered issues? Issues are best served by an approach that questions and interrogates the taken-for-granted view of the particular subject. Rather than a move to solve problems, an in-depth analysis of issues includes an exploration of barriers that makes visible the complexity of the issue. This exploration moves us past the notion that any one strategy could move an issue to resolution. To articulate an issue fully means to consider the political, historical, social, and economic realities on and through which issues are constructed.

The nursing shortage is an excellent example of how we might distinguish between issue analysis and resolution, and problem solving. If we think of the shortage as a problem of not enough nurses—a problem of numbers—the shortage could be solved by producing more nurses. If we think of the shortage as reflecting nurses' dissatisfaction with their work, we might move to improve nurses' salaries and other contractual issues. However, regardless of what might be accomplished by addressing these individual problems in the short term, studies have shown that it is not one but many problems, and the relationships between them, that contribute to the shortage (Baumann et al., 2001). The recurrence of the nursing shortage over time suggests that it would be more beneficially analyzed and addressed as a complex issue including many overlapping and interconnected problems.

Analyzing the nursing shortage as a political issue raises many questions. How might we account for the cycle of surplus and shortages historically? What constitutes a shortage of nurses? Who is the authority on what counts as a shortage? How do the prevailing attitudes in society about what it means to be a nurse contribute to the shortage? What of the status of nurses' work and nursing knowledge in the recruitment and retention of nurses? Is it possible that nursing shortages are created? Who might benefit from such a shortage? Who suffers? What are the economic implications of a shortage for nurses, for the healthcare system, and for the health of Canadians? Moving the shortage past the idea of individual problems to be solved to the depth and scope of a political issue illuminates the potential barriers for resolution. Barriers to resolving the nursing shortage include the incongruity between the complex nature of nursing practice and the lesser status attributed to nurses' work and nursing knowledge, the reality that many decisions made about nurses' work are not made by nurses, and the use of nurses as temporary workers prepared to fill a gap in services. Strategies that emerge from such an analysis would necessarily include the multiple stakeholders involved and consideration of these barriers so that solutions are long term.

SIGNIFICANCE FOR THE PROFESSION

The significance of clear articulation of issues for the profession goes beyond the individual nurse to include the organization of nurses and their ideas into a larger collective. To be effective in supporting political action within the profession, nurses need to speak in unison on issues and organize themselves to act provincially and territorially, nationally, and internationally. In 1977, Mussallem (1977, p. 156) claimed what is still true today: In the context of state-provided healthcare, the link between healthcare and political action is inseparable. The *raison d'être* of nursing is healthcare. The quality of healthcare depends to a large extent on the nature of the nursing component determined by four elements:

- Standards of education and preparation for those entering the profession
- Quality of care provided by the practitioner—a quality closely associated with education and preparation
- Number of nurses available—a determination considered in modern times largely by the social and economic status the profession offers its members
- Milieu in which care is offered.

If nurses are concerned about healthcare, they must accept responsibility for safeguarding these four dynamic elements of nursing practice. This safeguarding can be achieved only by the participation of nurses in political action. By political action we refer to the idea that nurses, because of what they know, are well positioned to speak or to act on behalf of people/patients/clients, who have less knowledge or are not in a position to act on their own behalf. It is useful to note that political action is not without risk. There are, throughout nursing history, examples of serious consequences for nurses who have made their voices heard on behalf of others.

NURSING PRACTICE AS POLITICAL ACTION

The need for problem solving and decision-making abilities has been ingrained in the discipline of nursing since its inception. We recognize that many problems are amenable to deductive thinking and problem solving. Deductive thinking can be understood as the application of general rules and laws to a specific concrete situation in nursing practice. For example, a deductive approach might lead a person to think that a rule, such as do no harm, could be applied, at face value, to every situation without considering the increasingly complex issues in a continually expanding array of practice settings. And so, although nursing practice and education have historically relied on a deductive approach to decision making, the changing world in which practice occurs and the advancing education level of nurses underscore the need for more inductive, interpretive approaches. By inductive approaches we mean those that take into consideration the particularities of the context from local to global and specific details of situations.

In recent years, there has been an increased focus on nurses' advocacy. Legislative changes in the scope of practice and in the code of ethics have contributed to the politicization of nursing practice. While once many nurses self-identified as non-political, today political awareness, political action, and social justice are increasingly—and necessarily—embedded in nursing education and nursing practice. The advancement of nursing education underpins the movement of nurses into leadership positions in the healthcare system and in education. Concurrent with their increasing social consciousness, nurse leaders experience an awareness of the limitations of approaching complex social–political issues with short-term approaches to change. Canadian Nurses Association (CNA) "Code of Ethics for Registered Nurses (CNA, 2008 Centennial Edition)" explicitly states that "there are broad aspects of social justice that are associated with health and well-being and that ethical nursing practice addresses. Nurses should endeavor as much as possible, individually and collectively, to advocate for and work toward eliminating social inequities" (p. 20).

In the face of a healthcare system in which there are seemingly continual therapeutic and technologic advances, it is easy to think of healthcare and indeed of nursing practice as progressively advancing. However, the reality for many Canadians is diminished access to nursing and healthcare services. Perhaps more than ever before, nurses are in a position to bring attention to the healthcare needs of underserved populations. Increasing numbers of nurses are employed in the community, in home-care work, and in agencies and institutions providing care to elderly individuals (CNA, 2004). In these work environments, nurses face issues of health and healthcare that are mediated by the social and material realities of the lives of the people to whom they provide care. Community and home-care nursing magnifies our awareness of the realities of poverty, lack of education, inadequate housing, and isolation and their influence on the health of Canadians. Although we can expect that many people would have intellectual awareness of these impoverished circumstances within our society, nurses, through their privileged access to underserved populations in the provision of care, live alongside this knowledge in practice. Nurses are caught in the tension of knowing what is needed, yet also knowing that these resources are not forthcoming. This disparity is what incites the political will to challenge existing structures and processes that limit access to health and healthcare for underserved Canadians.

FRAMING THE TOPIC

To begin examining and acting on an issue, one identifies the topic of interest and from this selects a particular issue and articulates it clearly. An issue can be expressed as a dilemma, conundrum, question or series of questions, or a simple statement. Box 1.2 summarizes the steps used in articulating and analyzing an issue.

Situating the Topic

One situates the topic by gathering information about the topic and identifying beliefs, views, and assumptions about the topic. An assumption is an idea that is held to be true without any support or substantiation; all of us operate from day-to-day under assumptions. Gathering information includes looking to the literature to find out what is known about the topic within the discipline and in some cases, in literature outside the discipline. The literature review will help establish the particular issue that will be addressed within the topic. For example, within the topic of the nursing shortage, one might articulate the issue for analysis as the particular way in which the nursing shortage has been conceptualized or presented to the public.

The following are some questions to ask when situating the topic:

- What is already known about this topic?
- Who has generated this knowledge?
- What assumptions are held about this topic?
- What issue within this topic would you like to explore?

Articulating the Issue

Although the separation between the topic and the issue can seem artificial, the broader topic area will contain or lead to more than one issue. For example, nurse's work is a topic, under which a

---

BOX 1.2   Articulation and Analysis of an Issue

1. Identify the topic and any assumptions or beliefs you hold about the topic of interest.
2. Select a particular issue and articulate it clearly.
3. Proceed with the analysis by addressing appropriate frameworks.
4. Identify barriers to resolution.
5. Explore strategies for resolution.

number of issues can be explicated. One issue of nurse's work is who decides what constitutes nurse work. Once the issue to address has been identified, ask the following questions:

- What makes this issue a nursing issue?
- In what ways are nurses involved in the issue?
- Who are the other participants and what is their involvement in the issue?
- Who first became concerned with the subject?
- Who began to raise the subject as an issue and why?

ANALYZING THE ISSUE

Once the issue is articulated clearly, the analysis may proceed as outlined in the following section. Some issues call for a particular approach to analysis, but most issues benefit from more than one approach. However, it is unlikely that all approaches to analysis would be undertaken with every issue. Each of the approaches to analysis, described below, is intended to generate rather than limit possibilities for discussion. The purpose of asking these questions is to increase understanding of all aspects of the issue and to move the discussion toward resolution.

Historical Analysis of the Issue

A historical analysis of issues provides the opportunity to reopen nursing and healthcare history. This reopening is more than a return to the history that has been recorded by the culturally or politically dominant group; rather, it can be seen as an opportunity to excavate the historical understandings that have been silenced, diminished, or erased. This approach to history reminds us that each telling of history is necessarily situated in the standpoint or the assumptions of the one who recounts the story. Each telling of our past is, in some sense, a partial and incomplete interpretation. In this way, history is understood as multiple histories; each account presents a reality, although only a limited depiction of our recorded past. McPherson (1996), a nurse historian, points out that events from nursing history are understood quite differently depending on who has been responsible for the documentation or analysis of the event. For example, in her discussion of the subordination of nurses, McPherson highlights the difference in viewing historical events through a lens of class analysis, gender analysis, or academic and professional analysis. The view of a particular issue through a different lens for analysis reveals different historical realities, each of which contributes to a full understanding of the issue. The questions below are intended to guide a historical analysis:

- When did the issue originate?
- What are the conditions that led to the development of the issue?
- How have these conditions changed over time?
- What is the source of the historical accounts of the issue?
- Who documented this account of history and what has contributed to the stance taken by this person(s)/organization?
- What might have influenced this perspective of the history?
- What contributes to your interpretation of this history?
- What have been the barriers to resolution?
- What strategies for resolution have already been tried?

Ethical and Legal Analysis of the Issue

The CNA's "Code of Ethics for Registered Nurses (2008 Centennial Edition)" outlines the responsibilities and obligations for the provision of professional practice of safe, compassionate, competent, and ethical care. In addition to the values and responsibilities, the "Code of Ethics" addresses broad aspects of social justice that are associated with health and well-being. For this reason, the code itself provides a framework for an ethical analysis of issues for nurses' professional relationships with individuals, families, groups, students, colleagues, and other healthcare professionals.

In addition to consulting the "Code of Ethics," you may ask the following questions:

- What are the laws that influence this issue?
- What professional codes or legislative acts mandate participants' responses to this issue?
- What professional, organizational, and governmental (municipal, provincial and territorial, and national) documents inform, constrain, or influence the issue? In addition to CNA's "Code of Ethics," possibilities include the provincial and territorial standards of practice, the British North America Act, the Health Professions Act, and the Canada Health Act.

Social and Cultural Analysis of the Issue

Every issue develops in a societal context that shapes the issue and influences the possibilities for resolution. An analysis of the social and cultural context explores the prevailing attitudes, the values and priorities, and the privileges of the dominant culture. The questions below provide guidance in analysis:

- What social and cultural factors influence this particular issue?
- What are the prevailing attitudes or assumptions in society about this issue?
- What values and priorities of the dominant culture influence this issue? In what ways, if any, do these values and priorities privilege the dominant culture over other members of society?

Political Analysis of the Issue

A political analysis asks questions that explore the location of power and influence within particular issues. In other words, whose knowledge, whose voice is able to influence either the barriers to or the strategies for resolution of an issue? Specifically, what is the relationship between knowledge and power in this situation? Questions to guide the political analysis include:

- Who benefits from the issue staying the same?
- Who is resisting change and satisfied to maintain the status quo?
- Who is advocating for change regarding this issue?
- Who benefits from the issue being resolved?
- Whose interests are being served?
- Are there hidden agendas or less visible influences affecting this issue?

Critical Analysis of the Issue (e.g., Feminist and Postcolonial)

A critical approach asks questions that challenge the taken-for-granted assumptions that are prevalent in society, such as assumptions of gender, race, and class. A critical postcolonial analysis asks questions about the effect of colonization, or domination of one group over another. In particular, this position challenges notions of race, racialization, and culture and provides "social mandates of uncovering existing inequities" (Kirkham & Anderson, 2002, p. 1).

In feminist analysis, the intention is not to privilege the position of one gender over the other but to question the way in which notions of gender have been attached to issues influencing nurses, patients and clients, and relationships with others in the healthcare system. More often than not, a critical feminist analysis does not relate to the gender of a particular person, but rather to the ways that traditional structures based on gender divisions of power have influenced or shaped issues or events. The following questions could be included in a critical analysis:

- Are there errors or myths about women's or men's abilities or realities contained in this issue?
- Is this issue influenced by the power inequities or the hierarchical or patriarchal structures of institutions over nurses or patients and clients?
- In this situation, is expert power given authority over personal power and the right to be the subject of one's own life?
- Is the issue influenced by discriminating discourses regarding age, ability, race, ethnicity, sex, genders, and sexualities?
- Could the disparities between cultures be attributed to the effects of colonization?

Economic Analysis of the Issue

In today's healthcare systems, questions of economics are prevalent in relation to nearly every identified issue. The discourses that we hear and repeat are replete with the language of economic constraint, efficiency and cost effectiveness, and scarcity of resources. An economic analysis asks difficult questions that challenge the source of these pervasive discourses and asks how things could be otherwise. Questions for the economic analysis might include:

- Who is the author of the economic discourses we hear?
- Are there hidden agendas that are obscured by the focus on economic goals?
- Who benefits from the dominance of economic discourses over other knowledge affecting this issue?
- How are institutional wastefulness and misuse of resources accounted for in the face of claims of economic austerity?

BARRIERS TO RESOLUTION

One of the most important strategies for moving an issue toward resolution is identifying barriers that may impede the resolution process. Once the barriers are identified, there may be an increased opportunity for resolution through mediation, collaboration, or negotiation. The following are some potential barriers to resolution of nursing issues:

- Limited access to resources, such as human and financial resources, knowledge, or expertise, may obstruct resolution.
- Issues are not clearly understood or are understood in a limited way. For example, a barrier to resolving the nursing shortage is conceptualizing the issue as only a problem of the number of nurses entering the profession.
- Irresolvable differences or competing interests between participants may block the resolution of issues.
- Circumstances in which some participants benefit from the issue remaining unresolved limit the opportunity for resolution.
- Power inequities between parties invested in the issue can contribute to resistance to resolution.
- Participants in the issue may experience unconscious resistance to change.
- Key stakeholders in the issue may lack tolerance for multiple viewpoints.
- Stakeholders may ascribe to different underlying assumptions or beliefs that influence the way the issue is understood and the way resolution is undertaken.

- Alienation from co-workers, hostility from bureaucratic and administrative officials, and fear of job loss may isolate nurses from the supports needed for resolution.
- Lack of time, energy, role models, and mentors seriously undermines possibilities for effective resolution.

DEVISING STRATEGIES FOR RESOLUTION

After an issue relevant to the profession of nursing or healthcare is articulated and analyzed, multiple strategies can be implemented to address and resolve the issue. Essential to the success of any effort is the communication of a well-developed plan of action. Strategies for resolution include, but are not limited to, the following:

- Use of electronic and social media
- Preparation of resolutions for presentation to agencies, associations, and organizations
- Establishment of a letter-writing campaign
- Involvement of the news media through letters to the editor and articles that solicit public support.

The use of any of these strategies depends on the following:

- People affected by the issue
- Interest that is generated
- Time available
- Human and financial resources available.

To generate the maximum amount of support, it is important to enlist the assistance of as many people as possible who are affected by the issue. A greater response and resolution can be anticipated if the affected parties are unified in their efforts to address the specific issue. The following sections include specific, detailed examples of strategies that have been employed by individuals from multiple segments of the population in their efforts to create change and to address issues of relevance to them.

LOBBYING STRATEGIES

Although lobby groups are usually associated with persuading elected officials to vote a certain way on an issue or to carry an issue forward for debate, change within an organization can be promoted by lobbying key individuals. Regardless of whether the issue is of national or international importance, or whether the issue affects nurses and healthcare on a particular unit or in a particular agency, the same techniques are available and applicable.

Lobbying may occur through direct contact with people who are in positions to address the issue and through indirect methods by which others influence the officials (Hood, 1998). Table 1.1 provides a comparison of direct and indirect strategies.

Nurses must keep several key points in mind when initiating a lobby and planning meetings with key officials, including the following:

- Become informed about the issue by reading newspapers, documents, scholarly articles and reports; searching the Internet; and knowing the professional associations' positions.
- Use simple statistics and avoid percentages. The clearer the statistics, the more attention they will generate. Then apply the numbers in human terms, and illustrate the statistics with personal stories.
- Be sure to articulate clearly why the issue is an issue and identify its importance.
- Know what other people are saying about the issue.

Table 1.1   Comparing Direct and Indirect Lobbying Strategies

DIRECT STRATEGIES	INDIRECT STRATEGIES
Engage in campaigns to elected officials or others in power using electronic communication, social media, letters, and phone calls	Blogs, reports, articles
Meeting with key people professionally	Enlisting the support of key people
Taking opportunities to meet key people socially either face to face or electronically	Using the media through news announcements on the radio and on television, in newspaper and magazine columns, and in advertisements
Submitting resolutions to professional organizations and unions	

- Keep in mind that the more people supporting the issue, the more effective the lobby.
- If you are lobbying government officials or bodies, remember to include members of the opposition parties.
- Follow meetings with written submissions that are accurate and succinct.

Electronic and Social Media

Access to electronic communication and social media sources provides innovative and timely lobbying strategies, unheard of only a decade ago. Using email, text messages, and Twitter, allow nurses not only to communicate readily with one another, but also to send messages of political importance to community, political, and institutional leaders. Video messages can be distributed through YouTube and Facebook, while online petitions provide access to thousands who might support a political cause. (See Box 1.3 for an exemplar using electronic lobbying strategies.)

Letters to Officials

One popular and well-used lobbying strategy is writing letters. Prepare the letter so that it outlines a selected issue and the possibilities for resolution. Send the letter to a public official such as the dean of your school or faculty, the unit manager in your facility or organization, a city councillor, members of the legislative assembly of your provincial government, or members of parliament of the government of Canada. Consider sending a copy of the letter to other stakeholders and interested parties, and keep a copy of letters for your own files.

CNA actively demonstrates political action through letter writing to officials; for example, in November 2010, a letter to the Prime Minister from CNA expressed many nurses' disappointment

BOX 1.3   Using Electronic and Social Media

In the early months of 2012, CNA president Judith Shamian took action to mobilize Canadian nurses and nursing students over the proposed development of a new RN entry exam. In the President's message in the *Canadian Nurse* (2012) March, Shamian stated "I cannot think of another single issue CNA has raised that has so utterly galvanized the nursing community as the decision by 10 RN regulators to choose the National Council of State Boards of Nursing (NCSBN)—an American organization—to develop a new computer based RN entry exam for Canada" (p. 3). Using social media, Shamian posted videos on YouTube viewed by over 20,000 nurses, and circulated an online petition, calling for a made-in-Canada exam reflecting the health needs of Canadians, signed by 7,500 nurses and nursing students. These timely communications inspired more than 1,300 nurses to write letters to health ministers and nursing regulators.

at the defeat of the *Climate Change Accountability Act* in the Senate. Similarly, CNA and territorial and provincial associations and colleges have written letters expressing outrage to the president of Virgin Mobile Canada at the negative and offensive portrayal of nurses in television advertisements. Other exemplars of letter-writing campaigns as well as open letters to use as templates can be found on CNA and Registered Nurses Association of Ontario (RNAO) Web sites listed at the end of the chapter.

Letters to the Editor

To be published, letters to the editor should comment on a public issue, and they usually are a response to a particular article or editorial published in the newspaper. An example may be a letter that responds to an editorial discussing the next federal budget, which is expected to be a "health budget." Keeping the letter short and punchy will enhance its chances of being published. Remember to sign the letter and add a daytime telephone number in case the editor wants verification or more information from you. Information on where to send letters is usually found in the letters section of the newspaper.

Media Releases

A news release is much like a letter but does not have a salutation. Information should include relevant facts—the who, what, when, where, why, and how of the issue that you want to highlight. The release should also include the name and telephone number of a person whom the media can contact for further comments or to arrange for an interview. The following example of a news release may be adapted to fit various needs:

In (*name of region*), registered nurses will be meeting with politicians and holding events, such as news conferences, to build support for the nursing investment. A meeting with (*name of politician*) will be held on (insert date) at (*insert place*). A photo opportunity and brief statement by the nursing group will follow at (*time and place*). The event is scheduled in response to a public meeting held (insert when and where), when nurses joined their voices with the growing number of Canadian nurses calling for a federal investment in healthcare. Canadian nurses are warning the government that Canadians will soon be deprived of care if action is not taken to avert a massive nursing shortage.

"Nurses make up 75% of health professionals. Without registered nurses at the bedside, who will care for Canadians?" asked (*insert name*). "You can't open beds in hospitals or deliver quality home care if there are no nurses."

Earlier, in Ottawa, in meetings with members of parliament and government officials, Canadian Nurses Association (CNA) called on the federal government to support recruitment and retention of registered nurses, nursing research, and the dissemination and uptake of evidence. The CNA estimates that the federal government investment should be $40 million a year over the next five years. "Our support of this is essential. We know firsthand the impact of the nursing shortage on patient care," said (*insert name*).

The RNAO Web site is a useful resource for nurses to become involved in political action. Notably, on the home page of this association, a viewer will find a link to *media releases* prepared by the RNAO as well as an Action Alert link, which provides access to the most recent political issues that directly or indirectly concern nurses. For example, in January 2011, the RNAO Web site featured an Alert to the Mayor of Toronto urging him to enforce plastic bag fees as a successful environmental strategy.

Resolutions

A resolution can be written for presentation at a professional organization's annual general meeting, such as one for a provincial association, a college of nursing, or CNA. A unified political position of many Canadian nurses on various issues is reflected in *resolutions* approved at the CNA annual meetings. These resolutions are prepared by individual nurse members of the CNA or by the provincial organizations. Any topic that is of concern to nurses nationally and that advances the mission of CNA to represent the voice of nurses and the profession can be prepared as a resolution and included for the discussion at the annual meeting. For example, in 2010, resolutions addressed such diverse national issues as equitable access to health services for all Canadians, an Integrated National Housing and Homelessness strategy, Human Rights Protection for Transgender and Transsexual Canadians, and Canada European Union Trade negotiations.

To be most effective, resolutions should be submitted in writing before the meeting date, so be sure to check deadlines, as resolutions received after the deadline may not be able to be considered by the resolutions committee. Although resolutions can usually be presented from the floor of the meeting, this means that time for consideration and discussion may be limited. You will be most effective if you allow participants time to formulate their own responses and opinions on the topic.

A resolution is an original main motion written with great formality. A resolution generally has two parts: A preamble (optional) and the resolution.

The preamble states the reasons for making the resolution and is the equivalent to debating the question before it is on the floor. Each paragraph begins with the word "*Whereas*"—underscored or in italics and followed by a comma—and each paragraph closes with a semicolon. In addition, the word after "*Whereas*" begins with a capital letter (i.e., "*Whereas,* The"). There is no limit to the number of times you use "*Whereas.*"

A resolution is introduced with the word "*Resolved,*" and, as with "*Whereas,*" the word is underscored or put in italics and followed by a comma. In addition, the word after "*Resolved*" *begins with a capital letter (i.e.,* "*Resolved,* That"). You may have more than one "resolved" sentence.

All proposed resolutions must include supporting documentation, including the financial implications relevant to the proposal. Also, it is helpful if the proposed resolution includes an implementation date. Each resolution is moved, seconded, and voted on.

An example follows of a resolution presented and voted on at the 2011 CNA annual meeting:

BE IT RESOLVED THAT CNA IN COLLABORATION WITH MEMBER ASSOCIATIONS

- Reaffirm support for the principles of the *Canadian Environmental Protection Act 1999* specifically the precautionary principle with respect to fuels, air, and water pollution.
- Promote a moratorium on construction of new nuclear power plants and the phasing out of present nuclear reactors.
- Lobby provincial/territorial and federal governments for funding to identify best practices for conserving and reducing energy consumption and for safer alternative energy resources.

CARRIED

Questions regarding the preparation of a resolution can usually be answered by contacting the association office to which you will be submitting the resolution.

SUMMARY

This chapter addresses the significance of nurses' understanding the inherently political nature of nursing and being able to articulate clearly the relevant issues in nursing, in healthcare, and in advocating for the health of Canadians. Articulation of an issue involves selecting the particular issue from a topic of interest. The nature of the issue is articulated by asking such questions as: Who are the participants in the issue? What makes this a nursing issue? Who first raised this as an issue and why?

Beliefs and assumptions inform an understanding of the issue, and the importance of articulating these assumptions is the first step of issue analysis. A framework for the analysis of issues includes raising questions of historical, ethical–legal, social–cultural, political, critical feminist, and economic natures. The purpose of asking these questions is to increase understanding of all aspects of the issue and to move the discussion toward resolution. The categories of analysis are, however, not intended to be exclusive; pertinent questions may arise during the analysis process.

Identifying barriers to the resolution of an issue is an important step in moving the issue toward resolution. Potential barriers to resolution include inaccessibility of resources, irresolvable differences or competing interests between participants, and differing underlying assumptions on the part of key stakeholders.

Essential to the success of any effort in issue resolution is the communication of a well-developed plan of action. Strategies for resolution include, but are not limited to, formation of lobby groups; establishment of letter-writing campaigns; submission of letters to the editor; distribution of news releases to print and Internet sources.

Add to your knowledge of this issue:		*Online*
Canadian Nurses Association—examples of open letters and resolutions can be found on this site.	**www.cna-aiic.ca**	
Canadian Nursing Students Association	**www.cnsa.ca**	
RNAO Political Action Resources	**www.rnao.org**	

R E F L E C T I O N S *on the Chapter...*

1 From your practice experience, identify examples of nursing as a political action.

2 There is evidence to suggest that nurses take a variety of stances in relation to using their knowledge and influence to address relevant issues in their practice. How might you account for these differences?

3 Identify at least one issue in your practice experience. Using the questions highlighted in the chapter, begin to explore the nature of this issue and possibilities for why it has remained an issue. Identify your own assumptions and beliefs that influence your interpretation of this issue.

4 What are the barriers to this issue being resolved?

5 Review the strategies for issue resolution offered at the end of the chapter, and discuss the advantages and limitations of each for the issue you have selected.

Want to know more? Visit thePoint for additional helpful resources:

- Journal Articles
- Learning Objectives
- Nursing Professional Roles and Responsibilities
- Bonus chapters:
  - Health and Nursing Policy: A Matter of Politics, Power and Professionalism
  - The NP Movement: Recurring Issues
  - When Difference Matters: The Politics of Privilege and Marginality

References

Baumann, A., O'Brien-Pallas, L., Armstrong-Strassen, B., et al. (2001). *Commitment and care: The benefit of healthy work places for nurses, their patients and the system. A policy synthesis.* Ottawa, ON: Canadian Health Research Foundation. Government of Canada.

Canadian Nurses Association. (2000). CNA today. *Canadian Nurse, 10*(2), 11.

_____. (2004). *Highlights of the 2003 nursing statistics.* Ottawa, ON: Author.

_____. (2008). *Code of ethics for registered nurses (2008 centennial edition).* Ottawa, ON: Author.

_____. (2012). Message from the President. *Canadian Nurse,* March, p. 3.

Ceci, C., & McIntyre, M. (2001). A "quiet" crisis in healthcare: Developing our capacity to hear. *Nursing Philosophy*, 2(2), 122–130.

Hood, L. (1998). The professional nurse's role in public policy. In S. Leddy (Ed.), *Conceptual bases of professional nursing* (4th ed., pp. 275–298). Philadelphia, PA: Lippincott Williams & Wilkins.

Kirkham, S., & Anderson, J. (2002). Postcolonial nursing scholarship: From epistemology to method. *Advances in Nursing Science, 25*(1), 11–17.

McPherson, K. (1996). *Bedside matters: The transformation of Canadian nursing 1900–1990.* Don Mills, ON: Oxford University Press Canada.

Mussallem, H. (1977). Nurses and political action. In B. LaSor & R. Elliott (Eds.), *Issues in Canadian nursing.* Scarborough, ON; Prentice Hall.

2

Canadian Healthcare

Janet L. Storch

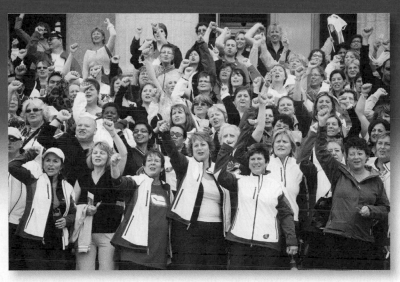

National nurses group rallies to influence change in the healthcare system. (Used with permission of Canadian Federation of Nurses Unions.)

Critical Questions

As a way of engaging with the ideas in this chapter, consider the following:

1. What views do you hold of Canadian healthcare and how have you come to hold those views?

2. In what ways does the healthcare system support the health of Canadians?

3. What are your thoughts about how the healthcare system structures nursing practice?

4. In your view, what is the major challenge facing those who manage the healthcare system?

Chapter Objectives

After completing this chapter, you will be able to:

1. Recognize the history of our current challenges in healthcare.

2. Appreciate the underlying tensions of issues in healthcare.

3. Understand the system's impact on Canadian nursing.

4. Recognize the need for nursing leadership in maintaining all that is good about healthcare and making changes to correct deficiencies.

5. Identify future possibilities for nurses in the healthcare system.

Nurses' practice is influenced by social, cultural, and historical realities worldwide, and Canadian nursing practice is no exception to this fact. These influences underlie the context within nurses' practice, a context that affects their everyday lives as nurses.

THE IMPORTANCE OF UNDERSTANDING CANADA'S HEALTHCARE "SYSTEM"

In 2007, the premier of British Columbia implemented a plan for public consultations focused on healthcare with the stated goal of making improvements to British Columbia's healthcare programs as informed by the residents of the province. At one of the many sessions held throughout the province, issues related to sustainability of the current healthcare system were raised by the facilitators, who were young men best acquainted with the forest industry. These facilitators questioned the value of Canada's approach to healthcare that uses tax dollars to fund medical care and hospital services for all individuals who are residents of Canada. They supported the idea of opening these same services to a market-based system, in which individuals and families could choose from a range of services, including private, public, and quasi-governmental services.

In response to their comments, one participant in the conference said that he recalled that his parents (prior to the implementation of Medicare and hospital insurance programs in Canada) raised funds for a neighbor who required surgery. The young facilitators responded with disbelief, wondering why his parents would have been involved in such fundraising. Even when the reasons were explained to them (i.e., that the family could not afford to pay for the surgery and hospital stay because they had no health insurance coverage), the facilitators were puzzled, seemingly unable to imagine such a situation.

The reality is that for anyone under the age of 60, living in Canada without full coverage of medical and hospital care has not been part of their experience. Canada's national Medicare program came into being between the late 1960s and the mid-1970s and was reaffirmed in the Canada Health Act (CHA) of 1984. That means that national health insurance programs in Canada are about 45 years old. It is no wonder, then, that the majority of younger adults have limited or no understanding of what life without national healthcare insurance programs would look like. In 1987, Malcolm Taylor (1987), a rigorous historian's writing about Canada's healthcare programs, stated:

> It is impossible for anyone under the age of forty today, protected as we now are with a full panoply of social insurance programs, to appreciate, or perhaps even to comprehend, the threats to individual and family independence and integrity that characterized the thirties and extended, to a declining degree, into the forties and fifties. But to millions the threats had been real and, for hundreds of thousands, had come to pass (Taylor, 1973, p. 2).

This chapter aims to provide nurses with an understanding of the healthcare system in which they work. To do so, reference will be made to the CHA. This act replaced two key federal acts in effect previously: The Hospital Insurance and Diagnostic Services Act first introduced by the Canadian government in 1957 and the Medical Care Act introduced in 1967. It was designed to affirm the four principles of the Medicare program and to add a fifth principle, "access to care" or accessibility. The CHA also placed a ban on physicians charging their patients extra money for medical services provided (i.e., charging patients funds over and above what the provincial government paid per patient visit). Such "extra billing" of patients is forbidden (Rice & Prince, 2000).

THE CANADA HEALTH ACT (CHA)

As a way of examining the strengths and limitations of Canada's approach to healthcare, the principles of the CHA (1984) will be used to frame this analysis. Each of these five principles will be examined, beginning with *comprehensiveness,* followed by *universality* and *portability, accessibility,* and *public administration.* It is hoped that by using these principles as a framework for discussion, readers will be attuned to the strengths of our healthcare system, the challenges involved in preserving the best of the system, and be better informed and equipped to work to make changes and improvements to address its limitations. Readers will be reminded about nursing's involvement in healthcare reform (past and present) and the nursing leadership needed to make a difference in this complex federal–provincial healthcare system.

As each principle is highlighted, its definition in the CHA (1984) will be provided. This definition will be followed by an analysis and discussion focusing on assessing the adequacy of Canadian healthcare in conforming to the principles as well as those areas of healthcare that are not covered by the act (based upon its definitions).

We begin with the principle of comprehensiveness. Is the Canadian healthcare system comprehensive? Does it meet the needs of Canadians? If not, what services are privileged, and what services are missing?

Comprehensiveness

> *. . . The health insurance plan of a province must insure all insured health services provided by hospitals, medical practitioners or dentists, and where the law of the province so permits, similar or additional services rendered by other health care practitioners.*
>
> Canada Health Act, 1984, c.6, s.9

The wording of what constitutes comprehensive in the CHA, with its focus on "medically necessary" services, spells out some of the limitations of this principle and explains some of the fragmentation of current healthcare. Excluded from the specified services in the definition, for example, are nursing services, public health services, communicable disease control, home care, pharmacare, chronic care, residential care, and any number of other health services, as well as a focus on primary healthcare.

The original *draft* of a comprehensive health and social insurance plan for Canada was much broader in concept and design. As long ago as the mid-1940s, while the country's efforts were focused on World War II (WWII), a broad plan was developed to include unemployment insurance, health insurance, and a full range of services for prevention, diagnosis, treatment, and care. This plan was in response to evidence that by the time Canada had entered WWII, healthcare needs continued to exceed the supply of any type of comprehensive healthcare. Infant and maternal mortality rates were high, and morbidity and mortality from communicable diseases were of grave concern (Taylor, 1973, p. 5). One third of the men who were examined for military service were unfit for service, with one third of that group rejected because of "psychiatric disorders" (Cassidy, 1947, p. 51). There was also a growing sentiment that Canada owed a comprehensive package of social programs to its returning troops (Rice & Prince, 2000), and that some type of publicly funded health insurance was inevitable. After all, Canadian soldiers returning from abroad had come to know that other countries were developing these types of programs.

The draft plan or *blueprint* for Canadian health and social programs reflected a postwar idealism fostered by international influences such as the freedoms outlined in the Atlantic Charter (Marsh, 1975; Taylor, 1973). This plan recognized that all are deserving of adequate social supports for living (Marsh, 1975). However, due to economic realities and political dissension, this comprehensive plan was not approved by Parliament, and what followed was a piecemeal implementation of programs and services over a 20-year period using the draft plan (blueprint) as a general guide. The effect of this piecemeal, politically expedient approach led to a poorly integrated health system that can scarcely be called a "system." Thus, in the 21st century, *poor integration of services* remain highly problematic (Leatt et al., 2000).

National Health Grants and the Public's Health

Some of the first programs the Canadian government took from the blueprint were designed to bolster health and healthcare in the provinces. Thus, the federal government began to offer targeted cost-sharing grants to the provinces to enable them to enhance their health services. To accept the federal government's offer, each province would have to agree to pay roughly 50% of the costs. Needs in these postwar years (1945 and onwards) are quite clear, based upon the named grants offered. These annual grants included general public health, venereal disease control, mental health, tuberculosis control, cancer control, crippled children funds, professional training, public health research, and grants for hospital construction (Taylor, 1973, p. 163). Organizational charts in provincial ministries of health reflected these grant categories, showing a deputy minister in charge of a string of programs aligned with the grants and with seemingly limited attempts to integrate program services (Defries, 1962).

The hospital construction grants that constituted part of the 50–50 offer set in motion an agenda of building hospitals, and, by default, minimizing attention to primary healthcare in Canada. Some have speculated that if the original comprehensive plan developed in the 1940s had been implemented, Canada would have set in motion a different course of action, one with an emphasis on basic health services that would have included primary healthcare.

Primary Healthcare

There are important distinctions to be drawn between primary care and primary healthcare: "*Primary care* is a medical concept referring to a situation wherein the physician provides diagnosis, treatment, and follow-up for a specific disease or problem" (Canadian Nurses Association [CNA], 2000b). In contrast, *primary healthcare*, as adopted by WHO in 1978 as the basis for the delivery of health services, most effectively involves both "a philosophy and an approach" to the way health services are delivered. It includes health promotion, disease prevention, curative services, rehabilitative care, and supportive or palliative care (CNA, 2000b). Primary healthcare involves a shift from traditional practices and power dynamics in healthcare to a system in which all health professionals are utilized to their maximum potential to affect good patient outcomes in care. Nurse practitioners, advanced practice nurses, and staff nurses alike are able to practice to their full scope of practice in this model.

There was a strong background for *primary healthcare* in Canada. Between World War I (WWI) and WWII, public health activities, carried out mainly through the work of competent nurses, increased significantly in an attempt to address deficiencies in health services (Hastings & Mosley, 1980, pp. 149–150). But this growth threatened many physicians and was opposed by them because "these nurses worked semi-independently in the community" (Coburn, 1988, p. 443). The continuation of this structured medical profession dominance led to significant delays in full implementation of expanded roles for nurses, such as the role of nurse practitioner (NP). For example, Angus and Bourgeault (1999) described the rise and fall of NPs in between the late 1960s and mid-1980s. Their rise occurred largely due to a perceived physician shortage; however, once that supply was replenished, organized medicine stood in opposition toward urban-based NPs in particular (p. 63). Over the past decade, progress has been made in the preparation and utilization of NPs; yet there continue to be barriers to NP extended practice (MacDonald et al., 2006).

In implementing interdisciplinary primary healthcare, similar barriers exist today. The concept of a primary healthcare center was widely discussed and debated in the 1970s, when a community health center project was underway in Canada. John Hastings (1972) described a model of *primary healthcare* and provided examples of its application. In essence, he and his colleagues were promoting interdisciplinary healthcare as a point of first contact as well as continuing care. His concept of healthcare involved different members of the healthcare team taking leadership, contingent upon the needs of the person seeking assistance. The opposition by organized medicine to this team-care model was widespread, and for a period of time this community health-centered approach to primary healthcare waned. In the late 1990s, the federal government again attempted to stimulate development of primary healthcare, using ideas similar to those proposed in the community health center report. Unfortunately, in some provinces moneys intended for pilot projects involving interdisciplinary team members were utilized instead to augment primary care services provided by physicians, and this development again faltered.

Organized nursing, largely through the Canadian Nurses Association (CNA), has been a steady, informed advocate of primary healthcare. In 1979, for example, in response to a federal commission called the Health Services Review, CNA developed a submission entitled "Putting Health Back into Health Care" (CNA, 1980), recommending that:

- The existing legislation underlying the hospital and medical insurance programs be revised to allow the emergence of a health insurance program that would stimulate the development of primary health services, permit the introduction of new entry points, and promote the appropriate utilization of qualified health personnel.
- Provincial legislation be revised to enable qualified nurses and other prepared health personnel to undertake activities currently defined as medical acts.
- Remuneration of all health personnel be salaried.
- The Health Services Review '79 strongly support the initiation of better preventive, diagnostic, and ambulatory care programs through various community-based points of entry.
- The federal government be requested to reinstitute a national health survey that would provide the necessary information on which to build and evaluate a healthcare system to meet the needs of the people of Canada.
- All governments and health profession organizations be urged by this Health Services Review to adopt, as a priority, better and broader health education programs to sensitize consumers to the cost of acute-care services.

The CNA's input was well received by the commissioner and constituted a major part of his report. However, this more comprehensive approach to healthcare and healthcare insurance has continued a slow development. In the late 1990s, CNA focused renewed attention on primary healthcare in publications, position statements, and "backgrounders" about primary healthcare. *Primary care* was described as "provider-driven; based in clinical diagnosis and treatment; institutionally oriented; individually focused; and emphasizing service provision" (CNA Backgrounder, 2005). In contrast, *primary healthcare* was described as offering a continuing and organized supply of essential health services available to all people without unreasonable geographic or financial barriers (or, "accessible"); involving public participation; focusing on health promotion to enable people to increase control over and to improve their health; utilizing appropriate technology; and involving inter-sectoral cooperation (i.e., commitment from all sectors) (p. 1).

Care of the Chronically Ill

Another sector of healthcare not covered adequately through the CHA definition of *comprehensive* is the care of the chronically ill, both institutional care and home care. In 2007, an entire issue of *Healthcare Papers* was devoted to the topic of the inadequacy of the healthcare system to address the multiple chronic diseases that those who are living longer endure. With the majority of attention in healthcare focused on acute, episodic care, those citizens needing continuing and comprehensive care to manage a chronic disease commonly "fall through the cracks" or are "lost in transition" (Morgan et al., 2007, p. 8). As Morgan et al. note, "Canadians with chronic illness deserve a transformed healthcare system that provides coordinated, comprehensive care—a system that results in fewer visits to the emergency departments, fewer complications and a better and longer quality of life (p. 21)."

One important approach to optimizing health and reducing hospital admissions for chronically ill patients is self-management education. Recognizing the contribution that patients and clients with chronic conditions can make to their own healthcare is a significant step forward in addressing chronic illness. This approach is neither simply "passing the buck" to the patient nor is it simply providing patients with information. It is about providing both information and support in an intensive and interactive manner by training patients to monitor themselves and by using written care plans that are tailored to individual lifestyles and needs. But, as researchers caution, "self-management education programs should be seen as part of a larger strategy for improving care for people with chronic disease" that includes a team of coordinated health professionals. Only in this way can patients be given the tools and treatments they need to lead better and healthier lives (Canadian Health Services Research Foundation [CHSRF], 2007a; Fierlbeck, 2011).

"Superbugs" and Patient Safety

Communicable disease control and patient safety has rapidly become another critical issue for Canadian healthcare. Topping the headlines in many current daily newspapers is the emergence of "superbugs" (Harnett, 2008; Priest, 2008). For example, the incidence of hospital-acquired *Clostridium difficile,* methicillin-resistant *Staphylococcus aureus,* and other such infectious microorganisms is alarming. It has been noted that many adverse events might be prevented by appropriate staffing with well-educated nurses, rather than reducing nursing staff to a minimum due to cutbacks in healthcare (Storch, 2005). In a similar manner, there is reason to believe that cutbacks and contracting out poorly supervised cleaning services in hospitals can lead to an increase in these organisms flourishing in hospitals and nursing homes. Hand washing alone in a filthy environment will not likely effect the decrease in these microorganisms needed to ensure that patients who are chronically ill, as well as those in acute care, are protected from the invasions of these superbugs.

Influenced by a major report from the Institute of Medicine in the United States (1999), attention has been focused on all manners of hospital-acquired injury or infection. Many Western countries have established organizations to focus on this new threat to the health status of their citizens. In Canada, the establishment of the Canadian Patient Safety Institute (CPSI) was announced by the federal government in December 2003 and became operational in 2005, with its headquarters in Edmonton, Alberta. The purpose of CPSI is "to provide national leadership in building and advancing a safer Canadian health system" (Canadian Patient Safety Institute, 2007, p. 1). Within a short time, CPSI engaged in a campaign to decrease adverse events in healthcare through involvement of teams of health professionals across Canada. Although initiatives started in acute care, CPSI has widened its gaze to include safety in home care (Lang et al., 2009) and in primary care (Kingston-Riechers et al., 2010) as well as supporting research that probes numerous specific concerns in patient safety and seeks to influence policy.

The Resurgence of Communicable Disease and Public Health Services

Initially, public health interventions were considered to be the domain of the state since clean water, safe food supplies, etc. were regarded as matters of local concern (Feldberg et al., 2010). The BNA (British North America) Act of 1867 "...overlooked private practice and curative medicine" (p. 281). Not surprisingly, the focus of the CHA to address these "oversights" separated them from public health funding.

Thus, despite the influx of federal money to the provinces through the cost-shared programs instituted in the late 1940s, attention to public health services has lagged behind acute care in its continuing development. The rise of communicable diseases and the threat of outbreaks, epidemics, and pandemics highlights the vulnerability of Canadians. This awareness has given rise to federal and provincial actions to enhance public health services. The outbreak of sudden acute respiratory syndrome in Toronto in the spring of 2003 served as a "wake-up call" to restore public health services. One might correctly guess that the lack of specific mention of public health services in the statement of comprehensiveness in CHA, and the fact that most Canadians take public health services for granted until some major public health problem develops, had allowed opportunities to reduce budgets in public health. If ever there was a call for a universal approach to health, threats of diseases that cross all borders and the threat of pandemics surely have emphasized that need.

In 2004, the Public Health Agency of Canada (PHAC) was created as a national presence to address some of these pressing issues. Their mission is "to promote and protect the health of Canadians through leadership, partnership, innovation and action in public health" (www.phac-aspc.gc.ca). PHAC has been effective in uniting Canadian efforts in pandemic planning, as well as in addressing other national issues, and serves as a prime contact for the World Health Organization (WHO) for such international work. "The creation of the Public Health Agency of Canada marks the beginning of a new approach to federal leadership and collaboration with provinces and territories on efforts to renew the public health system in Canada and support a sustainable health care system" (www.phac-aspc.gc.ca). However, even with PHAC in place, the ability of this federal body to take action can still be impeded by Canada's constitutional provisions for federal and provincial responsibilities in healthcare. Thus, we move on to discuss the CHA's principles of universality and portability.

Universality and Portability

> ...*In order to satisfy the criterion respecting universality, the health care insurance plan of a province must entitle one hundred per cent of the insured persons of the province to the insured health services provided for by the plan on uniform terms and conditions.*
> Canada Health Act, 1984, c.6, s.10

> ...*In order to satisfy the criterion respecting portability, the health care insurance plan of a province must not impose any minimum period of residence in the province, or waiting period, in excess of three months before residents of the province are eligible to insured health services...*
> ...[The healthcare insurance plan] *must provide for and be administered and operated so as to provide for the payment of amounts for the cost of insured health services provided to insured persons while temporarily absent from the province...*
> Canada Health Act, 1984, c.6, s.11

One of the challenges in maintaining and sustaining Canadian healthcare is the difficulty the federal government encounters in influencing national policy and national standards. This difficulty tends to be a puzzling matter for many who study Canadian healthcare but only until they recall or realize that Canada's constitution dictates that health is the major responsibility of the provinces. This means that the principles of the CHA, including universality and portability, cannot easily be enforced by the federal government.

Barriers Imposed by the British North America Act

The Fathers of Confederation, who were the developers of Canada's constitution, are notable mainly for what they did not know—and what they could not have known—about future healthcare needs. When these leaders set out the terms of the BNA Act of 1867, which continues to form a part of Canada's current Constitution Act, they had no idea how trends in industrialization and urbanization would affect healthcare needs (Cassidy, 1947; Hastings & Mosley, 1980; Wallace, 1950). Thus, they wrote of what they knew and outlined very basic responsibilities of the federal government, leaving wide room for the provinces to be the key players in the provision of healthcare and believing that individuals could and should be self-reliant.

The federal and provincial responsibilities influencing healthcare (and universality in health programs) were stated in Section 91 (federal responsibilities) and Section 92 (provincial responsibilities), and included the following (Van Loon & Whittington, 1976):

> Sec. 91—taking of the census, . . . collecting statistics (birth, marriage, death), establishing quarantine regulations and hospitals for those in quarantine, and taking responsibility for Canada's native peoples.
>   Sec. 92 (7)—The Establishment, Maintenance and Management of Hospitals, Asylums, Charities, and Eleemosynary Institutions in and for the Province, other than Marine Hospitals.

This division of federal and provincial responsibilities has created permanent tension between the federal government, which collects most of the taxes, and the provincial governments, which have seen their mandate for the provision of health services growing each year (Feldberg et al., 2010; Fierlbeck, 2011; Lindenfield, 1959). Much of what might be titled "federal–provincial wrangling" over healthcare funding is based upon this distribution of powers.

The result of Sections 91 and 92 in relation to healthcare is that the federal government has limited ways to introduce national health and social service programs. Only three ways are open to them. They can change the constitution for a specific program they wish to introduce, they can offer cost-sharing programs that allow them to establish initiatives (as they did with the 50–50 cost-sharing health grants in 1947–1948), and they can set national standards with penalties for lack of adherence to such standards (as in the case of the CHA). Inevitably, this limitation requires some compromise on the part of the federal government as well. For example, the federal government compromised some of the blueprint for federal programs by developing a single-payer system (the public) utilizing the tax base to pay for health services (health insurance) that would be supplied by autonomous or semiautonomous "private" providers such as physicians and hospitals (Fuller, 1998).

Since each province still has a *choice* about joining a cost-shared program or forfeiting penalties to maintain its autonomy, it typically took several years before all provinces bought into various national programs, including hospital insurance, medical care insurance, and any number of other social programs. The consequence was, for example, that residents of Quebec were late beneficiaries of many of the national programs. In Quebec, the longstanding tradition of Catholic charity (Cassidy, 1947), ties to the "Old World," a commitment to maintaining an identity, and a lag in industrial development (Lindenfield, 1959) were some of the barriers that precluded easy adoption of federal programs.

With such potential and real diversity in provincial uptake of health and social programs (or not), issues such as universality and portability remain contingent upon a province's "buying in" to national initiatives. The Health Council of Canada, a national body created in 2003 as part of the First Ministers' Accord on HealthCare Renewal to monitor and report on healthcare towards improving the health status of Canadians, continues to highlight the disparities across provinces in terms of national initiatives. For example, their 2005 report titled "Health care renewal in Canada: Accelerating change," contains information tables that summarize by jurisdiction the status of initiatives in home care, primary care reforms, drug programs, human resources, and other areas of comparison (pp. 49–95). These tables exemplify the disparities across provinces (Health Council of Canada, 2005). The Health Council's 2010 Report stresses the urgent need to find a "better balance between investing in the acute care system and investing in the determinants of health" (Health Council of Canada, 2010, p. 28).

Frameworks for Health Promotion

Despite the limitations of the BNA Act, Canada has made unique contributions to public health worldwide. Just before WWI, the president of the Vancouver Medical Society, J. W. McIntosh

(1914), delivered a paper at the Royal Sanitary Conference in Vancouver on the topic of the inter-relationship of physician, citizen, and state to public health. He provided a conceptual framework to describe the disabilities affecting many Canadians, classifying them as hereditary, personal or self-imposed, or environmental—"the gift of our neighbors and surroundings" (McIntosh, 1914, p. 454). Years later, his framework would resonate with the writing of a federal civil servant named Laframboise (1973). Laframboise's article was the basis of a prominent Canadian report known as the Lalonde Report (1974), named after the Minister of Health, Marc Lalonde, during whose tenure this report was released.

The Lalonde Report, titled *A New Perspective on the Health of Canadians,* marked Canada as a leader in formulating a four-point policy framework that considered heredity, environment, lifestyle, and health services as critical to health. This report was considered an attempt to break away from the medical approach to health and move toward a more holistic approach (LaBonte, 1994, p. 74). Almost 10 years later, the new concept of public health began to focus on healthy policies and healthy cities and communities. The concept of healthy cities and communities was designed to incorporate citizen participation and to press local governments to cooperate in bringing about healthy outcomes.

In 1986, a compelling framework for health promotion was developed under the leadership of Jake Epp (1986) in a document titled, *"Achieving health for all: A framework for health promotion."* With the goal of achieving health for all Canadians, three key areas were identified: Health challenges, health promotion mechanisms, and implementation strategies (Rootman & O'Neill, 1994, p. 141). Health challenges called for a reduction in inequities, increasing prevention, and enhancing coping. Health promotion mechanisms included self-care, mutual aide, and healthy environments. Implementation strategies involved fostering public participation, strengthening community health services, and coordinating health public policy (p. 141).

With the cutbacks to healthcare in Canada in the late 1980s and early 1990s, implementation of these ideals of public health was seriously impacted. By the mid-1990s, cutbacks to the public health system had created a high degree of vulnerability for all Canadians. For example, the quality of the water supplies in many cities and towns in several provinces was found to be faulty (Pike-MacDonald et al., 2007). As the years have progressed, many municipalities have had to put their citizens on an "unsafe water supply alert" for a temporary period. The advent of mad cow disease (bovine spongiform encephalopathy), West Nile virus, and many other threats to public health found the system wanting.

As some of the earliest advances in maintaining health and preventing disease in early Canadian history had to do with improving water supply, sanitation, and conducting meat inspections, it is somewhat alarming to think that we may have returned to situations somewhat akin to pre-confederation days. When basic pillars for health promotion and preservation are removed from the health system, there are bound to be serious threats to health. Public health measures such as these have been taken for granted by most Canadians, and the warnings are clear: A public health system cut to the bone is not able to safeguard the health of Canadians.

Government Studies and Agreements

In 1994, the federal government established a National Forum on Health Care (1997) to make recommendations about the "crisis in healthcare." This eight-member committee studied various aspects of healthcare and came out in strong support of the merits of current Canadian health programs, adding to them the need to enhance home-care services as well as to improve coverage of pharmaceutical costs. Most of the forum's recommendations have yet to be implemented as other political agendas shift the emphasis in healthcare reform.

In 1999, the federal and provincial governments signed the Social Union Agreement, the purpose of which was to define the principles "for the design and development of social policies and programs" (CNA, 2000a). The principles include citizen engagement and accountability, and the agreement *reconfirmed* the conditions (principles) of the CHA of 1984.

Yet regional variations in the availability and caliber of services remain problematic within each province. Further, data released by the Canadian Institutes for Health Information indicate mounting evidence of wide gaps in healthcare benefits across the provinces. Further evidence of regional variation is seen in the erosion of the principle of portability of the CHA.

As noted earlier, pharmacare or reimbursement for outpatient prescription drugs is not mandated by the CHA or any other federal legislation. In a recent Canadian study, researchers compared provincial prescription drug plans and their impact upon patients' annual drug expenditures. Wide variations were found across the provinces, including drug plans with different criteria for reimbursement, deductibles, copayments, premiums, and maximum annual beneficiary contributions (Demers et al., 2008, pp. 405–406). Researchers concluded, "Given the differences in reimbursement according to age, income level, marital status and province of residence, prescription drug reimbursement in Canada is manifestly un-equal. Although current provincial drug plans provide good protection for isolated groups, most Canadians still have unequal coverage for outpatient prescription drugs (p. 409)."

In this case, adherence to both the principles of universality and portability is unenforceable in this highly costly, but typically medically necessary, healthcare need.

Accessibility (and Sustainability)

…The health care insurance plan of a province must provide for insured health services on uniform terms and conditions and on a basis that does not impede or preclude, either directly or indirectly whether by changes made to insured persons or otherwise, reasonable access to those services by insured persons…

Canada Health Act, 1984, c.6, s.12

From the outset, concerns about rising costs, about socialized medicine interfering with doctor–patient relationships, and any number of other reasons were put forward to promote the private operation of health services. In Alberta in particular, physicians moved to bill patients extra for the care they received based on the premise that limited Medicare funds restricted their right to adequate compensation for services. This practice, known as *extra billing* or *balance billing,* set the stage for a national drama as the federal health minister, Monique Begin, took a highly public stance against the Alberta government on this issue. With a change in the funding formula from the federal to the provincial governments (i.e., the transfer of tax points to the provinces), the federal government had lost some leverage in its insistence that the provinces adhere to the national standards for Medicare. The outcome was the passage of a new federal act meant *to enforce the principles* of Medicare, namely, the CHA.

In early April 2001, Roy Romanow, a former premier of Saskatchewan, was commissioned by an Order in Council of the federal government to inquire into and undertake policies and measures respectful of the jurisdictions and powers in Canada required to ensure, over the long term, the sustainability of a universally accessible, publicly funded health system that offers quality services to Canadians and strikes a balance between these investments in prevention and health maintenance and those directed to care and treatment (Commission on the Future of Healthcare in Canada, 2002, p. iii).

The report was tabled in November 2002 after one of the most extensive public consultations in Canadian history. Through these consultations Romanow was able confirm that:

- Canadians remain attached to the values at the heart of the system
- Medicare has served Canadians extremely well
- The system is as sustainable as Canadians want it to be

- Canadians want and need a truly national healthcare system
- Canadians want and need a more comprehensive healthcare system
- Canadians want and need a more accountable healthcare system
- The Canadian system is based on values (Commission on the Future of Health Care in Canada, 2002, pp. xvi–xix).

Romanow offered numerous recommendations in his 356-page report, almost all supported by strong research evidence secured through commission staff and commissioned papers. His key recommendations centered on the need for an infusion of funds into healthcare with calls for a dedicated health transfer payment to the provinces; a Canadian healthcare covenant; modernizing the CHA; a home-care transfer for postacute, palliative, and mental healthcare; a catastrophic drug transfer; and a rural and remote access fund. He also recommended the formation of a Health Council for Canada (mentioned earlier), reminiscent of the Dominion–Provincial Health Council formed in the 1940s, and he advised *against* for-profit delivery of health services.

Meanwhile, the Senate of Canada was also busily engaged in parallel activity by authorizing a committee led by Senator Michael Kirby to examine the fundamental principles on which Canada's publicly funded system is based, its historical development, the pressures and constraints on the system, and the role of the federal government in Canada's healthcare system. Kirby recommended no change to the CHA and to set funding priorities on service-based funding for hospitals. He also urged that greater responsibility be given to regional health authorities for delivering or contracting out publicly insured health services. As priorities, he recommended primary healthcare reform, a healthcare guarantee, coverage of catastrophic prescription costs, and home care. Kirby did not address Canadian values, and he left the door open to more private-sector involvement (Roberge, 2003). Whereas Romanow's findings were based on public consultation with over 40,000 Canadians, Kirby could only boast 400 voices. Some argue that portraying Kirby as the proponent of privatization and Romanow as the champion of a public system creates a false polarity (Chodos & MacLeod, 2004), but both Kenny (2004), an ethicist, and Deber (2004), an economist, disagree. Kenny suggests that the difference lies in Kirby's suggestion to let the market decide for itself, while Romanow sees *healthcare as a moral enterprise,* not a business venture. Deber concludes that very limited benefits are likely to arise from an increase in the delivery of for-profit clinical services. She suggests that, "This does not mean that they should be outlawed, or that one should be comfortable with the status quo. But neither does it present any reason why they should be encouraged...Improving care delivery, particularly more careful attention to best practices, communication and coordination, appears essential (pp. 59–60)."

In part as a consequence of these two reports, in February 2003, a Healthcare Renewal Accord was passed by the First Ministers' conference to reaffirm their commitment to the five principles of health insurance in Canada (the principles of the CHA). In this accord, they called for a standard of care that would include:

- Access to a healthcare provider 24 hours a day, 7 days a week
- Access to diagnostic procedures and treatments
- Reduction in duplication of patient histories and testing for every provider they visit
- Access to quality home and community care services
- Access to quality care no matter where they live
- A healthcare system that is efficient, responsive, and adapting to changing needs (Health care Renewal Accord, 2003).

To reach these goals, the federal government established a long-term (10-year) Canada Health Transfer to include a portion of the current cash and tax points corresponding to provincial expenditures and with predictable annual increases. This Health Transfer (Health Renewal Accord) is due for renegotiation in 2013–2014. The federal government has already signaled that present levels of funding would be reduced in future years (Picard, 2011).

Preceding and subsequent to this accord, surgical wait lists became the pressing problem of healthcare professionals and government officials as well as private entrepreneurs. The latter offered their services of surgical day care settings, as a solution to the problems of accessibility. Once again, the provincial and federal governments challenged physicians who were seen to be extra-billing patients through these surgical for-profit centers.

In late spring 2004, the case of *Jacques Chaoulli et al. v. Attorney General of Quebec* raised the issue of "whether there is an infringement of Charter rights that occurs when the public system is unable to provide timely access to needed services while simultaneously prohibiting individuals from purchasing these services using their own resources" (Chodos & MacLeod, 2004, pp. 24–25). Two years later, "the Supreme Court of Canada decided in a 4–3 judgment to invalidate Quebec's prohibition against the sale of private insurance for core medical services provided through Medicare on the grounds that it violated the guarantee of rights to life and to personal inviolability in Quebec's Charter of Human Rights and Freedoms" (Crawford, 2006, p. 92). This, if adopted by other provinces, would in effect negate the accessibility clause in the CHA that protects consumers from paying extra (either through private insurance or out-of-pocket expenditure) for publicly funded services. Some question the impact of this decision on other provinces and its impact on free-trade agreements. Since the Canadian government did not negotiate the exclusion of private health insurance from the terms of the North American Free Trade Agreement (NAFTA), market access might become open to other insurers beyond public health insurance (Crawford, 2006, pp. 93–95).

Considerable attention has been focused on wait times and wait lists, often with limited outcomes. In 2006, HealthcarePapers (2006) was devoted to wait-time strategies, with reports of some success in reducing wait times in select areas of surgical treatment and related diagnostics. Those commenting on these successes reminded readers that excluded from these wait-time considerations are wait times for home care (Shamian et al., 2006) and many other less dramatic services. In British Columbia, Priest et al. (2007), writing for the Canadian Centre for Policy Alternatives, analyzed the issue of wait lists. They highlighted the main reasons for wait lists and recommended attention to these barriers to time-appropriate surgeries. These recommendations include having a single common waiting list, improving current organizational processes, focusing on team-based care, offering pre-surgical programs, and using electronic information systems. In that many of these recommendations involve changes in ways of practice by many people (from surgeons to operating-room nurses, to administrators and the public), implementation of solutions to the problem of wait lists has taken some time to be realized. Delays in the introduction of electronic patient records and other patient information systems to allow healthcare providers ready access to information for care provision and planning is considered to be a major need for best practices in the Canadian healthcare system. But many provinces have been seriously delayed in adopting these innovative approaches.

Other issues of substance in late 2007 were those related to errors in pathology and histology laboratories. The main impetus for this news was the inaccurate results of lab tests in Newfoundland and Labrador, but the concerns about potential error rates in laboratories soon spread across Canada (Peritz, 2008; Porter, 2008). Accessibility to accurate test results, as well as the human cost of inaccurate lab results, became alarming concerns for most Canadians. Questions about national standards and supervision to ensure adherence to these standards were paramount in these discussions (e.g., see Gregory and Parfrey, 2010).

By 2010, concerns about wait-lists (while ongoing) were pre-empted in the healthcare literature by concerns for long-term care. Reichwein (2011) observed that "…what long term care used to mean and what it means presently is a challenge; new labeling of services keeps evolving and changing and causes confusion for professionals and the public at large" (p. 52). Others have urged that integrated approaches to home and community care become priority concerns in healthcare (Petch & Shamian, 2009; Williams et al., 2009).

In early 2012, a new concern emerged in the form of a looming shortage of drugs in Canada due to reliance on a sole drug supplier's inability to continue production of these drugs. But worldwide shortages of pain killers, sedatives, and antibiotics were also becoming a reality, causing cancellations of elective surgeries and other disruptions (Tam, 2012).

These are only a few examples of the many issues arising in healthcare in Canada. Some of these issues can be linked to previous and current cost-cutting measures and inattention to quality assurance, all leading to undesirable patient outcomes. Many of these issues are being used to question the sustainability of the Canadian healthcare system, particularly the financing of our publicly insured programs. Despite evidence to the contrary, many believe that the problem with the Canadian healthcare system is due to *public funding* and *public administration,* which they see as the problem rather than the solution (CHSRF, 2007b, p. 1).

Canadian Doctors for Medicare (2011) present a very different picture, showing through facts and figures that the costs of Medicare "...are not growing significantly and can easily be sustained" (p. 1). They note that rises in expenditures are a function of increases in costs in the private sector, pointing to pharmaceuticals and private insurance costs as the most significant drivers (p. 4). They continue to favor a single-party payer.

Public Administration

...The health care insurance plan of a province must be administered and operated on a nonprofit basis by a public health authority appointed or designated by the government of the province...

Canada Health Act, 1984, c.6, s.8

Canada does, in fact, have a mix of public and private for-profit care, with the private for-profit element normally linked to certain sectors of care. Roughly 70% of total health expenditures in Canada are paid by public-sector funding, with 30% financed privately through supplementary insurance, employer-sponsored benefits, or direct out-of-pocket expenditures (Health Canada, 2002). For example, dental and orthodontic care falls outside the publicly funded health services in most provinces. There are also numerous private for-profit nursing homes because these are outside the acute care and medically oriented emphasis of Canada's health programs, and complementary medicine is not normally covered. Many of the fastest rising expenditures in healthcare fall outside of Medicare. Drug expenditures are paid for by combinations of private insurance plans and public funds, often with added out-of-pocket expenditures. These costs have often tripled their share of the gross domestic product over the last 20 years (CHSRF, 2007b).

Calling Canada a "learning disabled nation," Lewis (2007) comments on our obsession with sustainability when the facts based upon 2007 data from the Organization for Economic Cooperation and Development are so clear. He states that when comparing Canadian financial figures in healthcare to 19 other nations, that "our cumulative rate of spending increases has been unexceptional; our fiscal houses are in order; and our economy is humming. It's hard to imagine a less daunting sustainability situation" (p. 21). Lewis maintains that preoccupation with sustainability arises from "three sources of inspiration" (p. 22). One is the growing proportion of provincial dollars consumed by healthcare, the second is that the aging population will bankrupt the healthcare system, and the third is the ideology of those who want to privatize the system.

Many Canadian families have a strong historical bias toward privatization. After the two world wars ended, and Canada began to prosper in the 1950s, many private medical insurance plans were developed by the provinces. With the popularity of these private medical insurance plans (particularly in the eyes of physicians and business leaders), and with hospitals available for use, the federal government was reluctant to rush to introduce the long-promised Medicare program that was the final part of the blueprint. At that point, another study (a Royal Commission) was conducted on the feasibility of introducing a Medicare program. Contrary to governmental expectations, when the commissioners considered the total package of healthcare services needed by a Canadian family, they recommended that it was cost effective to subsidize the ten health-insurance programs in Canada (Taylor, 1973). With that recommendation, the final plank of Canadian healthcare, a national Medicare program, was then put in place in the mid-1960s.

Following implementation of the major programs featured in the Canadian blueprint, governments began to study the effects of the Canadian Health Insurance programs. The economic downturn in the late 1980s (noted earlier with respect to public health services) began to seriously threaten Canada's federal–provincial healthcare programs. The political climate of the Western world was strongly influenced by the dominant neo-conservative ideology of political leaders in England, the United States, and Canada. The development of large corporations, a concentration of wealth, and free trade were outcomes of this ideology, which included adopting *a business model* for healthcare delivery, identifying people as deserving and undeserving, and the growing attempts of governments to withdraw from involvement in comprehensive public programs and to promote private-sector providers. Several provinces, Alberta and Quebec in particular, took the lead in downsizing healthcare through sudden and severe budgetary cutbacks.

Thus began massive layoffs of hospital workers—particularly nurses. Included in these cutbacks was the removal of one or two levels of nurse managers from the system, an action that ensured no one was there to advocate for professional nursing care. The effects of these actions are most evident today in serious nursing shortages and the serious shortage of clinical nurse leaders to mentor and support nurses entering practice and those changing practice settings (Broughton, 2001; Canadian Nursing Advisory Committee, 2002; Shamian & LeClair, 2000).

Part of the downsizing strategy included a push toward healthcare reform that promoted healthcare as just another "business" and promoted greater regionalization of health services. In regionalization, the downsizing of the provincial health departments was one consequence because centralized policies and services were considered to be no longer required. The loss of intellectual ability, experience, and wisdom in public-sector management and in healthcare policy development was immeasurable. Alberta is notable in a reversal of the trend to de-centralize with its sudden decision to centralize health services on April 1, 2009 (Duckett, 2010).

Many health regions also implemented program management, an approach adopted from the business world that is built on product-line management strategies. The goal in program management is the integration of care through "seamless systems" that would be devoted to one similar focus of care, such as heart health, to include the spectrum from prevention to tertiary care (Leatt et al., 1994). However, adopting this business way of thinking overlooks the unique aspects of healthcare, including the fact that patients, for example, do not fit into neat categories like product lines such as shoes or cars. This view might be described as the "false simplification of human life" (Saul, 1995). Although there is a cry for evidence-based practice, the evidence to support dismantling many good systems that were put in place to promote high-quality care is lacking.

The CHSRF (2004, 2007a, 2007b) has regularly pointed out that drawing money from another source additional to government funding does not make the system more affordable, because Canadians still have to pay for it. Further, sustainability is not only about money. Included in measures to sustain the system are changes that must be made in the system and are typically changes that have been resisted, such as a greater focus on primary healthcare, better home-care services, more focused preventive services, more interdisciplinary teamwork, and salaried physicians. As Kenny (2002, p. 29) points out, if these and similar recommendations to sustain the system are "eminently sensible and obviously necessary for maximum efficiency, why have they not been implemented? Who benefits from the status quo?" Another very serious question in this decade is who benefits from the push toward greater private health insurance? As has been noted, "When governments cut taxes, any public program, including health services, can be unsustainable. Fiscal sustainability, therefore, is a matter of government's choice, but more fundamentally the public's choice...Medicare is as sustainable as Canadians want it to be" (CHSRF, 2007b).

SO WHAT DOES THIS MEAN?

Despite its flaws, Canada's "system" of healthcare is well worth saving. While respecting its limitations, one can make a few general statements about the system's virtues. People in Canada do not have to be as fearful about their access to care and about the devastating costs of an illness or surgery as do many in the United States. Also, Canadian patients have considerably more choice in the selection of their doctors—and even their hospitals—than many of their neighbors to the south. Many managed care plans in the United States, for example, offer extremely limited choices to consumers, reserving considerable choice for the managers of the plans whose goal is to purchase the most cost-efficient services for their patient groups.

Physicians in Canada have freedom to choose their practice locations without restriction and they can set their work pace and manage their scheduling. Canadian national programs have also allowed for an enviable collection of data about hospital stays, patients' conditions, and physician services. And the programs still have the support of the majority of the public. Access to healthcare based solely on need is the core value that gave rise to and sustains Medicare, and the advent, through Medicare, of universal, publicly funded physician and hospital services substantially reduced disparities in access to, and outcomes of, healthcare based on socioeconomic status. But despite those gains, disparities remain—factors other than need continue to influence access to and use of services (Hutchison, 2007; Bryant et al., 2010).

The serious pressures on the system in the 21st century need to be carefully considered both in relation to our historical legacy and to the wider context of international capital in which our healthcare system and other countries' healthcare systems are embedded (Coburn & Rappolt, 1999). Problems arising from this legacy are our failure to develop a comprehensive system of care and our failure to recreate, re-energize, and renew our systems based on known evidence. These problems also represent our failure to change traditional practices, to move to primary healthcare, and to utilize all health professionals well. All of these problems might well be included in what Coburn and Rappolt (1999) describe as the "logic of Medicare."

So what has our history—our heritage—told us about our current situation in healthcare and the need and potential for change?

1. We continue to operate under the terms of the BNA Act provisions (now incorporated into the Constitution Act) for determining federal and provincial responsibilities in healthcare, meaning that we still operate with the same division of federal and provincial responsibilities in healthcare as seemed appropriate in 1867. Such a division of responsibility leaves room for provinces to assert their authority when it suits their particular situations, and it forces the federal government to work through three main alternate approaches to influence healthcare. More importantly, it leaves room for each level of government to blame the other for failure to take action (e.g., in areas such as pollution or home care) and to leave the public waiting—and often lobbying—for the impasse to be overcome.

2. We continue to talk about social determinants of health but have yet to deal with those determinants in a comprehensive and committed way. Governments and the public both are responsible for the lack of attention to these matters, yet conditions like full employment, a guaranteed annual income, stamping out poverty, and other such fundamental health-promoting conditions could have a significant effect on improving the health status of all and decreasing expenditures in tertiary healthcare.

3. Medicare continues to enjoy a high level of public support, although that level is slipping as corporate claims of better, more efficient care by for-profit medicine woo the public to their way of thinking. This persuasion is often accomplished by scare tactics, which distort the facts about current and projected public healthcare spending (CHSRF, 2007b).

4. As our history shows, in implementing federal and provincial programs, we have continued to compromise on what should be included and how the systems should operate. In the mid-1940s, we did not adopt a comprehensive approach to health and social security as had been suggested by Marsh and Heagerty. Instead, we chose to implement publicly appealing programs selectively (Armstrong et al., 2000). This approach had the effect of setting us up for rising costs because many of these programs were oriented toward high-technology medicine (e.g., the hospital insurance and diagnostic services program) and took the focus away from holistic patient care. Further, these programs excluded funding for many services, such as nursing homes, home care, and pharmaceutical coverage, and thereby disadvantaged elderly and poor people. Later, during the introduction of Medicare, Saskatchewan and then the federal government abandoned the concept of all-on-a-salary and gave in to doctors' demands for fee-for-service payments instead. This capitulation also paved the way for cost increases for healthcare and closed the door to a more level playing field in power relationships among physicians, nurses, and other health professionals, which has had a serious effect on women and on nursing.

5. The majority of nurses work in hospitals or other institutions where their autonomy is more limited than that of their counterparts working in the community. Relationships between physicians and nurses are not ideal, and this does not create the best environment for high-quality care.

6. The promise of health reform has yet to be realized; in fact, reforms such as regionalization may have added to the shortfall in comprehensive care as different regions make different decisions about what services they are prepared to offer.

7. Canada has failed to manage the growth of medical technology in a rational way. We have been unable to set limits on professional desires and public expectations.

8. We have yet to develop primary healthcare services, to make better legislative provisions for new entry points to the system, or to promote better use of qualified health personnel. Health promotion and disease prevention are key recommendations critical to current population needs.

9. We need to question whose interests are being served in keeping the system relatively unchanged since the 1960s. We need to ask what effect free trade and increased moves to globalization have had on maintaining a system characterized by medical dominance, an emphasis on technology without limits, unequal access to care, and marginalization of many health professionals and patient groups.

10. It is also necessary to ask what effect ideologies of individualism and egalitarianism have had on our inability to see the socioeconomic barriers that prevent patients from taking personal responsibility for their health (Anderson & Reimer-Kirkham, 1998).

11. There is no question about the need to work toward greater coordination and efficiencies in healthcare, as in any line of work. But, at the end of the day, the questions remain: Where else is the money going? What other corporate demands are driving healthcare? Who is profiting by maintaining the status quo in healthcare?

WHAT LIES AHEAD?

Several analysts (Armstrong et al., 2000; Coburn, 2010; Coburn & Rappolt, 1999) provide insights for understanding the context of healthcare today and prospects for tomorrow. They suggest that the gradual rise in medical dominance over the past decades in Canada and the implementation of Medicare by the governments in Canada were the last keys in the welfare state. In their analysis, Coburn and Rappolt (1999) see this as representing the triumph for labor and for the state (the government). However, they suggest that the gradual decline of medical dominance in healthcare and a decline in government involvement in healthcare have occurred as the result of a "major transformation of national and international political economies towards the internationalization of capital" (p. 142). This transformation has led to an increase in business power and a decrease in the relative autonomy of the state.

Coburn and Rappolt (1999) suggest that the "welfare state, and particularly anything to do with labour-market policy, is brought under fierce attack from a newly united right and its international and national agents in the business community, in neoliberal international institutions such as the International Monetary Fund, in national neoconservative policy institutions and think tanks, as well as the conservatively skewed media" (p. 152). Labeling these relatively recent phenomena as the "internationalization of capital" or "global capitalism," Coburn and Rappolt note how the International Monetary Fund, the World Bank, and the new ideologic unity between large and small businesses have had substantial influence on domestic business interests. This influence has enhanced the power of business with Canadian governments (both federal and provincial) and has particularly strengthened the hand of American influences on governments. Thus, free trade agreements are viewed as the inevitable costs of keeping Canada competitive, even though they have the potential to undermine Canadian social programs.

The potential scenario here is that governments' gradual undermining of social programs causes the public to see these programs as inadequate or outdated for 21st century needs. One has only to cut costs to particular services for so long before the public comes to believe that there must be no more money and, therefore, there is "no choice" except to welcome private, for-profit healthcare services. The effect has been one of the transformation with new "structures of class, state, welfare state, healthcare, health profession interaction [taking] one form under the particular dynamics of monopoly capitalism and [assuming] a new form under the somewhat different structure of global capitalism" (Coburn & Rappolt, 1999, p. 160). The overall impact has been designed "to produce powerlessness…making citizens powerless within their own countries" (p. 160). Coburn (2010) has focused on historical materialism to show how income inequalities and health inequalities have developed across countries and within Canada.

Yet when Coburn and Rappolt (1999) examine how "global" globalization really is, they point out that within the three major trading blocs in the world, the greatest influence on Canada is from the United States; and the effect on healthcare is that we are harmonizing downward toward this partner (p. 161). (This strong United States influence has become even more apparent since the September 11, 2001 terrorist attacks on the World Trade Center in New York, as many cherished Canadian policies in areas outside of healthcare, such as border guards carrying firearms in Canada, changed because of United States demands.) By altering the balance of power in Canada, the Free Trade Agreement (the agreement between the United States and Canada for free trade) and NAFTA (the free trade agreement that includes Mexico) have far-ranging consequences for Canada's social fabric and its social policies (p. 161). But even Coburn argues that there are "degrees of freedom and openings for resistance to neoliberal doctrines" (p. 160). To suggest that there is no choice left and that we cannot expect our social programs to continue is to adopt a fatalistic view that flies in the face of the power of individual and collective action to make a difference. The history and current status of Canadian healthcare make it clear that many of the important ideas and services in healthcare came about through struggle and persistence. A commitment to change is a commitment to engage in a political struggle that accompanies the change (Anderson & Reimer-Kirkham, 1998). One Canadian reality worth remembering is that the Canadian Constitution establishes that the federal government is responsible for making "Laws for the Peace, Order and good Government of Canada" (Van Loon & Whittington, 1976, p. 480). This concept is in contrast to that of the U.S. Constitution, which centers on individual liberties and freedoms. This difference set the stage for enacting Canadian legislation that emphasized the common (collective) good evident in values that promote Canada's social programs.

NURSES LEADING TO INFLUENCE CHANGE

If nurses are to be effective leaders in influencing change both individually and through collective action, some homework is needed. Nurses need to understand the history and structures of the healthcare system in Canada, to educate themselves to the needs of their patients, and to set goals and work together to achieve those goals.

What Nurses Need to Know

Individually, there is a need for nurses to know about the development of Canadian healthcare, or at least to be aware of basic programs and structures that have been put in place over time. This awareness includes some understanding of the historical ideologic debates and how those same debates continue to play out in healthcare today. This knowledge and understanding should not only give nurses confidence in stating their case, but also ensure that they are not susceptible to being silenced by others' rhetoric. In addition, nurses must be clear about some of the international and national pressures on the healthcare system and be ready to push against the perceived inevitability of a greater uptake of the business orientation that might diminish the effectiveness of healthcare delivery.

Second, nurses need good—and updated—information, including keeping up to date with public debates in the media and elsewhere and also digging deeper to uncover reliable facts and other viewpoints. Professional nursing associations, educational institutions, public libraries, and the Internet can be helpful resources for nurses. CNA's development of NursingOne can be a useful Internet access for all nurses.

Other information needed by nurses includes keeping abreast of the influence of trade agreements on healthcare and professional practice as well as on basic needs for the public's health, such as an adequate supply of clean water, clean air, security, and other essentials of life. Knowledge of ethics in nursing practice is critical to reflection on these issues (Storch et al., 2013). Nurses also need to know about their professional associations and professional colleges, including the freedom and responsibilities of self-regulation and the importance of collective action.

What Nurses Need to Be

Above all, nurses need to be well educated, good listeners, and sensitive caregivers. Nurses need to see and respond to the people who are marginalized in society: Aboriginal people, immigrants, different ethnic groupings, women—particularly single mothers and their children—those living in poverty, elderly people, and so forth.

We also need to see and critically think about the dominant players in healthcare and seek to understand their views as well as direct our attention toward ways to broaden and influence their thinking (e.g., Pauly, 2004; Varcoe, 2004). Despite the difficulties nursing faces today with regard to being valued, we need to keep on caring without regard for race, color, creed, religious persuasion, or political alignments. In short, we need to continue to be role models of caring practices. It is not surprising that the CNA chose "be the change" as the slogan for their Centennial Year.

What Nurses Need to Do

Collectively, nurses need to be willing to work together to reach good outcomes for their patients and for themselves. Canada has fine examples of nurses involved in collective action to make a difference through both provincial nursing organizations and through the CNA, including specific foci during provincial and federal elections.

Nurses also need to use the knowledge gained through nursing education and nurse–patient relationships to focus attention on the determinants of health. Frank and Mustard (1994), and many before them, demonstrated the relationships between illness and socioeconomic factors. In addition to noting how the job hierarchy influences health, these authors suggested that "an individual's sense of achievement, self-esteem, and control over his or her work and life appears to affect health and well-being" (p. 9). As nurses come to know their patients, they see the effects of these variables on patient well-being and on their own health. That is important knowledge to be utilized in dialogue with politicians or bureaucrats.

Working collectively toward the goal of primary healthcare for all is also critical work for nurses today. Nurses in advanced nursing practice make a difference in patient care and can improve the health system overall. The persistence of nurses in moving toward patient-centered goals continues to make a difference within specific areas and has a spillover effect over time (Pauly et al., 2004).

Individually, nurses can also be ready to speak, to question, and to spread hope (Broughton, 2001). As nurses, we may not have all the answers but we do know most of the questions. With regard to information about the political economy discussed in this text, an individual nurse may not have complete knowledge but can question politicians and government bureaucrats, as well as other civil servants, neighbors, friends, and colleagues to make them think and potentially to influence their actions however large or small they may be. This is to move against a place of powerlessness.

SUMMARY

Nurses need to understand what drives today's healthcare system, particularly in regard to the underpinnings of Medicare, the international economic manipulation of resources available for healthcare, and the related disempowerment of healthcare professionals.

The same value conflicts that we see today were inherent in the development of Canadian policies and programs since their inception: A focus on individual responsibility and self-reliance versus collective responsibility; a free market system versus more socially oriented collective policies and programs in healthcare (the privatization debate); an emphasis on scientific discovery and technologic imperatives versus humanism and care for the disadvantaged; and those who believe that all have equal opportunities to healthcare versus the reality that gender, race, and class differences affect the way in which healthcare is delivered (Anderson et al., 2009).

Canadian nurses have sought for almost three decades to promote primary healthcare, and it continues to be a model worth pursuing. In fact, it is one of the CNA's two key goals in this millennium; the other goal is achieving improved quality of work environments for nurses.

Nurses can influence change by attending to the history, current status, and future projections for healthcare; by being caregivers who both listen and care; and by taking action individually and collectively to promote greater attention to social determinants of health and better healthcare provision for their patients.

As nurses, we need to be clear about our own values and opinions and be able to stand by them so our voices can help shape better approaches to healthcare. If we are not prepared to do so, nursing and nurses will have little to say in the healthcare system of tomorrow.

Add to your knowledge of this issue:

Online

Canadian Nurses Association	**www.cna-aiic.ca**
Health Canada	**http://www.hc-sc.gc.ca**
Canadian Health Services Research Foundation	**www.chsrf.ca**

R E F L E C T I O N S *on the Chapter…*

1 In what ways do you think the Canadian healthcare "system" would have been different and subject to less political influence if the Fathers of Confederation had chosen to assign principal responsibility for healthcare and education to the federal government rather than to the provinces?

2 If medical care insurance had been introduced before the introduction of hospital insurance, what differences might we have seen in the formation of health facilities? What contributions do you think this might have made in controlling the costs of technology? Would primary healthcare likely have become the norm?

3 Do you believe that healthcare costs are out of control? Why or why not?

4 In reflecting on what you know about nurses' individual or collective actions to influence better healthcare, what types of knowledge have they utilized to influence change?

5 To what degree have you felt powerless or powerful against business interests in healthcare? Why have you felt that way?

Want to know more? Visit thePoint. for additional helpful resources:

- Journal Articles
- Learning Objectives
- Nursing Professional Roles and Responsibilities
- Bonus chapters:
  - Health and Nursing Policy: A Matter of Politics, Power and Professionalism
  - The NP Movement: Recurring Issues
  - When Difference Matters: The Politics of Privilege and Marginality

References

Anderson, J., & Reimer-Kirkham, S. (1998). Constructing nation: The gendering and racializing of the Canadian health care system. In V. Strong-Boag, J. Anderson, S. Grace, & A. Eisenberg (Eds.), *Painting the maple: Essays on race, gender, and the construction of Canada* (pp. 242–261). Vancouver, BC: UBC Press.

Anderson, J., Rodney, P., Reimer-Kirkham, S., Browne, A.J., Khan, K.B., & Lynam, M.J. (2009). Inequities in health and healthcare viewed through the ethical lens of critical social justice. *Advances in Nursing Science, 32*(4), 282–294.

Angus, J., & Bourgeault, I.L. (1999). Medical dominance, gender and the state: The nurse practitioner initiative in Ontario. In D. Coburn, S. Rappolt, I. Bourgeault, & J. Angus (Eds.), *Medicine, nursing and the state* (p. 55). Aurora, ON: Garamond Press Ltd.

Armstrong, P., Armstrong, H., Bourgeault, I., Choiniere, J., Mykhalovskiy, E., & White, J. (2000). *"Heal thyself": Managing health care reform.* Aurora, ON: Garamond Press.

Broughton, H. (2001). *Nursing leadership: Unleashing the power.* Ottawa, ON: Canadian Nurses Association.

Bryant, T., Raphael, D., & Rioux, M. (Eds.). (2010). *Staying alive* (2nd ed.). Toronto, ON: Canadian Scholars' Press.

Canada Health Act. (1984). c.6. Ottawa: Minister of Justice.

Canadian Doctors for Medicare. (2011). *Neat, plausible, and wrong: The myth of health care unsustainability.* Toronto, ON: Author.

Canadian Health Services Research Foundation (CHSRF). (2004). *Mythbusters–Myth: For-profit ownership of facilities would lead to a more efficient health care system.* Ottawa, ON: Author.

_____. (2007a). *Evidence Boost for Quality: Self-management education to optimize health and reduce hospital admissions for chronically ill patients.* Ottawa, ON: Author.

_____. (2007b). *MythBusters–Myth: Canada's system of healthcare financing is unsustainable.* Ottawa, ON: Author.

Canadian Nurses Association. (1980). *Putting "Health" back into health care.* Submission to the Health Services Review '79. Ottawa, ON: Author.

_____. (2000a). *The Canada health act.* Ottawa, ON: Author.

_____. (2000b). *The primary health care approach.* Fact sheet. Ottawa, ON: Author.

_____. (2005). *CNA backgrounder: primary health care: A summary of issues.* Ottawa, ON: Author.

Canadian Nursing Advisory Committee. (2002). *Our health, our future: Creating quality workplaces for nurses.* Final report. Ottawa, ON: Health Canada.

Canadian Patient Safety Institute (CPSI). (2007). *Patient safety: New heights, higher standards.* Edmonton, AB: Author.

Cassidy, H.M. (1947). The Canadian social services. *The Annals of the Academy of Political and Social Sciences, 253*(September), 190–201.

Chodos, H., & MacLeod, J.J. (2004). Romanow and Kirby on the public/private divide in healthcare: Demystifying the debate. *HealthcarePapers, 4*(4), 10–25.

Coburn, D. (1988). The development of Canadian nursing: Professionalization and proletarianization. *International Journal of Health Services, 18*(3), 437–456.

Coburn, D. (2010). Health and health care: A political economy perspective. In T. Bryant, D. Raphael, & M. Rioux (Eds.), *Staying alive: Critical perspectives on health, illness, and health care* (2nd ed., pp. 65–91). Toronto, ON: Canadian Scholars' Press Inc.

Coburn, D., & Rappolt, S. (1999). The "logic of medicare": Variants of capitalism and medical dominance. Contextualizing profession-state relationships. In D. Coburn, S. Rappolt, I. Bourgeault, and J. Angus (Eds.), *Medicine, nursing and the state* (pp. 139–167). Aurora, ON: Garamond Press.

Commission on the Future of Healthcare in Canada. (2002). *Building on values: Final report.* Commissioner R.J. Romanow. Ottawa, ON: National Library of Canada.

Crawford, M. (2006). Interactions: Trade policy and healthcare reform after Chaoulli v. *Quebec. Healthcare Policy, 1*(2), 90–102.

Deber, R.B. (2004). Cats and categories: Public and private in Canadian healthcare. *HealthcarePapers, 4*(4), 51–60.

Defries, R.D. (1962). *The federal and provincial health services in Canada.* (2nd ed.). Toronto, ON: Canadian Public Health Association.

Demers, V., Melo, M., Jackevicius, C., et al. (2008). Comparison of provincial prescription drug plans and the impact on patients' annual drug expenditures. *Canadian Medical Association Journal, 178*(4), 405–409.

Duckett, S. (2010). Second wave of reform in Alberta. *Healthcare Management Forum, 23*(4), 156–158.

Epp, J. (1986). *Achieving health for all: A framework for health promotion.* Catalogue No. H39-102/1986E, Health and Welfare Canada, Ottawa ON, November.

Feldberg, G., Vipond, R., & Bryant, T. (2010). Cracks in the foundation of the Canadian and American health care systems. In T. Bryant, D. Raphael, & M. Rioux (Eds.), *Staying alive: Critical perspectives on health, illness, and health care* (pp. 267–285). Toronto, ON: Canadian Scholars' Press Inc.

Fierlbeck, K. (2011). *Health care in Canada.* Toronto, ON: University of Toronto Press.

Frank, J.W., & Mustard, J.F. (1994). The determinants of health from a historical perspective. *Daedalus*, Fall, 1–19.

Fuller, C. (1998). *Caring for profit: How corporations are taking over Canada's health care system.* Vancouver, BC: New Star Books.

Gregory, D.W., & Parfrey, P.S. (2010). The breast cancer hormone receptor retesting controversy in Newfoundland and Labrador, Canada: Lessons for the health system. *Healthcare Management Forum, 23*(3), 114–118.

Harnett, C.E. (2008). Superbug spreading in hospitals, communities. *Times Colonist*, March 3, A1, A4.

Hastings, J.E.F. (1972). *Report of the community health centre project to the health ministers.* Toronto, ON: Canadian Public Health Association.

Hastings, J.E.F., & Mosley, W. (1980). Introduction: The evolution of organized community health services in Canada. In C.A. Meilicke & J.L. Storch (Eds.), *Perspectives on Canadian health and social services policy: History and emerging trends* (pp. 145–155). Ann Arbor, MI: Health Administration Press.

Health Canada. (2002). *Canada's health care system.* Retrieved from http://www.hc-sc.gc.ca/

Health Care Renewal Accord. (2003). *First ministers accord on healthcare renewal.* Retrieved from http://www.hc-sc.gc.ca/english//hca2003/accord.html

Health Council of Canada. (2005). *Health care renewal in Canada: Accelerating change.* Ottawa, ON: Author.

Health Council of Canada. (2010). *Stepping it up: Moving the focus of health care in Canada to a healthier Canada.* Ottawa, ON: Author.

HealthcarePapers. (2006). *New models for the new healthcare, 7*(1):4–74. Entire issue.

Hutchison, B. (2007). Editorial: Disparities in healthcare access and use: Yackety-yack Yackety-yack. *Healthcare Policy, 3*(2), 10–13.

Institute of Medicine. (1999). *To err is human: Building a safer health care system.* Washington, DC: National Academics Press.

Kenny, N. (2002). *What good is health care?* Ottawa, ON: CHA Press.

Kenny, N. (2004). Value(s) for money? Assessing Romanow and Kirby. *HealthcarePapers, 4*(4), 28–34.

Kingston-Riechers, J., Ospina, M., Jonsson E., Childs, P., McLeod, L., & Maxted, J.M. (2010). *Patient safety in primary care.* Edmonton, AL: Canadian Patient Safety Institute and the BC Patient Safety & Quality Council.

LaBonte, R. (1994). Death of program, birth of metaphor: The development of public health in Canada. In A. Pederson, M. O'Neill, & I. Rootman (Eds.), *Health promotion in Canada: Provincial, national and international perspectives* (pp. 72–90). Toronto, ON: W.B. Saunders Canada.

Laframboise, H.L. (1973). Health policy: Breaking the problem down into more manageable segments. *Canadian Medical Association Journal, 108*(February), 388–393.

Lalonde, M. (1974). *A new perspective on the health of Canadians.* Ottawa, ON: Information Canada.

Lang, A., Macdonald, M., Storch, J., et al. (2009). Home care safety perspectives from clients, family members, caregivers and paid providers. *Healthcare Quarterly, 12*(Sp), 97–101.

Leatt, P., Lemieux-Charles, L., & Aird, C. (1994). *Program management and beyond: Management innovations in Ontario hospitals.* Ottawa, ON: Canadian College of Health Service Executives.

Leatt, P., Pink, G.H., & Guerriere, M. (2000). Towards a Canadian model of integrated healthcare. *HealthcarePapers, 1*(2), 13–35.

Lewis, S. (2007). Can a learning-disabled nation learn healthcare lessons from abroad? *Healthcare Policy, 3*(2), 19–28.

Lindenfield, R. (1959). Hospital insurance in Canada: An example in federal–provincial relations. *Social Services Review, 33*, 148–160.

MacDonald, M., Regan, S., Davidson, H., et al. (2006). Knowledge transfer to advance the nurse practitioner role in British Columbia. *Healthcare Policy, 1*(2), 80–89.

Marsh, L. (1975). *Report on social security for Canada 1943.* Toronto, ON: University of Toronto Press.

McIntosh, J.W. (1914). Inter-relation of physician, citizen and state to public health. *The Public Health Journal, 5*(July 14), 451–455.

Morgan, M.W., Zamora, N.E., & Hindmarsh, M.F. (2007). An inconvenient truth: A sustainable healthcare system requires a chronic disease prevention and management transformation. *HealthcarePapers, 7*(4), 6–23.

National Forum on Health Care. (1997). *Canada health action: Building the legacy.* Ottawa, ON: Health Canada.

Pauly, B. (2004). Shifting the balance in funding and delivery of health care in Canada. In J. Storch, P. Rodney, & R. Starzomski (Eds.), *Towards a moral horizon: Nursing ethics for leadership and practice* (pp. 181–208). Toronto, ON: Pearson Education Canada.

Pauly, B., Schreiber, R., MacDonald, M., et al. (2004). Dancing to our own tune: Understandings of advanced nursing practice in British Columbia. *Journal of Nursing Leadership, 17*(2), 47–57.

Peritz, I. (2008). Technician faces trial over false blood-test results. *The Globe and Mail*, February 6, A7.

Petch, T., & Shamian, J. (2009). Adding value while saving dollars: Unleashing the potential of a national, integrated approach to home and community care. *HealthcarePapers*, 9(4), 41–46.

Picard, A. (2011, November 22). "Days of blindly topping up medicare over". *The Globe and Mail*, p. A5.

Pike-MacDonald, S., Best, B.G., Twomey, C., Bennett, L., & Blakeley, J. (2007). Promoting safe drinking water. *Canadian Nurse, 103*(1), 15–19.

Priest, L. (2008). Ottawa targets hospital superbugs. *The Globe and Mail*, February 4, A1, A6.

Priest, A., Rachlis, M., & Cohen, M. (2007). *Why wait? Public solutions to cure surgical waitlists.* Vancouver, BC: Canadian Centre for Policy Alternatives BC.

Reichwein, B.P. (2011). Alberta's long-term care services are in crisis: Government's relentless pursuit to privatize long-term care. *HealthcarePapers*, 10(4), 51–56.

Rice, J.J., & Prince, M.J. (2000). *Changing politics of Canadian social policy.* Toronto, ON: University of Toronto Press.

Roberge, G. (2003). *A four part paper on health policy and management implications of the Romanow and Kirby reports.* Unpublished paper. Faculty of Human and Social Development, University of Victoria, Victoria, BC.

Rootman, I., & O'Neill, M. (1994). Developing knowledge for health promotion. In A. Pederson, M. O'Neill, & I. Rootman (Eds.), *Health promotion in Canada: Provincial, national and international perspectives* (pp. 139–151). Toronto, ON: W.B. Saunders Canada.

Saul, J.R. (1995). *The unconscious civilization.* Concord, ON: Anansis.

Shamian, J., & LeClair, S.J. (2000). Integrated delivery systems now or…? *HealthcarePapers, 1*(2), 66–75.

Shamian, J., Shainblum, E., & Stevens, J. (2006). Accountability agenda must include home care and community based care. *HealthcarePapers, 7*(1), 58–64.

Storch, J.L. (2005). Patient safety: Is it just another bandwagon? *Nursing Leadership, 18*(2), 39–55.

Storch, J.L., Rodney, P., & Starzomski, R. (Eds). (2013). *Towards a moral horizon: Nursing ethics for leadership and practice* (2nd ed). Toronto, ON: Pearson Education Canada.

Tam, P. (2012, March 9) Drug shortages could last a year: Expert, *The Times Colonist*, p. A12.

Taylor, M.G. (1973). The Canadian health insurance program. *Public Administration Review, 33*(January–February), 31–39.

Taylor, M.G. (1987). *Health insurance and Canadian public policy* (2nd ed.). Montreal, QC: McGill Queens University Press.

Van Loon, R.J., & Whittington, M.S. (1976). *The Canadian political system: Environment, structure and process* (2nd ed.). Toronto, ON: McGraw-Hill Ryerson.

Varcoe, C. (2004). Widening the scope of ethical theory, practice, and policy: Violence against women as an illustration. In J. Storch, P. Rodney, & R. Starzomski (Eds.), *Towards a moral horizon: Nursing ethics for leadership and practice* (pp. 414–432). Toronto, ON: Pearson Education Canada.

Wallace, E. (1950). The origins of the social welfare state in Canada, 1867–1900. *Canadian Journal of Economics and Political Science, 16*, 383–393.

Williams, A.P., Lum, J.M., Deber, R., et al. (2009). Aging in home: Integrating community-based care for older persons. *HealthcarePapers, 10*(1), 8–21.

Nursing Education and Healthcare in Québec

Jacinthe Pepin

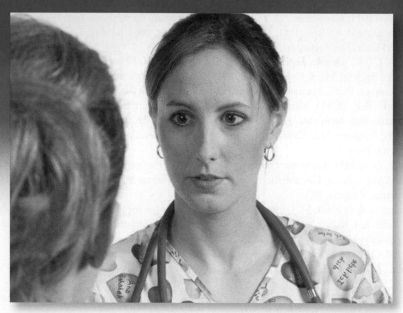

Québec nurses challenge the persistence of two levels of educational preparation for new Registered Nurses. (Used with permission Canadian Federation of Nurses Unions.)

Critical Questions

As a way of engaging with the ideas in this chapter, consider the following:

1. What do you know of nursing education in Québec?

2. How does language influence nursing knowledge?

3. How important is the issue of preparation of new nurses for healthcare?

Chapter Objectives

After completing this chapter, you will be able to:

1. Discuss the significance of higher education of nurses for healthcare.

2. Identify factors that delayed the decision to prepare all new nurses at the baccalaureate level.

3. Compare Québec nursing education with education in another province or territory.

In the opening chapter of this text, McIntyre and McDonald outline the significance of the profession for healthcare:

> The quality of healthcare depends to a large extent on the nature of the nursing component determined by four elements: standards of education and preparation for those entering the profession; quality of care provided by the practitioner—a quality closely associated with education and preparation; number of nurses available—a determination considered in modern times largely by the social and economic status the profession offers its members; and milieu in which care is offered. (2013, p. 6)

This chapter addresses these four elements in the context of Québec, with particular attention paid to the first two: Nursing education and healthcare. Nursing students across Canada might well ask about the differences in the way nursing education and healthcare has developed across various provinces. In this chapter, the evolution of nursing education and healthcare in Québec are explored, highlighting both the similarities and the uniqueness of the situation for nurses in this province. Although historically, events unfold differently in various provinces, the issues for Québec nurses reflect some of the key challenges that are important for all nurses to consider.

Canada is diverse in both education and healthcare systems, and Québec exemplifies this diversity. For example, Québec education and healthcare systems are organized into French-speaking services and English-speaking services. Healthcare professionals must demonstrate sufficient mastery of French because 86.3% of the population is French-speaking (Statistics Canada, 2006). Québec's unique position in Canada dates from the New-France Era (1608–1759), a period in which nursing developed within a French–Canadian model designed by religious communities, particularly by the Sisters of Charity, also named Grey Nuns (Cohen et al., 2002; Paul & Ross-Kerr, 2011). It is only with the establishment of the first nursing schools in Québec in English hospitals, starting in 1875, that the secular Nightingale model and the Catholic French–Canadian model began inter-influencing one another toward professionalization (Mansell & Dood, 2005). Today, Québec contributes to the development of Canadian nursing and Canadian nursing education while maintaining its uniqueness.

Nursing education and research in Québec will first be described. From this description, one major issue—the persistence of two levels of preparation for new registered nurses—will be further discussed including an exploration of the significance of the issue for nurses, the profession, and healthcare. An in-depth analysis of this issue will include historical, socio-cultural, and political perspectives. A discussion of barriers to resolution and current as well as potential strategies to address this issue will conclude the chapter.

NURSING EDUCATION AND RESEARCH

This first section describes the existing nursing education programs in Québec that prepare those entering the profession and those pursuing graduate studies. The standards of education and the ways in which Québec nurses participate in setting those standards are presented. Finally, the topic of knowledge development as central to nursing education is addressed, and leads the way to stating the major issue being discussed: The persistence of two levels of preparation for new registered nurses.

The Programs

The Québec Ministry of Education (2008) describes its education system as being "made up of public and private French and English educational institutions" (p. 1). Education in public schools is free at the first three levels: Elementary (which also includes preschool), secondary, and college. The fourth level is university education. In Québec, a person who wants to become a nurse must attend a total of 11 years before making a decision about which path to follow to enter a nursing program. This person will then go into college education either in the 2-year preuniversity education path or in the 3-year technical training path. This technical training path leads to the job market with a College Education Diploma, after a total of 14 years of schooling. Alternatively, the preuniversity path will necessarily be followed by 3 years in the Bachelor of Science Degree program in Nursing (BScN) that also leads to the job market, this time after 16 years of schooling. The university educational path is comparable to the required initial preparation of Registered Nurses to practice as generalists elsewhere in Canada (CNA & CASN, 2004).

Since 2004, a person choosing the technical path may continue for an additional 2 years to achieve the same or equivalent BScN. This continuum agreement between colleges and universities, where the university recognizes the college nursing program toward the degree, was implemented within nine consortia university colleges. The college portion, includes 65 units* of specific nursing education (preparation to provide care for patients of all ages in medical–surgical and mental health wards as well as perinatology and long-term care facilities) plus six units of general education (French, English, and Philosophy) linked to nursing (e.g., ethics is the main topic of the philosophy course). This is 71 of the 91 2/3 units of the 3-year program, and the rest is general education (Ministère de l'Éducation, du Loisir et du Sport [MELS], 2007). The university portion adds the science and research components, as well as the preparation for family and population foci, interprofessional collaborative practices, critical care, community nursing, and quality of care assessment; it strengthens the preparation to mental healthcare (*Comité des spécialistes,* 2000). This continuum can be compared to the collaborative programs in the rest of the country, except for the entry to practice with a Diploma, which is still in place in Québec.

While it is often thought that undergraduate education is mainly theoretical, today, all nursing education units in colleges and universities in Québec have access to well-equipped labs to help students develop psychomotor and relational skills, including sophisticated mannequins for the simulation of nursing patient care. All education units in Québec also have access to sufficient clinical placements of their students, which is monitored by collaborative groups in the Regional Health Agencies.

Hence, a person entering nursing will have developed professional competencies to a certain point at the college or university level, and will register as a nurse after the successful completion of the Order of Nurses in Québec's (ONQ) professional examination or the Canadian Registered Nurse Examination (CRNE). Other potential paths to develop the nursing professional competencies before completing one of these examinations include Direct-Entry Master of Science (Applied) in Nursing offered at McGill University to university graduates with a general degree, and a professional integration program tailored for applicants who received their nursing diploma or degree outside of Canada.

In Québec, only people who have sufficient knowledge (verbal and written comprehension and expression) of French can practice their profession (Office Québécois de la langue française [OQLF], 2009). Therefore, nurses who studied in English have to write the OQLF French exam before they can obtain their practice license, and this is a challenge for some nurses. It is of particular interest that in 2010, Québec and France signed a unique agreement of mutual recognition of registered nurses who have a degree (BScN) in Québec and a State Diploma (License since the Bologna Accord) in France. An integration period of 75 days and an evaluation precedes the right to practice, without a nurse having to write the professional exam of the other country (Ordre des infirmières et infirmiers du Québec [OIIQ], 2010a).

Graduate programs in nursing are offered in all Québec universities with nursing schools. McGill University, Université Laval, Université de Montréal, and Université de Sherbrooke have Masters and Doctorate programs in nursing or Doctorate programs with a major in nursing, while the five constituents of *Université du Québec* share a Masters' program (Abitibi-Témiscaminque,

---

*1 unit = 45 hours of learning activities

Chicoutimi, Outaouais, Rimouski, Trois-Rivières). Much like in the rest of Canada, the 2 to 3 year Master's programs prepare nurses for advanced practice, either as clinical nurse "specialists" (CNS), specialized nurse practitioners (SNP), nurse educators, or nurse administrators. With the rest of Canada, in September 1994, the Faculty of Nursing of the Université de Montréal and the School of Nursing, McGill University began offering a joint bilingual doctoral program (PhD).

In summary, except for the two levels of preparation of new nurses and the predominance of the French language, much of the Québec nursing education is similar to that in other regions of Canada, and in many ways Québec nurses participate in setting Canadian education standards.

The Standards

Québec faculties and university schools of nursing are members of the Canadian Association of Schools of Nursing (CASN), whose mission is to be the national voice for nursing education, research, and scholarship and to represent baccalaureate and graduate nursing programs in Canada. Therefore, university nursing units are eligible to participate in the voluntary CASN Accreditation peer-review program. CASN Accreditation promotes excellence in nursing education by setting and revising the standards, by evaluating the programs in their context at least every 7 years, and by maintaining a philosophy of continuing improvement (CASN, 2011). At the moment, most Québec university baccalaureate nursing programs have "accredited" status. As far as accreditation of graduate programs is concerned, CASN is not yet offering an evaluation process. The other nursing educational programs (in colleges, and Masters and Doctorate in universities) are subjected to a variety of quality evaluation processes, within the respective institutions. These processes usually include self-evaluation and external review.

Québec nurses have made an outstanding contribution to the development of standards and national accreditation through their central participation in the CASN. In 1942, representatives of four nursing university programs participated, along with colleagues of seven programs from other provinces, in the founding of CASN (Kirkwood & Bouchard, 1992). Québec nurses also participated in the establishment of CASN's accreditation program, first published in 1987. Québec continues to be represented on the CASN Board of Directors, and over the years many nurses from Québec have chaired the board and its committees.

Not only did Québec nurses take part in defining what would be taught to prepare new nurses, they have innovated and influenced how new nurses learn and integrate knowledge into practice. For example, Evelyn Adam of the Université de Montréal and Moyra Allen of McGill University are among the Canadian nurse scholars who proposed Canadian conceptualizations of nursing and nursing education (Pepin, 2008; Thorne, 2011). The relevance of these frameworks continues to this day, both in French and in English (Gottlieb, Feeley & Dalton, 2006; Pepin et al., 2010). Moreover, professors from the Université de Montréal are among the Canadian nurses to shift nursing education to a research focus (Goudreau et al., 2009). Grounded in a constructivist educational perspective, these authors described what they called a second generation of the competency-based approach to nursing education and presented its application in their 2004 version of the Université of Montréal's baccalaureate program. Moving away from task orientation, this competency-based approach is centered on knowledge integration and on the development of competencies.

Nursing Knowledge

Currently, nursing knowledge is being developed and implemented largely through interuniversity nursing research groups, nursing chairs and intra or interprofessional teams in partnerships with professional practice. For example, the Québec Interuniversity Nursing Intervention Research Group (GRIISIQ), created in 2003 by the School of Nursing at McGill University and the Faculty of Nursing at Université de Montréal, is "unique by being involved exclusively in developing and evaluating nursing interventions and in measuring their clinical outcomes" (http://www.griisiq.ca). More recently the group has grown to include four universities and other partners with in Québec. Similarly, the interuniversity FERASI center focuses on training and expertise in nursing administration and research. Finally, the Centre for Innovation in Nursing Education (CIFI) was established in 2007 at the Université de Montréal with the goal of fostering leading-edge educational programs at every level of education, including continuing education, that enhance the quality of care. With colleagues from other universities, CIFI closes the gap between well-implemented research for nursing interventions and nursing administration.

Nursing research flourishes in Québec, as in the rest of the country, with national and international knowledge contributions in both French and English and with scientific breakthroughs, characterized by Donaldson (2000) as nursing work that brings a "transdisciplinary change in thinking" (p. 247) for the benefit of patients and their families. Care of the elderly and of family members is an example of such fields where change is visible: Healthcare professionals now consider caregivers as a focus of care and financial relief has recently been granted to caregivers (Ducharme, 2009).

It is beyond the scope of this chapter to present a complete picture of the nursing research activities and their impact in Québec. This cursory look reflects the active involvement of many researchers in interuniversity partnerships, and with nurse clinicians, other professionals and decision-makers, in three main areas of nursing practice: Care and health, administration, and education.

If the implementation of graduate programs shows formal recognition of the discipline of nursing, the support by research funding agencies and the impact of research results on clinical and political decisions attest to the quality of nursing's scientific activities. In this rich context of knowledge production and implementation, one might wonder why a university education has not yet been required in Québec for all new nurses.

The Persistence of Two Levels of Preparation for Newly Registered Nurses

Thirty years after Québec nursing's regulatory body, the Order of Québec Nurses (ONQ) agreed in 1982 that a baccalaureate degree should be the entry requirement for the profession (CASN/CNA, 2005), the topic remains sensitive and the process is not yet complete. The other Canadian provinces and territories took the same standpoint on the entry requirement and they have reached their goal by 2000 for some and 2010 for others, not without having to overcome obstacles along the way. In Québec though, the two levels of preparation for new registered nurses still give access to the profession. As pointed out earlier in this chapter, the entry-to-nursing-practice exam can be written after obtaining either a diploma or a degree in nursing. It is a unique situation in Canada and the French-speaking world (together with Lebanon) since nursing education in Europe was raised to the undergraduate level after the Bologna Accord was signed in 1999 by the ministers of education (CIFI, 2010).

In the last decade, many changes occurred in Québec nursing education and healthcare system that led to a recent step in the direction of university education requirement for all new nurses. In education, collaborations between colleges and universities have been strengthened through the implementation of the continuum that allows students to transfer from colleges to universities to complete their BScN.

Hence, the step forward taken by Québec nurses was supported by the vast majority of delegates at the 2011 annual meeting of Québec nurses regulatory body of a motion put forth to request action by the regulatory body toward the requirement of university education for the nursing profession (Ordre des infirmières et infirmiers du Québec [OIIQ]). The Annual Conference that followed this annual meeting was on nursing education: Where does Québec stand in relation to the rest of the world? It became an occasion to bring together the conference participants and the whole population of nurses as one unified voice for university education.

The issue of the persistent continuation of two levels of preparation for registered nurses will be analyzed through different lenses in the last section of this chapter. Questions will be raised to better understand the complexity of Québec nursing education and to suggest strategies for resolution. First, we will explore the significance of this issue for nurses, the nursing profession, and healthcare.

Significance of the Issue of Two Levels of Preparation for New Nurses

For nurses, the issue of two levels of preparation of new colleagues is very important as it places nurses in a position of having to defend their own preparation as a healthcare professional. For new nurses with a diploma, it means having been recognized by the Québec regulatory body as a professional who can provide safe care, while being encouraged to continue studying at the baccalaureate level. Duchscher (2008), who conducted studies on the experiences of newly graduated registered nurses, reported that over 30% of graduates going through their initial transition period "expressed concerns about being placed in clinical situations beyond their cognitive and experiential comfort zone" (p. 7).

In 2004 and 2005, the Québec government created distinct titles, job descriptions, and revised salary ladders for the diploma-prepared nurse and for the degree-prepared nurse with additional responsibilities. On the one hand, this creation recognizes the distinct preparations; on the other hand, it formalizes two different nursing groups in practice and tends to take degree-prepared nurses away from the bedside. Nursing managers in the healthcare system are challenged in their attempt to work with nurses prepared at both levels and to find ways to support the ongoing development of nursing competencies for each.

The issue of two levels of preparation brings into question how to recognize the nursing profession as an autonomous discipline with its own body of knowledge. Similarly, nursing education is challenged to deliver a contemporary nursing education in line with the changes to the field of practice. Rodgers (2005) points out that nurses often find themselves answering the question, "what do nurses do" and that many valid answers to that question exist. The author argues that the importance of nurses' contributions is not what nurses do but rather what they know. It is the knowledge on the basis of nurses' interventions that distinguishes their contribution to the patient, family, community, and population health. Rodgers (2005) reminds all nurses to be aware of the knowledge on which they build their practice, to question it, and to participate in its development.

The persistence of two levels of preparation is then important to the profession because only part of the nursing workforce is prepared to participate in knowledge questioning and development and consequently in the evolution of nursing practices. This is acknowledged by the Ministry of Health and Social Services (MSSS) (2004) in its description of benefits of the degree-prepared nurse. In Québec, 33% of the nursing workforce holds a nursing degree (OIIQ, 2011a, 2011b), in comparison to more than 40% in Canada (Canadian Institute for Health Information, 2010), and about 40% of new nurses in comparison to 100% in the rest of Canada. Moreover, all members of other healthcare professions hold at least an undergraduate education and expect everyone in the team to keep up with new knowledge for the benefit of interprofessional work and ultimately patient and family care and health.

In 2010, CASN reports in its white paper that:

> A growing body of North American research over the last decade has clearly shown that patient safety and outcomes are directly related to the overall level of nursing knowledge within a health care agency (Ellis et al., 2006). Patient outcomes are significantly better when patients are cared for by registered nurses who are baccalaureate prepared. The risk of death is decreased, fewer adverse reactions to treatment occur, there are fewer procedural violations, and there is a reduction in medication errors. (McGillis Hall et al., 2004; Tourangeau et al., 2006, p. 4)

Hence, the issue of the preparation of new nurses is of the utmost importance for healthcare, for nurses and for the nursing profession. The complexity of care and the level of decision making in nursing calls for university preparation for all new nurses. Research has shown that patient outcomes are linked to this preparation and the baccalaureate requirement is supported through a consensus among international nurses associations (International Council of Nurses [ICN], 2010; Secrétariat international des infirmières et infirmiers de l'espace francophone [SIDIIEF], 2011; World Health Organization [WHO], 2009).

ANALYSIS OF THE ISSUE

Now that a picture of the education and healthcare context has been sketched and the significance of two levels of preparation of new nurses has been made explicit, the issue will be analyzed using the framework introduced in Chapter 1 of this text. Historical, socio-cultural, and political questions will be raised following a brief statement of salient elements for each.

HISTORICAL QUESTIONS

Up until the 1960s, basic nursing education in Québec was located in hospitals and advanced education for nurses (administration, public health, and teaching) in universities. Practice knowledge was formalized by the publication of nursing journals and manuals as early as the 1920s (Cohen et al., 2002). University courses in nursing were offered in 1923 at the Institut Marguerite d'Youville (IMY) and in 1934 by the Grey Nuns and affiliated with Université de Montréal.

A dual approach to the preparation of new nurses originated when nursing education shifted from the hospital system to the colleges in 1967 during the secularism movement in Québec education and in the hope of standardizing preparation. Yet, entry-to-practice university education for nurses had already been established in the French sector in 1962 and in the English sector in 1957 (Cohen et al., 2002; Paul & Ross-Kerr, 2011). Moreover, nurses were the first women to access and direct a complete university education, in public hygiene, at the Université de Montréal in the first half of the 20th century (Cohen et al., 2002).

Then a back and forth movement crystallized the issue. In 1972, 5 years after opening the technical program in the colleges, the problems, particularly regarding the insufficient preparation of the teachers, were not resolved. An important revision of the program was to be undertaken, and in 1977, the regulatory body took the position in favor of the entry-to-practice preparation at the college level while new university programs opened across Québec. In 1979, in light of these opposite positions, the Ministry of Education requested an investigation of all nursing programs. This review supported the view where the entry to practice is at the college level. Understandably, this recommendation met with universities' opposition (Cohen et al., 2002), and in 1982, under a new president and in line with the rest of Canada, the Québec regulatory body took a position in favor of the entry-to-practice preparation at the university level. This position was felt as a thunder stroke by the college nursing teachers who had struggled to raise education to the regulatory bodies expectations (Frenette-Leclerc, 2010). This was 15 years after the opening and the distribution of the technical program in colleges across Québec under the Ministry of Education governance.

Today, 30 years later, after threats of closing university entry-to-practice programs, two rounds of harmonization, and integration of the colleges' and universities' programs, the process to entry-to-practice preparation at the university level has yet to be completed. Nevertheless, Québec nurses are closer to completion since the 2011 annual meeting vote by the delegates requesting representations toward the requirement of university education for the nursing profession.

This glance at the recent history of nursing education in Québec raises these questions:

• Why, after being the first women to access and direct a complete university education in Québec in the first half of the 20th century, do nurses still have to claim university education for their entry to practice in the beginning of the 21st century?
• What role did seeking a uniform nursing education and the unique college structure play in the process to carry out entry-to-practice preparation at the university level?
• What is now in place for Québec nurses to carry out entry-to-practice preparation at the university level?

SOCIO-CULTURAL QUESTIONS

In Canada, nursing can be learned and practiced in the French language, among an increasingly diverse population. Over seven million Canadians are French-speaking, which is 24.1% of the total population, located in Francophone Québec (QC), representing 86.3% of its population; bilingual New Brunswick (NB), representing 33.1% of its population; and all Anglophone provinces and territories, with Ontario (ON) having the highest percentage, 4.7% of its population (Statistics Canada, 2006). Hence, nursing educational programs are offered in French at eight of the nine Québec university units and at 39 of the colleges in Québec, at the various campuses of the University of Moncton, in New Brunswick, at Laurentian University and the University of Ottawa in Ontario, at The University College St-Boniface, in Manitoba, and at the University of Alberta, St-Jean Campus, in Alberta (CIFI, 2011).

Although there has been an increase in available scientific literature in the last three decades, learning in French means that students have access to nursing literature in French, which is less abundant than the nursing literature in English, although several organizations have promoted knowledge transfer in French since the beginning of the 1980s. Québec universities require students to be able to read in both French and English; this is not true of the other levels of the educational system. This also poses a challenge, although not insurmountable, for the integration of new knowledge into nursing practice. Not reading French or any other language apart from English is a limitation; not reading English or any other language apart from French is, at the moment, a greater limitation to accessing new nursing knowledge.

The *Rapport Parent* in 1965 stressed the importance of democratizing education, including regional access to free education, such as that offered in colleges. Hence, in the 2000s, the nursing programs have been strengthened and integrated into university baccalaureate programs, for which students have to pay tuition. If tuition is perceived as a barrier, one should know that Québec students pay about half the average undergraduate fees as other Canadian students (Statistics Canada, 2011).

The technical programs, included in higher education and preparing students for the job market, have many attributes; for example, they are recognized as giving graduates very good psychomotor skills preparation. On the contrary, university programs have the reputation of not sufficiently preparing their graduates to this dimension of practice, but rather of being too theoretical. However, like everywhere, the reality in Québec universities has changed in the last 10 years. Nursing students are practicing psychomotor skills, decision making, and teamwork among themselves and with other healthcare professionals in impressively equipped labs. Moreover, the new generation of students welcomes active learning, challenging programs, and recognition of their technologic fluency.

In the process of carrying out entry-to-practice preparation at the university level, nurses have to overcome perceptions and lasting images as barriers: Access to nursing knowledge in French, accessibility of university education to all, and professional practice preparation at the university level.

At this point, one cannot help but notice a parallel between the women's right-to-vote movement and the nurses' right to education at the university level. In the first part of the 20th century, women around the world demanded the vote to express their political preferences and partake in decision making for the improvement of their societies. Women from New Zealand (1893), Australia (1902), Finland (1906), Iceland (1915), Canada, Germany, Ireland, and United Kingdom (1918) were among the first to be granted the right to vote (IPU, 2005). Nurses, the majority of who are women, claim that a university education of future generations of professionals is needed to benefit the population's healthcare and to further the knowledge of the discipline. CNA (2011) reports that, as in Canada, "in Australia, Iceland, Ireland and New Zealand, RNs must have a baccalaureate degree to practise" (p.1). The pioneer countries for the women's right-to-vote movement then overlap with those who promote nurses' right-to-education at the university level. Other countries are working to establish baccalaureate education as an entry-to-practice requirement for registered nurses.

To continue the parallel, women were divided during the right-to-vote movement; some had doubts about the necessity to obtain the vote and about their readiness and capability. It appears that nurses, through the process of claiming education at the university level, still had some doubts about its necessity. It is worth noting that the preparation of school teachers, another "women's profession," adopted the requirement of a university education between 1968 and 1971.

Women's right to vote across Canada (except for Québec and the Territories) was obtained over a 9-year span (1916–1925). Nurse's education at the baccalaureate level was formalized across Canada (except in Québec) within a 12-year span (1998–2010). Table 3.1 compares the Canadian jurisdictions on those two important processes. In Québec, after many attempts to gain the right to vote, the winning strategy was an alliance with the opposition party. Despite the opposition of the Roman Catholic Church, women's right to vote was won in 1940 (Dumont, 2008); 15 years after the other jurisdictions.

This overview of the socio-cultural dimension of nursing education, including a brief parallel between women's right to vote and the issue of university education raises these questions:

- In a knowledge world and economy, what assumptions do Québecers hold about nursing and higher education, assumptions that may prevent them from choosing a university education for nurses?
- What can the parallel of the women's right to vote movement teach Québec nurses in their deliberations to carry out entry-to-practice preparation at the university level?

POLITICAL QUESTIONS

The Québec government created the college education programs in the 1960s as a strategy to advance education and economy in all its regions; nursing was among the first technical programs to be implemented. To this day, the college administrations are proud of their professional/technical programs that give their graduates direct access to the job market (MELS, 2007). They are willing to participate in continuum programs but the request by nurses that their nursing graduates continue at the university level without direct access to work seems contrary to the college education programs' founding principles. The incentive that college programs obtain through immediate access of graduates to the job market is stronger than the continuum that will lead all nursing graduates to complete an undergraduate-level degree before practicing. The shortage of nurses, together with this incentive, creates a barrier for the long-term view of baccalaureate entry to practice preferred by all other provinces and territories. For the Québec regulatory body and the universities, choosing the baccalaureate as the entry-to-practice education for future nurses does not mean the end of nursing education in the colleges but rather an extension of the continuum between colleges and universities.

Searching for a solution to the problem of underfunding, universities have promoted the idea that a well-educated population will be a healthier population (Conférence des recteurs et des

Table 3.1   Comparison of Canadian Jurisdiction on the Women's Right to Vote and the RN Baccalaureate Education. Data from: Parliament of Canada

JURISDICTION	YEAR WOMEN'S RIGHT TO VOTE	YEAR RN BACCALAUREATE EDUCATION
Manitoba	1916	2005 completed (last diploma program did not take new students in September 2011)
Saskatchewan	1916	2000 completed
Alberta	1916	2009 completed
Canada	1917: Women who had close relatives in the armed forces could vote on behalf of their male relatives 1918: All women, in effect: January 1, 1919	1982: All provincial and territorial nurses associations in Canada have agreed that a baccalaureate degree in nursing should be the entry requirement for the profession
British Columbia	1917	2006 completed
Ontario	1917	2005 completed
Nova Scotia	1918	1998 completed
New Brunswick	1919	1998 completed
Yukon	1919	Yukon has no entry-level educational programs
Prince Edward Island	1922	1998 completed
Newfoundland and Labrador	1925	1998 completed
Québec	1940	Québec continues to offer a diploma program while supporting the development of continuum DEC-BAC
Northwest Territories	1951	2010 completed

Source: http://www.parl.gc.ca/parlinfo/Compilations/ProvinceTerritory/ProvincialWomenRightToVote.aspx and The Canadian Nurses Association (CNA), Public Policy Department, June 2009: http://www.cna-nurses.ca/cna/nursing/education/baccalaureate/table/default_e.aspx

principaux des universités du Québec [CREPUQ], 2011). However, basic professional programs are still costly. The balancing of tuition costs between basic and integrated nursing baccalaureate programs would be welcomed by universities as well as the Québec government. Hence, nursing faculties together with the Québec regulatory body support the two models of university education (basic and integrated) that would lead to the same degree.

At the Ministry of Health, Québec nurses recently obtained the nomination of a Chief Nursing Officer (OIIQ, 2011a, 2011b) and are increasingly in a better position to participate in decisions for the continued improvement of nursing services and to foster the nursing profession and nursing education as part of an improvement of quality care.

After 30 years of working on the process of entry-to-practice preparation at the university level, including years of building an integrated education, the fruits of the efforts invested are yet to be fully realized. In the national arena, the Québec regulatory body left Canadian Nurses Association, even though it shared its view regarding the baccalaureate as entry-to-practice requirement. University programs continue to be CASN members and many other national partnerships activities persist. On the international scene, the Québec regulatory body is a founding member of SIDIIEF, a

French-speaking association that has the potential to influence nurses at large as well as politicians. The European position in favor of university preparation for all professionals, including nurses, influenced the Québec 2011 vote and could facilitate the completion of the process in Québec.

Reflecting on the political dimensions of this issue raises these questions:

- How can Québec nurses take advantage of the unique CEGEP and university structures as they approach resolution toward university education for all new nurses?
- How would the strengthening of international collaborations be a stepping stone for nursing higher education and improvement of quality care?

SUMMARY

This chapter raises important questions for nursing education and healthcare in Québec. One major issue—the two levels of preparation of new nurses—was discussed, highlighting the significance of the issue for nurses, the profession, and healthcare. Although presented separately, the historical, socio-cultural, and political dimensions of this issue of the persistence of two levels of preparation for new nurses are intertwined. Questions are raised following a brief statement on salient elements for each of these dimensions. Although Québec is closer than ever to carrying out entry-to-practice preparation at the university level, strategies for resolution are presented throughout the analysis while others remain to be developed. Major points are the necessary recognition of nursing knowledge in the discipline of nursing and the need for a common voice on a nursing education that affirms the importance of quality patient care.

Online

Add to your knowledge of this issue:

Canadian Nurses Association (CNA),   **http://www.cna-nurses.ca**
Public Policy Department, June 2009:

Parliament of Canada: **http://www.parl.gc.ca**

Want to know more?   Visit the Point for additional helpful resources:

- Journal Articles
- Learning Objectives
- Nursing Professional Roles and Responsibilities
- Bonus chapters:
  ◦ Health and Nursing Policy: A Matter of Politics, Power and Professionalism
  ◦ The NP Movement: Recurring Issues
  ◦ When Difference Matters: The Politics of Privilege and Marginality

References

Assemblée nationale du Québec. (2002). *Projet de loi no 90, chapitre 33. Loi modifiant le Code des professions et d'autres dispositions législatives dans le domaine de la santé.* Québec: Éditeur officiel du Québec.
Canadian Association of Schools of Nursing (2011). *CASN and Accreditation.* Retrieved September 2 2012 from www.casn.ca/en/21

Canadian Association of Schools of Nursing & Canadian Nurses Association (2005). *Student and Faculty Survey Report.* Retrieved September 2 2012 from www.casn.ca/en/Surveys_112/items/7.html

Canadian Institute for Health Information. (2010). *Regulated nurses: Canadian trends.* Ottawa, ON: Author.

Canadian Nurses Association. (2011). *RN education, registered nurses and baccalaureate education.* Ottawa, ON: Author.

Canadian Nurses Association & Canadian Association of Schools of Nursing (2004). Promoting continuing competence for Registered Nurses. Retrieved from http:/www2.cna-aiic.ca/CNA/documents/pdf/publications. Retrieved on September 2 2012.

CIFI (Pepin, J. & Ha, L. 2011). *Analyse et mise en contexte des profils de formation infirmière dans différents pays francophones.* Rapport rédigé pour le Secrétariat international des infirmières et infirmiers de l'espace francophone. Montréal: Centre d'innovation en formation infirmière, Faculté des sciences infirmières, Université de Montréal.

Cohen, Y., Pepin, J., Lamontagne, E., & Duquette, A. (2002). *Les sciences infirmières, genèse d'une discipline.* Montréal: Les Presses de l'Université de Montréal.

Comité des spécialistes. (2000). *Projet de formation infirmière intégrée. Rapport du comité des spécialistes soumis au comité directeur sur la formation infirmière intégrée.* Québec: MELS.

Conférence des recteurs et des principaux des universités du Québec (CREPUQ). (2011). *Projet de loi no 127: l'importance de préserver la mission universitaire des établissements de santé.* Retrieved from http://www.crepuq.qc.ca/spip.php.article 1305

Desrosiers, G. (2009). Libérer les talents. *Perspective infirmière, 6*(2), 33–48.

Donaldson, S.K. (2000). Breakthroughs in scientific research: The discipline of nursing, 1960–1999. *Annual Review of Nursing Research, 18*(1), 247–311.

Ducharme, F. (2009). Summary of current research, policy and practice initiatives in the field of family care in Canada. *Bulletin of the International Advisory Board of the National Competence Centre in Sweden for Family Care Issues.* Retrieved September 2 2012 from www.chairedesjardins.umontreal.ca/fr-bibliotheque/autres.html

Duchscher, J.B. (2008). Transition shock: The initial stage of role adaptation for newly graduated Registered Nurses. *Journal of Advanced Nursing.* vol. 65(5) p. 1103–1113 doi: 10.1111/j.1365-2648.2008.04898.x.

Dumont, M. (2008). *Le féminisme québécois raconté à Camille.* Montréal: Les Éditions du remue-ménage.

Ellis, J., Priest, A., MacPhee, M., Sanchez McCutcheon, A., on behalf of CHSRF and partners. (2006). *Staffing for safety: A synthesis of the evidence on nurse staffing and patient safety.* Ottawa, ON: Canadian Health Services Research Foundation.

Fondation de recherche en sciences infirmières du Québec. (2009). *Programme MELS-Universités: Bourses d'études de maîtrise et de doctorat pour les sciences infirmières.* Montréal: Author.

Frenette-Leclerc, C. (2010). Reseau Collegial du Quebec. Newsletter Archives. Retrieved September 2 2012 from www.lescegeps.com

Gottlieb, L., Feeley, N., & Dalton. C. (2006). The Collaborative Partnership Approach to Care: A Delicate Balance. Toronto: Mosby.

Goudreau, J., Pepin, J., Dubois, S., Boyer, L., Larue, C., & Legault, A. (2009). A second generation of the competency-based approach to nursing education. *International Journal of Nursing Education Scholarship, 6*(1), art. 15, 1–15.

International Council of Nurses (ICN). (2010). *Global issues and trends in nursing education.* Genève: ICN-CII.

International Organization of Parliaments (IPU) 2010. Women's Suffrage. Retrieved September 2 2012 from www.IPU.org/wmn-e/suffrage.htm

Kirkwood, R., & Bouchard, J. (1992). *"Take counsel with one another". A beginning history of the Canadian Association of University Schools of Nursing 1942–1992.* Ottawa, ON: CASN.

Lacoursière, J., Provencer, J., & Vaugeois, D. (2011). *Canada-Québec. Synthèse historique 1534–2010.* Québec: Les éditions Septentrion.

Lambert, C. (1979). *Historique du programme des techniques infirmières. 1962–1978.* Rapport présenté à la DGEC en vue de l'évaluation du programme des techniques infirmières. Québec: DIGEC, p. 164.

Mansell, D. & Dood, D. (2005). Professionalism and Canadian Nursing. In: C. Bates, D. Dood & N. Rousseau (ed.) On All Frontiers: Four Centuries of Canadian Nursing. (pp. 197–212). Ottawa: University of Ottawa Press.

Martin-Misener, R., Bryant-Lukosius, D., Harbman, P., et al. (2010). Education of advanced practice nurses in Canada. *Canadian Journal of Nursing Leadership, 23*(Special Issue), 61–84.

McGillis Hall, L. Doran, D. & Pink, G. (2004). Nurse staffing models, nursing hours, and patient safety outcomes. *Journal of Nursing Administration, 34*(1), 41–45.

Ministère de l'Éducation, du Loísìr et du Sport. (2004). *La main d'œuvre infirmière de formation universitaire au Québec. Orientations ministérielles.* Québec: Gouvernement du Québec.

———. (2005). *Nomenclature des titres d'emploi, des libellés, des taux et des échelles de salaires du Réseau de la santé et des services sociaux.* Québec: Gouvernement du Québec.

———. (2007). *180. A0 Soins infirmiers.* Québec: Gouvernement du Québec.

———. (2008). *L'Éducation au Québec* (Québec School System). Québec: Gouvernement du Québec.

Office Québécois de la langue française. (2009). *Le français, un tremplin pour exercer une profession au Québec.* Montréal: Author. Retrieved from www.oqlf.gouv.qc.ca

Ordre des infirmières et infirmiers du Québec (OIIQ). (1982). *Rapport préliminaire du cheminement d'une étude éventuelle sur la formation professionnelle initiale des infirmières et infirmiers au niveau universitaire.* Montréal: Author, p. 95.

———. (2010a). *Arrangement de reconnaissance mutuelle France-Québec (ARM).* Montréal: Author. Retrieved from http://www.oiiq.org/admission-a-la-professìon/ínfirmiere-formee-hors-quebec/arm-france-quebec

———. (2010b). *Agrément des programmes de formation d'infirmière praticienne spécialisée (IPS).* Montréal: Author.

———. (2011a). *Infostats.* Récupéré à www.oiiq.org 27.01.2011

———. (2011b). *InfOIIQ.* Récupéré à http://www.oiiq.org/uploads/infOIIQ/5avril/index.htm

Ordre des infirmières et infirmiers du Québec (OIIQ), Relive the 2011 Conference retrieved Septmeber 2 2012 from www.oiiq.org/evenements

Ordre des infirmières et infirmiers du Québec (OIIQ), Collège des médecins du Québec (CMQ) (2008). *Soins de première ligne: étendue des activités médicales exercées par l'infirmière praticienne spécialisée en soins de première ligne,* document conjoint. Westmount, QC: Author. Retrieved from http://www.oiiq.org; http://www.cmq.org

Paul, P., & Ross-Kerr, J. (2011). The origins and development of nursing education in Canada. In J. Ross-Kerr & M. Wood (Eds.), *Canadian nursing issues & perspectives* (5th ed., pp. 327–358). Toronto, ON: Elsevier Canada.

Pepin, J. (2008). L'évolution du savoir infirmier au Québec, dans C. Dallaire (dir.), Le s*avoir infirmier au cœur de la discipline et de la profession infirmière* (chapitre 4; pp. 71–91). Montréal: Gaëtan Morin.

Pepin, J., Dubois, S., Girard, F., Tardif, J., & Ha, L. (2011). A cognitive learning model of clinical nursing leadership. *Nurse Education Today, 31*(3), 268–273. doi: 10.1016j.nedt.2010.11.009.

Pepin, J., Kérouac, S., & Ducharme, F. (2010). *La pensée infirmière.* (3e éd.). Montréal: Chenelière Éducation.

Rodgers, B.L. (2005). *Developing nursing knowledge: Philosophical traditions and influences.* Philadelphia, PA: Lippincott Williams & Wilkins.

Secrétariat international des infirmières et infirmiers de l'espace francophone (In Press, 2011). *La formation universitaire des infirmières et infirmiers, une réponse aux défis des systèmes de santé.* Montréal: Author.

Statistics Canada. (2006). *Population by mother tongue, by province and territory and Statistics on official languages (2006 Census).* Retrieved from www.statcan.gc.ca

Statistics Canada. (2011). *Average undergraduate tuition fees for Canadian full-time students, by province.* Retrieved from http://www.statcan.gc.ca/daily-quotidien/091020/t091020b1-eng.htm

Tardif, J. (2006). *L'évaluation des compétences: Documenter le parcours de développement.* Montréal: Les Éditions de la Chenelière Inc.

Thorne, S. (2011). Theoretical Issues in Nursing. In J. Ross-Kerr & M. Wood (Eds.), *Canadian nursing issues & perspectives* (5th ed., pp. 85–104). Toronto, ON: Elsevier Canada.

Tourangeau, A. Doran, D., McGillis Hall, L. et al. (2006). Impact of hospital nursing care on 30 day mortality for acute medical patients. *Journal of Advanced Nursing, 57*(1), 32–44.

World Health Organization (WHO) (2009). *Global standards for the initial education of professional nurses and midwives.* Retrieved from http://www.who.int/hrh/nursing_midwifery/hrhglobalstandardseducation.pdf

Wood, M.J., & Ross-Kerr, J.C. (2011). The growth of graduate education in nursing in Canada. In J. Ross-Kerr & M. Wood (Eds.), *Canadian nursing: Issues & perspectives* (5th ed., pp. 388–409). Toronto, ON: Elsevier Canada.

Young, L.E., & Paterson, B.L. (2007). *Teaching nursing: Developing a student-centered learning environment.* Philadelphia, PA: Lippincott Williams & Wilkins.

4

Stepping into the Future: Challenges with Health Transfer in First Nations Communities

Fjola Hart Wasekeesikaw

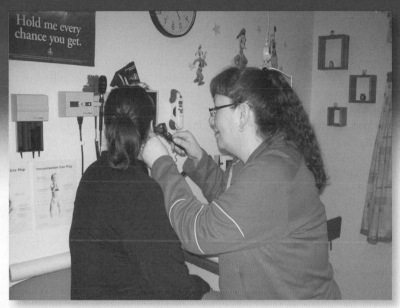

Graduate of the University of Manitoba BN Program, Norway House site, provides care at the Public Health Unit at Norway House. (Used with permission University of Manitoba.)

Critical Questions

As a way of engaging with the ideas in this chapter, consider the following:

1. Begin to think about the assumptions that you hold about nursing in First Nations communities.

2. How have you come to hold these assumptions?

3. What might be the influence of these assumptions and beliefs on the provision of healthcare to First Nations people?

Chapter Objectives

After completing this chapter, you should be able to:

1. Describe the relationship between the colonization of First Nations people and health-related issues.

2. Analyze the significance of concepts of population health in addressing issues of inequity.

3. Examine some of the different views of health held by First Nations individuals, families, and communities.

4. Interpret the significance of cultural resurgence, community development, and the expressed need to widen the scope of health and transfer of healthcare services to First Nations communities.

5. Evaluate the role of nurses and nursing in the delivery of healthcare services to First Nations communities in Canada.

(continued on page 54)

6. Examine the following issues confronting nurses in the provision of healthcare services to First Nations people:
- population demographics and the relationship to the healthcare needs

- transfer of healthcare services in relation to nursing issues
- need for cultural competence
- educational needs for nurses working in First Nations communities.

This chapter introduces the reader to issues related to health, healthcare, and nursing for First Nations people in Canada and presents basic information to facilitate greater understanding of First Nations community members. Key to understanding is recognition of the great diversity among First Nations communities and the views of health held by First Nations. Also discussed are the relationship between the historical attempts for enfranchisement of First Nations people and health-related issues and the significance of cultural resurgence among First Nations in community development. How these factors influence the practice of nursing in Canada and how, in turn, nurses can potentially influence the healthcare of First Nations people will be explored. In addition, current issues related to the nursing and delivery of healthcare to First Nations people will be identified.

DIVERSITY OF THE FIRST PEOPLES

The 634 First Nations in Canada constitute a diverse population of descendants of the First Peoples of North America (Aboriginal Affairs and Northern Development Canada, 2010). Many of these nations are further grouped into tribal councils, which provide unity and greater political power as well as combined resources among nations. Each First Nation has its own reserve land base, traditional territories, culture, and language.

First Nations are part of a larger group of Aboriginal people. As defined in the Canadian Constitution Act of 1982, the term *Aboriginal* refers to First Nations, Inuit, and Métis. All Aboriginal people originate from 11 different language families (Kerr & Beaujot, 2011, p. 151): Eskimo-Aleut, Algic, Nadene, Haida, Wakashan, Salishan, Tsimshienic, Kootenai, Siouan-Catawba, Iroquoian, and Beothuk.

According to the Indian Act, an act of the Canadian Parliament, First Nations members are legally defined as "Indians." The Indian Act, first passed in 1876, was designed to administer programs to Indians for the purpose of assimilating them into Canadian society; the act also determined who was legally defined as an Indian. There have been many revisions to the Indian Act since its inception, but the purpose remains the same. Each person who is deemed to be legally Indian has a registration number to reflect her or his population number within her or his band or First Nations community.

Many First Nations people are also referred to as having "treaty Indian status." Treaty Indians are persons who belong to a First Nation that signed a treaty with the Crown (Aboriginal Affairs and Northern Development Canada, 2008). First Nations conducted negotiations with the British government or with Canada in the right of the Crown, before and after Confederation in 1867, resulting in the signing of treaties. Through this treaty process, certain rights and benefits are provided to the Treaty First Nations. For example, the Natural Resources Transfer Agreements of 1930 guarantee that First Nations people residing in Manitoba, Saskatchewan, and Alberta have the right to hunt, trap, and fish except for commercial purposes. Treaties continue to be developed in the new millennium where First Nations' rights and benefits are set out in these agreements. These may include, for example, ownership of certain lands; wildlife harvesting rights; participation in land, wildlife and environmental management in specific areas; financial payments; resource revenue sharing; self-government; and measures to participate in the economy (Aboriginal Affairs and Northern Development Canada, 2008). Treaty rights vary between First Nations. The First Nations leadership through the treaty process guaranteed the right to be born and live as First Nations people.

The term *Indian* originates from early explorers to North America who thought they had discovered India. First Nations members assert that the roots of this term are inappropriate and serve to reflect a history of colonialism. To reflect more appropriately that they are descendants of the First Peoples on this continent, the First Nations have determined that they would be identified accordingly.

EUROPEAN RELATIONSHIP WITH FIRST NATIONS

What is the significance of the impact of colonization on the lives and ways of living of First Nations families and communities in Canada? *Colonialism* involves the settlement of territory, the exploitation or development of its resources and the attempt to govern the indigenous peoples of the occupied lands (Boehmer, 1995, p. 2). Colonization was formidable to the First Peoples' way of life. Their economic and political systems were destroyed; worldviews were trivialized; overt expressions of cultures, such as spiritual and traditional healing ceremonies, were desecrated, degraded, and labeled as devil worshipping; and, feasts, give-aways, singing, and dancing were deemed sinful (Aboriginal Nurses Association of Canada, 2009, p. 6). The indigenous peoples' connection to the land was considered an expression of their primitiveness.

Before contact with European colonizers, the First Peoples had their own systems of government, trade, and healthcare. After confederation, Canada began to displace the First Nations from their traditional territories to make room for the ever-increasing influx of European settlers. Government policies were developed to protect, civilize, and assimilate the First Peoples into Canadian society. The process undertaken to achieve this end would greatly affect the mental, physical, and spiritual health of First Nations. The inherent oppressive and suppressive nature of these policies has had, and continues to have, far-reaching negative effects on First Nations governance and cultural identity.

Because of its extensiveness and the length of time during which colonization took place, this chapter presents no more than a brief overview. The risk in attempting to discuss the historical highlights is the potential to oversimplify the European relationship with the First Nations and the long-lasting negative effects on the population. With this in mind, the history will briefly cover the following key phases: Cooperation, nation to nation; Colonization and its effects on the health of First Nations people and their communities; and First Nations' cultural resurgence.

Cooperation Among Nations

Colonization did not begin at the point of original contact between the Europeans and First Nations. Unlike the history between the First Peoples and European settlers in the United States, in which wars established the dominance of European culture, the initial relationship between the First Peoples and first the French, and then the British in Canada was one of mutual tolerance and respect. The social, cultural, and political differences between these societies were maintained. This tolerance reflected how First Nations related to each other. The newcomers came to a continent that was already inhabited by diverse nations of indigenous people who formed alliances and good relations with one another to access and distribute their tribal resources (Dickason, 1994, p. 76).

The First Peoples had their own economic, health, political, and social systems that were developed within their communities according to their traditions and the need imposed by their environments (Dickason, 1994). When the first Europeans came into contact with the First Nations, each thought of the other as distinct and autonomous. Each nation continued to govern its internal affairs. Nations cooperated in areas of mutual interest and were connected in various trading relationships and other forms of nation-to-nation alliances.

The Royal Proclamation of 1763 demonstrates that the partnership between First Nations and the British Crown was one of cooperation and protection. In exchange for cooperation in the partnership that characterized the relationship between them at that time, the king of England extended royal protection to the First Peoples' lands and political autonomy. When Canada was formed in 1867, a legislative basis for dealing with the Indian people as nations had already been established. At this juncture, it is important to identify the underlying assumptions held by the British Crown that formed the basis for passing laws to govern the First Peoples.

Colonization and the Effect on First Nations People

The written word reflects an author's attitudes and beliefs, and so it was that the plans of action or policies to carry out the government laws reflected the attitudes of the people who wrote these policies. The Indian Act was the legislative vehicle for implementing policies to civilize, protect, and assimilate the Indian people (Tobias, 1991). No single event marked the beginning of these colonial practices. Rather, they began with the attitudes of the time and laid the foundation for a series of actions that deemed the Indian people as inferior beings. Government laws still reflect these attitudes today; in doing so, these laws perpetuate a colonialist attitude.

A series of actions led to the proclaiming of the Indian Act. This was one act of many that laid the foundation for the civilization program that was developed in 1828 and gave rise to the reserve system that became a social laboratory designed to enable Indian communities to adopt European values (Tobias, 1991). This program established Indians in isolated, fixed locations where they could be educated, converted to Christianity, and transformed into farmers. The goal was to eradicate the First Peoples' values through education, religion, new economic and political systems, and a new concept of property. Not only was the distinct cultural group to disappear but so, too, was the laboratory where these changes were brought about. It was assumed that each Indian person who became enfranchised would also take his share of the land from the reserve.

The Assembly of the United Canadas of the Gradual Civilization Act of 1857 provided the criteria for determining whether an Indian person qualified to become enfranchised. A special board of examiners determined each applicant's merit based on whether the person was educated, free from debt, and of good moral character. If so, the person was awarded 20 hectares of land within the colony and "the accompanying rights" as a citizen of the Dominion (Milloy, 1991, p. 147). One of the accompanying rights was the opportunity to vote in the country's elections. It was assumed that Indian people would sever ties with their communities and embrace colonial living and values.

The British North America Act of 1867, establishing the Canadian nation, also contained the forerunner of the Indian Act and placed First Nations, and lands reserved for them, under the legislative authority of the Canadian federal government. The Indian Act was amended almost every year to address unanticipated problems in carrying out the government policies. The need for policy revision also reflected resistance by First Nations people to changing their values and cultural ways (Milloy, 1991). The amendments persisted on a course to erode the land base of First Nations, wipe out traditional political governance, and smother traditional ways of expression and living. Some effects of the amended Indian Act include the following:

• **The erosion of the protected status of reserve lands.** In 1894, the government took over reserve land held by physically disabled Indian people, widows, orphans, and others who could not cultivate it, and then the government leased these tracts of land to European settlers (Royal Commission on AboriginalPeoples [RCAP], 1996a). Later, in 1918, the government broadened its leasing policy to take over Indian reserve lands that were uncultivated. Only

Indian people who cultivated their land were allowed to keep tracts of reserve land. The First Nations people did not surrender these tracts of land nor was their approval obtained in order for the government simply to take over the land and lease it to European settlers. This government practice was in violation of treaty obligations connecting Canada to the Royal Proclamation of 1763, in which Indian title to land and the need to obtain proper surrender of Indian lands were stated.

- **The undermining of traditional political processes used by First Nations communities.** The federal government determined how First Nations community leadership was to be elected and interfered with the decision-making processes of the communities' affairs. For example, the superintendent of Indian Affairs determined the time, place, and manner in which the elections took place (Milloy, 1991). In addition, a governor could remove a chief or councilor from office if he thought the leader was dishonest, intemperate, or immoral. The interpretation of these terms and how they were applied to each case was left to the governor's advisors and departmental agents. The extent to which community members participated in the elections was limited to all males over the age of 21 years. The chief and council were forced to function within a foreign-designed and foreign-controlled system. Federal authority also set a bureaucratic system of controlling the communities' affairs. The nature of the concerns in which the chief and council could make decisions was preset. Furthermore, each decision was subject to confirmation by the governor (Cassidy & Bish, 1989). The chief and council functioned within a narrow, federally controlled context. The government controlled First Nations' affairs by making bylaws for a variety of purposes including band membership; provision of public health; regulation of commerce, traffic, construction, and buildings; assurance of the observance of law and order; prevention of disorderly conduct and nuisances; construction and maintenance of water supplies, roads, bridges, and other public works; regulation of animal populations; and removal of trespassers from reserve land. By interfering with the governing processes of First Nations communities, the federal government undercut the authority of the First Nations communities' leadership.
- **The suppression of the traditions and values of First Nations.** In a concerted effort to extinguish any traditional beliefs and practices in the First Nations community, laws were enacted to ban all traditional ceremonies and to control Indian movement from one reserve to another (Milloy, 1991). It was thought that intertribal gatherings, celebrations, and ceremonies were the primary obstacles to Indian people becoming Christians. In 1884, the potlatch and the Tamanawas dance were prohibited, with a jail term of 2 months to 6 months for any Indian who was convicted of engaging in or assisting with these dances. In later years, further amendments banned the practice of other traditional dances such as the Blackfoot Sun Dance. In part, the system was an attempt to control discussion between political and spiritual leaders living on various reserves. In 1885, Indian people were prohibited from traveling off their reserves without written authorization of the Indian agent on the reserve. These laws were designed to suppress historical, social, and political organization of First Nations societies and governments.

Government laws and policies have systematically assaulted First Nations in their spiritual practices and in their social organization, governance, and economic activities. For many First Nations, the residential school system in which the state and church attempted to capture and socialize First Nations children was the sharpest cut of all (Aboriginal Healing Foundation, 2002; RCAP, 1996b). The residential school experience left in its wake dislocation and a strong sense of loss for individual students and their families, with rippling, cumulative, intergenerational effects on First Nations communities (Aboriginal Healing Foundation, 2004). Dislocation from one's community effected many losses, including culture, language, spirituality, identity, pride, self-respect, and ability to parent. As a result of these experiences, many First Nations individuals, families, and communities were trapped between what remained of traditional ways of doing things and the fear of importing too much more of mainstream Canadian cultural values into reserve life.

The residential school system insult to the spirit of the First Nations people has had, and continues to have, destructive effects on many individuals, families, and communities (Aboriginal Healing Foundation, 2003, 2007). It is important to recognize, however, that colonization processes have not been successful in eliminating First Nations. Rather, they have propelled First Nations to embark on reviving traditions, proclaiming their identities, and developing healthcare systems, for example, that reflect their populations' cultural needs. Attitudes and policies reflecting the colonial system continue today because the present healthcare and government systems exist on a foundation of protection, civilization, and assimilation (Smylie, 2000). This fact has repercussions for the relationships between the First Nations people and their healthcare providers.

CULTURAL RESURGENCE OF FIRST NATIONS AND COMMUNITY DEVELOPMENT

The First Nations cultural resurgence and community development share similar roots and are closely intertwined. In the 1960s, First Nations people demanded the right to set their own cultural course. They spoke out about indigenous perspectives on development. Their voices were significant in creating a pathway on which community development could be used to bring about economic and social changes in First Nations communities.

Until 1951, when the Indian Act was revised, laws banned First Nations members from attempting to organize themselves. With the revisions to the Indian Act, First Nations members began the enormous task of developing political organizations to strengthen and improve the situations of First Nations people (Assembly of First Nations [AFN], 2011b). Members began traveling from community to community, discussing issues and potential actions to change the conditions within the communities. Over the ensuing decade, tension between First Nations and the government of Canada developed. The early 1960s was a time when government control was so deeply entrenched that policy controlled almost every aspect of First Nations people's lives, interests, and concerns. For example, the Indian Act affected the family unit in that it provided for arbitrary enfranchisement of an Indian woman who married a person who was not registered as an Indian. Within a family unit, women's status as band members could cease depending on whom the female siblings married. Concomitant with this example, the Wildlife Act prohibits any Indian person from giving meat to a non-Indian. The non-Indian person in this case could be a sister who is enfranchised.

First Nations people set out to challenge policies reflecting a belief that Canadian institutions alone could prescribe solutions to the problems faced by First Nations people. They had different ideas about dealing with their own issues. Provincial organizations were developed to deal with concerns facing the status of Indian people. Nationally, the first status Indian organization, the National Indian Brotherhood, was started in December 1968. (*Note:* The term *status Indian* is applied to an Indian person who is registered under the Indian Act.) The National Indian Brotherhood, now known as the Assembly of First Nations, gave a single voice to all status Indian people in Canada (AFN, 2011b). Of particular significance was the First Nations response to the White Paper, a Canadian government policy statement in 1969 that aimed to abolish all First Nations rights, including rights to reserve lands. The First Nations' response shifted the nature of the relationship the First Nations would have with the government of Canada; the response would be a key in moving away from a relationship whereby Indian people were the wards of the state. First Nations governing their own affairs would provide a basis for developing community-specific health and healing systems.

The Truth and Reconciliation Commission of Canada

In 2008, the Truth and Reconciliation Commission of Canada (TRC) was established to make the history of the Indian Residential Schools (IRS) and its effects on generations of Aboriginal people known to Canadians. A second goal of the TRC is to "guide a process of reconciliation between and within Aboriginal families, communities, churches, governments and Canadians" (www.TRC.ca). An effort toward reconciliation began with Prime Minister Stephen Harper's June 2008 apology to the more than 150,000 former Aboriginal residential school students, on behalf of all Canadians, in which he acknowledged the policy of the IRS was to "kill the Indian in the child" (www.TRC.ca). Most recently, the reconciliation process has included National and regional gatherings to hear and gather statements from survivors of the residential schools, which will be used to educate Canadians about the IRS experience and the long-term effects of this tragic history on the health of Aboriginal people in Canada.

MIYUPIMAATISSIIUM: BEING ALIVE WELL

Miyupimaatissiium, or "being alive well," is seen as an interdependent relationship people have with the natural world and with keeping one's spirit strong (Adelson, 1991). Culture, language, and traditions used to express concepts similar to that of *being alive well* vary from one First Nations community to another. For example, to the members of a First Nations Eastern Ininiwuk—or "human beings"—community, also known as the Cree people, in the province of Quebec, Ininiwuk food is essential to miyupimaatissiium. Game and fish are requirements for miyupimaatissiium and symbolize essential aspects of Ininiwuk life.

To the people in this community, "eating well" means that one has been eating bush food, or food from the land and from this, it can be assumed that there has been a good hunting season. In turn, a good hunting season signifies that one has the physical strength required to work in the bush. Miyupimaatissiium is evidence of an experienced hunter and of a woman who has the skills and ability required for preparing the meat and hides. The spiritual aspect of eating well is at the moment when the animal chooses to give itself to the hunter. The relationship between an Ininiwuk hunter and the animals hunted for food is based on mutual respect. A cyclical affinity between the Ininiwuk (human being), hunting, the land, and food incorporates all aspects of life and so, too, being alive well. Miyupimaatissiium is a holistic concept encompassing people in relation to their environment. The natural world is viewed as a source for life and extends the view of health beyond the biomedical or social lens and recognizes connections between ecosystems, equity, and health. As such, holism is an integral part of Aboriginal health, well-being and healing systems (Parkes, 2011).

Health Status of the First Peoples

The First Peoples enjoyed good health in the Americas; then, as result of European contact, the decimation and extinction of many First Peoples followed. The effects of infectious diseases, such as smallpox, were devastating to the health and cultures of the First Peoples. They suffered many losses, ranging from decreased community sizes to a strong sense of personal and collective loss. The epidemics resulted in declining fertility rates because infected women were unable to conceive or carry their pregnancies to term and also in decreased chances of conceiving as a result of population loss and subsequent lack of partners. Loss of relatives and large numbers of community members resulted in loneliness, grief, and depression. Loss of leaders, warriors, and hunters, and the reduced size of communities, made it difficult to protect territorial boundaries (Ray, 1974). This resulted in migratory shifts in the tribal territories and the modification of economic roles from trappers to middleman traders. Canadian historian Olive Dickason presented to the members of the Royal Commission of Aboriginal Peoples reasons for the impressive state of good health of the First Peoples and then related the impact of infectious diseases on their health and well-being:

> Some analysts argue that disease agents themselves were rare in pre-contact America until the tall ships began to arrive with their invisible cargo of bacteria and viruses. What is more likely is that Aboriginal people had adapted well to their environment; they had developed effective

resistance to the micro-organisms living along side them and had knowledge of herbs and other therapies for treating injury and disease . . . some . . . died prematurely. But more stayed well. Or recovered from illness, and thus lived to raise their children and continue the clans and the nations. Aboriginal populations fluctuated largely in relation to food supply.

Hundreds of thousands . . . died as a result of their encounters with the Europeans . . . infectious diseases were the greatest killer. Influenza, measles, polio, diphtheria, smallpox, and other diseases were transported from the slums of Europe to the unprotected villages of the Americas. . . . Aboriginal people were well aware of the link between the newcomers and the epidemics that raced through their camps and villages. During the eighteenth and nineteenth centuries, their leaders sought agreements or treaties with representatives of the British Crown aimed at ensuring their survival in the face of spreading disease and impoverishment. In the expectation of fair compensation for the use of their lands and resources and in mounting fear of the social and health effects of Euro-Canadian settlement, many Aboriginal nations, clans and families agreed to relocate to camps, farms, villages or reserves distant from sites of colonial settlement. Many did so in the belief that the Crown would guarantee their wellbeing for all time. Given the gulf that separated Aboriginal and non-Aboriginal cultures, it is not surprising that the meaning of those oral and written agreements has been a matter of conflicting interpretation ever since. (RCAP, 1996c, p. 112)

Access to Healthcare: A Fiduciary Responsibility

The federal government recognizes the existence of a fiduciary relationship and that fiduciary obligations are owing to First Nations Peoples (Boyer, 2004, p. 5). However, the nature and scope of this fiduciary relationship and the political, legal, and financial implications stemming from this relationship have been the source of debate among First Nations, the Crown, and the courts (AFN, 2011a, 2011b, 2011c; Boyer, 2004). The federal government takes the position that the provision of health services to First Nations Peoples is done as a matter of policy only and not because of any fiduciary obligation, or treaty right.

HEALTHCARE IN NORTHERN AND ISOLATED COMMUNITIES

From the end of the 19th century, semi-trained government agents, members of the Royal Canadian Mounted Police, and missionaries provided healthcare services. Graham-Cumming wrote in 1967 that the first Department of Indian Affairs, established in 1880, was not originally concerned with First Nations health problems (as cited in Waldram et al., 2006). Then, after decades of ignoring the health of First Nations people, the government of Canada began to develop a system of primary care clinics, a public health program, and regional hospitals. This was done primarily to avoid the threat of tuberculosis epidemics spreading to the general Canadian population. Traditional indigenous healing practices were absent from this healthcare system. Western medical personnel devalued the practice of indigenous medicine by determining it to be nothing more than witchcraft and sorcery. As a result of this, and the government policy, the people who practised traditional indigenous medicine feared persecution and went underground with their skills and knowledge.

Nurses and doctors, employees of the federal government of Canada, were integral to delivering healthcare to First Nations. Nurses have served as entry to this Western model of healthcare in First Nations communities since the beginning of the 20th century (Young, 1984). In response to the healthcare needs of the First Peoples, the Department of National Health and Welfare established the nursing station model as the center for providing medical services in northern communities (Waldram et al., 2006). In 1922, a mobile nurse–visitor program was implemented to provide both medical and nursing care services in communities. The first nursing station was opened in 1930 on the Fisher River Cree Nation in Manitoba. By 1935, the Medical Branch of the

Department of Indian Affairs employed 11 field nurses who joined a team of medical officers and Indian agents with medical training to provide services to First Nations communities. Nurses in these stations provided all primary care with only radio contact with physicians, and clients were evacuated to southern urban hospitals for more comprehensive treatment. By the mid-1950s and into the 1960s, a total of 37 nursing stations in northern Canada had become essential to accessing healthcare in First Nations, Inuit, and Métis communities.

In the new millennium, nurses work in rural, remote, and isolated First Nations settings where they provide service at 76 nursing stations and over 195 health centers (Health Canada, 2011c). Nurses continue to be the communities' main point of contact with the healthcare system. In about half of these health facilities, registered nurses are employed by Health Canada. In the other communities, nurses are employed by the First Nation Council (i.e., band council) as these communities have responsibility for healthcare services through a transfer agreement. Many function collaboratively within a community-based health and social system comprising of community support workers and social service workers.

Widening the Scope of Health: A First Nations Perspective

In 1978, First Nations protested when the government attempted to reduce non-insured health benefits, such as prescription drugs and eyeglasses, dental work, and transportation costs for medical services (Health Canada/Assembly of First Nations, 2011; RCAP, 1996b). They argued that treaty rights were being violated because changes were being made without negotiation with First Nations. The subsequent debate gradually widened to include all aspects of federal policy on healthcare for First Nations people. As result, and in acknowledgement of its responsibility in the area of First Nations health, a new federal *Indian Health Policy* was released recognizing the importance of First Nations involvement in the provision of health services to their communities. The federal government had acknowledged the following three pillars:

1. Community development as a key strategy for improving First Nations health.
2. The continuing special responsibility of the federal government for the health and well-being of First Nations people.
3. The essential contributions of all elements of the Canadian healthcare system, including (but not limited to) the federal, provincial/territorial, municipal, First Nations jurisdictions.

It is important to note that also in the *Indian Health Policy* the federal government made a commitment to greater participation by First Nations in planning and delivering their own health services (Health Canada, 2011a). A new era in First Nations and government relations was to come about relative to healthcare; the First Nations people remained vigilant.

Justice Thomas Berger (1980), in his *Report of the Advisory Commission on Indian and Inuit Health Consultation,* proposed mechanisms that included First Nations consultation in the development of community-controlled health and healing systems. However, despite these proposed changes, First Nations were cautious of the federal government initiatives on transfer of healthcare services. They expressed their unease at the federally initiated Community Health Demonstration Program, which began in 1981. Why should First Nations have to prove to the federal government that they could manage their own community affairs? Community health projects were implemented to provide information about costs for First Nations control of health services (Health Canada, 1999). When the demonstration projects were completed in 1987, First Nations communities participated in the federal initiatives for transfer process to administer the control of federally sponsored healthcare programs. Many First Nations participated in the transfer program even though it was laden with controversy; they saw health transfer as a means to achieve some of their own communities' health objectives.

Waldram et al. (2006) related some of the controversy. The Assembly of First Nations suggested in 1988 that "the transfer program was ultimately designed to assist the government in reducing its spending on First Nations health and, therefore, abrogated treaty rights and its fiduciary relationship to Indians (p. 269)." Waldram et al. also related Culhane Speck's (1989) critical analysis of the health transfer program. In addition to being an assimilations process, the health transfer policy did not represent a positive departure from the past or a fundamental change in position by the federal government regarding First Nations healthcare. Furthermore, the federal government continued to refuse legal responsibility for Indian health and the policy was an attempt to ultimately transfer the responsibility to the provincial governments. This was seen as being reflective of the White Paper of 1969 which was a proposal to terminate Indian "status" and turn over program administration to the provinces.

Transfer of Healthcare Services to First Nations

As of March, 2008, 83% ($n = 501$) of eligible First Nations communities are involved in the First Nations control process and have taken on the administrative responsibility for healthcare services—either individually or collectively—through multi-community agencies or tribal associations (Health Canada, 2008). Of the 46% of First Nations that have assumed greater responsibility for their healthcare resources through transfer agreements, 139 have signed community-based transfer agreements representing 279 First Nations communities and 19 Agreements for treatment programs, hospitals, and second/third level services. In addition, 33% of First Nations communities have signed integrated community-based health services contribution agreements. Lastly, 4% ($n = 23$) of First Nations have signed self-government agreements. Communities that have completed the transfer process are employers for nurses and other healthcare personnel in their communities.

Since the health transfer policy was first introduced, First Nations communities have developed different approaches to managing healthcare services (Smith & Lavoie, 2008). One of these approaches was the development of collaborative networks involving a number of First Nations communities, often organized through affiliation with tribal councils or health authorities. When multiple communities join together, they have the opportunity to share available expertise and utilize resources that otherwise may not be available.

The key to restoring well-being among Aboriginal people originates from within First Nations cultures (RCAP, 1996c) and proposed that new Aboriginal health and healing systems embody the following four essential characteristics:

1. Pursuit of equity in access to health and healing services and in health status outcomes
2. Holism in approaches to problems and their treatment and prevention
3. Aboriginal authority over health systems and, where feasible, community control over services
4. Diversity in the design of systems and services to accommodate differences in culture and community realities.

There could be as many variations of healthcare delivery systems as there are First Nations communities in Canada. Self-determination is integral to the development of community healthcare systems.

CLIMATE FOR CHANGE: NURSING IN FIRST NATIONS COMMUNITIES

Nurses have played a vital role in the delivery of health services in First Nations communities over the past century. Nursing continues to have a critical role in addressing the healthcare needs of people living in First Nations communities. Improving the overall health status of First Nations people is the impetus for creating more effective ways of delivering nursing care services that reflect the health and healing systems determined by each community or tribal council.

Nursing services are an integral part of a First Nations community's health and healing system. A community's processes for economic development and participation in transfer of healthcare services can serve as vehicles for making these changes. This would require nurses to learn how the First Nations community or tribal council in which they work views health and healing, whether community development is being used, what is being planned, and what changes have been made. Having this information will provide nurses with context and an understanding of the healthcare priorities selected by the community. These are important elements of a population health approach and the use of community development principles in providing nursing care in First Nations communities.

Lavoie et al. (2005), in an evaluation of the First Nations and Inuit health transfer policy, found that a majority of respondents in a telephone survey agreed that either the transfer or the integrated model improved service responsiveness, flexibility, and control over programs and service delivery. However, many First Nations communities face challenges, and some of these are barriers to the delivery of effective healthcare services. Some of the barriers include the following:

1. **Recruiting and retaining nursing staff.** MacIntosh (2008) succinctly describes why this is an issue for First Nations and refers to Lavoie, Forget, and O'Neil's discussion of the 2005 *National Evaluation of the Health Transfer Policy* findings to support her statements. Transfer agreements include "non-enrichment clauses" that results in funding being based on expenditures the year before the community initially entered into a transfer agreement. As result, First Nations are "locked into a level of funding based on historical expenditure" and even though First Nations have different per capita funding depending upon the year they entered into their agreement, their funding is such that they are unable to compete with the increases in salary or other recruitment incentives that are offered to healthcare professionals who work as federally or provincially funded employees (MacIntosh, 2008, p. 74). Consider the following: If the provinces face recruitment and retention challenges, then this issue is compounded for First Nations communities.

2. **Jurisdictional roles and responsibilities.** Lavoie et al. (2005) related that unresolved jurisdictional issues continue to undermine the ability of First Nations people to reasonably access services (p. 12). There is lack of clarity in roles and responsibilities between many First Nations organizations, the province/territory, and First Nations and Inuit Health Branch of Health Canada. Allec (2005) explains, "To a large degree, jurisdictional issues . . . stem from the decades of a 'tug of war' over which level of government is responsible for services (p. 13)." The provincial government under the Canada Health Act is required to provide equal access to healthcare services for all provincial residents including First Nations living on reserves. However, some provincial organizations and health authorities take the position that the federal government is responsible for certain health services to First Nations people who are Status Indians under the Indian Act. As a result, some health services not covered by the Canada Health Act but otherwise provided by the provinces through the provincial health authorities may or may not be provided to First Nations communities. As a result of this, lack of clarity in roles and responsibilities of First Nations communities are faced with program fragmentation, problems with coordinating programs, under-funding, inconsistencies, service gaps, and lack of integration.

   Gaps in health services. Many First Nations experience difficulties in accessing health services for their community members as a result of jurisdictional issues. There are over 600 First Nations in Canada located across Canada; each could draft its own list of health services gaps. The First Nations, Inuit and Aboriginal Health (Health Canada, 2011b) Aboriginal Health Transition Fund (AHTF) from 2006 to 2011 supported Aboriginal projects to address issues related to jurisdictional ambiguity. Some First Nations communities were among the projects that promoted the integration of federally funded health services within First Nations communities with those funded by provincial and territorial governments. Some of the overall AHTF results included: (1) an increase in partnerships among Aboriginal groups and different levels of government in the health system; (2) increased awareness on behalf of provincial/territorial governments regarding Aboriginal health issues; (3) increased awareness of provincial/territorial health services by Aboriginal organizations; (4) increased participation of Aboriginal people in the design, delivery and evaluation of health services; (5) improved integration and adaptation of existing health services; and (6) improved access to certain health services available to Aboriginal people. The 311 projects across all provinces and territories piloted different approaches to better coordinate and adapt health services in areas such as e-health, substance abuse, child and youth care, mental health, chronic disease, public health, home care, and governance.

3. **Emphasis on curative services and physical health.** The Canadian health system's focus on curative services ignores holistic health and culturally based health programming. The limited health resources are focused on treatment services in many First Nations communities and subsequently there are few resources for innovative health promotion and prevention.

Many First Nations face obstacles in delivering healthcare services to their community members. Subsequently, each of these barriers produces challenges for nurses and nursing. Current issues in the provision of nursing care to First Nations in Canada include the following:

- Population health approaches to address inequity in health among First Nations people.
- Population demographics in relation to the healthcare needs of First Nations people.
- Transfer of healthcare services and community development as a climate for change in providing nursing care to First Nations, including issues faced by nurses.
- Impact of colonialism in providing meaningful nursing care to First Nations.
- First Nations perceptions about accessing health services.

Use of a Population Health Approach to Address Inequity

Population health is based on the understanding that health is determined as much or more by social, economic, environmental, and cultural factors than it is by genetic or medical factors (Senate Committee on Population Health, 2009). It includes a study of the determinants of health and disease, health status, and the degree to which healthcare affects the health of the community (Public Health Agency of Canada, 2008). An examination of the determinants of health helps to identify and then address inequities using an intersectoral (i.e., beyond that of the health sector) approach (Reuters & Kushner, 2010). Many First Nations have identified clean drinking water and safe, uncontaminated food (Chan et al., 2011; Parkes, 2011); reliable sanitation; comfortable housing (First Nation Information Governance Centre, 2011a) and workplaces, and adequate employment as essential to the health of the population (RCAP, 1996c). Health inequities result from the external environment and other social and economic conditions that, while largely outside the control of the individuals and families affected, are amenable to mitigation by the implementation of well-crafted public policy that is referred to as population health policy (Senate Committee on Population Health, 2009).

Human poverty is any fundamental need that is not adequately satisfied. Some First Nations communities have come to know many faces of poverty as it relates to marginalization, poor education, lack of support and recognition, inadequate resources, and the imposition of alien values on local and regional cultures (Aboriginal Nurses Association of Canada, 2009). Health involves more than physical integrity of the body; it includes social and political concerns and the relationship of individuals to the environment in which they live. Community development is an avenue for facilitating active participation of each member in a community in accordance with the values, attitudes, and aspirations of that community (Reading et al., 2007). Resources—both personal and social in nature—to improve the health and social conditions of people may be at first hidden from the health professional. One of these resources is First Nations' determination in obtaining community control and adequate resources to design health, social, and political systems that are of their choosing and reflective of their communities' cultures. Self-determination is one of the most important determinants of health among First Nations—they must be equal participants in political decision-making and have control over their lands, economies, education systems, and social and health services (Reading & Wien, 2009). The Royal Commission on Aboriginal Peoples articulated in *Gathering Strength* (1996c) that Aboriginal people want to access health and healing services and to achieve health status equal to that of the general Canadian population.

Population Demographics

First Nations people are demographically distinctive from the Canadian population. Compared to the Canadian population, significant growth of the registered Indian population (First Nations) is projected well into the future (Aboriginal Affairs and Northern Development Canada, 2010). Under the medium-growth scenario, the total population in Canada entitled to Indian registration is expected to increase by 40% (from 7,643,000 to about 1,069,600) during the period from 2004 to 2029. In addition, the First Nation population will remain extremely youthful in comparison to the Canadian population (Aboriginal Affairs and Northern Development Canada, 2010, p. 5). Declining fertility and improvements in life expectancy are expected to result in shifts in the age structure of the registered Indian population during the period from 2004 to 2029. The projections indicate a significant drop in the share of the population less than 15 years of age (from 32% in 2004 to 24% in 2029), resulting in a substantial growth in the share of the registered Indian population aged 45 or more (from 21% in 2004 to 32% in 2029). In comparison, about 49% of the Canadian population will be aged 45 years or more in the year 2029. In addition, during this same period, the registered Indian population living on-reserve is projected to rise by about 62%, whereas the registered Indian population living off-reserve is projected to increase by about 12%. The contrast between First Nations and the general population within the scope of current and projected population growth provides a basis for developing an understanding about the healthcare needs of First Nations people.

Regional variations exist in projected population growth among First Nations communities (Aboriginal Affairs and Northern Development Canada, 2010). The overall expected population growth is most prominent in the Prairie Provinces, whereas declining off-reserve First Nations population are projected in British Columbia and the provinces east of Manitoba. In addition to regional variation, knowledge about the migration patterns of young First Nations women to and from reserves can affect the nature of healthcare services provided both on and off the reserves. Demographic profiling serves as a valuable frame of reference within which to determine appropriate healthcare programming now and in the future.

Creating First Nations Health Services

Many First Nations communities took part in the health transfer program because it was viewed as an opportunity to set priorities at the community level and to design programs to meet these priorities (Lavoie et al., 2005, p. 5). According to an evaluation of the First Nations and Inuit health transfer policy in 2005, community level decision-making has improved program responsiveness and changing community needs can be accommodated without lengthy approval processes by First Nations and Inuit Health Branch of Health Canada. This section relates some areas where First Nations are involved in as they create health services based on their communities' needs. Each community is unique in its health services development.

1. First Nations health organizations (Lavoie et al., 2005), largely those that signed "integrated" agreements, had been able to develop administrative, management, service delivery, and programming skills. Provincial and private resources were utilized to adapt training to sessions

at the community level; the First Nations and Inuit Health Branch of Health Canada was not seen as a source of support for capacity development.

2. Health Services Accreditation through the Canadian Council on Health Services Accreditation is one avenue in which First Nations are pursuing to assist them in the development of their organizational infrastructure. It is one element of a quality assurance program.

3. Membership with the First Nations Health Managers Association (NDa, NDb), a national organization, provides leadership in health management by promoting standards, research, certification, and professional development. This association was created as a result of a joint Assembly of First Nations and First Nations and Inuit Health Branch meeting in March 2005. Senior management agreed that increasing capacity of First Nations health managers was important to improving First Nations health service delivery at the community level. The competency standards have been developed (First Nations Health Managers Association [2011]) and for the basis for the professional program, examination, work experience requirements, and maintenance of certification policies have been administered.

When the administration of healthcare services is transferred from Health Canada to a First Nations community, nursing service delivery also becomes the responsibility of that community. Issues that have been identified for nurses working in First Nations communities include:

• Some band-employed nurses do not believe they have the respect of the community in which they are employed. This lack of respect is evident when there is interference with the nurses' decisions.

• The retention of nurses in First Nations communities is related to the quality of the practice environment (Hart Wasekeesikaw, 2011). What are some key elements that would ensure quality is retained in the community workplace?

• In many First Nations communities, the nurse's ability to create linkages is necessary in order to facilitate client accessibility to health services, both within and outside the community. How might the new nurse establish linkages to various health and social services and develop processes to facilitate client service delivery?

Nursing and Effective Healthcare Programming

For many nurses, working with First Nations presents an opportunity to provide nursing care in cultures that differ from their own. This opportunity, in turn, creates other opportunities to positively affect nurse–client relationships. Community development principles (World Health Organization, 2009) can advance relationships with a First Nations community's leadership, health manager, and membership. Nurses who see themselves as partners with a community recognize that the strengths of the community will form a basis for organizing and improving the health of that community. Also, integral to the formation of these relationships is cultural competence (AFN, 2011c). Cultural competence is the application of knowledge, skills, attitudes, or personal attributes required by nurses to maximize respectful relationships with diverse populations of clients such as individuals, families, and communities (Canadian Nurses Association, 2010). However, it is important to recognize that cultural competence may overlook colonialism. Nurses need to understand how colonialism affected, and continues to affect, the lives of First Nations people to understand First Nations health today (Aboriginal Nurses Association of Canada, 2009). The development of a partnership relationship based on the understanding of colonialism could help to convey an attitude that will foster the kind of relationship First Nations clients would find helpful as they manage their healthcare needs.

Postcolonialism is one of the critical theories that provides a theoretical lens that allows access to the everyday experiences of marginalization, as structured by: (1) use of formal and informal power by individuals and groups to achieve their goals within organizations; and (2) the dynamics within organizations, institutions, and systems including the history of these dynamics (Kirkham & Anderson, 2002). Nurse–client relationships are affected by the perceptions that community members have about nurses and the nursing profession. First Nations people consider nurses and other healthcare providers to be a part of a healthcare system rooted in colonization. Postcolonialism may be useful in gaining insights into the issues that First Nations people face in healthcare. Indeed, elements of colonization continue today and affect nurse–client relationships, in turn positively or negatively affecting access to healthcare services by First Nations members.

First Nations Perceptions—Access to Services

Access to health services is an important determinant of health among Canadians. The Regional Health Survey (RHS) Phase 2 (2008/2010) provides some insight as to how adult First Nations people residing on-reserve view their access to health services. First Nations adults who felt they had the same access to health services compared to the general population increased from 2002 to 2003 (40.8%), with almost half (49.1%) of respondents reporting such access in the current survey (First Nations Information Governance Centre, 2011a, 2011b, 2011c). In addition, just over 12% (12.4%) rated their access to health services as better than the general Canadian population. This is a decrease as 23.6% of the respondents in 2002 to 2003 RHS rated their access to health services as being better than the general Canadian population. This downward trend requires caution in how data are used as these findings are self-reported perspectives about accessing health services. Subsequently, the findings are not indicative of actual access to health services. However, it may be useful to explore why these trends are occurring among First Nations peoples. One possible consideration is that First Nations people may be developing more awareness of disparities.

According to the preliminary results of the RHS Phase 2 (2008/2010), the perceived level of healthcare access (compared to the general Canadian population) is correlated with geographic remoteness (p. 19). For example, of First Nations people living in a community in which there is no year-round road access to a service center (i.e., special access community), 64.9% perceived themselves as having less access. Not surprisingly, this proportion decreases as geographic remoteness is minimized (32.7% living on reserves located in urban areas). Likewise, the proportion of First Nations adults indicating better access is highest among those living in an urban community (14.6%) and this proportion deceases as remoteness increases (6.7% in special access areas). Please note that in some areas of Canada, some First Nation communities or reserves are adjacent to or within large cities. For example, within the cities of Vancouver and North Vancouver are reserve communities such as Musquem, Squamish, and Tsleil-Watuth First Nations.

Gender is also a determinant of health status (First Nations Information Governance Centre, 2011a, 2011b, 2011c). First Nations women were more likely to report difficulties accessing traditional medicine and accessing NIHB services than First Nations men. The RHS on healthcare access relates an important point by Wilkins et al. (2008) that it is important to understand "whether variations in effectiveness are rooted in differing patterns of services use between men and women or are caused by the way services are structured—or by some combination of the two." The RHS recommends that further research on gender and help-seeking behavior, and gender and experience of services are required to better tailor health programs to First Nations adults.

S U M M A R Y

Nursing in First Nations communities presents many challenges. At the forefront is the need to understand indigenous history, starting from the time when only First Peoples inhabited North America. The relationship of First Nations with the Crown of England and, later, the government of Canada beginning with the treaties and then the Indian Act, the goal of colonization to obliterate First Nations peoples' cultures and assimilate them into mainstream society, and First Nations' cultural resurgence and determination to obtain self-government are important parts of this history.

Both community development and transfer of healthcare services are integral to the development of culturally specific community health and healing systems. Population health is a way of identifying determinants of health to address inequities in healthcare. Nurses are also challenged to understand the relationship between population demographics and the development of relevant health programs. Nursing issues related to the transfer of healthcare services to First Nations communities will require critical analysis and collaborative efforts to affect optimal resolutions.

Add to your knowledge of this issue:

Aboriginal Canada Portal – Health & Social Services	http://www.aboriginalcanada.gc.ca
Aboriginal Affairs and Northern Development Canada (formally known as Indian and Northern Affairs Canada)	www.ainc-inac.gc.ca
Aboriginal Healing Foundation	www.ahf.ca
Aboriginal Nurses Association of Canada	www.anac.on.ca
Assembly of First Nations	www.afn.ca

Online

R E F L E C T I O N S *on the Chapter...*

1 How have teachings regarding First Nations healthcare been included in your nursing program? Where can you obtain further information?

2 Before reading this chapter, were you aware of the work of the Truth and Reconciliation Committee of Canada? Based on reading this chapter and a review of the TRC.ca website, consider how Canadians will know when reconciliation has taken place?

3 Using the determinants of health, examine the impact on the health of First Nations members and their communities.

4 Name four healthcare needs in First Nations communities. What are some strategies for dealing with them?

5 Using First Nations demographic data, determine two health issues that could become priorities by the year 2020.

6 Identify four approaches that will enhance nurse–client communication with a First Nations person.

Want to know more? Visit thePoint for additional helpful resources:

• Journal Articles
• Learning Objectives
• Nursing Professional Roles and Responsibilities
• Bonus chapters:
  ○ Health and Nursing Policy: A Matter of Politics, Power and Professionalism
  ○ The NP Movement: Recurring Issues
  ○ When Difference Matters: The Politics of Privilege and Marginality

References

Aboriginal Affairs and Northern Development Canada. (2008). *Treaty negotiation.* Retrieved from http://www.ainc-inac.gc.ca/al/hts/tng/index-eng.asp

———. (2010). *Registered Indian demography – Population, household and family projections, 2004–2029.* Retrieved from http://www.aadnc.gc.ca/eng/1100100016838

Aboriginal Healing Foundation. (2002). Indian residential schools. An overview. In *The healing has begun. An operational update from the Aboriginal Healing Foundation* (pp. 3–7). Ottawa, ON: Author.

———. (2003). *Aboriginal people, resilience and the residential school legacy.* Ottawa, ON: Author. Retrieved from http://www.ahf.ca/downloads/resilience.pdf

———. (2004). *Historic trauma and Aboriginal healing.* Ottawa, ON: Author. Retrieved from http://www.ahf.ca/historic-trauma.pdf

———. (2007). *Addictive behaviours among aboriginal people in Canada.* Ottawa, ON: Author. Retrieved from www.ahf.ca/publications/research-series

Aboriginal Nurses Association of Canada. (2009). *Cultural competence and cultural safety in nursing education: An integrated review of the literature.* Ottawa ON: Author. Retrieved from: http//www.cna-nurses.ca/CNA/documents/pdf/publications/Review_of_Literature_e.pdf

Adelson, N. (1991). "Being alive well": The praxis of Cree health. *Arctic Medical Research, 50*(Suppl.), 230–232.

Allec, R. (2005). *First Nations health and wellness in Manitoba. Overview of gaps in service and issues associated with jurisdictions. Final report.* Prepared for the Intergovernmental Committee on First Nations Health. Retrieved from www.gov.mb.ca/ana/publications/1st_nations_health_final2005.pdf

Assembly of First Nations (AFN). (2011a). *Annual general assembly. July 12, 13 & 14, 2011. Moncton, NB. Resolution no. 04/2011. Making First Nations health a priority.* Ottawa, ON: AFN. Retrieved from http://www.afn.ca/uploads/files/aga-2011-resolutions.pdf.

———. (2011b). *Assembly of First Nations. The story.* Retrieved from http://www.afn.ca./index.php/en/about-AFN/our-story

———. (2011c). *Health and social secretariat. Key issues and activities.* Retrieved from http://www.afn.ca/index.php/en.policy-areas/health-and-social-secretariat

Berger, T.R. (1980). *Report of the Advisory Commission on Indian and Inuit Health Consultation.* Indian and Northern Affairs. Ottawa, ON: Government of Canada.

Boehmer, E. (1995). *Colonial and postcolonial literature: Migrant metaphors.* New York: Oxford University Press.

Boyer, Y. (2004). *Discussion paper series in Aboriginal health: Legal issues. No. 2 First Nations, Métis and Inuit health care. The Crown's fiduciary obligation.* Ottawa, ON: National Aboriginal Health Organization.

Canadian Nurses Association. (2010). *Position statement: Promoting cultural competence in nursing.* Retrieved from www.cna-aiic.ca/CNA/documents/pdf/publications/PS/14_Cultural _Competence_2010_.e.pdf *Code of ethics for registered nurses.* Ottawa, ON: Author.

Cassidy, F., & Bish, R. (1989). *Indian government: Its meaning and practice.* Lantzville, BC: Oolichan Books.

Chan, L., Receveur, O., Sharp, D., Schwartz, H., Ing, A., & Tikhonov, C. (2011). *First Nations food, nutrition and environment study (FNFNES): Results from British Columbia (2008/2009).* Prince George, BC: University of Northern British Columbia. Retrieved from http://www.fnfnes.ca/images/uploads/docs/FNFNES_report_BC_FINAL-PRINIT-v2.pdf

Dickason, O.P. (1994). *Canada's First Nations: A history of founding peoples from earliest times.* Toronto, ON: McClelland & Stewart.

First Nations Health Managers Association. (N.D.a). *Competency standards.* Retrieved from http://www.fnhma.ca/content.php?doc=27.

———. (N.D.b). *The First Nations health managers association has been established.* Retrieved from http://www.fnhma.ca/content.php?sec=1

First Nations Information Governance Centre. (2011a). Housing. *RHS Phase 2 (2008/10) preliminary results. Adult. Youth. Child* (Revised Ed., pp. 17–18). Ottawa, ON: First Nations Information Governance Centre.

———. (2011b). Access to services. *RHS Phase 2 (2008/10) preliminary results. Adult. Youth. Child* (Revised Ed., pp. 19–21). Ottawa, ON: First Nations Information Governance Centre.

———. (2011c). Healthcare access. *RHS Phase 2 (2008/10)*. Chapter 5, Adult. Ottawa, ON: First Nations Information Governance Centre.

Hart Wasekeesikaw, F. (2011). *Creating healthy workplace environments for nurses working in First Nations communities.* A presentation. The quality worklife – quality healthcare collaborative's 5th annual summit. Mississauga, ON. March 2–3, 2011 Retrieved from www.qwqhc.ca/documents /03-F. Hart-Wasekeesikaw.pdf

Health Canada. (1999). *Ten years of health transfer. First Nation and Inuit control. April 1989–March 1999.* Ottawa, ON: Minister of Public Works and Government Services Canada.

———. (2008). *First Nations and Inuit health. Transfer Status as of March 2008.* Retrieved from http://www.hc-sc.gc.ca/fniah-spnia/finance/agree-accord/trans_rpt_stats-eng.php

———. (2011a). *About health Canada. Indian health policy 1979.* Retrieved from http://hc-sc.gc.ca/ahc-asc/branch-dirgen/fnihb-dgspni/poli_1979-eng.php

———. (2011b). *First Nations, Inuit and Aboriginal health. Aboriginal health transition fund.* Retrieved from http://www.hc-sc.ca/fniah-spnia/services/acces/ahtf-eng.php

———. (2011c). *First Nations, Inuit and Aboriginal health. Health care services. Nursing.* Retrieved from http://www.hc-sc.gc.ca/fniah-spnia/services/nurs-inform/index-eng.php

Health Canada/Assembly of First Nations. (2011). *Your benefits. A guide for First Nations to access non-insured health benefits.* Retrieved from http://www.hc-sc.gc.ca/fniah-spnia/alt_formats/pdf/pubs/nihb-ssna/yhb-vss/nihb-ssna-yhb-vss-eng.pdf

Kerr, D., & Beaujot, R. (2011). Aboriginal demography. In D. Long & O. P. Dickason (Eds.), *Visions of the heart, Canadian aboriginal issues* (3rd ed.). Don Mills, ON: Oxford University Press.

Kirkham, S.R., & Anderson, J.M. (2002). Postcolonial nursing scholarship: From epistemology to method. *Advanced Nursing Science, 25*(1), 1–17.

Lavoie, J.G., O'Neil, J., Sanderson, L., et al. (2005). *The evaluation of the First Nations and Inuit health transfer policy. Final report: Volume 1, Executive summary.* Winnipeg, MB: Manitoba First Nations Centre for Aboriginal Health Research.

MacIntosh, C. (2008). Envisioning the future of aboriginal health under the health transfer process. *Health Law Journal.* Retrieved from www.law.ualberta.ca/centres/hli/userfiles/file/HLJ/Visions/05_MacIntosh.pdf

Milloy, J.S. (1991). The early Indian Acts. In J.R. Miller (Ed.), *Sweet promises: A reader on Indian–White relations in Canada* (pp. 145–154). Toronto, ON: University of Toronto Press.

Parkes, M.W. (2011). *Ecohealth and Aboriginal health: A review of common ground.* Prince George, BC: National Collaborating Centre for Aboriginal Health.

Public Health Agency of Canada. (2008). *What is the population health approach?* Retrieved from http://www.phac-aspc.gc.ca/ph-sp/approach-approche/index-eng.php

Ray, A.J. (1974). *Indians in the fur trade: Their role as trappers, hunters, and middlemen in the lands southwest of Hudson Bay 1660–1870.* Toronto, ON: University of Toronto Press.

Reading, J. L., Kmetic, A., & Gideon, V. (2007). *First Nations wholistic policy and planning model. Discussion paper for the World Health Organization Commission on social determinant of health. April, 2007.* Ottawa, ON: Assembly of First Nations. Retrieved from ahrnets.ca/files/2011/02/AFN_Paper_2007.pdf

Reading, C.L., & Wien, F. (2009). *Health inequities and social determinants of aboriginal peoples' health.* Prince George, BC: National Collaborating Centre. Retrieved from www.nccah-ccnsa.ca/docs/social determinants/NCCAH-loppie-Wien_report.pdf

Reuters, L., & Kushner, K.E. (2010).'Health equity through action on the social determinants of health': Taking up the challenge in nursing. *Nursing Inquiry, 17*(3), 269–280.

Royal Commission on Aboriginal Peoples (RCAP). (1996a). *Report on the Royal Commission on Aboriginal Peoples. Vol. 1, Chap. 9.1: Protection of the reserve land base* [Online]. Ottawa, ON: Government of Canada. Retrieved from http://www.ainc-inac.gc.ca/ch/rcap/index_e.html

———. (1996b). *Report on the Royal Commission on Aboriginal Peoples. Vol. 2: Restructuring the relationship* [Online]. Ottawa, ON: Government of Canada. Retrieved from http://www.ainc-inac.gc.ca/ch/rcap/index_e.html

———. (1996c). *Report on the Royal Commission on Aboriginal Peoples. Vol. 3: Gathering strength.* Ottawa, ON: Government of Canada. Retrieved from http://www.ainc-inac.gc.ca/ch/rcap/index_e.html

Senate Committee on Population Health. (2009). *A healthy, productive Canada: A determinant of health approach.* Standing Senate Committee on Social Affairs, Science and Technology. Final Report of Senate Subcommittee on Population Health. Retrieved from http://www.parl.gc.ca/content/SEN/Committee/402/popu/rep/rephealth1jun09-e.pdf

Smith, R., & Lavoie, J.G. (2008). First Nations health networks: A collaborative system approach to health transfer. *Healthcare Policy, 4*(2), 101–111.

Smylie, J. (2000). Society of Obstetricians and Gynaecologists policy statement. A guide for health professional working with Aboriginal peoples: The sociocultural context of Aboriginal peoples in Canada. *Journal for Society of Obstetricians and Gynaecologists, 100*, 1070–1081.

Tobias, J.L. (1991). Protection, civilization, assimilation: An outline history of Canada's Indian policy. In J.R. Miller (Ed.), *Sweet promises: A reader on Indian-White relations in Canada* (pp. 127–144). Toronto, ON: University of Toronto Press.

Truth and Reconciliation Commission of Canada. Retrieved from www.TRC.ca May 9 2012

Waldram, J., Herring, D.A., & Young, T.K. (2006). *Aboriginal health in Canada: Historical, cultural, and epidemiological perspectives.* Toronto, ON: University of Toronto Press.

Wilkins, D., Payne, S., Granville, G., & Branney, P. (2008). *The gender and access to health services study.* Final report. Men's Health Forum. University of Bristol. Retrieved from http://www.dh.gov.uk/prod_consu_dh/groups/dh_digitalassets/@dh/@en/documents/digitalasset/dh_092041.pdf

World Health Organization. (2009). *Milestones in health promotion. Statements from global conferences.* Geneva: World Health Organization.

Young, K. (1984). Indian health services in Canada: A sociohistorical perspective. *Social Science and Medicine, 18*(3), 257–264.

5

Issues in Contemporary Nursing Leadership

Gail J. Mitchell and Joy Richards

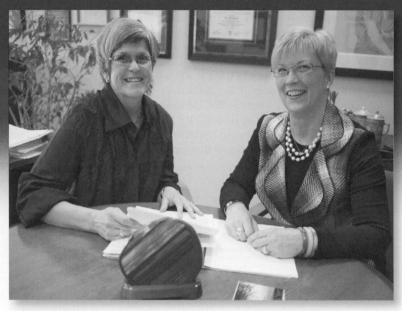

Chapter authors Gail Mitchell (left) and Joy Richards (right). (Used with permission. Photographer Nicholas Brudnicki.)

Critical Questions

As a way of engaging with the ideas in this chapter, consider the following:

1. Drawing on your student experience in nursing practice, how do you understand leadership in nursing?

2. In what ways do you provide leadership with others?

3. How might you enable the potential for leadership in others?

Chapter Objectives

After completing this chapter, you will be able to:

1. Identify relevant concepts in relation to nursing leadership and complexity theory.

2. Describe relationships between leadership and change.

3. Identify opportunities for leadership in your nursing work.

4. Describe how ethics and leadership are inextricably linked and lived out in relationships with others.

The premise of this chapter is that leadership is about the potential to make a difference and this potential is present in every nurse. While some formal roles are afforded specific leadership responsibilities, all nurses are called, morally and professionally, to make a difference to the quality of patient care and to organizational and community culture. In order to consider the various ways of being and becoming a leader, we will consider specific terms describing leadership and delve in some depth into the importance of relationships for inspiring and enabling change. The practice of nursing is predominantly housed in institutions, agencies, and organizations that are under increasing pressures to deliver health services with less cost, enhanced safety, and greater efficiency. These performance pressures exist within mounting consumer concerns for timely, quality care that is both personalized and meaningful. This picture, with all of its pressures and expectations, provides a glimpse into the reality and complexity of contemporary nursing practice and leadership.

Throughout this chapter, you will have opportunity to reflect on your own potential for leadership, as well as your capacity to participate with and support others who are in leadership positions. Leaders are called to inspire and enable others to contribute and work toward a shared vision or for a compelling purpose (Kouzes & Posner, 2003). Leaders work to create networks and network to complete their work. Leaders know how to be in challenging situations and they are comfortable with ambiguity, uncertainty, and possibility. As you begin reading this chapter, take a moment to reflect on your own life; who has exemplified leadership qualities that you value? What is it about those qualities that you hold as important? What leadership qualities would you like to develop?

It can also be helpful to think of leaders you have known who exemplify what you do not want to become. Some leaders, for instance, do not encourage open discussion of issues, or some may make judgments that shut down communication or embarrass people. Considering actions or behaviors that have the potential to harm or silence others is a way to put unwanted actions in a spotlight in order to avoid them.

COMPLEXITY THEORY AND LEADERSHIP

Complexity science provides a constellation of concepts that are informing critical thinking and research scholarship in multiple disciplines and professional groups—including organizational development, education, medicine, physics, biology, and nursing (Uhl-Bien, 2007; Westley et al., 2006). The main concepts that will be discussed in this chapter on leadership are complex adaptive systems (CAS), emergence, unpredictability, and relationships. Each of these is considered from a leadership perspective. We encourage you to pursue particular ideas that appeal to you in your own scholarship and practice. Complexity science offers a theoretical perspective, and like all theories, it provides a way to think about reality and day-to-day life. If you find the concepts interesting and useful, you may choose to continue thinking about them in your own practice and development as a nurse and leader.

To offer a broad view of complexity thinking, consider the following. Reality, including the many realities where nursing happens, is inherently complex, relational, full of paradox, pressures, opportunities, obstacles, expectations, hopes, inspirations, fears, values, and concerns. The inherent complexities of life require thinking about concepts that help people to organize, strategize, collaborate, and move ahead with others to achieve goals and to meet expectations. Bottomline—there are no simple answers in complex situations. Leaders cannot control nurses and nurses cannot control patients. However, leaders can inspire and enable nurses to rally around a goal or purpose that they care about and nurses can inspire and enable patients to rally around a goal or purpose that they care about. Control and command, as well as their companions predict and prescribe, are not meaningful or effective ways of being with complex situations. This is true even though there are times when command and control is useful and effective. Complexity theory eliminates *either–or* and *right–wrong* thinking. There are multiple ways of knowing and understanding the world and people benefit from being able to move or jump from level to level, or perspective to perspective, when required, by changing situations. There is no simple cause and effect in complexity thinking (Westley et al., 2006). A large and costly initiative can leave nothing changed and very small changes can sometimes create strong and powerful transformation. So how then can you begin to think about complexity concepts in ways that enable your own leadership potential and the potential of others? Let us look more closely at some important ideas.

The first concept relates to the idea that human beings and even organizations are living, changing systems that continuously transform with shifting circumstances and emerging situations (Westley et al., 2006; Wheatley, 2006). There is an interplay or mutual exchange among people such that we both change and are changed by involvement in life. Human beings are always trying to make sense of what is happening. What is the meaning of what is going on? What do I have to do? How do I prioritize among competing demands? And, how am I going to act? Groups of people are also continuously shifting and changing according to what is going on. Complexity theory has a term—complex adaptive system (CAS)—to represent this living, self-organizing activity of persons and groups of persons. Self-organizing activity can be seen among all kinds of patterns; consider the patterns of fractals that look like the patterns of living plants—that look like the patterns in our living universe. Families have patterns when they live day-to-day priorities and establish rituals that become important for holidays and vacations. Living things organize in patterns and the patterns formed are influenced by what is going on, what is important, and by what opportunities and risks predominate.

Two other ideas from complexity theory are important to our current consideration of leadership. First, amid the continuous shifting and sensemaking about what is going on is the belief that things are not linear or predictable and what we think and want to happen can influence what emerges. Our intentions and attentions have an influence in the world. Second, relationships are critically important—the quality of our relationships enables change, innovation, collaboration, and growth. It is interesting to note that many leaders who have worked with nurses and other organizational leaders for decades promoting various leadership approaches (such as, transformational leadership and servant leadership) now attest to the critical importance of relationships and possibility (see e.g., Maxwell, 2008; Westley et al., 2006; Wheatley, 2006; Wheatley & Kellner-Rogers, 1998).

SITUATING THE TOPIC: THE NATURE OF THE ISSUE

Although there are many ways to talk about or understand leadership, one distinction that seems important to point out is the difference between the idea that leadership is something that *happens to us,* rather than something that *each of us participates in* (Cashman, 2008; Maxwell, 2008; Wheatley, 2006). We would suggest that not only is it possible for us to participate in nursing leadership, but that professional nursing leadership is a shared project in which we participate through our words, actions, attitudes, and relationships. We will use three stories here as a way of showing how you might participate in nursing leadership—for better or worse. These stories will provide a rich context for examining a leadership issue from a position of social activism and change.

The first story is called *Crossing the Line* and nurses participate in this kind of leadership practice from their first days as a student. Indeed, this kind of leadership practice is one of the most important issues in nursing practice. Choosing to cross a line, or not, will have layers of consequences. Please read the story and think about a similar situation you may have experienced or witnessed at this point in your career. After reading the story, think about the questions and jot down your answers in the margin of the book.

Story and Reflection—Crossing the Line

Hansen had just started working as an Registered Nurse (RN) and was 3 months into a full-time role as primary nurse in a long-term care facility affiliated with a university in a large Canadian city. She was pleased to get a full-time position and was extremely anxious to learn all the skills and routines that would help her to fit in and become an accepted member by the other nurses on her unit. The work that happens on a nursing unit is very complex. In addition to all the skills and routines, there are relationships and power struggles, friendships and tensions among some individuals, and rumor mills and expectations from leaders and colleagues. Hansen was really trying to be a quick study and learn the ropes so she could settle in like the other more experienced nurses. At the 6-month mark Hansen felt more secure with the routine and role expectations. She had established excellent relationships with her primary patients and had set up family meetings once a month for all her residents. Things were going very well, but as often happens, life was about to present a new and very challenging situation that would require Hansen to reflect and make a decision about how to act when her colleagues and issues started *crossing the line.*

The trouble started on night shift. Hansen noticed that her teammates stopped offering to help her with her more complex residents when they needed to ambulate or be repositioned. There was no explicit talk about a change. Hansen just felt something was wrong and she was disturbed about having to ask for help all the time when previously, her colleagues had just automatically helped each other. Hansen let a week or two go by to see if things changed, but the absence of help and collegiality continued. When her team switched shift a week later, Hansen decided to broach the topic with one of the senior RNs she liked and trusted. The senior RN was kind but the news was not what Hansen expected. The senior nurse told Hansen that her teammates were unhappy with the way she was working with residents and their families. Apparently, family members were talking among themselves and those not in Hansen's group went to the manager to request that their primary nurses also begin to have family meetings to address questions and concerns and to give families an opportunity to contribute to care practices for their loved ones. Hansen's colleagues were angry at her for practicing in ways that shed light on others who were not practicing the same way. Hansen was shocked and dismayed. When she asked what her colleagues expected, the senior RN said, "They want you to stop the family meetings." Hansen was very upset and distressed. She had some decisions to make that would change her situation in a major way.

Hansen did not get the support she hoped for from the senior RN. Indeed, the message she received from the senior RN was to fit in or her life would be miserable on the unit. Hansen realized she was being bullied but was fearful of going against her teammates. She did not want to leave the unit and she really cared for the residents and families with whom she had quality relationships. She spoke with a few close friends who were also new grads, one of whom had just left an oncology unit because of a command-and-control manager, and they both advised Hansen to quit the unit and find a new job. As a new nurse, Hansen was deeply troubled. She tried to speak with the manager, who knew about the issue, but the manager did not have time to meet with her. Weighing the pros and cons and advice from her friends, Hansen decided to resign. She started a new job 2 months later in a different facility with the hopes of making it with a new group of colleagues.

Reflection

This story was called *Crossing the Line* for several reasons. First, the more experienced nurses exerted power against Hansen and the change in practice she introduced with

(continued on page 76)

Story and Reflection—Crossing the Line (continued)

families on the long-term care unit. How is their action to withdraw assistance to Hansen an example of crossing the line? How many lines did the nurses cross with their withdrawal of help? Second, the senior RN who spoke kindly with Hansen about the other nurses also crossed a line—how so do you think? What are your thoughts about the knowing manager who did not have time to meet with Hansen? What line did the manager cross? And Hansen, what do you think of her choice to resign? Did she cross a line from your perspective? What are some of the other ways the situation could have turned out—recognizing that there are always many possibilities for how things might unfold?

As a nurse and a leader, you will be called on to act in ways that will test your values and your courage to risk things that are important. Hansen is a young nurse and, as occasionally happens, she was not treated very well by more senior colleagues. The concept of *crossing the line* surfaces many times in a leader's life. There are always pressures to conform, to not rock the boat, and to step in line with what others want. Choices on either side of the line have consequences. Thinking ahead about these times of crossing the line may help you prepare for the times you will make a choice to cross the line, or not. How might you have acted in Hansen's situation? What is the line in the sand that you would not cross in order to protect the quality of patient care? What could Hansen have done differently to demonstrate leadership in this situation? What leadership actions and attitudes from others could have shown up in this situation?

A second way to participate in leadership endeavors is to engage with the vision and authority of a designated leader. Nurses have many opportunities to discuss ideas, participate in projects and committees, and work to advance a vision or purpose linked with patient care, governance, or quality of work life. Nurse leaders need the energy and commitment of all nurses on a unit or in an organization to bring a vision to life. Leaders often lead by asking questions and this is a powerful way to spark dialogue about possibilities and obstacles to change. Consider the following story and reflection about a manager of a busy medical unit.

Story and Reflection—Critical Questioning: What will it Take?

Kai-Lee graduated from a BScN program 5 years ago and worked primarily in critical and emergency care areas. She is intelligent, committed to quality patient-centered care, and motivated to take more responsibility and contribute to nursing leadership in her organization. Nurses with commitment and motivation are always noticed in organizations—organizational leaders are always scanning the horizon for *bright lights*. It was not long into her career that Kai-Lee was invited to become a project leader on her unit and a nursing council representative for the critical care program. In her 5th year, a director asked Kai-Lee to consider applying for a manager role in the Emergency Department (ED)—a busy community hospital with approximately 40,000 visits a year. The unit had high staff turnover, falling patient satisfaction scores, increasing pressures to see more people in less time, and pressures to generally improve quality of care—especially for admitted patients in hallways. Kai-Lee was very well aware of the issues in the ED—she had been a full-time nurse there for 2 years and she had a good understanding of some of the pressures from nurses in other areas of the hospital. On the one hand, she was overwhelmed with the enormity of the job of manager. On the other hand, she wondered what it would take to try to improve the situation for patients, families, and nurses. Armed with important questions and the intention to try, Kai-Lee applied and was accepted into the role of manager.

It was not long before Kai-Lee learned that one of the most important leadership actions is to listen to the concerns and issues of persons you are working with. Kai-Lee listened to nurses, other health professionals in the ED, patients and families, her director, and others who approached her with multiple requests and projects. She listened intently and purposefully for a number of reasons. First, she was in a new role and wanted to learn as much as possible. Second, she knew that being listened to is one of the fundamental practices of respect, and respect is essential for building relationships. And third, she listened to try to figure out the right questions to ask in order to promote dialogue among the people she worked with. Kai-Lee had a list of issues and priorities identified by colleagues in the ED and she had a list of priorities and issues identified by nurses and others who did not work in the ED. In her many meetings with individuals and groups, Kai-Lee decided to tackle one shared issue for both ED staff and nurses working on units who received patients from the ED. The ED staff complained bitterly about the floor nurses who did not understand the pressures on the ED and the need for the floor nurses to accept patients immediately upon request. The floor nurses complained bitterly that the ED nurses did not understand what it was like to have six or seven very ill patients, with some emergencies, distraught family members, people admitted to hallways, and the constant worry of making an error. Both groups of nurses wanted more respect and understanding about what was happening, as well as more help when the situations were dangerous—which, was pretty much most of the time.

Kai-Lee knew she could not "fix" this one important issue. Both groups of nurses had legitimate fears, concerns, and desires. So how does a leader proceed? Kai-Lee met with nurses in both areas and asked them: What will it take to help change this situation? She believed that if any possibilities existed for change, it would need to start with the people involved in the issue. When Kai-Lee met with each group, they identified small initiatives that would be a first step to breaching the gulf of bitterness and misunderstanding. Dialogue led to a program called, *Walk a Day in My Shoes*. Kai-Lee met with the managers and the director in the medical–surgical programs, areas where most ED patients need admission, and presented the issues and proposed the program. The cost for the program was doable for managers who agreed to find funding for one RN for three shifts a week where nurses from each area worked with a colleague to develop understanding and additional recommendations for how to support each other. Kai-Lee had her first success with one simple question and a lot of respect and belief in the possibility of people to organize and change.

It may be evident to you that Kai-Lee was an excellent leader who also happened to be a manager. Some authors draw clear distinctions between leadership and managerial roles (e.g., Kotter, 1996). Kai-Lee and many others do not fit in such distinct categories because there are nurse leaders who are excellent managers with large operational budgets, but who are not viewed as nursing leaders and vice versa. Leadership is not defined by or contained in a label. As noted above, leadership is viewed as relationship-enhancing actions that enable and inspire change, and nurse leaders in all roles may have the knowledge and skill to invite and enable dialogue and possibility with others.

Story 3 is about a nurse, Nazilla Kessam, in the role of Vice President and Chief Nurse Executive (VP/CNE). This nurse is an experienced leader and she has been in the role for several years when a critically important issue is brought to her attention. The issue, as you will read, requires an extensive inquiry and analysis before the nurse chooses her plan of action. After reading the story *Ethical Drift and the Emergence of Moral Courage,* we will provide the highlights of the VP/CNE's analysis and invite you to consider the issues and the decisions you might make if you found yourself in a similar place.

Story and Reflection—Ethical Drift and the Emergence of Moral Courage

Nazilla is a nurse leader with more than a decade of experience in progressive nursing leadership roles—including president-elect of a local chapter of an international scholarly association, practice leader consultant for her provincial nursing association, professional practice leader for a large cardiovascular program, and director of nursing at a teaching hospital. Nazilla had achieved a master's degree in nursing and had worked as an advanced practice nurse before becoming a director of nursing. She is currently enrolled in a doctoral program and is very interested in the politics of nursing as a female profession, critical theory, and the social politics of professionalism—including professionalism in nursing.

Nazilla is VP/CNE in a 600-bed teaching hospital. From a practice perspective, her leadership has primarily focused on helping create an environment to support excellence in patient-centered nursing, best practice applications, and a patient safety culture. Nazilla is familiar with best practice evidence and regularly looks to research to examine relevant issues in her role as a leader. Her own leadership role includes a program of research where she uses appreciative inquiry to work with nurses creating innovative practices to enhance the quality of care. The teaching hospital is affiliated with two universities with nursing and other health professional programs. Research is extremely important to the hospital because it helps create new clinical knowledge to improve quality of care, it brings in research dollars for supporting infrastructure, and it attracts philanthropists who give money to support hospital programs. Nazilla is a research consumer, advocate, and educator. One day a staff nurse enters her office to discuss a concern about research and patient care.

Nazilla was not expecting the story that she was hearing from one of the experienced nurses from the Oncology Department. The nurse was distraught and felt she and other nurses were becoming unethical in their practices. Many physicians had treatment and drug protocols that the Oncology RNs were asked to assist with. Decision trees helped the Oncology staff to decide if a patient might be a candidate for a study. Some of the medical residents affiliated with particular physicians, or sometimes research assistants, were called if a patient was eligible to hear more. The problem was that this nurse indicated that she saw and heard patients being coerced to join studies. Patients were being told things, such as, "If you do not enter the study, we cannot guarantee that you will get the best drugs" or "only patients in the study have a chance for the newest treatment." Some patients indicated they wanted more time to think but they were discouraged to take time to think about the consequences. The nurse also described times when treatment was delayed in order to follow research protocols. For instance, a patient having angina was not treated in the usual way to relieve pain because another test or intervention of the research protocol was needed first. The third thing the nurse identified was the concern that she and her colleagues were performing more and more aspects of the research protocols. The research work was not considered part of their job descriptions and time to complete research protocols was eating into their time with patients. The nurse detailed specific examples of the issues as indicated above and then handed Nazilla a detailed report with the signature of 20 Oncology nurses.

ARTICULATING THE ISSUE

The issue identified in Nazilla's story begins with a concerned group of nurses who have raised serious concerns about quality patient care and its interface with research protocols on the in-patient Oncology unit. Nazilla must carefully consider the concerns and the report provided by the Oncology nurse and proceed to make and take actions to enable change that will diminish the threats to patient care. The magnitude and potential messiness of the issue is daunting. Even as the nurse was speaking, Nazilla wished that she could stop the disclosure of what she knew immediately to be a critical and perhaps career and life-altering issue. There are times as leaders when you wish you did not have to hear certain truths. Nazilla knew she would not ignore the issue, but she had no idea then what might happen next. She thanked the nurse for bringing the issues and the report and stated that following some thought and inquiry, she would meet with the nurses involved. In keeping with the format of this text, a multilevel examination of the issue is presented.

Historical Analysis

A historical analysis asks the questions: Under what conditions did the current situation originate and what has contributed to the evolution of the issue over time? In a historical analysis it is also useful to ask: What has influenced the positions that people have taken on this issue? Thinking about the issue facing Nazilla, we first considered the rapid growth of research activity in large teaching hospitals that began in the early 1990s. The growth of research brought opportunities for advancement of knowledge and healthcare delivery, but also increased risk for patients involved in experimental treatments and drug trials. Large research programs bring prestige and competition among hospitals and hospital budgets often benefit from overhead costs affiliated with space and other resources. Most health professionals experience pressures to be evidence-based and to follow best practice guidelines. It is hard to imagine that anyone could or should question the value of research in healthcare settings where patients are vulnerable and ill, but experience has taught us that nurses need to have the courage to ask questions, even when there is a risk to one's own position. The courage to question and the risks that might be affiliated with the questioning are connected to the social and cultural dimensions of the organization.

Social and Cultural Analysis

We considered what social and cultural contexts shaped this particular issue about research and ethics, as well as the prevailing attitudes and assumptions in society and in the particular hospital and unit where the issue surfaced. It is our view that the prevailing attitude among health professionals about research is that it is good and needed for quality patient care. A predominant assumption in society is that research generates knowledge. There is also a commonly held view among healthcare consumers that teaching/research hospitals provide better "cutting or leading edge" care. At the same time, many people fear being used as an experimental object or a *guinea pig* where one feels used for others' purposes. In some specialty hospitals, there is an explicit expectation voiced to patients about the research culture and the need to help improve care—patients in some organizations are expected to agree to research in order to receive best care. The pressure of the research culture is a reflection of the value placed on contemporary *science*. There is still, we believe, a general fascination with quick cures or magic bullet solutions to eradicate serious health issues, in spite of the reality that poverty (socioeconomic status) is the leading cause of global disease and illness (Raphael, 2006).

We know, as do many nurses in practice and academia, that a particular kind of science is ranked highest. The randomized control trial (RCT) is the gold standard for clinical and drug trials. This is true, even though the RCT is not the preferred approach for studying human experiences or processes of care that tend to be far too complex to be amenable for the controls required in a sound RCT. Physicians Jaded and Enkin (2007) have written a compelling text on the most suitable place for RCTs in healthcare. To quote the authors, "Most RCTs focus on clinical questions and management of disease. Many of the major determinants of health or illness, such as absolute or relative poverty, social class, literacy, transportation or other infrastructure, are not amenable to medical interventions. RCTs can only answer questions for which quantitative results are applicable . . . many things that really count cannot be counted" (p. 9). The open discussion of the rightful place for the RCT is not a common occurrence in healthcare settings. We wonder if review boards and ethics committees sanction the RCT under the assumption that it is the best approach in health research? The distinct kinds of knowledge found helpful by different health workers have not, to our knowledge, been addressed in modern healthcare institutions. Perhaps it is time. As well, there are other issues affiliated with the dominant culture—the politics of power and position.

Political Analysis

A political analysis asks questions that explore the location of power and influence within particular issues. In other words, whose knowledge, whose voice is able to influence either the barriers to or the strategies for resolution of an issue? Specifically, what is the relationship between knowledge and power in this situation? Nurses are typically expected to obey orders and to be *good* (obedient) team members when decisions are made about how to provide care. Nurses are expected to do the work delegated by the dominant group, as well as often picking up work technically handled further down the organizational hierarchy. This means that nurses are often expected to *add on* additional tasks without complaint (move beds, mop up soiled floors, assist with research protocols). Involvement in research can be expected of nurses even though the language used in research can be quite abstract and inaccessible to those (professional and nonprofessional) not involved in specific research traditions. This inaccessibility may be one reason why many nurses do not feel prepared to question research protocols. Physician researchers who are the Principal Investigators (PIs) of a program of research are often world renowned and highly regarded. The power of the physician researcher is undeniable. Consider the additional position of power when English is not the first language of patients (or nurses) or when persons have physical challenges like blindness, deafness, and disability. As the VP/CNE in the organization, Nazilla needs to think about the overall relationship between nurses and doctors in her organization. She needs to anticipate how her voice and the voices of the Oncology nurses will be heard when she begins to discuss issues with hospital leaders. Nazilla anticipates that some will hear her, but that there will also be strong pressures to not rock the research boat. She also needs to consider her own power in the organization. Do senior leaders and physicians typically listen to her? Does she have the political weight and support of the CEO? These realities will all come into play. And, once started, as is often the case in very complex situations, issues will come forth in fits and starts, with feelings of fear and courage, in the midst of clarity and obscurity.

The question of who benefits from research being conducted in hospitals is multilayered and complex. First, one would hope that members of society will benefit from the new knowledge and treatment being tested and it is reasonable to expect that in the long term, this expectation will be realized. However, the risks to the persons who are current participants/subjects may outweigh the potential gains. The question of risk in these situations surfaces the concern: Are persons being used as means to an end in contemporary healthcare studies, especially when they come to a hospital for emergency and/or unexpected situations such as chest pain, paralysis, trauma, or life-saving chemotherapy?

Resistance to change in the situation of research in healthcare may be considered from multiple perspectives. First, the researchers conducting particular studies are heavily invested in the work being done. Typically, the researchers have been granted external funds to conduct the studies and there are multiple pressures to complete work and report findings. The pressures come from the funding agencies as well as from academic institutions that are increasingly judging the value of work according to the number of grants and dollars allotted. Resistance may also come from hospital administrators who benefit from research dollars that support staff and infrastructure in both service and academic institutions. Plus, there is a prestige associated with the dollar amount of research funding and whole departments can be staffed with individuals whose sole purpose is to help administrators and researchers to secure more funding. It is necessary to consider the view that research has become a huge enterprise, a massive turbine of activity, and the pressure to support research activity is felt by healthcare staff and patients. Some nurses, like those who came to see VP/CNE Nazilla, are participating more in research than in relational practice and the outcomes. The Oncology nurses believed patient care was being compromised and they offered at least five examples of typical situations when they experienced ethical distress and when they witnessed compromised care and treatment. The nurses also described times when they did raise questions about what they were experiencing with their unit manager and some physicians, but their issues where typically dismissed as unfounded since the research protocol was approved by at least one ethical review committee. They escalated their concerns to the CNE because they were not able to get a satisfactory change in the research practices within their Oncology unit/program.

The two most obvious groups to benefit from resolving the issues, at least in the short-term, are the direct care providers who are charged with participating in the research protocols and the patients/persons who are being coerced or denied usual care in order to execute the research protocol. Longer-term benefits to others are possible, but must, in Nazilla's analysis, take a second order of importance. The issue of who benefits from current healthcare research has been addressed to some degree—the researchers, the future public (possibly), and the hospital. Perhaps the less visible forces are the corporations, especially drug and supply conglomerates that grow their profits from business with healthcare providers. The challenge for whistle-blowers to go public with a charge of unethical behavior involving drug companies was front page news in Toronto when a physician, Nancy Oliveri, went to the press about research and ethical concerns (see http://www.careeractivist.com/my-articles/whistleblowing-the-right-way.htm for story on whistle blowing). Politics, power, punishment, conformity—all these ideas clear the way for a critical analysis of the research ethics issue facing Nazilla.

Critical Analysis (Feminist and Postcolonial)

A critical approach asks questions that challenge the taken-for-granted assumptions that are prevalent in society such as assumptions of gender, race, and class. A critical postcolonial analysis asks questions about the effect of colonization or domination of one group over another. In particular, this position challenges notions of race, racialization, and culture and provides "social mandates of uncovering existing inequities" (Kirkham & Anderson, 2002, p. 1). In feminist analysis, for example, the intention is not to privilege the position of one gender over the other, but to question the way in which notions of gender have been attached to issues influencing nurses, patients, and clients, and relationships with others in the healthcare system. More often than not, a critical feminist analysis does not relate to the gender of a particular person, but rather to the ways that traditional structures based on gender divisions of power have influenced or shaped issues or events.

A critical analysis of the situation involving nurses' concerns about research protocols and quality of care on the inpatient Oncology unit are influenced by issues of power and gender. One myth about gender that comes to mind is that women and nurses can be labeled as emotional, too involved, and/or not objective enough. The Oncology nurses may be viewed as oversensitive to patients and their ethical concerns minimized or dismissed. We mentioned above that the dominant values for expert or scientific knowledge over experiential and personal knowledge is a prominent reality in healthcare culture and ethical concerns or moral residue could be judged as subjective and unfounded.

The culture of an organization influences the expression of contrary views, the freedom to dialogue and debate important issues, as well as the processes for addressing conflict and diversity. Many organizations state that they value diversity—but sometimes it is welcome only if views do not question authority. Nazilla must be able to think about her organization through this cultural lens, and the critical analysis may help her prepare for how best to begin the dialogue about the issues raised by nurses. Does the organization employ an ethicist or ombudsman that Nazilla could seek out to assist with raising critical issues for discussion? And Nazilla is herself a fairly new immigrant to Canada; how will her own ethnicity influence the unfolding dynamic?

The power inequities between physicians and others can be a serious threat to staff and to patients/families—the latter being perhaps at the very bottom of the healthcare hierarchy. Just as nurses have been discouraged from questioning a physician's judgement, patients too have been silenced and expected to comply with authority and privilege. There is no doubt that the issue of personal voice, whether patient or nurse, is a legitimate concern. The structures and processes of modern healthcare relentlessly reinforce the expert voice, the evidence-based voice, the physician or researcher voice. For instance, patient rounds are typically the place where care planning is conducted. Yet patients and often the nurses who care for the patients (and one could argue, who knows them best) are not often present at the meetings discussing care.

Economic Analysis

Economic challenges are not new to nurse leaders. "Since the post-war years, at least nurses in Western industrial countries have had to negotiate among the sometimes-conflicting demands and obligations of their employers, healthcare organizations and those for whom they care" (Ceci, 2006, p. 56). And, as economic constraints intensify, nurses in practice settings find themselves with diminishing resources and a "limited capacity to exercise control over their practice" (p. 56). Nurse leaders, in turn, are caught in the tension between professional practice needs and the economic demands of the institution or organization.

In the context of this story, an economic consequence for the organization is a possible outcome once the issue is fully disclosed. One thing that has become clear to us over years of leadership is that sometimes all one has to do to be a leader is to speak truthfully about an issue with passion and respect for all involved. It is likely that protocols will be reviewed and research delayed if issues concerning quality of patient care are raised. A long-term economic impact is unlikely in our analysis. However, we do expect significant pushback from the involved researchers and possibly the funders. Recall the issues with drug companies funding research to consider other economic implications. The more invisible implications may issue from companies or governments who punish groups or organizations for embarrassing, public disclosure of ethical issues.

Ethical Analysis

Nursing ethics is concerned with the delivery of professional nursing practice and the influence of broad societal issues on the health and well-being of Canadians (Canadian Nurses Association [CNA], 2008). The CNA code of ethics is intended to serve as "an ethical basis from which nurses can advocate for quality work environments that support the delivery of safe, compassionate, competent, and ethical care" (p. 2). An ethical analysis surfaces relevant points for addressing the issue. First, the nursing ethical codes of both the College of Nurses of Ontario (CNO) and CNA clearly state that patients are never to be used as a means to an end. Even if significant benefits for future patients were possible, the care and service for current patients should not be compromised in any way. Second, the moral distress of nursing and other staff participating in research protocols that they perceive to be unethical must be addressed. The possibility of additional patient outcomes linked with adverse events, coercion, additional pain and/or suffering all relate in direct and important ways with ethics. There are three other concepts worthy of brief mention here. We encourage you to pursue these concepts in additional study if you find them of interest. The three ethical concepts we want to briefly cover are ethical drift, moral residue, and moral courage.

Ethical Drift has been written about by Kleinman (2006) who broaches the reality that sometimes ethical people can stray from their values and guiding principles. The current issue of ethical violations in research is a good example of a concern that is so big and messy that it is hard to tackle. Research protocols have often been scrutinized by whole committees of experts, right? Maybe the nurses are just overreacting, right? Maybe if Nazilla just waits awhile, this issue will blow over—like so many issues tend to do in our busy lives. Watch out for ethical drift and trust your gut if something is troubling you. *Moral residue* is a term used by an ethicist Webster and his colleague Baylis (2000) to describe what happens for nurses and health workers who participate in care or research processes that are less than the standard they expect, and where, in some situations, the actions are outright harmful. We have listened to many nurses telling their painful stories of moral residue, questioning why they did not speak up or why they kept going when they knew it was not right. Sometimes it is moral residue that spurs a nurse to resign, or even leave nursing. *Moral courage* is defined as "the quality of mind and spirit that enables one to face up to ethical challenges firmly and confidentially, without flinching or retreating" (Kidder, 2005, p. 72). It is a commitment to moral *principles,* an awareness of the *danger* involved in supporting those principles, and a willing *endurance* of that danger (Kidder, 2005). Moral courage enables us to face up to problems—not necessarily to resolve them, and certainly not to promise that we will master them, but to address them squarely, head on, and with determination. Moral courage is considered as an everyday aspect of experience; as a challenge to be authentic and honest in one's self-appraisals and self-expressions; and a commitment to act in accordance with one's own values in spite of fear, threats of physical danger, or social consequences (Richards, 2008). Threats to self are often a fear that keeps nurses from acting. Nazilla has faced the fear and is prepared to act, but first, she must consider the barriers—in addition to fear—that stand before her.

BARRIERS TO ADDRESSING THE ISSUE

The most obvious barrier to addressing the issue for the nurse leader is that she will be required to take a stand that questions current research being conducted in her organization. The questions raised will, we suspect, be initially challenged by researchers (and/or senior management) who will perceive these messages as unfounded. We appreciate that accusations of coercion and intimidation may be taken as personal assaults and the subtlety of both can be difficult to share with others outside of the actual situation. As nurse leaders, we have both experienced pressures to keep silent, keep the party line, and cease making disclosures that might embarrass and harm the organization. Ridicule and threat are first-line attacks from colleagues who do not want you to persist on the path you have chosen. It is not easy to be isolated, publicly embarrassed, or silenced. Sometimes, the only thing that you can do is keep breathing and speaking your own truth. One thing that has helped us over the years is to imagine the consequences if you do not do what you believe is right. What do you imagine will happen? Who will be harmed? Are the imagined consequences worth your silence?

Another more hopeful thing we have learned is that others will see the truths you are bringing to light and some brave souls will support you. The higher the stakes, the greater the passion, the more intensity you will be asked to engage and lead. Only you can answer the question of whether or not it is worth the risk to take action as a leader. The other truth is that there will be some battles that cannot be fought—at the time or place. We hope that we have given some food for thought so that you can think about all the angles and formulate a plan of action. We turn now to Nazilla's strategies and actions to address the serious issues raised by nurses on the inpatient Oncology unit within her organization.

STRATEGIES FOR ADDRESSING THE ISSUE

The following is a representation of Nazilla's plans and strategies. We invite you to think about her plan and what you might do similarly and differently. There is no specific blueprint for being a leader—just possibilities.

- Meet with nurses, leaders, and physicians in the Oncology program/unit to listen to their issues and concerns linked with research activities.
- Meet with research assistants involved in data gathering on the Oncology unit. Spend time with them as they are speaking with patients and families about participation. Privately ask patients and families on the unit about their experiences, concerns, and issues relating to research participation.
- Conduct analysis to determine if this trend is localized to the Oncology unit or more widespread. Do nurses in other research intensive areas have similar or additional ethical concerns? Are there themes around one particular PI or is it every study?
- Gather details, facts, specific times, dates, names, study particulars, testimonials; try to avert a dismissal and accusations of emotional overlay; focusing on the facts helps to ground the discussion.
- Meet with research director, ethicist, chair of ethics committee.
- Following meetings and clarifications with nurses and other staff, prepare a brief statement of the issue (a one-page handout that clearly presents the issue, its scope, and consequences for patients and staff).
- Speak privately with the CEO, and share the one-page document to give him/her the "heads up" and to get a sense of whether or not there will be support at the top.
- Speak privately with the VP of research, the Chiefs or VP of medicine to gain their perspective and see where possible tension points are. Do not air issues publicly before speaking with key players one-on-one.
- Share a draft of the one-page statement of issue and ask for input and comments from other leaders—include their thoughts in the revised document. This way, it is no longer just Nazilla's voice.
- Share the one-page document with the senior executive team and develop a plan to address the issue with the Medical Advisory Committee (MAC), the Patient Care/Quality Care Committee of the Board (PCC), the Research Ethics Board (REB), the Professional Advisory or Interprofessional Care Committee, and the Nursing Council.
- Collaborate on defining a short-term strategy to limit threats to patient care, as well as a longer-term strategy with MAC, PCC, and REB to initiate plans to address the more systemic issues relating to research, staff involvement, and patient care.
- Conduct interviews or focus groups with patients participating in research and involve patient representatives and an ethicist.
- Create a support structure—such as a discussion group or arts-based project with staff nurses to provide additional opportunity for conversation on the issues as well as to provide a place to try out different responses when coercion or intimidation is experienced or witnessed.
- Recognize that this may be a long journey and not a quick fix. As you have seen in thinking about complexity theory, often change comes in an instant when you least expect it. Keep on top of each incident that happens and bring the stories back to the senior team. This creates a sense of urgency and moral distress that cannot be overlooked long term.
- Breathe and stay true to yourself.

Celebrating and Learning From our Nursing Leaders

Your task, should you choose to complete it, is to complete a web quest (see Table 4) on Canadian nurse leaders and examine how the leaders you select connect with the three themes of the stories included in this chapter. The themes are: Crossing the line, asking, what will it take, and emergent moral courage. For example, the only recipient of the highest level of the Order of Canada is Dr. Helen K. Mussallem. If you Google Dr. Mussallem's name and title, you will be taken to websites such as the following: http://en.wikipedia.org/wiki/Helen_Mussallem There are other sites and content areas you might explore about Dr. Mussallem or other Canadian nursing leaders that might interest you. When you Google Canadian nursing leaders, you will find many names and awards. Follow your own path to complete the web quest.

Web Quest on Nursing Leadership

Web quests, also called learning quests, are ways of engaging students to go to the web to look for some specific ideas of points of interest. You have read the three stories of leadership in this chapter and considered the leadership ideas of: Crossing the line, critical asking, and emergent moral courage. In the web quest, you are asked to go searching for examples of how Canadian nursing leaders have lived these concepts in their own careers. Start with the website on Dr. Mussallem's at: http://en.wikipedia.org/wiki/Helen_Mussallem and go on your search from there. Specifically, you are asked to:

1. Identify three Canadian nursing leaders from the web
2. Read about their lives, careers, and awards
3. Identify at least one connection between a Canadian nursing leader and each of the leadership concepts Crossing the Line, Critical Asking, and Emergent Moral Courage

S U M M A R Y

In this chapter, we have offered three narratives intimately related to nursing leadership that we hope enables conversation and critical debate for students in nursing programs across Canada. The three stories address issues and questions about: Crossing the line, critical questioning, and emergent moral courage. Our views have been shaped by experience, education, nursing knowledge, and complexity science. We believe that ideas aligned with complexity offer a meaningful way to think about nursing, leadership, and organizations. These ideas inspire us to look to the quality of our relationships for inspiring change and transformation. It is our hope that you find the content in this chapter interesting and provocative enough to discuss with your colleagues and classmates. There are many excellent nursing leaders in Canada and so we will close with an invitation for you to conduct a web quest on nurse leaders in Canada. We have much to learn from them.

Add to your knowledge of this issue:	
Canadian Nurses Association	**www.cna-nurses.ca**
Canadian Association of Schools of Nursing	**www.casn.ca**
Health Canada	**www.hc-sc.gc.ca**
Canadian Nursing Students' Association	**www.cnsa.ca**

Online

R E F L E C T I O N S *on the Chapter…*

1 What ethical issues, other than the one focused on in this chapter, can you identify for nurse leaders?

2 In your practice experience this far, what qualities can you see in yourself as a nurse leader?

3 In your experience, what barriers can you identify to effective leadership?

4 What concepts from the chapter do you find particularly relevant and why?

5 What personal experiences came to mind when reading this chapter?

Want to know more? Visit thePoint for additional helpful resources:

- Journal Articles
- Learning Objectives
- Nursing Professional Roles and Responsibilities
- Bonus chapters:
  - Health and Nursing Policy: A Matter of Politics, Power and Professionalism
  - The NP Movement: Recurring Issues
  - When Difference Matters: The Politics of Privilege and Marginality

References

Canadian Nurses Association. (2008). *Code of ethics for registered nurses* (2008 centennial edition). Ottawa, ON: Author.

Cashman, K. (2008). *Leadership from the inside out: Becoming a leader for life* (2nd ed.). San Francisco, CA: Berrett-Koehler.

Ceci, C. (2006). Impoverishment of practice: Analysis of effects of economic discourses in home care case management. *Canadian Journal of Nursing Leadership, 19*(1), 56–58.

Jaded, A.R., & Enkin, M.W. (2007). *Randomized controlled trials. Questions, answers, and musings* (2nd ed.). Malden, MA: Blackwell.

Kidder, R.M. (2005). *Moral courage: Taking action when your values are put to the test.* New York: HarperCollins.

Kirkham, S.R., & Anderson, J.M. (2002). Postcolonial scholarship: From epistemology to method. *Advances in Nursing Science, 24*(1), 1–17.

Kleinman, C.S. (2006). Ethical drift: When good people do bad things. *JONA's Healthcare Law, Ethics & Regulation, 8*(3), 72–76.

Kouzes, J. & Posner, B. (2003). *The Leadership Challenge.* San Fransisco: Wiley.

Kotter, J. (1996). *Leading Change.* Watertown, MA: Harvard Business Press.

Maxwell, J.C. (2008). *Leadership gold. Lessons I've learned from a lifetime of leading.* Nashville, TN: Thomas Nelson.

Raphael, D. (2006). Social determinants of health: Present status, unanswered questions, and future directions. *International Journal of Health Sciences, 36*(4), 651–677.

Richards, J. (2008). The development and practice of courageous leadership: A phenomenological inquiry of female leadership within the Canadian health care system. *Dissertation Abstracts International,* (UMI number 3306690).

Uhl-Bien, M. (2007). Complexity leadership theory: Shifting leadership from the industrial age to the knowledge era. *The Leadership Quarterly, 18*(4), 298–318. doi: 10.1016/j.leaqua.2007.04.002.

Webster, G.C., & Baylis, F.E. (2000). Moral residue. In S.B. Rubin & L. Zoloth (Eds.), *Margin of error: The ethics of mistakes in the practice of medicine* (pp. 217–230). Hagerstown, MD: University Publishing Group.

Westley, F., Zimmerman, B., & Patton, M.Q. (2006). *Getting to maybe.* Toronto, ON: Random House.

Wheatley, M. (2006). *Leadership and the new science: Discovering order in a chaotic world* (3rd. Ed.). San Francisco, CA: Berrett-Koehler.

Wheatley, M., & Kellner-Rogers, M. (1998). *A simpler way.* San Francisco, CA: Berrett-Koehler.

6

Policy: The Essential Link in Successful Transformations

Judith Skelton-Green, Judith Shamian, and Michael Villeneuve

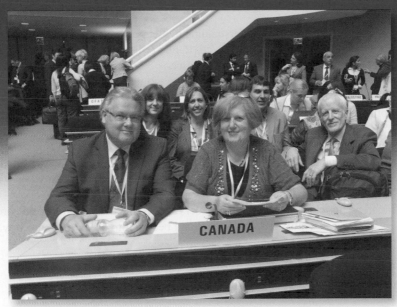

The power of representation is illustrated in political action. This photo shows Canadian Nurses Association president, Dr. Judith Shamian, as a member of Canada's delegation to the World Health Assembly (WHA) 2011. Nearly 200 countries meet annually at WHA to set policy for the World Health Organization. (Used with permission of the Canadian Nurses Association.)

Critical Questions

As a way of engaging with the ideas in this chapter, consider the following:

1. What have you observed to be links between nursing and/or health policy and the delivery of healthcare?

2. What is your understanding of the influence of policy on health system change?

3. What are your assumptions about how effective policy comes into being?

4. What do you assume to be the link between policy and research?

Chapter Objectives

After completing this chapter, you will be able to:

1. Define policy, and appreciate the role of politics in policy development.

2. Identify the steps in the policy cycle and give examples of ways these steps might play out with a real-world issue of concern to nurses.

3. Identify three key aspects of change leadership and illustrate how they can be applied in advancing a new policy.

4. Describe the relationship between research and policy, and explain why credible research is insufficient to effect policy change on its own.

(continued on page 88)

5. Understand the importance of strategic relationships for successful policy change.

6. Identify ways that political acumen may be leveraged to influence policy.

The importance of nurses understanding public policy—its development, implementation, and evaluation—cannot be overemphasized. Public policy decisions directly affect the way that nurses practice, and the outcomes of that practice.

This chapter discusses nursing and healthcare policy, and nurses' roles and responsibilities in influencing policy. Policy is introduced as a process, as a political act, and as a professional responsibility. The history of nurses' involvement in healthcare policy is briefly described. A conceptual framework is introduced to illustrate the steps in the policy process, and a model for change leadership is offered to provide practical advice regarding how to move a policy initiative forward. Five essential components of effective policy development are identified and discussed. Ways in which nurses have been active, influential, and successful in the policy arena are highlighted throughout the chapter.

Ultimately, this chapter aims to help readers understand the importance and process of policy, and to encourage every nurse to think about and become involved, in some way, in influencing health policy.

POLICY, POLITICS, AND PROFESSIONALISM

Policy: What Is it and Why Does it Matter?

At the most basic level, policies guide "the way things are done around here," particularly when they are explicitly stated. The Canadian Nurses Association's (CNA's) *Influencing Public Policy* workshop (2007 and following years) describes *policy* as: "...a statement of direction resulting from a decision-making process that applies reason, evidence, and values in public or private settings." Each phrase in this definition bears examination. A *statement of direction* guides us to an end point. Decision making helps us decide what direction to take, and *decision-making processes* guide the manner that we come to a decision, for example, collectively, individually, through organizational processes, voting, etc. *Reason, evidence, and values* are the principles that inform the action and the decisions taken to support that action. Policies guide the actions we take in our daily lives. They are based upon values and choices that support our interests as individuals, families, and communities.

Public policy is defined as the "directives that document government decisions....the process of taking problems to government agents and obtaining a decision or reply in the form of a program, law, or regulation" (Milstead, 1999, p. 1). Public policy involves a conscious choice of action, inaction, decisions, and/or non-decisions directed toward an end—a deliberate choice between alternatives. It gives direction for action and is usually expressed as a regulation or law.

Health policy, one aspect of public policy, includes "the principles, plans, and strategies for action guiding the behavior of organizations, institutions, and professions involved in the field of health, as well as their consequences for the healthcare system" (West & Scott, 2000, p. 818). Healthy public policies make healthy choices possible or easier for citizens. And they make social, work, and physical environments (including healthcare facilities) health enhancing.

It is important to understand that many public policies affecting health exist outside the health sector. Examples include housing, social security, minimum wage laws, traffic control, the food and tobacco industries, and the environment. As nurses we need to have a strong knowledge of the broader environments and determinants that impact health, as well as the key legislation and those who influence it.

Nursing policies exist as part of the everyday practice of nursing. They arise from several sources (Taft & Nanna, 2008):

- **Public sources:** Authoritative decisions, laws, or operational rules determined by government (e.g., what agencies will be funded to operate and what budget will be allocated).
- **Organizational sources:** Developed by healthcare institutions to govern work places and direct behaviors (e.g., who can undertake which procedure and how it is to be done).
- **Professional sources:** Discipline-specific and multidisciplinary organizations that establish standards, guidelines, and research-based recommendations (e.g., practice standards and competencies).

In the first part of this chapter we focus on public/health policy, and in the latter part on organizational policy—the kind of policy that staff nurses deal with in their day-to-day practice.

Politics—What Is the Relationship to Policy?

If we think of health as something broadly defined and influenced, we begin to arrive at the inescapable conclusion that to be concerned with health is to be concerned with the social context, and that nursing is, indeed, a political act.

(Canadian Nurses Association (CNA), 2000)

In determining how to participate in shaping any type of policy, one needs first to distinguish between political strategies and policy agendas. *Policy* deals with *shoulds* and *oughts*. *Politics* deals with *conditions,* and sometimes impedes or accelerates the policy process. People perceive politics in different ways. For some, the term evokes images of clandestine meetings, influential lobbyists, or power in the hands of a few. For others, the images are of vigorous but reasoned debate and the playing out of our democratic processes. Whatever the perception, politics is the art of understanding relationships between groups in society, and using that understanding to achieve particular outcomes (Clarke, 2006).

As a phenomenon, politics is often reactive. Policy, on the other hand, is more proactive, involving give-and-take in negotiation. When values are in conflict, as they often are in the health and nursing policy arenas, politics often shapes the content and process of policy development.

It is important that nurses recognize the importance of developing political skills, whether for use in their everyday working environments or in formal policy arenas. Articles designed to encourage nurses to develop their political skills are routinely published in a range of professional journals. Universities and professional associations offer policy and politics courses, seminars, workshops, and toolkits. CNA has published several helpful documents—for example, *Nursing Is a Political Act: The Bigger Picture* (2000). Provincial and territorial associations are also on the bandwagon with such tools and resources as the Registered Nurses Association of Ontario's (RNAO's) political action kit *Nurses as a social force: Using evidence, politics & media to shape health policy* (2006). A number of non-nursing organizations have also published excellent "how to" resources that are well worth reviewing (e.g., Smith, 2003; YMCA Canada, 2003).

Professionalism: Why Should Nurses be Involved in Influencing Policy?

Why should nurses be concerned with health policy?

Consider the impact that nursing has on cost, quality, and access to care, and it becomes apparent why there is a definitive role for nursing to play . . .

(Ridenour & Trautman, 2009, p. 360)

Influencing policy is a professional obligation. The *raison d'être* of any profession is the contribution it makes to society. The nursing profession contributes to the delivery of care and the health status of the population. The ultimate reason for enhancing nurses' political influence, be it in the workplace, community, government, or professional organization, is to improve the healthcare received by individuals, communities, and populations (Clarke, 2006).

Nurses contribute to healthy public policy in a number of ways: They have expertise in a range of health-related topics and issues; they help explain individuals' and communities' needs; they conduct health research that contributes evidence to policy development through nursing knowledge and experience; and they interpret and use the results of research.

As a profession, nursing is increasingly aware that all health issues, no matter how seemingly remote from nursing, can have an impact on the direction of health policy and eventually on nursing and nurses. For example, today's nursing shortage is the result of policy decisions made in the mid-1990s to reduce the number of hospital beds and at the same time reduce the number of students accepted into nursing schools. Other policy decisions, such as regionalization, reduction in funds for certain services, redefined scopes of practice, and decreased funding for equipment, have direct effects on nurses' practice in direct care, education, administration, and research (Clarke, 2006).

HISTORY AND BACKGROUND: PERSPECTIVES ON POLICY

From the beginning of organized nursing, our leaders have used their political strength to make needed policy changes in the healthcare system. Florence Nightingale was a consummate politician who used evidence to influence policy (Mason et al., 2007). While she was famous in the 1860s as the "lady of the lamp" in the Crimean War, her lasting contributions to modern healthcare were as a social reformer and political activist, a sanitarian, and an authority on the management of hospitals and the training of nurses (Allemang, 2000).

Although nurses successfully influenced policy in the century after Nightingale, professional nursing associations have taken up the cause with renewed vigor over the past 30 years. A 2009 paper by Fyffe undertakes a critical review of British and American literature relevant to *Nursing shaping and influencing health and social care policy.* Fyffe notes that the first nursing Political Action Committee (in New York) was established in the 1980s. Since then we have seen exponential growth in activities designed to prepare nurses for effective policy intervention, to the point where the American Nurses Association today is a recognized leader in the formulation of effective healthcare and public policy in the United States. Similarly, Fyffe notes that it was a paper by Clay (1987), entitled *Nurses: Power and politics,* that provided momentum for the recent growth in the awareness of, and preparation for, effective nursing influence in policy in the United Kingdom. In the 1990s the UK Royal College of Nurses established a policy unit "to ensure a strategic focus for policy development in nursing and health that reflected and influenced wider social, economic, and political developments" (Fyffe, 2009, p. 702). In 2000 the International Council of Nurses formally stated that preparation for nurses "should include the development of knowledge and skills for influencing change, engaging in the political process....forming coalitions and working with the media and other means of exerting influence" (International Council of Nurses, 2000).

Professional nurses and nursing organizations across Canada have a long history of targeted policy activities. As far back as the late 1800s, Canadian nurses lobbied successfully for establishment of provincial and territorial nurse registration acts that gave them control of and accountability for standards of nursing practice, education, and continuing competency as well as protection of the use of the titles *nurse* and *Registered Nurse (RN)* (Clarke, 2006). CNA produced its first nursing human resources report—describing statistics, trends and issues, and concerns about recruitment and attrition and the need to better deploy nurses—in 1926. And the 1932

"Weir Report" commissioned by CNA and the Canadian Medical Association influenced national policy in nursing education for a generation. More recently:

1. The recommendations in the 1980 CNA submission to the federal government's commission for the review of national and provincial health programs, entitled *Putting "Health" Back into Healthcare* served as the basis for the major 1984 lobbying efforts of nurses across Canada to influence amendments to the Canada Health Act. The new enabling legislation allowed nurses and health professionals other than physicians to be fully used in a reformed healthcare system inspired by primary healthcare.

2. In 1998, a nursing task force was established to address concerns regarding the future supply and retention of RNs and Licensed Practical Nurses (LPNs) in Ontario. In 1999, in response to one of the two key recommendations of the task force, the Minister of Health and Long-Term Care (MOHLTC) created a $375 million Nursing Enhancement Fund (NEF). Over the next 2 years, the NEF supported more than 12,000 new nursing positions in the province, and the rate of full-time work increased significantly (Joint Provincial Nursing Committee, 2001, 2004). As of July 2011, a total of 479 Advanced Clinical Practice Fellowships had been awarded (RNAO personal correspondence, August 2011), and development of a broad slate of Best Practice Guidelines (BPG) was well under way. See the RNAO BPG website for more information.

3. In Quebec, the Ordre des infirmiéres et infirmiers du Québec (2000) actively used its political clout to obtain government adoption of a regulation enabling second-year nursing students to be hired as "externs" for summer and holiday season vacation relief work. This regulation resulted in nearly 1,200 students being hired by 50 institutions in its second year of operation.

4. In January 2000, the Saskatchewan government said it could not support the Saskatchewan Registered Nurses Association's (SRNA) position on baccalaureate education as entry to practice for RNs and was going to look again at diploma programs. Backed by SRNA, student nurses sent postcards to every member of the legislative assembly and to the premier and appeared in person on the steps of the legislature, asserting that reverting to diploma education was a "Band-Aid" solution that would do nothing for nursing recruitment and retention in the long term. Eventually, the government dropped its plan.

5. In 2002 nursing professional organizations and unions worked closely together with federal, provincial, and territorial governments on the Canadian Nursing Advisory Committee *(CNAC),* which culminated in a final report and recommendations, *Our Health, Our Future: Creating Quality Workplaces for Canadian Nurses,* that was extremely influential in focusing attention on the need for workplace changes for nurses in this country.

6. More recently, the nursing profession has been successful in obtaining legislation and educational and employment opportunities for nurse practitioners (NPs) as a strategy for increasing choice and accessibility to healthcare in Canada. New legislation in many provinces and territories will permit employers to engage the services of NPs wherever there is felt to be a need. That outcome reflects the culmination of a careful, collaborative process spearheaded by the CNA, its members, and its partners over many years. One of the outcomes of all this work has been a significant increase in the number of NPs practicing in Canada.

7. In recent years, CNA has been providing leadership for the national discussion on the future of healthcare in Canada, and nursing's contributions to that future. In 2006, CNA published *Toward 2020: Visions for Nursing* (a document laying out future scenarios for nursing in a variety of areas) and engaged thousands of nurses across the country in discussion of its provocative ideas. In 2011, CNA launched a National Expert Commission entitled, *The Health of Our Nation—The Future of Our Health System.* Timed to release recommendations during the lead-up to negotiations on the successor to *The First Minister's 10-Year Plan to Strengthen Health Care* (2004–2014), commonly called "the Health Accord," or

"the Accord," which expires in 2014, the Commission will recommend ways in which the system can be transformed to put the patient and family first, with a renewed focus on quality care in both community and institutional settings. The Commission's website is one that nurses will want to follow closely. http://expertcommission.cna-aiic.ca

These are just a few among dozens of success stories showing that Canadian nurses can make a difference in the development of healthy public policy! But to be successful, we need senior nurses in positions that have legitimate roles in policy development. Fortunately, since the turn of the century, we have seen significant progress in this regard. In 1999 federal health minister Alan Rock created the Office of Nursing Policy (ONP) within Health Canada. Since then, the majority of provincial and territorial governments, and health regions and authorities, have instituted offices or positions for nursing policy and strategic planning.

INFLUENCING POLICY

Policy making is complex, and many factors play into it. It is often a bewildering process to comprehend, and daunting to undertake. Several theories, models, and conceptual frameworks have been developed in an attempt to make the policy process more understandable (Dobbins et al., 2002; Kingdon, 1995; Milstead, 1999; Tarlov, 2000). A theory offers an explanation of *why* things happen the way they do. A model or conceptual framework attempts to provide a map that suggests *how* to proceed.

The Policy Cycle

The ONP was established in 1999 to provide input and advice to Health Canada and the Canadian healthcare system on a wide range of issues. (Judith Shamian, one of the authors of this chapter, was the inaugural Executive Director of the ONP.) To provide systematic, high-quality, evidence-based policy advice, the ONP needed a framework to guide its work and its partnerships—both inside and outside of governments, and with other stakeholders. After careful review of the available models at the time, the ONP chose to adapt a conceptual framework developed by Tarlov (2000).

Figure 6.1 illustrates the eight-step policy cycle of (1) values and cultural beliefs, (2) emergence of problems or issues, (3) knowledge and development of research, (4) public awareness, (5) political engagement, (6) interest group activation, (7) public policy deliberation and adoption, and (8) regulation, experience, and revision.

The policy cycle has two distinct phases, each of which is anchored by a particular step in the cycle. We will discuss the eight steps in detail, using *quality professional practice environments* as an example of the way(s) a policy problem was moved from idea to action. That is, each step described theoretically is followed by a corresponding entry from the quality professional practices environment example.

Getting to the Policy Agenda

The first phase of the cycle, *getting to the policy agenda,* is anchored by beliefs and values. If society and its representative structures do not value and believe in the issues that are put forth in the policy arena, the issues will have no energy to support them and they will fail to be advanced.

Values and Cultural Beliefs

Action on any policy issue must be firmly grounded in a supportable set of values and cultural beliefs. Identification, validation, and articulation of these basic values are important not only at the outset of the initiative (to ensure that the agenda is value based) but also in moving forward

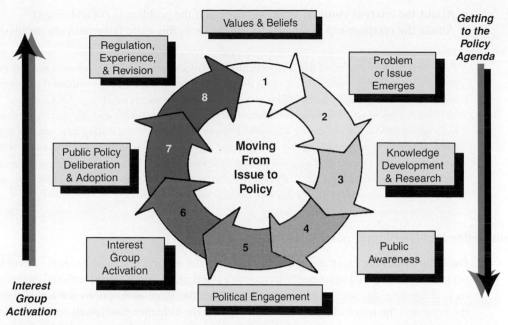

FIGURE 6.1 The policy cycle. (Adapted from Tarlov, 2000.)

(to connect others who share the values). Examples of core values and beliefs relevant to nursing include the following:

- Nurses matter; they are valuable to and highly respected by citizens.
- Nurses are an essential part of the healthcare delivery system, necessary to delivering access and quality care.
- Nurses should be treated fairly and work in healthy work environments.

> *In the example of the Healthy Nurses, Healthy Workplaces agenda, four basic, yet powerful, beliefs or values were dominant:*
>
> - *Canadians firmly support the principles of the Canada Health Act.*
> - *Nurses are an essential part of the healthcare delivery system.*
> - *To offer both access and quality, the healthcare system needs nurses.*
> - *The public trusts nurses.*

Emergence of Problem or Issue

Kingdon (1995) makes the point that an issue can come from anywhere and that in some ways its source or origin does not matter. Rather, it is essential that the issue lands on fertile soil and is nurtured. That is to say, it is not sufficient for an issue just to exist; it must have some urgency. To have traction, it must be a problem that is visible and important to others, not just to those immediately affected. Nurses in senior policy positions have also learned that the windows for advancing policy agendas may not open infrequently nor stay open long (MacMillan, 2007). It is important, therefore, for those who wish to advance policy initiatives to be alert to opportunities.

Issue identification begins with gathering the information and evidence we need to support our rationale for pursuing a specific issue and selected solutions. To define the problem and surrounding issues, we need to ask a series of questions:

- **About the problem:** What is the problem and whom does it affect?
- **About the policy solutions:** What are the various options for action?

- **About the current context:** What will happen if the problem is not addressed?
- **About the relationship to our organization:** Does this issue fall within our mandate?

> *For years, nurses complained that aspects of their workplaces were negatively affecting not only their productivity and performance but also their personal health. During the 1990s and into this century, they were vocal in articulating the effects of organizational downsizing and restructuring on their workloads. They made it plain that the situation was becoming intolerable and that it was contributing to increased absenteeism by driving down job satisfaction and morale and driving up illness and injury rates. Most importantly, by noting that shortages and high workloads were chipping away at the vigilance function that lies at the heart of excellent nursing care, nurses began to tie their working conditions to patient outcomes and patient safety. By 2000, the frustration boiled over, with highly emotional and visible job action surrounding labor contract negotiations in many provinces.*

Knowledge and Development of Research

Once the issues are clear and pressing, research and evidence should be used to provide solid support for the desired outcome. Information gathering, research, and situational analyses enable us to determine our needs; ask questions; analyze the issue and options for action; understand the issue and the range of policy options; examine the evidence base; analyze the costs of taking or not taking action; and anticipate barriers and challenges, and pro-actively develop mitigating strategies. Research can propel an issue into the spotlight, but at the same time, it can be used as factual evidence to support anecdotal perceptions.

> *Data from the Statistics Canada Labour Force Survey showed that in 2002, the rate of RN illness- and injury-related absenteeism stood at 8.6%, up from 5.9% in 1987—the equivalent of paying 10,808 full-time nurses to stay off the job for a full year (Canadian Labour and Business Centre [CLBC], 2002). RNs' illness and injury rate was 83% higher than the Canadian average. Furthermore, in 2002, 26% of RNs worked overtime each week. This rate had more than doubled between 1997 and 2002, and was higher than the average reported among all other workers. Indeed, the number of nurses working overtime in 2002 was equivalent to 8,643 full-time RNs (CLBC, 2002).*
>
> *Around this time the ONP began to push for the establishment of a national survey of nurses' health that would more fully explain the dynamics of absenteeism, and would include all the regulated nursing groups, not just RNs. The result of years of lobbying was the 2005 National Survey of the Work and Health of Nurses (NSWHN)—a collaborative effort involving the Canadian Institute of Health Information (CIHI), Health Canada, and Statistics Canada, and the first nationally representative survey of its kind. Nearly 19,000 RNs, LPNs, and registered psychiatric nurses (RPNs) across the country were interviewed on topics including the conditions in which they practice, the challenges they face in doing their jobs, and their physical and mental well-being. The impact of the RN overtime and absenteeism situation—not only on costs to the healthcare system but also on quality of patient care—was found to be significant and unsustainable.*
>
> *The positive relationship between care by RNs and patient outcomes had also become increasingly well established (Aiken et al., 1998; Organization for Economic Cooperation and Development, 2004).*
>
> *Finally, multiple studies and reports—from the late 1970s through more than two decades of magnet hospital research (Scott et al., 1999) and recent studies of Ontario's Nursing Health Services Research Unit, to Commitment and Care, a synthesis paper commissioned by the Canadian Health Services Research Foundation (Baumann, O'Brien Pallas, Armstrong-Stassen, et al., 2001)—clearly, consistently, and repeatedly described the conditions that make a difference to nurses' satisfaction with the quality of their workplaces.*

Public Awareness

The last step of the first phase in the policy cycle is the creation of broad-based awareness—both of the issue and of the potential solutions or strategies for addressing it. There is always an ongoing competition among the proponents of a set of issues to gain the attention of media professionals, the public, and policymakers. Problems require exposure—coverage in the mass media—before they will be considered public issues and thus of sufficient importance to be addressed through policy. The Center for the Advancement of Health (2001) suggests the following tips for researchers in interacting with the media:

- Get their attention (be strategic!).
- Write an engaging news release.
- Think like a reporter.
- Prepare for and conduct successful interviews.

Creating buy-in is one of the main goals of this step. In this quest, it is important to identify as many potential supportive audiences as possible and to customize the message for each audience. When customizing the message, one needs to think as the target group thinks, identifying how they would benefit from change. For example, when speaking to the funders, the message of improved efficiency should be portrayed; when speaking to patient advocacy groups, the message of higher-quality care should be emphasized.

> *Although additional research might have proved valuable in supporting the need for policy action related to nurses' workplaces, it was more important to show that the existing results were accessible and compelling. The ONP set out to do just that, creating tight, succinct, emotionally engaging messages (based on facts such as absenteeism statistics) that could be easily articulated, easily repeated, and easily reported. Messages were customized for specific target audiences, and speaking engagements for the executive director were used as opportunities to present these messages. To add emphasis and credibility to the case, the many sources supporting the key messages were cited.*

Moving into Action

The second phase of the cycle, *moving into action,* is anchored by political engagement. To advance an issue to policy and then to action, political engagement is required. Without the engagement of political sponsors, policy issues can be "out there" and acknowledged by various stakeholders but they will not result in policy change.

Political Engagement

Kingdon (1995) says that for an issue to be placed on a political agenda, it must have been "softened up." The softening-up process refers to the fact that people have to get used to the idea so that support and acceptance for the proposed solution or strategy can be built. This process of political engagement should be designed to initiate a ripple effect that can grow into a wave of support for the proposed strategy. In planning for political engagement, it is critically important to accomplish the following:

- Know the government structure, committees, caucus, and key members of Parliament (those in power, those in opposition, and the non-elected players who have informal power).
- Target individuals with interest, information, passion, or influence regarding your topic.
- Utilize carefully considered, person-to-person contacts.
- Customize the message for each contact person.
- Keep these individuals regularly updated regarding your activities, your progress, and your specific needs for ongoing support.

Milstead (1999) adds the importance of using personal stories gained from professional nurses' experiences to forge an emotional link connecting the listener with the proposed strategies.

The ONP utilized many strategies to secure political engagement in the healthy workplaces agenda. In the late 1990s the Federal/Provincial/Territorial Advisory Committee on Health Human Resources had set up a working group to develop a Nursing Strategy for Canada. ONP quickly become involved, and had an influence on the report. The establishment of a national CNAC—the first recommendation of the Nursing Strategy for Canada—represented an important step forward in the policy cycle. ONP provided the secretariat for CNAC, which offered 51 recommendations to improve quality of nursing work life (CNAC, 2002).

As a complementary activity, ONP gained the support of the federal Minister of Health for a fall 2000 Toronto meeting on healthy workplaces for nursing—a meeting designed to garner the support and subsequent lobbying efforts of a number of key stakeholders. The timing of all of this action was exceptionally fortuitous, in that governments across the country were seeing the impacts of the early 1990s playing out among nurses and impacting patient care.

Interest Group Activation

Once public awareness and political engagement have been sparked, it is important to deliberately exploit every opportunity to repeat the message and, if possible, to build ripples of interest into a tidal wave. Interest groups are some of the key stakeholders in this part of the process. They provide the opportunity for the issue and potential policy solution to be repeated over and over again, through every medium, in addition to meeting with and pressuring politicians and influential others.

Actions taken by the ONP to engage other interest groups in the healthy workplaces agenda included the following:

- *Direct mail from the office (e.g., "Here is the basic message; please spread and respond.");*
- *Publications (e.g., the ONP electronic newsletter, and pieces in other publications);*
- *Word of mouth (e.g., speeches, regional visits, and interviews);*
- *Bringing key people together (e.g., a National Policy Forum hosted by the ONP in February 2003 immediately following the release of Health Accord 2003), and*
- *Direct dialogue with key nursing and other health organizations.*

Public Policy Deliberation and Adoption

When the wave of interest and support is great enough, the agenda needs to be deliberately moved to tables where it can be debated and policy can be formulated. At this point, the potential solution and policy formulation should be thoroughly and thoughtfully deliberated. If the policy is not able to reach this point, then the success of the previous steps should be evaluated and assessed. Kingdon (1995) says that once an issue is on the political agenda, it must meet five criteria if it is going to survive: technical feasibility, value acceptability within the policy community, tolerable cost, anticipated public agreement, and a reasonable chance for elected officials to be receptive to it.

The "Healthy Nurses, Healthy Workplaces" agenda appeared on public and government agendas, including the First Ministers' meeting (February 2003), in the national level health system reviews conducted by Kirby (2002) and Romanow (2002), in similar reviews conducted in each of the provinces and territories, and in the Nursing Strategy for Canada and CNAC reports.

When the 2003 Health Accord was being negotiated by federal, provincial, and territorial governments, Health Canada was invited to generate ideas for the federal government to bring to the discussion table. As a result of ONP's involvement in the many activities described above, the Office was able to bring forth critical perspectives regarding nursing practice and nursing working conditions across the country. Ultimately, the 2003 Health Accord included a specific focus on national health and human resources (HHR) planning, recruitment, and retention; healthy workplaces; and interprofessional education for collaborative clinical practice. Nearly $90 million was targeted for 2004–2008 to strengthen Canada's HHR, and the ONP was given oversight for several aspects of that funding.

Regulation, Experience, and Revision

In the final step of the policy cycle, the proposed action becomes a formal policy, law, or regulation. This entity, in turn, becomes a new cultural value or norm, which is routinely experienced and revised until the next issue comes along. During this phase, policy implementation and evaluation also take place, and these processes may, in turn, generate new information to continue the cycle. To have an optimal policy evaluation, the data elements to be assessed should be decided during Steps 1 and 2 to the policy process.

It is in this final step that the "Healthy Nurses, Healthy Workplaces" agenda found itself in 2008— after nearly a decade of work. By 2004, based on progress achieved, the ONP was able to move parts of the agenda on to other important players. The CNA, for example, took on much of the leadership around development of quality worklife indicators by 2004–2005 and continues to play an important role in the agenda.

Along with other partners, CNA was a founding member of the Quality Worklife Quality Healthcare Collaborative (QWQHC)—a national interprofessional coalition of healthcare leaders whose vision is that all Canadian healthcare providers will work in healthcare settings that demonstrate leadership in healthy workplaces and management practices. QWQHC unambiguously takes the position that "it is unacceptable to work in, receive care in, govern, manage, and fund unhealthy healthcare workplaces" (Quality Worklife Quality Healthcare Collaborative, 2007).

Workplace quality indicators have now been developed and integrated into Qmentum, Accreditation Canada's new accreditation program (Accreditation Canada, 2008). As the standards for healthcare settings across the country, these indicators compel employers to monitor and address working conditions and their impact on employees and patients. And Health Accord 2003 put in place accountability mechanisms that require provinces and territories to report on access to health professionals by the public to reduce waiting times and lead to better care.

However, the current Health Accord will come to an end in 2014. Even if a new accord is negotiated (which all political parties promised in the 2011 federal election), there is no guarantee that health human resources—never mind the matter of healthy nursing workplaces—will be included. Implementing a plan that will continue to advance the progress made on HHR is a current and important imperative for nurses and nursing organizations across the country.

Sometimes world events can accelerate the policy cycle in ways we could never have anticipated. The creation of a national Public Health Agency for Canada was such a case. As problems and concerns about public health emerged during the 1990s and into this decade, it became clear over time that there would be value in establishing a federal Public Health Agency that could oversee national issues including water safety and communicable diseases. Some knowledge had emerged, and research was underway. Then in the fall of 2002, severe acute respiratory syndrome (SARS) broke out in Asia and was carried to Vancouver and then to Toronto, resulting in hospital admissions and deaths, worry, fear, and outright panic in some areas. By April 2003, there were global travel advisories warning the world against travel to Canada and especially Toronto. The crisis went on until the summer of 2003, and it became clear that a strong political response was expected. SARS accelerated the public health policy agenda so dramatically that the remaining steps of Tarlov's policy cycle were essentially skipped right over, and the Public Health Agency of Canada was proposed, structured, established, and staffed within 1 year.

> *At other times world events can bring a policy agenda to a halt. By August 2001, the Quality of Professional Practice Environments agenda had so much traction that Canadian nurse leaders were quietly talking about proposing development of a $1 billion fund for a decade of renewal of the Canadian nursing workforce. Attention to nursing by governments was unprecedented. The events of September 2001 collapsed that agenda completely, setting it back nearly to its own "ground zero" and threatening to render the broader agenda unrecoverable. Discussions about the $1 billion fund went silent. In the end, $85 million was allocated by governments for 5 years for all health human resources, of which about a third was earmarked for "healthy workplaces."*
>
> *As the Canadian public began to grow weary of our participation in wars in the Middle East, its attention was turned to climate change and the broader environmental agenda. Dire pronouncements about the climate sealed the fate of "health" as the public's leading concern, dropping it for the first time in a decade to a "top five" issue. By the time the federal government announced its agenda and budget priorities in February 2008, there was no further mention of work environments and barely a mention of "health" outside the context of environmental health. The work to strengthen both workforces and workplaces continues, but it has never again had the momentum and attention it had captured by the summer of 2001.*

A Framework for Leading Change

Change is a fact of life. We can engage in it or ignore it, but we can't stop it. In this section we're going to talk about change, because policy development and implementation is all about change.

Since 2001, Skelton-Green, Simpson, and Scott have been lead developers and facilitators for the Dorothy Wylie Nursing Leadership Institute. As part of the Institute's program, participants plan and advance a change initiative or project within their home organizations. In designing this learning experience, the authors identified three typical approaches to leading change within an organization: a strategic approach, an organizational development or people-driven approach, and a project management approach. They also noted that many writers (and indeed many leaders) tended to emphasize one approach over another. It was Skelton-Green, Scott, and Simpson's belief that no one approach was sufficient. Accordingly, they developed a framework that incorporates all three approaches, illustrated in Figure 6.2 below (Skelton-Green et al., 2007).

Figure 6.2, Change Leadership Framework, incorporates three major elements, each of which is required in order to successfully introduce change. The first requirement for success is being strategic—in the choice of a project and the timing of it, the ability to be clear about the need for change and the desired outcomes, and the ability to develop an articulate and engaging vision of what the world will be like when the change is realized. The second requirement is engaging people in the change—not only those affected by your change, but also those whom you hope might favorably influence the change, and those you need to help you get there. The third requirement is managing the change. This is more of a methodological phase where you develop the action plan, monitor progress, implement the change, and evaluate the results. Note that the framework is not static and the elements overlap. In order to introduce change successfully you need to attend to all three areas.

Subsequently, in their developmental work for the CNA's Influencing Public Policy workshops (2007), Villeneuve and Skelton-Green recognized how closely the three phases of the

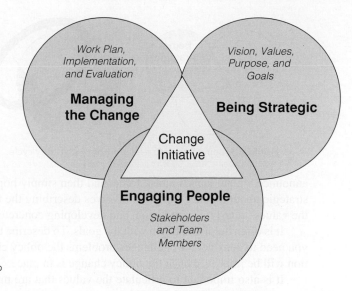

FIGURE 6.2 Change Leadership
Framework.

change framework aligned with the steps in the policy cycle, and how helpful the change framework could be in providing practical advice in how to move policy changes forward.

The balance of this section will examine policy development from the perspective of change management utilizing the Change Leadership Framework, and illustrating it with the following case study:

Case Study

You are working as a staff nurse on the medical-surgical unit in the only acute care hospital in Fredericton, New Brunswick. In your 3 years on the unit you have seen many patients admitted with fractures as a result of falls, and indeed, have had several patients who experienced falls while in the hospital. At a local nursing association chapter meeting, you become involved in a discussion with colleagues who work in home care and long-term care and become excited about the idea that if an inter-agency program (and enabling policies) could be developed to prevent falls in the first place, and to follow up better when patients are discharged post-fall, the elderly in your community would be healthier, and you could save the system money.

Being Strategic

Figure 6.3, Being Strategic, aligns with policy cycle steps 1 (Values and Beliefs), 2 (Problem or Issue Identification), and 3 (Knowledge Development and Research). Being Strategic ensures that we address such questions as the following:

- What challenges/problems need to be addressed? How will the situation be improved if a policy change is enacted?
- What values would motivate people to want to address the issue?
- To what extent is the proposed policy initiative consistent with current strategic plans or priorities?
- Is the timing good to embark on this initiative?

Kanter (2000) states that the most important things a leader can bring to a changing organization are passion, conviction, and confidence in others. She comments that too often leaders

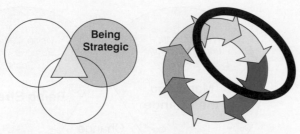

1. Values and Beliefs
2. Problem or Issue Identification
3. Knowledge Development and Research

FIGURE 6.3 Being Strategic—relationship with policy cycle.

announce a plan, launch a task force, and then simply hope that people find the answers. Being strategic about a policy initiative involves describing the future you envision, being clear about the values underlying that vision, and developing concrete goals for the change.

It is often helpful to begin with the goals. To describe the goals for a proposed policy change, you need to consider the challenges/problems the policy change will address, and how the situation will be improved once the policy change is in place.

It is also important to articulate the values that are most important to the successful implementation of the policy change. Values are the underlying principles behind the need for change; clear values serve as the glue to hold stakeholders together, and motivate people to want to move the policy forward.

Once the goals and values are clear, you will want to craft a vision statement for your preferred future. If you want to get people excited you need a vision that is compelling—that describes a unique and ideal image of what the future will look like when the policy is implemented and how everyone will benefit from it (Kouzes & Posner, 2007).

Kouzes and Posner (2007) emphasize that the most powerful visions use metaphor or visual analogy to change abstract notions into tangible and memorable images. Accordingly, if possible, it would be good to select a metaphor, slogan, or symbol for your policy change, something pithy that will capture the essence of the vision in a way that is clear and engaging.

Case Study

In our case study, your problem is clear: "Preventable falls are causing unnecessary pain and suffering in the elderly, and resulting in unnecessary hospitalization and health system costs." You and your colleagues develop the following goal statement: "To develop an integrated program (with enabling policies) that brings together the efforts of hospital, home care, and long-term care nurses to prevent initial and recurring falls in the elderly." Key values underlying your initiative include: "The elderly can be spared the pain and suffering of falls through timely assessment and prevention; nurses can play a value-added role in falls prevention; preventing initial or recurrent falls will save hospital days and dollars." Your vision statement might be, "As a result of nursing collaboration, fewer people suffer falls in Fredericton than in any other city in Canada." And your metaphor might be a picture of a group of nurses holding a safety net under an elderly couple out for a stroll with a cane and walker.

To complete the Being Strategic Phase, you will want to assess the feasibility and timeliness of your proposed policy change. This involves determining whether or not the time is ripe to move this initiative forward, and whether you can mobilize the resources to actualize your dream. Your best chance of success will exist when your proposed policy initiative is consistent with other strategic priorities that already have people's attention. When considering resources—in addition to money and people—you will want to consider such things as leadership and experience, the reputation of the organizations and individuals likely to be involved, opportunities to develop coalitions, access to information, and research.

> ## Case Study
>
> In assessing the timeliness of your proposed initiative, you note that patient safety is a major priority in your hospital's current strategic plan. Moreover, there have been frequent stories in your local paper about people waiting in the emergency department for a hospital bed, and rumors that funding for hospital and home care may be cut as part of the upcoming provincial budget. Finally, all three of your employers have very active quality and safety programs in place, and are regularly inviting staff to come forward with ideas for improvement. It seems to you that your falls idea could be interesting to a lot of players just now.

Engaging People

Figure 6.4, Engaging People, aligns with policy cycle steps 4 (Public Awareness), 5 (Political Engagement), and 6 (Interest Group Activation). Engaging People turns our focus to the following questions:

- Who are the key stakeholders (persons, groups) who are likely to be affected by, or influential in, the success of this policy initiative?
- Who are our potential allies? Are there any highly placed opponents?
- How can we leverage the support of our allies and mitigate the resistance of our opponents?
- How will we create the necessary project team to move the initiative forward?

The Engaging People element of the change framework consists of two distinct aspects: engaging key stakeholders and developing a project team.

Kanter (2000) emphasizes that for change to succeed, leaders need the involvement of people who have the resources, knowledge, and political clout to make things happen. In Figure 6.4, Engaging People, it is extremely important, therefore, to deliberately identify your stakeholders; to determine whether they are likely to be influential, supportive, neutral, or resistant to the proposed change; and to craft deliberate strategies to leverage support or mitigate resistance.

Influential and supportive stakeholders have the potential to promote and direct the adoption and dissemination of your proposed policy change. They are your best allies, and can do a great deal to ensure your success. They will need attention and information in order to maintain their commitment and endorsement. Your approach will be to leverage their support, by engaging them in the change process, keeping them informed, and providing opportunities for them to be publicly supportive (Skelton-Green et al., 2007).

Regrettably, you will encounter opponents to the policy change you wish to advance. Resistant stakeholders have the potential to impede the project's adoption and dissemination. Many experts have suggested strategies to address resistance. The particular strategy chosen will need

4. Public Awareness
5. Political Engagement
6. Interest Group Activation

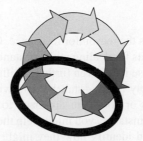
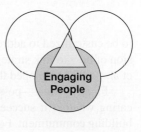

FIGURE 6.4 Engaging People—relationship with policy cycle.

Table 6.1   Strategies for Dealing with Resistant Stakeholders

REASON FOR RESISTANCE	GENERAL APPROACH	STRATEGIES
Not in their interest to change OR violates their beliefs or values	Explain, persuade, negotiate, or remove	• Recognize their needs. • Identify how they might benefit from success in the project; link their needs to the benefits. • Help them to see how the status quo is shortchanging them, and how supporting the project will help them achieve their particular agenda. • Involve them at some level.
Not enough time or resources	Resource, prioritize, stop doing things!	• Stop something before starting anything new. • Intentionally neglect non-essential projects. • Rethink support structures. • Restructure daily activities. • Invest early in help, internal (coaching and mentoring) or external (consultants). • Build internal competence and capacity.
Think the change is stupid, ill-conceived, wrong-headed, or not relevant	Explain	• Build strategic awareness among key leaders; link project goals to overall business strategy and realities. • Explicitly raise questions about relevance. • Make more information available. • Revisit relevance regularly.
Fear and anxiety due to a lack of understanding of why the change is necessary or what change is required, or they don't think they will be able to change	Expose the "rocks beneath the water"; encourage and coach	*(Note: Fear is a healthy response to change, but may be demonstrated in various ways, including defensiveness, ridicule, silence or superficiality.)* • Start small and build momentum. • Avoid frontal assaults. • Use breakdowns as opportunities for learning. • Ensure that participation in pilot groups is a matter of choice rather than coercion. • Assist people in developing skills of openness, inquiry and self-awareness.

From Skelton-Green, J., Simpson, B., & Scott, J. (2007). An integrated approach to change leadership. *Canadian Journal of Nursing Leadership, 20*(3).

to be customized to address the reason for resistance. Gantz (2005) provides an excellent discussion of how to link strategies for dealing with resistance to the underlying causes. Skelton-Green et al. (2007) developed these ideas even further, as illustrated in Table 6.1.

Finally, some—possibly many—stakeholders will be neutral about the project, not really caring whether it succeeds or not. Your approach to these individuals needs to be focused on building commitment. For instance, you might help them to see how the status quo is shortchanging them in some way, and identify how they might benefit from the policy change (Skelton-Green et al., 2007).

Case Study

In analyzing your stakeholders, you and your colleagues identify that the nurse manager of your medical-surgical unit can be one of your most strong and influential allies in this process. She has a long history of leading successful patient-centered change in the hospital, and is an executive member of the local professional association chapter where she is well connected and well respected. You decide to approach her to be the honorary chair of your planning group, and to meet with her at every stage of your process to get her advice. You will also look for opportunities for her to be the cheerleader for your initiative and, perhaps, to assist you in convincing others who are less enthusiastic.

On the other hand, knowing that your eventual plans are likely to have some up-front costs before savings can be realized, you anticipate resistance from the finance officers of all three organizations. You believe that the main reason for their resistance is that, given the current tight financial climate, it will be difficult to justify spending money on any new initiative. You resolve that you need to do some research to (a) quantify the current costs of caring for patients with falls in your community, and (b) find examples of other cross-institutional falls programs, and document the fiscal as well as the health benefits. After that you anticipate that you will need to put together a business case for your proposal.

Many excellent initiatives fail because of ineffective or insufficient communication. As you are identifying their key stakeholders and strategies, plan for how you will communicate with each of these individuals. In formalizing your communication plan, it is helpful to think about how the project could benefit each stakeholder, or how each might be negatively affected if the project does not go ahead. Then determine who would be the best person to lead communication with each stakeholder, how best to frame the message and the best means and timing for doing so. Remember, an effective message is short, simple, clear, and compelling; it is based on evidence and reinforced by statistics and anecdotes; it is meaningful and relevant to the target audience; it is communicated in plain language; and it provides a clear opportunity to take action (CNA Influencing Public Policy Workshops, 2007).

Case Study

Your communication plan for dealing with the medical-surgical nurse manager seems straightforward. You won't have to convince her of the problem; rather your emphasis will be on gaining her support for a broader-based solution than has been in place to date. You determine that you will seek a group meeting with her to share your excitement and your ideas to date, and to request her assistance. In your preliminary research, you discover the following key facts: "falls account for up to 84% of inpatient incidents," "all injuries pose a significant burden in terms of loss of life, reduced quality of life and economic cost"(Registered Nurses Association of Ontario [RNAO], 2005). You realize that you can build upon these facts to persuade your financial leaders. However, given your positions as staff nurses in your respective organizations, you feel that the financial argument will be better received if it is put forth by someone higher up the chain of command, so you decide to seek advice from the nurse manager regarding how and by whom the message would be best conveyed.

Successful change is rarely effected by one person alone. The second activity in Engaging People is to enlist others in your effort by engaging a project team. When you are ready to create your team, there are a number of questions they will want to consider:

- What size do you want this team to be? A smaller team is generally easier logistically, but a larger one offers the opportunity to get more perspectives and stakeholder commitment.
- What skills and experiences do you need for success? Who needs to be involved? Who has high influence with the target audience?

Be purposeful in establishing your project team. Document your decisions using a "team launch" table with the following headings: team member; major contribution; and enabling actions (what you need to do to enable each member to make the optimal contribution).

Case Study

Of course you and your colleagues will be core members of the team you put together to realize your dream. And you have agreed that you will ask the medical Nurse Manager to be your honorary chair. In your preliminary discussions you have determined that you need good data on the current situation, information about what may have already been accomplished elsewhere, financial and analytic skills to develop a business case, and some vocal and visible champions to carry the message to those who may be involved or affected by the change. Accordingly, you decide to approach the following individuals regarding potential participation: A geriatric researcher from the kinesiology department at the university; data support staff from the hospital and the local health authority; a well-respected local entrepreneur who is active in the Chamber of Commerce; the health advocate from the community chapter of the Canadian Association of Retired People (CARP), and the local gerontologist. As you speak to each of them, you intend to ask what additional expertise they believe will be required, and who can help. Your overall plan is to keep the core team relatively small and nimble, and to find a variety of ways to acquire expertise as you need it.

Managing the Change

And finally, Figure 6.5, Managing the Change, aligns with policy cycle steps 7 (Public Policy Deliberation and Adoption) and 8 (Regulation, Experience and Revision). Managing the Change ensures that we attend to questions such as:

- How, specifically, will we proceed with the policy work?
- How will we gather and deploy our resources to bring this policy initiative to fruition?
- How will we know whether the policy change has been successful?

7. Public Policy, Deliberation, and Adoption
8. Regulation, Experience, and Revision

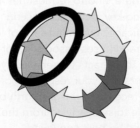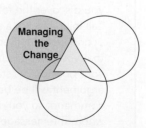

FIGURE 6.5 Managing the Change—relationship with policy cycle.

The Managing Change part of the framework is designed to assist change leaders to develop a clear idea of how they are going to operationalize the change process. It includes, at a minimum, a project plan and an evaluation strategy.

The project plan maps out the pacing and timing of change, those who will be responsible for project elements, and key deliverables. The first step in the project plan is to identify key milestones and target dates. Focus on the major steps that need to be undertaken, keep in mind small wins you might be able to achieve. The next step is to list the major activities required to achieve each milestone, and attach an accountable team member's name to each milestone or activity. In planning your activities, it is useful to think about activities that are internal to your organization and those that are done outside (externally). While details are important, we strongly encourage change leaders to avoid becoming obsessed with planning every detail. Don't make a project out of the project plan! Rather than trying to control the entire change process, let it evolve over time (Auster et al., 2005).

Case Study

In your preliminary research, you have discovered a number of suggested goals, components, and steps for implementing a falls prevention program. Building on this information, your team decides that the key milestones in your policy initiative will be the following:

- Determine current annual cost of falls for (at least) the clients of your three agencies.
- Research examples of successful integrated inter-agency falls prevention programs.
- Describe the ideal components of a "made in Fredericton" program (including the organizational policies that will need to be implemented).
- Develop a business case for the proposed program.
- Develop a communication and advocacy strategy to carry the plan forward.

Once these milestones are determined, you will be able to develop an action plan with key steps and accountabilities, as well as how you will evaluate your success.

There are a number of tools and strategies that you may wish or need to use as part of managing the process. They include:

- **Resolutions:** A resolution is a motion that is submitted to an organization or association and voted on by its members. If it receives an affirmative vote, it becomes an expression of the organization's stand on certain policies, issues, or programs. Nursing groups can share resolutions with decision makers to illustrate the collective view and voice of nurses on particular issues.
- **Position papers:** A position paper or statement presents a viewpoint on a particular health issue or program and provides documented background data on the issue. It is often used to explain, justify, or recommend a particular policy.
- **Business plans:** If your proposed policy change has significant financial implications, you may be required to develop a business case to secure commitment from key decision makers. There are lots of online resources available for business plan development.
- **Lobbying:** Lobbying is the process of making your views and those of your association known to elected representatives and other policy makers with the intent of influencing their decisions. A good lobbyist presents credible information to officials in an interesting and relevant way, listens to the viewpoint of the officials, and identifies areas of common ground.

- **Use of the media:** Working with the media is essential when you want to disseminate your message to a broader audience. One of the most effective ways to work with media is to find a local champion—a reporter, news anchor, producer, or radio host who supports your issue and is interested in its success. Other tips for working with the media have been discussed earlier in this chapter.

In today's healthcare climate, there is an increased requirement to ensure that accountability is woven into the work we do. The final consideration in Managing the Change is the development of an evaluation plan in order to provide indicators of the project's success. Kanter (2000) states that one of the mistakes leaders make is to launch changes and then leave them. It, developing your evaluation plan, will be important to be specific about what it is that you are going to measure, who will be accountable for the evaluation components, and the timing. Evaluation steps and measures should be written into the project plan wherever they are needed.

KEYS TO SUCCESS

It has been our experience that five basic factors greatly enhance the likelihood of success in influencing policy: high-quality evidence, effective research–policy linkages, strategic relationships, political acumen, and relevant and conscientious evaluation. Each of these is discussed in the following section.

High-Quality Evidence

No leader in the healthcare system today would admit to entering into decision making, whether for clinical aspects of healthcare, management, education, or policy formulation, without first being informed by evidence and leading practices (Weinick & Shin, 2003).

Essentially, three basic kinds of information or evidence are needed to make meaningful policy decisions about nursing recruitment, retention, and role optimization:

1. Information about nurses themselves. What are the demographics of today's nurses? What will attract the right candidates into the profession? What resources do nurses need to perform their work most effectively? What is required to keep them in the workforce?
2. Information about the context within which nursing is practiced. What are the health and healthcare needs of Canadians? What are the most significant determinants of health? What changes are occurring and anticipated in the Canadian healthcare system? What are the plans, initiatives, and political agendas of those in power?
3. Information about the effects of nursing practice. Where has nursing made a difference for patients, families, communities? What outcomes have been improved? What are the cost implications of quality nursing interventions?

Progress is being made in all three areas of research. Provincial nurse registries and nursing associations now track and publish key information about their members (see, e.g., the RNAO Backgrounder on RNs, 2011). Numerous studies clearly identify the conditions that will attract, retain, and satisfy nurses. The CIHI regularly releases papers summarizing what we know and what we do not know about factors affecting the supply, demand, education, health, and work lives of healthcare providers in Canada (e.g., CIHI, 2005).

More information is emerging every month to answer the second set of questions. For example, in 1999 Statistics Canada published a comprehensive Statistical Report on the Health of Canadians, and CIHI's website includes a section on Factors Influencing Health. Good data on the effects of nursing interventions are also becoming available. Take for example Gina Browne and her colleagues' randomized control trial to assess the effects and costs of an interdisciplinary team approach to fall prevention compared with usual home care for frail older people at risk for falls (Markle-Reid et al., 2007). Or consider the benefits of the Canadian Health Outcomes for Better Information and Care (C-HOBIC) initiative. C-HOBIC, which has been implemented in three Canadian provinces, comprises a set of clinical patient data that can be collected by nurses on admission and discharge in acute care (and on admission and quarterly intervals in other sectors). By comparing serial data on a patient across multiple time points, C-HOBIC can generate nursing-sensitive patient outcome reports (Hannah et al., 2009).

While evidence is certainly essential, Hewison (2008) raises the caution that an over-emphasis on gathering evidence can deflect attention from more practical approaches to policy involvement on the part of nurses. Shamian agrees: "Don't wait for perfect data; rather use solid data that will persuade others to join you in moving forward with a shared agenda" (personal communication).

Effective Research–Policy Linkages

If the necessary evidence regarding nursing practice is growing, why is it that those in decision-making positions are not acting on the information? Numerous authors have written about the importance of building linkages between all steps of the research and decision-making processes (Canadian Institute for Health Information, 2001; Campbell et al., 2009; Chunharas, 2001; Feldman et al., 2001; Gold, 2009; Hinshaw & Grady, 2010; Lavis et al., 2003; Lavis et al., 2002; Lomas, 2000a, 2000b; Pope et al., 2006). What follows is a summary of their observations and advice.

There are three main stakeholders in the research–policy interface: researchers, decision makers, and members of the community. Unfortunately, their values and priorities are not always aligned. Researchers' bias for methodologic purity can limit the practical utility of their findings, whereas decision makers' push for speed and output can compromise the quality of the research. Decision makers may be more likely to use research results if researchers involve them in formulating questions and problems. Researchers may be more interested in conducting needed research if they are consulted about the appropriate approach and methodology. Finally, members of the community—the putative subjects and targets of research and decision making (and who are often intimidated by both researchers and decision makers and are forgotten in the processes)—can contribute much to both the issues that need investigating and the appropriate application of results.

Researchers must learn how to tease out from complex methods and findings a limited number of clear, concise, and relevant messages. To accomplish this, researchers need to be aware of popular themes and priorities, and learn how to make the connection between "our findings" and "their priorities." Bridging the gap between researchers and policy makers can also benefit from the use of knowledge brokers—who have been described as specialists with effective communication skills, the ability to educate and report, and familiarity with differing approaches and research methods—a hybrid of journalist, teacher, and researcher.

Timing is critical. Policy windows open and close at their own pace, having more to do with election cycles, public opinion, and fiscal years than with the emergence of research findings. Even when a study has been directly commissioned and competently performed, it will have to compete for attention with other priorities and influences at the time that it is completed.

Strategic Relationships

West and Scott (2000) highlight the importance of relationships in the policymaking process. They describe policy networks as formal or informal groups of politicians, civil servants, policy analysts, experts, and professionals who use their relationships to influence the formation and implementation of policy. Nurses must maneuver to be included in policy networks as insiders; they can be successful in achieving this status on the basis of either their specialized knowledge or their ability to promote the aims and objectives of the policymakers.

In the past decade, recognizing the importance of leveraging strategic relationships, the CNA board and staff have held regular meetings with senior federal officials, including the health minister, and on some issues, have collaborated strategically with partners such as the Canadian Medical Association, Canadian Pharmacists Association, and Canadian Healthcare Association in their lobbying efforts.

CNA has also joined forces with other organizations in formal coalitions whose specific role is to influence policy in various areas of health systems and healthcare delivery. For example:

- CNA is a founding member of The Health Action Lobby (HEAL)—a coalition of national health, healthcare, and consumer organizations dedicated to protecting and strengthening Canada's health care system. Initiated in 1991 to respond to cuts in federal funding for healthcare, a total of 38 organizations have now joined HEAL; half a million Canadians are represented by these organizations.
- CNA is a founding member of the QWQHC—a national network developed to address and resolve ongoing issues related to the health of practice environments, those who work in them and those who receive care in them. In 2007, QWQHC released Within Our Grasp: A Healthy Workplace Action Strategy for Success and Sustainability in Canada's Healthcare System. This initiative is a call for action at all levels of our system to improve health system delivery and patient outcomes, by nurturing and supporting health human resources.
- CNA is also a founding member of Canadian Health Leaders Network (CHLNet)—a group of allies with a common interest in strengthening leadership in the healthcare system. The most significant accomplishment of CHLNet has been the adoption of LEADS in a Caring Environment (Dickson, 2010), a framework representing the key skills, abilities, and knowledge required to lead at all levels of the health system, which has subsequently been endorsed by a number of organizations involved in the education and development of healthcare leaders across the country.

Political Acumen

It is important to keep in mind that policymaking is not always—in fact, it is seldom—the rational, step-by-step process portrayed in the previous discussions. Policy formulation may be driven by factual data or logical process, but it is more often a value-driven, dynamic, and at times chaotic cascade of influences and decision-making behaviors. Economist Robert Evans points out that policy making occurs because someone (or some group) determines that a certain action is the best solution that can pragmatically be attained at a given time. Indeed, the same factual data is often used in different ways by different interest groups, resulting in different policy positions (Evans, 2010). As Glassman and Buse say, "There is ample documentation that politics frequently trumps evidence as a driver of policy priorities and reforms" (Glassman & Buse, 2008, p. 163).

Policymaking is ultimately a process of social influence involving activities of persuasion, attitudinal change, decision making, and compromise (Abood, 2007; Glassman & Buse, 2008; Ridenour & Trautman, 2009), which is why a key requisite for influencing policy is political acumen. Florence Nightingale perhaps stands out as the ultimate role model for nurses' use of political skill to influence policy for the benefit of patients.

Abood (2007) and Glassman and Buse (2008) emphasize that as any health care issue moves from a proposal to an actual program that can be enacted, implemented, and evaluated, the policy process is impacted by the preferences and influences of elected officials, other individuals, organizations, and special interest groups. These different factions often do not necessarily view the issue through the same lens. Decision makers rely mainly on the political process as a way to find a course of action that is acceptable to the various individuals with conflicting proposals, demands, and values. Political interactions take place when people get involved in the process of making decisions, making compromises, and taking actions that determine who gets what in the health care system. There are political windows of opportunity where reform is feasible—at the beginning of political mandates, when a policy maker has a strong and narrow political coalition and when benefits outweigh costs for a government or a politician. Knowing and maneuvering through these windows requires knowledge and ability. Finally, in order for a policy initiative to be successful, decision makers need to see it as not only valuable, but also politically feasible. This means that the policy promoters need to be politically attuned to power structures, power brokers, and financial and media resources in order to frame the policy change positively.

Our nursing professional associations have, in recent years, become much more adept at flexing their political muscles, and some do it particularly well. For example, The College and Association of Registered Nurses of Alberta (CARNA) has an excellent member of legislative assembly (MLA) Mentorship Program, which encourages registered nurses to engage and interact with elected representatives to promote understanding of CARNA's positions and increase the individual nurse's understanding of ways that nurses can influence public health policy. RNAO meets quarterly with the Minister of Health and the Health opposition critics, holds an "Annual Day at Queen's Park" where professional association and political leaders meet together to explore issues of common interest, and promotes an annual "Take your member of provincial parliament (MPP) to Work Campaign," which allows political leaders to see and hear first hand from the nurses who care for people in many different ways in many different places. And in Saskatchewan the nurses' professional association, the union, and the government are working together in very proactive ways to engage the public in health system innovation.

Conscientious and Relevant Evaluation

> What is important to me is, are we getting the results that matter? Are we doing the right things to make an impact on the health of the populations that we are serving?
> (Margaret Chan (2007), Director-General, World Health Organization)

There is considerable risk that, once enacted, policies will continue in place indefinitely, whether or not they are truly making a difference. It is critical, therefore, that deliberate and careful attention be paid to evaluating whether or not the policy that is implemented actually makes a difference in addressing the problem that led to the policy development in the first place. Research and data play a very significant role in effective policy evaluation. Ongoing research and evaluation will help decision makers to determine if the problem has been resolved, if the policy instruments used are the correct ones to resolve the problems, and/or if further work is needed to resolve the problem. For evaluation to be most effective, thought should be given to identifying criteria and measures of effectiveness early on in the policy process, so that pre- and post-data can be gathered. It is also important to ensure that the criteria and measures are appropriate, and that, for example, they are not vulnerable to outside or intervening variables.

S U M M A R Y

Whether they acknowledge it or not, all nurses are touched by the policy and politics of the health care system (Abood, 2007). Nurses and the nursing profession are at the center of public health issues that are of tremendous and enduring importance—issues such as who has access to what providers and what makes a difference in quality and cost effectiveness of care. There are also issues crucial to the future of the nursing profession, such as who will be the gatekeeper in primary care and what the appropriate scope of practice is for RNs, LPNs, and RPNs across various service sectors.

The active engagement of nurses in shaping health policy is essential. Together, RNs, LPNs, and RPNs represent the largest proportion by far of the health workforce. They exert an enormous influence on the health of this nation. Nurses know about health and healthcare; they know about communities and people. The knowledge and experience of nurses shaped much of the public health history of this country and contributed significantly to the state of health that makes Canadians the envy of most of the world. It is the vigilance of nurses in hospitals, nursing homes, and long-term care facilities that continues to shepherd patients safely through their health challenges and transitions. The presence of nurses comforts, prevents disease, and improves health. And we know now that when the system creates conditions that result in too few nurses, the impact of work overload and fatigue on patients, families, and nurses themselves can be catastrophic.

A variety of strategies can be used to effect change and influence healthcare policy. They include conducting credible research, making effective links between research and policy, understanding how to initiate and manage change, understanding the policy cycle, crafting strategic relationships, and being politically savvy. A plethora of tools and resources is available to assist nurses to be active and influential in shaping policy.

Nurses' voices must be heard and their knowledge integrated as health and social policy is developed. And so, this chapter concludes with a challenge to all nurses to think about ways in which they can positively influence health policy, both individually and collectively, and wherever they practice.

Add to your knowledge of this issue:		
Canadian Institute for Health Information	**www.cihi.ca**	*Online*
International Council of Nurses	**http://www.icn.ch/**	
National Forum for Healthcare Quality Measurement and Reporting	**www.qualityforum.org**	
World Health Organization	**www.who.int/en**	

R E F L E C T I O N S *on the Chapter...*

1 Think of an existing healthcare policy that you consider successful. What kind of research, if any, do you think is linked to this policy? What factors do you think make the policy successful?

2 With a group of classmates, select a problem or an issue that you have encountered in your own experience as a nursing student. What kind of action plan do you think would be effective in building a policy to address the issue(s)?

Want to know more?   Visit the Point. for additional helpful resources:

- Journal Articles
- Learning Objectives
- Nursing Professional Roles and Responsibilities
- Bonus chapters:
  ○ Health and Nursing Policy: A Matter of Politics, Power and Professionalism
  ○ The NP Movement: Recurring Issues
  ○ When Difference Matters: The Politics of Privilege and Marginality

References

Abood, S. (2007). Influencing health care in the legislative arena. *The OJIN: Online Journal of Issues in Nursing, 12*(1), manuscript 2. Retrieved September 9, 2012 from www.nursingworld.org.

Accreditation Canada. (2008). *Qmentum.* Accreditation program. Author.

Aiken, L.H., Salmon, M., Shamian, J., Giovannetti, P., Muller-Mundt, G., & Hunt, J . (1998, April). *An international study of the effects of the organization and staffing of hospitals on patient outcomes.* Presentation at Outcomes/Indicators Session, WHO, CCNM, Korea.

Allemang, M.M. (2000). Development of community health nursing in Canada. In M.J. Stewart (Ed.), *Community nursing: Promoting Canadians health* (2nd ed., pp. 4–32). Toronto, ON: W.B. Saunders.

Auster, E., Wylie, K., & Valente, M. (2005). *Strategic organizational change: Building change capabilities in your organization.* New York: Palgrave Macmillan.

Baumann, A., O'Brien Pallas, L., Armstrong-Stassen, M., et al. (2001). *Commitment and care: The benefits of a healthy workplace for nurses, their patients and the system. A policy synthesis.* Ottawa, ON: Canadian Health Services Research Foundation and the Change Foundation.

Campbell, D.M., Redman, S., Jorm, L., Cooke, M., Zwi, A.B., & Rychetnik, L. (2009). Increasing the use of evidence in health policy: Practice and views of policy makers and researchers. *Australia and New Zealand Health Policy, 6,* 21. Accessed on line September 9 2012 doi:10.1186/1743-8462-6-21.

Canadian Institute for Health Information. (2001). An environmental scan of research transfer strategies. *Canadian Population Health Initiative,* February. Ottawa, ON: Author.

Canadian Labour and Business Centre. (2002). *Full-time equivalents and financial costs associated with absenteeism, overtime, and involuntary part-time employment in the nursing profession: A report prepared for the Canadian Nursing Advisory Committee.* Ottawa, ON: Author.

Canadian Nurses Association. (1980). *Putting "health" back into healthcare.* Submission to the Health Services Review '79. Ottawa, ON: Author.

———. (2000). Nursing is a political act: The bigger picture. *Nursing Now. Issues and Trends in Canadian Nursing* (Vol. 8). Ottawa, ON: Author.

———. (2006). *Toward 2020: Visions for nursing.* Ottawa, ON: Author.

———. (2007). *Influencing public policy: Strtategies and tactics.* Ottawa, ON: Author.

———. (2011). *The health of our nation–The future of our health system.* Final report of the National Expert Commission. Retrieved September 9, 2012 from http://expertcommission.cna-aiic.ca/

Canadian Nursing Advisory Committee (CNAC). 2002. *Our health, our future: Creating quality workplaces for Canadian Nurses.* Health Canada. Retrieved September 9, 2012 from www.hc-sc.gc.ca/hcs-sss/pubs/nurse-infirm/2002-cnac-ccsi-final/index-eng.psp

Center for the Advancement of Health. (2001). *Communicating health behavior science in the media: Tips for researchers.* Washington, DC: Author.

Chan, M. (2007). Interview on taking office as Director-General of the World Health Organization, 4 January.

Chunharas, S. (2001). Linking research to policy and action. In N. Neufeld & N. Johnson (Eds.), *Forging links for health research: Perspectives from the Council on Health Research for Development.* Ottawa, ON: International Development Research Centre.

Clarke, H.F. (2006). Health and nursing policy: A matter of politics, power and professionalism. In M. McIntyre & C. McDonald (Eds.), *Realities of Canadian nursing: Professional, practice and power issues* (3rd ed.). Philadelphia: Lippincott Williams & Wilkins.

Clay, T. (1987). *Nurses: Power and politics.* Oxford: Heinemann Nursing.

Dickson, G. (Ed.). (2010). *The LEADS in a caring environment capabilities framework* (Vols. 1–5). Victoria, VA: The Canadian College of Health Leaders; the Canadian Leadership Network, and leaders for life.

Dobbins, M., Ciliska, D., Cockerill, R., Barnsley, J., & DiCenso, A. (2002). A framework for the dissemination and utilization of research for health-care policy and practice. *The Online Journal of Knowledge Synthesis for Nursing, 9*(7).

Evans, R.G. (2010). The TSX gives a short course in health economics: It's the Prices, Stupid! *Healthcare Policy, 6*(2), 13–23.

Feldman, P.H., Nadash, P., & Gursen, M. (2001). Improving communication between researchers and policy makers in long-term care: Or, researchers are from Mars; policy makers are from Venus. *The Gerontologist, 41*(3), 312–321.

Fyffe, T. (2009). Nursing shaping and influencing health and social care policy. *Journal of Nursing Management, 17*(6), 698–706.

Gantz, J. (2005, April 15). *Leading change.* Presentation to the Alumni, UWO Ivey School of Business.

Glassman, A., & Buse, K. (2008). Politics, and public health policy reform. *International Encyclopedia of Public Health, 5*, 163–170.

Gold, M. (2009). Pathways to the use of health services research in policy. *Health Services Research, 44*(4), 1111–1136.

Hannah, K.J., White, P.A., Nagle, L.M., & Pringle, D.M. (2009). Standardizing nursing information in Canada for inclusion in electronic health records: C-HOBIC. *Journal of the American Medical Informatics Association, 16*(4), 524–530.

Hewison, A. (2008). Evidence-based policy: Implications for nursing and policy involvement. *Policy, Politics and Nursing Practice, 9*(4), 288–298.

Hinshaw, A.S., & Grady, P.A. (Eds.). (2010). *Shaping health policy through nursing research.* New York: Springer Publishing Company.

International Council of Nurses. (2000). *Participation of nurses in health services decision making and policy development.* Retrieved from http://www.icn.ch/pspolicydev00.htm

Joint Provincial Nursing Committee. (2001). *Good nursing, good health: A good investment. First progress report on the Nursing Task Force recommendations.* Toronto, ON: Ministry of Health and Long-Term Care.

———. (2004). *Good nursing, good health: Progress report November 2003.* Toronto, ON: Ministry of Health and Long-Term Care.

Kanter, R.M. (2000). The enduring skills of change leaders. *Ivey Business Journal,* May–June, 1–6.

Kingdon, J.W. (1995). *Agendas, alternatives, and public policies.* New York: Harper Collins College Publishers.

Kirby, M.J.L. (2002). *The health of Canadians: The federal role.* Government of Canada. The Standing Senate Committee on Social Affairs, Science and Technology. Ottawa, ON: Queen's Printer.

Kouzes, J., & Posner, B. (2007). *The leadership challenge* (4th ed.). San Francisco: John Wiley & Sons.

Lavis, J.N., Robertson, D., Woodside, J.M., McLeod, C.B., Abelson, J., & Knowledge Transfer Study Group. (2003). How can research organizations more effectively transfer knowledge to decision makers? *The Milbank Quarterly, 81*(2), 221–248.

Lavis, J.N., Ross, S.E., Hurley, J.E., et al. (2002). Examining the role of health services research in public policymaking. *The Milbank Quarterly, 80*(1), 125–154.

Lomas, J. (2000a). Using "linkage and exchange" to move research into policy at a Canadian foundation. *Health Affairs (Chevy Chase), 19*(3), 236–240.

———. (2000b). Connecting research and policy. *Isuma: Canadian Journal of Policy Research,* 140–144.

MacMillan, K. (2007). *Personal principles of leadership and leadership style.* Toronto, ON: Dorothy Wylie Nursing and Health Leaders Institute. Unpublished.

Markle-Reid, M., Henderson, S., Hecimovich, C., et al. (2007). Reducing fall risk for frail older home-care clients using a multifactorial and interdisciplinary team approach: Design of a randomized controlled trial. *Journal of Patient Safety, 3*(3), 149–157.

Mason, D.J., Leavitt, J.K., & Chaffee, M.W. (Eds.). (2007). *Policy and politics in nursing and health care* (5th ed.). St Louis, MO: Elsevier Saunders.

Milstead, J.A. (1999). *Health policy and politics: A nurse's guide.* Gaithersburg, MD: Aspen.

Ordre des infirmiéres et infirmiers du Québec. (2000). *Le financement et l'organisation des services de santé et des services sociaux.* Mémoire présenté á la Commission d'étude sur les services de santé et les services sociaux. Montréal: Author.

Organization for Economic Cooperation and Development. (2004). *Resolving nurse shortages in OECD member countries.* Paris: Human Resources for Healthcare Nursing Project.

Pope, C., Mays, N., & Popay, J. (2006). Perspectives on evidence, synthesis and decision-making. Informing policy making and management in healthcare: The place for synthesis. *Healthcare Policy, 1*(2), 43–48.

Quality Worklife Quality Healthcare Collaborative, (2007). *Within our grasp: A healthy workplace action strategy for success and sustainability in Canada's healthcare system.* Ottawa, ON: Author.

Registered Nurses Association of Ontario. (2005). *Falls prevention: Building the foundations for patient safety, A self-learning package."* Best Practice Guideline. Toronto, ON: Author. Retrieved from http://www.rnao.org/Storage/26/2035_168_Falls_Self-LearningPackage_FINAL.pdf

———. (2006). *Nurses as a social force: Using evidence, politics & media to shape health policy. Political action kit.* Toronto, ON: Author. Retrieved from http://www.rnao.org/Storage/18/1235_Appendix-_Doris_Framework.pdf

———. (2011). *Backgrounder on Ontario's registered nurses' workforce.* Toronto, ON: Author.

Romanow, R.J. (2002). *Building on values: The future of health care in Canada.* Final Report of the Commission on the Future of Health Care in Canada. Ottawa, ON: Queen's Printer.

Scott, J.G., Sochalski, J., & Aiken, L. (1999). Review of magnet hospital research. *Journal of Nursing Administration, 29*(1), 9–19.

Skelton-Green, J., Simpson, B., & Scott, J. (2007). An integrated approach to change leadership. *Canadian Journal of Nursing Leadership, 20*(3).

Smith, B.L. (2003). *Public policy and public participation: Engaging citizens and community in the development of public policy.* A workbook prepared by BLSmith Groupwork Inc. for Population and Public Health Branch, Atlantic Region.

Statistics Canada. (1999). *Statistical report on the health of Canadians.* Ottawa, ON: Author.

———. (2002). *Labour force survey.* Ottawa, ON: Author.

Taft, S.H., & Nanna, K.M. (2008). What are the sources of health policy that influence nursing practice? *Policy, politics and nursing practice,* 9(4), 274–287. Retrieved from http://ppn.sagepub.com/content/9/4/274.full.pdf+html

Tarlov, A. (2000). *The future of health in Canada: "The art of the possible."* Proceedings of the 69th Annual Couchiching Summer Conference, Geneva Park, August 10–13. Orillia, ON.

Weinick, R.M., & Shin, P.W. (2003). *Developing data-driven capabilities to support policymaking.* Washington, DC: George Washington University: The Agency for Healthcare Research and Quality's (AHRQ).

West, E., & Scott, C. (2000). Nursing in the public sphere: Breaching the boundary between research and policy. *Journal of Advanced Nursing, 32*(4), 817–824.

YMCA Canada. (2003). *Be H.I.P.P. Have influence on public policy. A manual and toolkit on how voluntary organizations can influence public policy.* Prepared with the assistance of Human Resources Development Canada.

The Influence of Organizational Structures and Regulation

2

7

Canadian Nurses Association and International Council of Nurses

Michael J. Villeneuve

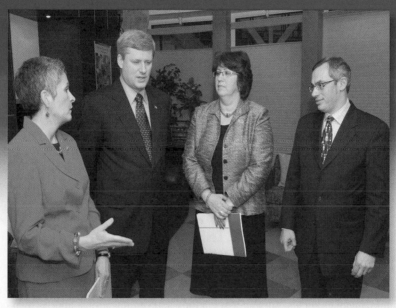

Nursing leaders meet with government officials. (Used with permission of Canadian Nurses Association.)

Critical Questions

As a way of engaging with the ideas in this chapter, consider the following:

1. What are the roles, purpose, and relevance of national and international nursing organizations to 21st century nurses, students, citizens, and global health outcomes?

2. What are the roles of your own provincial and territorial nursing association(s) and how do they support, benefit from, and contrast with the work of Canadian Nurses Association (CNA)?

3. How do national and international nursing organizations effectively bring the knowledge

and experience of nurses to bear on population health outcomes and the development of healthy public policy?

4. How do national and international nursing organizations contribute effectively to global agendas in key areas impacting health outcomes, such as aging, gender, diversity, disease transmission, poverty, the environment, technology, system delivery innovations, and safety?

Chapter Objectives

After completing this chapter, you will be able to:

1. Identify the types, roles, and purposes of professional and regulatory organizations and identify at least three leading pan-Canadian and international nursing organizations.

2. Describe four areas in which the power of representation of CNA and International Council of Nurses (ICN) have brought about changes to improve global health.

(continued on page 118)

3. Differentiate the elements of CNA's governance structure and describe three of its partnerships.

4. Identify five key issues, priorities, or challenges confronting CNA and ICN and their strategic responses as organizations.

This chapter provides an overview of the CNA and the ICN, and the contexts in which they exercise their respective roles and functions. Examples are used to highlight the complex kinds of issues confronting the CNA and the ICN, including the tensions and contradictions inherent in bringing about social change and improved health outcomes at national and international levels. The structure and governance of the CNA are described, examples of current priorities are discussed, and the challenges of balancing advocacy and regulatory functions are introduced. At the international level, the historical development of the ICN is highlighted to give context to its current objectives and the broader history of the evolution of organized nursing. The roles and influence of the ICN are discussed with regard to its contributions to global health and its initiatives to support the nursing profession within its member countries.

CANADIAN NURSES ASSOCIATION: THE NATIONAL VOICE OF NURSES IN CANADA SINCE 1908

During its milestone 100th anniversary in 2008, CNA celebrated the achievements and influence of individual Canadian nurses, nursing associations and organizations, and its own century-long history of leadership within Canada and internationally. The centennial year themes led CNA's Board of Directors, staff and partners, along with all Canadians and their nurses, to discuss, debate, and generate solutions in three key areas: Leadership, the future of nursing, and a healthy environment. As it moved into its second century in 2009, CNA undertook a governance and membership review, establishing a renewed vision and set of goals, to ensure it would be well positioned to meet the challenges ahead. To understand the organization, its strengths, and likely future struggles, it is important to understand the foundation on which the CNA and its centennial celebrations and themes were built.

Who and What Is CNA?

CNA is a federation of 11 provincial and territorial professional associations and regulatory colleges representing some 147,000 Canadian registered nurses (RNs) and nurse practitioners (CNA, 2012)—more than half of Canada's 268,000 employed RNs (Canadian Institute for Health Information [CIHI], 2011). With various mandates to protect the public, speak on behalf of the profession, or both, the federation includes the members named in Table 7.1.

Jurisdictional Members

While all of the provincial and territorial nursing organizations have at one time been members of CNA, the face of CNA membership continues to change. Missing from the CNA federation now are some Ontario nurses, some British Columbia nurses, as well as the nurses of Quebec.

Ontario. To practice in Ontario, its 95,000 employed RNs (CIHI, 2011) must register with the College of Nurses of Ontario (CNO), which has a mandate to protect the public. Ontario RNs

Table 7.1 Provincial and Territorial Members of the Canadian Nurses Association

CANADIAN NURSES ASSOCIATION'S PROVINCIAL AND TERRITORIAL JURISDICTIONAL MEMBERS	WEB SITE	MANDATE REGULATORY	PROFESSIONAL
The Association of Registered Nurses of Newfoundland and Labrador	www.arnnl.ca	☐	☐
The Association of Registered Nurses of Prince Edward Island	www.arnpei.ca	☐	☐
The College of Registered Nurses of Nova Scotia	www.crnns.ca	☐	
The Nurses Association of New Brunswick	www.nanb.nb.ca	☐	☐
The Registered Nurses Association of Ontario	www.rnao.org		☐
The College of Registered Nurses of Manitoba	www.crnm.mb.ca	☐	☐
The Saskatchewan Registered Nurses Association	www.srna.org	☐	☐
The College and Association of Registered Nurses of Alberta	www.nurses.ab.ca	☐	☐
The Association of Registered Nurses of British Columbia	http://www.arnbc.ca/		☐
The Registered Nurses Association of the Northwest Territories and Nunavut	www.rnantnu.ca	☐	☐
The Yukon Registered Nurses Association	www.yrna.ca	☐	☐

Individual nurses who are members of their provincial and territorial nursing association automatically become full members of the Canadian Nurses Association and the International Council of Nurses.

who voluntarily join the professional association, the Registered Nurses Association of Ontario (RNAO), become members of CNA and in turn, ICN.

Quebec. The Order of Nurses of Quebec/Ordre des infirmières et infirmiers du Québec (OIIQ), which has both regulatory and professional mandates, withdrew from CNA in 1985 at the height of the political separatist movement, citing long-standing concerns with the fee structure and lack of services in French. The OIIQ represents Quebec's 66,000 employed RNs (CIHI, 2011). Nurses in Quebec may join the Nurses Association of New Brunswick or the Yukon Registered Nurses Association, both of which offer associate memberships to non-resident nurses, giving them access to membership in CNA and ICN.

British Columbia. The 31,000 RNs employed in British Columbia (Source, 2011), must register with the College of Registered Nurses of British Columbia (CRNBC) in order to practice. In April 2010, CRNBC advised CNA of its intention to withdraw its long-standing membership over concerns regarding perceived conflicts with CRNBC's regulatory mandate. In June 2010, a motion to withdraw from CNA was approved at the CRNBC's annual general meeting and subsequently its jurisdictional membership was assigned back to the CNA. In July 2010, the emerging professional association, the Registered Nurse Network of British Columbia, now known as the ARNBC, became the CNA member for British Columbia. Nurses who voluntarily join ARNBC enjoy membership in CNA and ICN.

STUDENT MEMBERS OF CNA

Since June 2008, nursing students have been eligible to become individual members of CNA if they are enrolled in an education program for entry to practice as a registered nurse; are members in good standing of the Canadian Nursing Students' Association (CNSA); and are members of a provincial and territorial jurisdictional association. Quebec nursing students may become CNA members through the CNSA and the Nurses Association of New Brunswick.

CNA's Vision, Mission, and Goals

CNA is "the national professional voice of registered nurses, advancing the practice of nursing and the profession to improve health outcomes in a publicly funded, not-for-profit health system" (Canadian Nurses Association [CNA] Web site, 2012). Furthermore, CNA

> speaks for Canadian registered nurses and represents Canadian nursing to other organizations and to governments, nationally and internationally. It gives registered nurses a strong national association through which they can support each other and speak with a powerful, unified voice. It provides registered nurses with a core staff of nursing and health policy consultants and experts in areas such as communication and testing. CNA provides the exam by which all registered nurses, except Quebec, are tested to ensure they meet an acceptable level of competence before beginning practice. CNA's active role in legislative policy influences the health-care decisions that affect nursing professionals every day. (CNA Web site, 2012)

In 2011, CNA responded to its governance review by reorganizing and refocusing its vision, mission, and goals to better serve Canada's RNs. At the operations level, two nursing-led divisions were established: *Policy and Leadership* and *Professional Practice and Regulation*. The Policy and Leadership division leads CNA's efforts to advance nursing, health and health system policy by establishing strategic working relations with various levels of government, both in Canada and internationally. This division supports nursing leadership through governance and health system initiatives and engages in knowledge translation activities to advance evidence-informed policy and leadership.

The Professional Practice and Regulation division articulates the voice of nursing on a variety of current practice issues, maintains and promotes practice supports such as the Code of Ethics for Registered Nurses, and through a range of services available on CNA's portal NurseONE, connects nurses with each other and experts. The division also oversees the Canadian Registered Nurse Examination, Canadian Nurse Practitioner Examiniations, and the CNA Certification Program.

CNA's goals for 2010 to 2014 are:

- To promote and enhance the role of registered nurses to strengthen nursing and the Canadian health system.
- To shape and advocate for healthy public policy provincially/territorially, nationally, and internationally.

- To advance nursing leadership for nursing and for health.
- To broadly engage nurses in advancing nursing and health.
- To transform CNA governance structure and processes.

Governance Structure

A 19-member board of directors governs on behalf of the members and is accountable to membership. The board's main role is to govern the organization and set the goals. The three major governance roles of the board are policy development, advocacy, and visioning. The current president is Dr. Judith Shamian (Ontario 2010 to 2012). President-elect, Dr. Barbara Mildon (Ontario), will assume the presidency in June 2012 for a 2-year term at which time a new president-elect will be chosen. The chief executive officer (CEO) of CNA since 2009 is Rachel Bard. CNA's presidents and executive directors over the past quarter century are listed in Box 7.1.

The 19 board members include the president, president-elect, presidents of the 11 provincial and territorial jurisdictional members, two representatives of CNA's 40 Associate and Affiliate Members and Emerging Groups (see Members page on CNA Web site), two public representatives. The CEO of CNA and the president of the CNSA have ex officio (non-voting) seats at the CNA board table. The board's main role is to govern the organization, set goals, and monitor outcomes; in short, the board develops, sets, and monitors policy to help manage CNA. The three major governance roles of the board currently are in the areas of policy development, advocacy, and visioning.

CNA's board meets quarterly and reports at each annual general meeting on the business transacted. At the annual general meeting, delegates from each jurisdiction meet to fulfill their fiduciary responsibilities, such as electing a president-elect (biannually), choosing an auditor, changing bylaws, and giving guidance to the board of directors through voting on resolutions regarding the policy areas that they believe should be pursued. Although the board of directors is not bound by the resolutions on policy directives, a review of annual reports submitted to membership confirms that almost all resolutions have guided CNA and have been implemented.

BOX 7.1 Canadian Nurses Association Presidents and Executive Directors Since 1980

CNA Presidents	CNA Executive Directors
Dr. Shirley Stinson, 1980–1982	Dr. Helen K. Mussallem, 1963–1981
Dr. Helen Glass, 1982–1984	Dr. Ginette Lemire Rodger, 1981–1989
Lorrine Bessel, 1984–1986	Judith Oulton, 1989–1995
Helen Evans, 1986–1988	Dr. Mary Ellen Jeans, 1995–2001
Dr. Judith Ritchie, 1988–1990	Lucille Auffrey, 2001–2009
Dr. Alice Baumgart, 1990–1992	Rachel Bard, 2009-
Fernande Harrison, 1992–1994	
Eleanor Ross, 1994–1996	
Rachel Bard, 1996–1998	
Lynda Kushnir Perkul, 1998–2000	
Dr. Ginette Lemire Rodger, 2000–2002	
Rob Calnan, 2002–2004	
Dr. Deborah Tamlyn, 2004–2006	
Dr. Marlene Smadu, 2006–2008	
Kaaren Neufeld, 2008–2010	
Dr. Judith Shamian, 2010–2012	

CNA's board of directors decides on policy directions, priorities, and resources, ensuring that effective strategies are implemented by the CEO and staff. The board appoints the CEO, who has the authority and responsibility to implement the board policies, provide services to members, develop an appropriate network to fulfill the mandate, manage a team of staff members, and ensure linkage with CNA's subsidiary (i.e., Assessment Strategies, Inc.) and parallel organizations (i.e., the Canadian Nurses Foundation and the Canadian Nurses Protective Society).

The operational and staff structure complements the organization's goals, operating with a strong policy focus and programs delivered by the two nurse-led divisions cited earlier. The entire organization is supported with experts and operational programs in the executive office, administration and finance, information technology services, and communications and member outreach.

Partnerships

Nurses have always worked in partnership with others. Recognizing that successful "stand-alone" organizations and initiatives are now considered things of the past, CNA engages in a broad range of formal partnerships to increase the influence of nurses and other health providers.

For example, the Health Action Lobby (HEAL) is a coalition of national health and consumer organizations dedicated to protecting and strengthening Canada's healthcare system. The CNA was a founding member in 1991 and co-chaired the coalition. HEAL now comprises 35 organizations representing more than 500,000 providers and consumers of health care (Health Action Lobby, 2012).

CNA is a partner in several other initiatives that bring the collectivity of unified messages to bear in policy development. A founding member of the Canadian Health Leadership Network, the Quality Worklife—Quality Healthcare Collaborative, and the Canadian Consortium for Nursing Research and Innovation, CNA is also a partner in producing the annual "Healthcare in Canada" survey (led by Merck and POLLARA). Since the turn of the century, CNA has had a prominent role in diverse multistakeholder initiatives, for example, its own inauagural National Expert Commission, the Public Health Agency's Emergency Preparedness and Response, the Patient Safety Institute, the National Stakeholder Roundtable on Long-Term Care, Environmental Health Reference Group; and in partnership with the RNAO: Nurse Fatigue and Patient Safety, Nurses for Medicare, the Canadian Nursing Advisory Committee, the Canadian Nurse Practitioner Initiative, and *Building the Future*—the National Occupational/Sector Study of Nursing.

Multistakeholder partnerships also evolve around specific issues, such as patient safety or the need to have a strategy focused on healthcare human resources. In the latter case, CNA is part of an informal collective called the "G-4," comprised of the CNA, the Canadian Medical Association, Canadian Healthcare Association, and Canadian Pharmacists Association. The group meets on an ad hoc basis with the federal minister and/or deputy minister, and CNA staff contributes information and evidence to inform policy decisions through links with the federal, provincial, and territorial Advisory Committee on Health Delivery and Human Resources and through formal presentations to various federal committees. Given the strongly interdependent nature of so much of nursing and medical practice, CNA and the Canadian Medical Association have been particularly strategic in choosing to develop and speak with unified messages across a number of key policy areas. One example of shared messaging is found in the *Principles to Guide Health Care Transformation in Canada* (CNA & CMA, 2011), released by the two organizations in 2011 and subsequently endorsed by dozens of other national associations and organizations.

CNA also maintains relationships through regular formal and informal meetings with key national nursing partners, including Health Canada's Office of Nursing Policy and, in turn, the group of federal, provincial, and territorial principal nursing officers. CNA has many core nursing partners, for example, the Canadian Federation of Nurses Unions, Canadian Association of Schools of Nursing, and the Academy of Canadian Executive Nurses. Internationally, bilateral and joint meetings with the American Nurses Association (ANA), Sigma Theta Tau, the Commission on Graduates of Foreign Nursing Schools, and other national nursing associations are ongoing. ICN's membership structure encourages national nurse association member networking and collaboration among the diverse groups of nurses within the country (International Council of Nurses [ICN], 2001a).

How Does CNA Influence Policy?

Many national nursing organizations exist across the domains of nursing practice, representing interests in specific areas of practice and competence. While some functions overlap, the main purposes of organizations are grounded in their social roles. In nursing, these could be conceptualized as, (1) primarily protecting the public or society (e.g., a regulatory college), (2) primarily speaking on behalf of the profession (e.g., a professional advocacy association), and (3) primarily protecting the nurse or the individual practitioner (e.g., a union).

The ICN conducted a survey of its members in 1997 and found that 62% of its national nursing association members identified their major role as representing the profession; 31% of its members were unions that negotiate for nurses, and just 7% had a solely regulatory mandate (ICN, 2001a). Throughout the last decade Canada has seen the rise of nursing organizations in all these areas as well as hybrid organizations holding mixed functions. With its complex membership and mandates, CNA in 2012 is an example of such a hybrid organization.

CNA HISTORY

In 1908, under the leadership of Mary Agnes Snively of Ontario, the first national nurses association was formed in Canada so that nurses could (1) effectively and collectively exercise their professional responsibilities on behalf of the public, and (2) join ICN—for which a national association was required (CNA, 1968). During that year, representatives of 16 organized nursing bodies met in Ottawa to form the Canadian National Association of Trained Nurses. By 1911, the association included 28 affiliated member societies, including alumni associations of hospital schools of nursing and local and regional groups of nurses. By 1924, with the existing nine member provinces each having a provincial nurses organization, the group changed its name to the *Canadian Nurses' Association* (the apostrophe after "nurses" was dropped later in the century.)

Since its inception, CNA has been the national voice of nursing in Canada. CNA influences public policy, speaks and acts on behalf of Canadian nurses on health and nursing issues, and plays a role in the Canadian political process and in the development of nursing in Canada (CNA, 1958; CNA, 1968; MacPhail, 1996; Meilicke & Larsen, 1988). Over the past 20 years, the role of CNA has expanded in the areas of advocacy, strengthened nursing and the broader health system, and protected the public through its regulatory policy work.

While Florence Nightingale may be our most famous historical example of the impact of individual political activism and nursing advocacy, throughout history, many social movements were spearheaded by nurse leaders even if they did not consider their role (either individually or collectively as professionals) to be political activism. The power of representation is exercised most of the time through political action, meaning "a systematic series of actions directed toward influencing others into conformity with a pursued goal" (Lemire Rodger, 1999, p. 281). Since the early 1980s, CNA has promoted political action by nurses at the pan-Canadian level as a means of exercising the power of representation.

CNA RESPONDS TO THE CHALLENGES OF 21ST CENTURY NURSING

The national ideal for nursing in Canada is that nurses, as a collective and with partners, work to advance the health of Canadians. CNA has expressed its commitment to contribute to the health of the public in part through development of the profession and this commitment has been reiterated in corporate objectives, position statements, studies, speeches, and briefs to governments, health committees, and commissions. CNA's five goals do not represent all of the pressing issues that a national association has to address, but they help focus the policy work and resources of the organization. The CNA board further refines the directions and priorities of its work after continually scanning the environment. These ongoing scanning exercises include surveys of national, provincial, and territorial organizations and the larger world around them to identify trends and emerging issues that might impact the CNA or the larger nursing agenda. Let's turn to consider examples of CNA's work and influence in its various policy priority areas.

Public Policy and Leadership

This division is the lead for CNA's efforts to advance nursing, health and health system policy. To accomplish these goals, it establishes strategic working relations with various levels of government, both in Canada and internationally. This division also supports nursing leadership through governance and health system initiatives, including CNA's longstanding global health partnerships program. In addition, it engages in knowledge translation activities to advance evidence-informed policy and leadership. (CNA Web site, 2012)

CNA's public policy work is grounded in two fundamental sets of values: Those of primary health care and the Canada Health Act. Primary healthcare (Box 7.2) principles include health promotion and prevention of disease and injury, accessibility, public participation, multidisciplinary and intersectoral collaboration, and appropriate technology (World Health Organization, 1978). CNA includes in its thinking about primary health care the notion that there are many determinants of health and that its policy work (and nursing at large) should reflect those values. Second, the principles of the Canada Health Act include universality, portability, accessibility, comprehensiveness, and public administration (Government of Canada, 1984). All of these principles are central in the ongoing national debate about service delivery, funding, and system redesign—and are fundamental values grounding the work and thinking of CNA.

BOX 7.2   Primary Health Care

The definition of *primary health care* approved at the 1978 Alma Ata conference of the World Health Organization (p. 21) stated that:

> Primary healthcare is essential healthcare based on practical, scientifically sound and socially acceptable methods and technology made universally accessible to individuals and families in the community through their full participation and at a cost that the community and country can afford to maintain at every stage of their development in the spirit of self-reliance and self-determination. It forms an integral part both of the country's health system, of which it is the central function and main focus, and of the overall social and economic development of the community. It is the first level of contact of individuals, the family, and community with the national health system bringing healthcare as close as possible to where the people live and work, and constitutes the first element of a continuing healthcare process.

Nationally, a milestone for representation came in 1985, with the proclamation of the Canada Health Act. From coast to coast, many nurses participated for the first time in political lobbying that influenced changes in national legislation—changes that reflected nurses' values and beliefs about the future of the healthcare system. These beliefs were summarized in the brief, "Putting 'Health' Back into Healthcare" (CNA, 1980) that has guided pursuant changes by the CNA. CNA's impact on legislative changes to the Canada Health Act of 1984 ensured that national and provincial plans for the future of the healthcare system were guided by the principles of primary health care and the Canada Health Act (Mhatre & Deber, 1992). The nursing voice was part of the review of the Canadian healthcare system by the National Health Forum in 1997 and, into this century, the national health system reviews undertaken by Commissioner Romanow and Senator Kirby.

The launch in May 2011 of CNA's first National Expert Commission, mandated to develop evidence-informed recommendations to help shape the healthcare system into one better equipped to meet the changing needs of Canadians, heralded another new policy era for CNA. The commission is co-chaired by two exceptionally capable and respected Canadians: Nursing educator and researcher Dr. Marlene Smadu, and lawyer and rights advocate Maureen A. McTeer. A diverse roster of Canadians with complementary backgrounds, experience, and expertise, round out the commission. The commission is a strategy that has successfully placed CNA and the voices of nurses much more visibly and forcefully in arenas of dialogue around healthy public policy and system transformation. The commission's report, tabled with the CNA Board of Directors in June 2012, provides CNA with a framework of recommendations that could guide, inform, and support its policy work through the turbulent years of system transformation that lie ahead.

ADVANCING LEADERSHIP IN HEALTH HUMAN RESOURCES PLANNING

An example of the impact of CNA's public policy work can be found in the area of leadership in health human resources planning. CNA's position as the *go-to* place for nursing human resources data and information has been earned through more than a decade of work and planning in partnership with groups such as the Canadian Institute for Health Information and the Canadian Association of Schools of Nursing. CNA's 1997 report on the future supply of RNs in Canada (Ryten, 1997) predicted a serious shortage of nurses by 2011 if no strategic action was undertaken immediately. In the wake of that report, CNA made formal presentations to inform federal and provincial governments and associations of employers of the significant trend apparently unfolding (CNA, 1998; CNA, 1999; CNA, 2000; CNA, 2001) and undertook significant, informal political lobbying in Ottawa and nationally.

Further research (CIHI, 2005; Ryten, 2002) validated the projections, and attempts were made to engage governments in understanding that the situation was serious enough to undermine the sustainability of the Canadian healthcare system. A concerted lobbying effort with the provincial jurisdictions and other nursing and health associations was also needed to persuade governments and employers that action was required immediately. The issues of recruitment and retention were addressed in these representations—and retention and the quality of the professional practice environment soon became priority policy areas for CNA.

In 2009, CNA updated supply projections using utilization-based models and called on Canada's policymakers to address the RN shortage immediately or face shortages in the order of 60,000 full-time equivalent RNs by 2022. Since then CNA has sought to draw attention to the impact of continuing shortages. CNA collaborates with its members to ensure governments and the public understand the impact of shortages—long wait times, adverse effects on patient care, and untenable work situations for RNs.

CNA's formal presentations and behind-the-scenes lobbying helped to build and launch a pan-Canadian agenda in the area of nursing and health human resources still playing out in 2008. Emerging from the chaos of 1990s system downsizing, CNA approached Canada's federal government in 1998 with its brief entitled *The Quiet Crisis,* in which it made plain the association's growing concern about a looming shortage of nurses and the need to bolster the academic and practice foundations of nursing for what looked like a rocky journey ahead. CNA's lobbying helped prompt the establishment of the new federal Office of Nursing Policy at Health Canada in 1999, mirrored in the following years by the appointment of "chief nurses" and senior nurse advisor positions in the provincial governments of Newfoundland, Prince Edward Island, Nova Scotia, New Brunswick, Ontario, Saskatchewan, and British Columbia. Other provincial governments also employed nurse advisors under various titles.

That agenda soon gave rise to a roster of pan-Canadian nursing initiatives including advisory committees, studies, and the establishment of a decade-long, $25 million national nursing research fund. *The Nursing Strategy for Canada* and its offspring, the Canadian Nursing Advisory Committee, prompted the governments of several provinces and territories to develop comprehensive plans to address nursing human resources—and the topic of nursing recruitment and retention was established as a regular item on the federal, provincial, and territorial policy agenda for health ministers.

The importance of a broad health human resources agenda, including the issue of healthy work environments, was reflected in the 2003 First Ministers' Accord on Healthcare Renewal wherein some $90 million in funding was directed to the issue of health human resources with particular attention to healthy workplaces, interprofessional education and collaborative practice, and recruitment and retention. CNA urged a principles-based HHR planning framework as outlined in *Toward a Pan-Canadian Framework for Health Human Resources: A Green Paper* and in its position statement, *National Planning for Human Resources in the Health Sector.* CNA led the steering committee for the Diagnostic Phase for Internationally Educated Nurses national project. To keep in touch with policy decision makers and the larger healthcare community on key issues, CNA hosted a long-running *Knowledge Series*– a monthly, multistakeholder policy discussion to examine specific issues related to health human resources. As a result of ongoing leadership and collaborative actions of CNA, challenges related to the demand for nursing services and supply of nurses to provide them in 2008 are familiar not only to nurses but to employers, governments, other providers, and the public across the country.

The preceding examples represent just a sample of CNA's extensive public policy work at the national level over the past 10 years, which also included inverventions related to interprofessional collaboration, the *First Ministers' 10-Year Plan to Strengthen Healthcare,* primary health care, and its leadership of the Canadian Nurse Practitioner Initiative among many others.

INTERNATIONAL POLICY AND DEVELOPMENT

Since 1976, CNA has worked with national nursing associations (NNAs) in Africa, Asia, the Americas and Eastern Europe as well as with the Canadian International Development Agency (CIDA) and other funding organizations in Canada and abroad. CNA has built partnerships to increase NNAs capacities to strengthen the nursing profession and improve the quality of nursing and health services delivered in partner countries.

> *(Knowing No Boundaries: The Canadian Nurses Association and its International Health Partnerships, 1976–2006, CNA Web site, 2012)*

CNA is involved in international policy, development, and partnerships, maintains an active and formal relationship with the ICN, and links on an ad hoc basis with the World Health Organization (WHO), its nursing office, and a range of other international organizations.

FOSTERING CANADIAN LEADERSHIP WITHIN ICN

Through meetings such as the ICN Quadrennial Congress, Council of National Representatives, and ICN Socio-Economic Workforce Forum, CNA's membership in ICN provides the association and Canadian nurses with direct links to fellow nurses in 125 countries around the world. These links enable CNA to share nursing knowledge and best practices, collaborate on policy development, and contribute to strengthening the profession and the delivery of quality nursing care. Former CNA president, Dr. Marlene Smadu, is the third vice-president of ICN for the period 2009 to 2013.

INTERNATIONAL HEALTH PARTNERSHIPS

In its development work, funded by the Canadian International Development Agency, CNA has had nine long-standing projects impacting partner nations on four continents, including the "Strengthening Nurses, Nursing Networks, and Associations Program" (SNNNAP) (2007 to 2012), the "Canada-South Africa Nurses HIV/AIDS Initiative" (2003 to 2008), the "Ethiopian Nurses and Needle Stick Injury Research Project" (2006 to 2008), and the "Canada-Russia Initiative in Nursing" (2004 to 2008).

During the past decade, CNA's international policy and development work has also included responding to emergencies, contributing to gender equality, reinforcing institutional capacity, engaging Canadian nurses in global knowledge sharing, international liaising in HIV/AIDs prevention and care and WHO involvement, and contributing to global health and equity through a variety of organizations and initiatives. As its "Strengthening Nurses, Nursing Networks, and Associations Program" wraps up in 2012, CNA is evaluating directions where it could bring the most value in the next phase of building on its long history of international work.

Professional Practice and Regulation

This division provides a variety of supports to optimize the role of registered nurses, including nurse practitioners and clinical nurse specialists. The division articulates the voice of nursing on many current practice issues and maintains and promotes the Code of Ethics for Registered Nurses. It connects nurses with each other and with experts through a growing range of services on CNA's portal, NurseONE. The division also oversees the Canadian Registered Nurse Examination, Canadian Nurse Practitioner Examinations, and the CNA Certification Program.

(CNA, 2012)

PROVIDING LEADERSHIP TO PROMOTE QUALITY PROFESSIONAL PRACTICE ENVIRONMENTS

The power of representation was exercised by the CNA in recent years in response to a crisis in quality of practice environments. The socioeconomic environments of nurses were transformed by the events of the 1990s, when major cutbacks in healthcare funding exerted a devastating effect on nursing education, the nursing workforce, and practice settings. Thousands of nurses lost their positions when hospital and community services were curtailed by provincial governments across the country—and some 5,500 nursing leadership and administration positions disappeared. Workplaces saw increases in the number of patients or clients cared for by each nurse, and a loss of support structures for education and research. Since 2000, CNA has led and partici-pated in numerous studies and projects contributing knowledge to the growing understanding that quality practice environments, staffing, and staff mix are linked to outcomes. CNA held a strong leadership role, for example, in establishing the national Quality Worklife—Quality Healthcare Collaborative, which is building quality of worklife outcome indicators into the Accreditation Canada program—closing one part of a loop of work begun in partnership with the federal Office of Nursing Policy in the year 2000.

REGULATORY POLICY

CNA has always played a supportive role in regulation and regulatory policy. Its role has grown as regulation, licensing, ethics, and public protection grew in influence as policy priorities since the 1980s. Among its partnerships, the department works with the National Advisory Committee for Canadian English Language Benchmark Assessment for Nurses and the National Council of State Boards of Nursing in the United States, and has held the chair of the group of 19 organiza-tions who make up the Canadian Network of National Associations of Regulators. Examples of CNA's regulatory policy work during the past decade can be found in the areas of testing, spe-cialty certification, code of ethics, mutual recognition agreement, entry to practice, and nursing legislation. Short descriptions of CNA's work in each of these areas follow.

Testing

By 1969, CNA had established a testing service to prepare and administer the national registra-tion examination; that effort gave rise to the *Canadian Registered Nurse Examination* (CRNE) we know today. The CRNE helps to protect the public by ensuring that entry-level RNs possess the competencies required to practice safely and effectively; the level of competence of RNs in all provinces and territories (except Quebec) is measured in part by the CRNE. It is anticipated that the national examination may be provided by another organization by 2015. The most recent updates on the national examination are available on CNA website.

Specialty Certification

Recognizing the increasing specialization across the health system and demand for specialty recognition, CNA began developing specialty certification examinations during the mid-1980s. To date, more than 16,200 Canadian RNs have been certified in 19 nursing specialty certification programs (CNA, 2012). The voluntary process requires periodic renewal and certifies that an RN has demonstrated competence in an area of nursing practice by having met predetermined standards. Certification is intended to promote excellence in nursing care by establishing national standards of practice while providing an opportunity for practitioners to confirm their compe-tence in a specialty. The national nursing associations that are actively involved in, and endorse, the CNA Certification Program are listed in Table 7.2.

Code of Ethics

CNA's *Code of Ethics for Registered Nurses* offers "guidance for ethical relationships, respon-sibilities, behaviors and decision-making" and "serves as a means for self-evaluation and self-reflection for ethical nursing practice and provides a basis for peer review" (CNA 2012). Reflecting the impacts of changing social norms, constantly emerging health science, and new technologies on nurses and their practice settings, the code is reviewed on an ongoing basis and revised periodically. The code, updated in 2008, "informs other health-care professionals as well

Table 7.2 Canadian Nurses Association (CNA) Certification Programs

SPECIALTY	DESIGNATION	NATIONAL ASSOCIATION AFFILIATED WITH CNA
Cardiovascular Nursing	CCN(C)	Canadian Council of Cardiovascular Nurses (CCCN)
Community Health Nursing	CCHN(C)	Community Health Nurses Association of Canada (CHNAC)
Critical Care Nursing	CNCC(C)	Canadian Association of Critical Care Nurses (CACCN)
Critical Care Pediatric Nursing	CNCCP(C)	Canadian Association of Critical Care Nurses (CACCN)
Emergency Nursing	ENC(C)	National Emergency Nurses' Affiliation (NENA)
Enterostomal Therapy	CETN(C)	Canadian Association for Enterostomal Therapy (CAET)
Gastroenterology Nursing	CGN(C)	Canadian Society of Gastroenterology Nurses and Associates (CSGNA)
Gerontology Nursing	GNC(C)	Canadian Gerontological Nursing Association (CGNA)
Hospice Palliative Care Nursing	CHPCN(C)	Canadian Hospice Palliative Care Association (CHPCA)
Medical-Surgical Nursing	CMSN(C)	Canadian Association of Medical and Surgical Nurses (CAMSN)
Nephrology Nursing	CNeph(C)	Canadian Association of Nephrology Nurses and Technologists (CANNT)
Neuroscience Nursing	CNN(C)	Canadian Association of Neuroscience Nurses (CANN)
Occupational Health Nursing	COHN(C)	Canadian Occupational Health Nurses Association (COHNA)
Oncology Nursing	CON(C)	Canadian Association of Nurses in Oncology (CANO)
Orthopaedic Nursing	ONC(C)	Canadian Orthopaedic Nurses Association (CONA)
Perinatal Nursing	PNC(C)	Canadian Association of Perinatal and Women's Health Nurses (CAPWHN)
Perioperative Nursing	CPN(C)	Operating Room Nurses Association of Canada (ORNAC)
Psychiatric/Mental Health Nursing	CPMHN(C)	Canadian Federation of Mental Health Nurses (CFMHN)
Rehabilitation Nursing	CRN(C)	Canadian Association of Rehabilitation Nurses (CARN)

as members of the public about the ethical commitments of nurses and the responsibilities nurses accept as being part of a self-regulating profession" (CNA Web site, 2012). CNA also publishes *Ethical Research Guidelines.*

Mutual Recognition Agreement

The 12 nursing regulatory authorities in Canada (including Ontario and Quebec) have developed a "Mutual Recognition Agreement" for RNs in Canada in compliance with the obligations of Chapter 7 of the *Agreement on Internal Trade.* Since November 2006, the executive directors of all 12 provincial and territorial nursing regulatory authorities have met to develop an agreement that enables the unobstructed mobility of RNs in Canada, with CNA serving as co-chair of that group.

Entry to Practice

In 1982, CNA members took the position that entry to the profession would be at a baccalaureate level. Today, baccalaureate education is required for entry to nursing practice in all parts of the country except for Quebec and Manitoba. Quebec continues to offer diploma programs. Manitoba's two diploma programs no longer accept applicants and will end in 2012 and 2013, respectively.

Nursing Legislation

Nursing legislation has been substantially amended in most provinces and territories since 1980. With the exception of RNAO, all provincial and territorial nursing associations or colleges regulate the profession and approve entry to practice educational programs. Internationally, a forum regrouping national nursing associations involved in regulation was created. An international framework for the development of credentialing (ICN, 2001b) and a registry for credentialing research have been developed to guide the evolution of credentialing in nursing (ICN, 2001c). Credentialing indicates that an individual, program, institution, or product has met established standards; standards may be minimal and mandatory or above the minimum and voluntary (ICN, 2001b).

Communication, Information, and Administration

In support of its priority policy programs, CNA offers a wide range of communications, translation, and publication services. These teams provide and support programs such as Media Awards (in partnership with the CMA), National Nursing Week events and materials, CNA's own annual general meeting and biennial national convention, the biennial National Nursing Leadership Conference (along with partners), and the editing, translation, and publication of dozens of position statements, papers, studies, and pamphlets every year. They are also responsible for CNA's leading communication vehicles, *Canadian Nurse,* CNA's Web site, and the nurseONE portal. CNA has a financial and administration team that oversees the physical plant, human resources and finances, and finally an Information Technology Services division that supports the entire organization.

The Future of CNA

In the spring of 2006, CNA published *Toward 2020: Visions for Nursing* (Villeneuve & MacDonald, 2006) to lay out evidence about global and health system trends and to provoke dialogue and debate about scenarios that could shape nursing in the future. Thousands of nurses and health leaders across the country participated in workshops, lectures, and seminars focused on the futures document and its scenarios. The ideas in the *Toward 2020* document gave rise to *The Next Decade: CNA's Vision for Nursing and Health* (2010). Many of them mirror those of nurses, who for years have advocated, for example, for more and better services for Canadians in their communities, schools, homes, and non-acute institutional settings. They know that their practice can and should be expanded and elevated to provide better and faster access to care for the Canadians they serve. They are dissatisfied with working conditions in many practice settings and tired of *study* usurping *action* on the ground at real points of care and service delivery. Despite the plethora of the best-intended, high-level responses, many working nurses and other care providers see little relief in sight after years of climbing absenteeism, overtime, and soaring workloads. Nurses also expect a modern curriculum and education system that capitalizes on their education and prior learning, enabling them to move seamlessly to new and different levels of education. And they want to be able to move just as seamlessly around the country and even beyond, within and across jurisdictional borders. The futures document captured some of that same spirit.

CNA's futures work since 2004 has identified worrying global, health, and nursing trends and accompanying opportunities for nursing on many fronts. Going forward, CNA faces challenges in both its own membership and business roles and in its *de facto* stewardship of Canadian nursing at large. How will CNA balance this complex matrix of variables and competing priorities? What are the activities in which CNA must be engaged in the interests of its own members and for the nursing and the health system at large?

CNA FUTURE ISSUES AND PRIORITIES

To be sustainable and relevant, CNA will need to continue to address policy issues on many fronts. Any smart and proactive association is sensitive to the members it represents and the issues they and the profession are likely to face in the future. The future focus and high-level nature of an effective national association is likely to create tensions within the membership who live in the "here and now." Some member discontent is, in fact, a positive indicator of an organization fulfilling its role for the public, the profession, and the members. Too much discontent makes an organization dysfunctional and paralyzes action. CNA will need to continually seek balance and keep an eye on the tipping point.

A proactive nursing organization also seeks opportunities in the sociopolitical environment to pursue its objectives and takes advantage of these opportunities to inform and influence through a nursing lens. The ability to mobilize quickly is critical. At the same time, the finite resources, the challenge of information sharing in a vast country, the membership base represented, and the effectiveness of its spokespersons are part of this complexity and of CNA's ability to respond and influence.

Influencing policy and shaping change are required skills of professional associations such as CNA. In a complex environment where many agendas compete for attention, finding points of access to influence change and understanding the right policy levers and timing to do so is challenging. Nurses understand the importance of being prepared to take on this work: Among the most popular themes of conferences and meetings of provincial and territorial, national and international specialty groups are political action, power and influence, strategies, managing change, and leadership. The topic of political action is also becoming increasingly visible in the curriculum of many nursing education programs. Nurses will never speak with "one voice," but CNA could provide a valuable intervention by continuing to seek partnerships and mechanisms that allow the multitude of nursing voices to speak some common messages.

Key business and organizational challenges CNA faces internally include maximizing success within a competitive federated model; sustaining and growing membership in an era of slow growth of the nursing workforce; attracting new members; and generating strategies to both balance and take advantage of the strong and growing regulatory policy agenda on the one hand, and the equally strong need for professional representation and advocacy on the other.

NURSING AND THE HEALTHCARE SYSTEM: ISSUES AND PRIORITIES

As well as a strong professional nursing association, Canadians and their governments need a strong nursing profession to improve population health and ensure sustainability of the healthcare system. To support an effective workforce and health system, CNA will need to be closely involved in two key areas of growth over the short and the medium term—credentialing/regulation and leadership:

- **Credentialing and regulation**—internationally, the ICN framework will guide credentialing of individuals, programs, and products. In Canada, credentialing mechanisms have been developed for individuals in regard to registration for entry to practice and certification in a specialty, for example. We have credentialing for some programs, such as accreditation of a school of nursing or nursing services, but we have not developed credentialing for all products. CNA must continue to be involved in this area, especially as pressure continues to mount to dismantle traditional regulatory structures that are seen by some as unjustified barriers to practice and mobility.
- **Leadership**—the profession needs to continue to move toward a model of leadership and influence by all professionals so nursing values can be present in all disciplinary and multidisciplinary networks in health care. CNA's ability to boost leadership across all roles and domains of practice (e.g., by linking nurses to educational offerings or providing them directly) adds value for Canadian nurses.

Still unresolved and meriting the leadership and intervention of CNA are the areas of building healthy work environments, developing a base of support for Canadian nursing science, expanding public policy to address broad determinants of health, and working with governments to shift from acute care to provisions for universal access to community, long-term, and home care. Furthermore, CNA will need to work with governments, employers, educators, and other partners to reduce the mismatch between demand for and supply of nursing services; prepare for emergencies and pandemic communicable diseases at home and abroad; work with international partners to plan appropriate and ethical migration programs; and work with partners in nursing education and governments to maximize enrollment in nursing education programs and develop the models of learning, teaching, curriculum, and professional development needed to move nursing forward in the 21st century.

THE INTERNATIONAL COUNCIL OF NURSES: A HISTORICAL PERSPECTIVE

At its Centennial Conference in London in 1999, the ICN celebrated its 100th year as an international organization for nurses. For more than a century, the ICN has sustained its place as an important and meaningful beacon for nurses around the world. The overall goal of the ICN is to unite nurses worldwide by forming a confederation of national nursing organizations, while supporting national nursing organizations in their efforts to influence national health and nursing policy. Throughout the years, motivation, commitment, and enthusiasm banded nurses together despite turbulent social and economic changes, hardships of war, and profound cultural differences. Currently, the ICN represents national nursing organizations from more than 120 countries and has more than 1 million members. However, the ICN started out as a small organization within the broader context of the women's movement. It was founded in 1899 on the initiative of the British nurse and suffragist Ethel Gordon Manson, later Mrs. Bedford Fenwick, a prominent leader of the British Nurses Association.

Early Goals

From the outset, the professional welfare of nurses, the interests of women, and the improvement of human health were intertwined goals for the founders of the ICN. A small group consisting primarily of British, American, Canadian, Scandinavian, and German nurses, the ICN intended to unite nurses worldwide through an international organization. Nursing as a respected, paid, professional occupation for middle-class women was a new phenomenon at the end of the 19th century.

Health care profoundly changed as a result of industrialization and urbanization. Hospital reform and modern hospital development were important goals throughout Europe and North America at the time, and the foundation of hospital schools to train nurses followed in their wake. The women's movement sprung in part from the desire of middle-class women to make themselves more socially useful and to carve out respectable work opportunities in areas deemed appropriate for women—thereby extending women's traditional roles in the family, such as caring for the sick, teaching, and performing social work. The founding members of the ICN were part of the growing number of women who were active in social and healthcare reform and who simultaneously sought to improve women's social position and to obtain the right to vote.

ICN held its first meeting in 1901 in Buffalo, New York, at the Pan-American Exposition, and met again 3 years later in Berlin in conjunction with the congress of the International Council of Women. At the 1904 meeting, only Germany, Great Britain, and the United States were ready for confederation. Canada joined ICN at its next congress, held in 1909 in London, as did the Netherlands, Finland, and Denmark. By 1922, ICN represented 15 countries. Christiane Reimann (Denmark) became secretary, replacing Lavinia Dock, who had been in the position for 22 years. Reimann pushed publication of the *ICN Bulletin*—the small newsletter that evolved to become the *International Nursing Review*, the official journal of the ICN (published quarterly).

The ICN and World Health During the War Years and the Great Depression

From its founding, ICN was strongly committed to the improvement of world health. In the early decades of the 20th century, contagious diseases and high infant mortality exerted a devastating impact in the rapidly industrializing Western world. The years following World War I saw the expansion of public health services, especially in child welfare and tuberculosis care, and set a new public health agenda. During the 1929 ICN meeting in Montreal, massive changes in public health nursing dominated the agenda. Acceptable standards and conditions for general and public health nursing education provoked much debate. The powerful presence of Columbia University's Teacher's College graduates in the ICN influenced its position that science and research in nursing should be promoted as a way to strengthen the nursing profession. For most membership countries, this novel idea had limited immediate relevance, although the issue would never disappear from the ICN agenda.

By 1930s, the worldwide economic depression had exerted a significant impact on nursing and health systems, and soon the threat of war once again shaped the actions of ICN's leaders. The rise of national socialism in Germany ended the independence of the German Nurses Association, which dissolved into the Reich's Union of German Nurses and Nursing Assistants in 1939, and World War II (WWII) began the same year. The disruption, destruction, and political realignments of the two world wars resulted in profound social change and ultimately changed the identity of the ICN. The organization struggled to regain normalcy as many member associations had changed, others no longer existed, and some rejoined under new circumstances. After WWII, international initiatives to make health care "accessible for all" gained momentum. The momentous advent of antibiotics and innovative medical technology on a wider scale generally increased confidence that world health could be improved and should be considered a basic human right.

In 1948, the newly established WHO declared health to be "a state of complete physical, mental, and social well-being and not merely the absence of disease or infirmity" (Howard-Jones, 1981, p. 472). In many ways, the 50th anniversary meeting (1949) in Stockholm truly introduced the ICN's voice—and thus nurses' voices—on the international stage with other players all working toward the common goal of world health. Gradually, the ICN carved out the right to speak for nursing in an ever-wider sphere of influence, assuming more activist stances and linking with international organizations, such as the United Nations and WHO. The ICN implemented a new global agenda, addressing economic, racial, religious, and gender issues that continued to complicate the professional development of nursing in many countries.

The ICN's "official relationship" status with the WHO gave it new privileges and responsibilities. During this time, the ICN developed the "International Code of Nursing Ethics" (1973) and translated it into numerous languages. It still provides national nurses associations with a valuable resource to address ethical nursing issues; up until the 1980s, CNA, for example, relied on the ICN ethical standards for its own code of ethics.

In 1966, ICN relocated its headquarters to Geneva, reflecting the importance of the ICN's growing external relationships. At that time, Canadian Alice Girard was president (1965 to 1969). She was the founding dean of the Faculty of Nursing Education at the Université de Montréal, and the first bilingual president of the CNA (1958–1960). She is still the only Canadian ever elected to the presidency of the ICN, although many other distinguished Canadian nurse leaders—including Mary Agnes Snively, Jean Gunn, Grace Fairley, Helen Evans, Helen Glass, Alice Baumgart, Eleanor Ross, and Verna Huffman Splane—have served as ICN vice presidents. All except Huffman Splane also served as presidents of CNA. Dr. Huffman Splane's vice presidency (1973 to 1977 and 1977 to 1981) followed with her tenure as Canada's first federal government *principal nursing officer* (1968 to 1972).

Increasing Activism: Position Statements

During the 1980s, the ICN and the League of Red Cross and Red Crescent Societies collaborated in preparing a teaching kit on human rights and the Geneva Convention. The increasingly activist role of the ICN impacted its political course. At the international meetings, the ICN began to adopt position statements that publicly articulated the membership's point of view on nursing and health matters, such as "the nurse's role in family planning" or "smoking and health." Also, more political statements were accepted on topics, such as "activities of war and their influence on personality development of children and adolescents" (ICN, 2004a). Position statements had political implications; the aim was that national nursing organizations would strive to implement the suggestions made in the statements within their countries. In doing so, nurses at the national level would be better able to influence national health policy and to develop strategies for nursing action.

However, an increasingly political course created new dilemmas. Although the ICN claimed neutrality in the national affairs of its member countries, a profound internal conflict arose within the ICN over the membership of South Africa. The South African Nurses Association adhered to its country's apartheid directives, inhibiting non-White membership into the organization. Faithful to the ICN standpoint on racial matters, some member organizations insisted that South Africa open up membership to all nurses irrespective of racial background or national law. Eventually the Dutch and Swedish national organizations moved that the ICN accept a resolution to expel South Africa from membership; the resolution passed in 1974. By declaring itself against racism, the ICN also disapproved of the internal politics of one of its member associations. As a consequence, the ICN lost one of its earliest members (Rafferty & Brush, 1995). Today, a newly integrated South African national nursing organization, the Democratic Nursing Organization of South Africa, is an active ICN member and close partner of the CNA.

By 1985, the ICN represented 97 countries, and national nurses associations paid dues based on their number of individual members. "ICN membership grew 18% between 1980 and 1985, from 862,123 to 1,056,066 members" (Brush et al., 1999, p. 169). Despite the ICN's increasing diversity, however, 11 countries (Japan, United States, Canada, United Kingdom, Sweden, Denmark, Australia, Spain, Finland, Norway, and Switzerland) alone accounted for 86% of its members. As such, the agendas of industrialized countries disproportionately influenced policy directions within the ICN. However, the political point of view of the ICN changed from the past and now represented a more multinational vision. During the 1970s and 1980s, the ICN clearly spoke out against human rights violations and political suppression; the ICN considered health a basic human right for all.

Current Thinking: Issues for the ICN and the International Community

Many concerns facing the ICN in the 1990s had been issues throughout the organization's history, including professional service issues, economic stability, international relations, and global nurse representation. During the 1990s, the ICN sought new ways to address old and familiar problems. As the century drew to a close, more than 4,500 nurses from every region of the world gathered at the ICN Centennial Conference in London, where they accepted a new vision to lead the ICN and nursing into the 21st century.

REGULATING NURSING

With the many new national nurses associations joining the ICN in the 1970s and 1980s, regulation of nursing again became an agenda of the ICN. Many national associations facing difficult legal and cultural circumstances often called on the ICN for help in dealing with these complex matters. To assist leaders of national nurses associations to develop and implement national nursing regulatory systems that would meet international ICN guidelines, the ICN held six "Nursing Regulation: Moving Ahead" project workshops between 1988 and 1991. Through this project, the ICN helped prepare 161 nurses from 99 national nursing associations and 62 governments to take an active role in assessing and revising national regulations and laws controlling nursing practice and care delivery in their countries. At its 1995 meeting, the Council of National Representatives approved continued international examination of national nurse regulation and the W.K. Kellogg Foundation provided the ICN with funding for a 3-year nursing regulation study.

Korean Mo-Im Kim, elected ICN president in 1989, played an essential role in increasing political activities in regard to nursing regulation. Dr. Kim, who had previously served as the president of the Korean Nurses Association and as a member of the Korean Parliament (1981 to 1985), was keenly aware of the urgency for all nurses to become more politically involved in defining nursing's place in their countries' healthcare systems. Without an official position on international regulation of nursing practice, she argued, the ICN and its member associations were vulnerable to the ad hoc decisions of local government officials. Nurse education and practice varied widely among nations, which enhanced opportunities for politicians to create nurse practice acts based on their own political agendas rather than on professional nursing standards. Dr. Kim was followed as president by Margretta ("Gretta") Madden Styles (United States), elected at the Madrid, Spain meeting in June 1993, and then by Kirsten Stallknecht (Denmark), elected at the Vancouver, Canada meeting in 1997.

STANDARDIZATION AND CREDENTIALING

At the Centennial Conference in 1999, the Council of National Representatives proposed to expand nursing's role in professional standard setting and quality assurance in health care. It was believed that the time was right to develop a framework and criteria for international standardization and credentialing procedures for nursing and health care as a way to assure healthcare recipients of the competency of nurses and other health professionals.

Regulation became one of the key program areas of the ICN in addition to professional practice issues and the socioeconomic welfare of nurses. The ICN's long-standing goal to enforce standards for nursing education and practice provoked a renewed effort to develop universal guidelines for basic and specialty practice. In this way, the ICN sought to assist National Nurses Associations (NNAs) dealing with expanding roles of nurses, new educational standards, and the evolution of nursing specialties.

After WWII, membership countries faced the increased use of auxiliary and unlicensed personnel in a rapidly expanding healthcare system, making clear definitions and explication of boundaries of nursing practice all the more urgent. The ICN's recent involvement in an advisory and supporting role in credentialing is part of its strategy to respond to changing practice demands. The ICN's position on these issues and its effort to collect reliable data on nursing help NNAs to effectively represent nursing within national health policy debates and governmental politics (ICN, 2004b). The ICN has established the Web-based Registry of Credentialing Research, to make research findings on credentialing available to researchers and nurses, thereby assisting NNAs with their credentialing processes (ICN, 2004c).

THE GLOBAL SHORTAGE OF NURSES

The urgency of addressing issues related to regulation, credentialing, and classification of nursing care in the 1990s provoked a range of responses and strategies within ICN. However, critical nursing shortages emerging around the world compromised these initiatives at the same time. In its 1989 report to the 42nd World Health Assembly, the ICN urged WHO member states to develop strategies:

- To recruit, retain, and educate nurses and midwives.
- To elevate nurses to senior leadership and management positions.
- To support nursing research.
- To adopt policies to include nurses in primary care activities.

Factors that influenced decreasing numbers of nurses in many industrialized nations included declining lengths of hospital stays, increased nursing workloads through the use of technology and higher patient acuity, shift work, and attrition through marriage and childbirth. Low wages and layoffs resulting from health reform in the 1990s also played a role. Facing severe budget cuts in health care and consequent layoffs in nursing during the early 1990s, Canada, for example, saw many of its qualified nurses have their hours reduced or positions eliminated, and some crossed borders to nations like the United States. Simultaneously, nurses from developing countries were attracted to Canada. To balance their demand for nurses, many wealthier nations recruited nurses from developing countries. Higher salaries and better working conditions, coupled with high-powered recruitment strategies, attracted nurses to the United States, Canada, Great Britain, Australia, Israel, and other industrialized nations.

A case in point is the Philippines, which faced a severe "brain drain" of its qualified nurses during the 1980s. In 1989, about 65% of the country's 13,000 new nurse graduates emigrated abroad, mostly to the United States and Middle Eastern countries, leaving many healthcare facilities in the Philippines short of staff (Brush, 1999a). Among many other worried voices on the world stage, Beverly Malone, then general secretary of the United Kingdom's Royal College of Nurses, commented on the ethical dimensions of international recruitment, emphasizing the importance for governments, employers, and nurses alike of maintaining responsible recruitment and hiring strategies (Malone, 2003).

African nations have suffered severe shortages of nurses because of the increased demand for nursing and preventive care in the face of a rapidly spreading AIDS epidemic—set against the reality that so many nurses, doctors, and other providers were themselves infected. As of 2007, an estimated 33.2 million people are living with HIV globally—68% of them in sub-Saharan Africa (77% of all cases in women). Largely as a result of HIV/AIDS and its related complications, among the 25 nations having the lowest life expectancies on earth, only two—Haiti and Afghanistan—lie outside Africa. With economic prosperity directly correlated with spending on health care and, in turn, nurse density, it is no surprise that despite the widespread need for nursing care, African nations fall far short of the supply they need. Nurse density varies as much as a 100-fold across the member states of WHO.

WHO noted in 2006 that "57 countries, 36 of which are in sub-Saharan Africa, have severe shortages of health workers. More than four million additional doctors, nurses, midwives, managers, and public health workers are urgently needed to fill this gap" (2006). In Europe, reports on nursing shortages are varied. The Netherlands and Norway, for example, had more than 2.5 times as many nurses per capita as did Canada in 2000, but their nursing workforces, too, were aging and not being adequately replenished with new graduates. Other members of the European community also reported increasing national shortages of nurses. The United States and Canada reported similar, and sometimes even worse, current and looming shortages.

Nurse migration compromises local and international efforts to improve short-term nurse recruitment and retention as well as long-term personnel planning. The ICN seeks to assist member associations in studying nursing personnel needs and resources, sharing information pertaining to nursing's worldwide employment status, and continuing discussions of the international impact of nurse shortages (Brush, 1999a). A new global partnership, the Global Health Workforce Alliance, was launched by the WHO in 2006 to address the worldwide shortage of nurses, doctors, midwives, and other health workers. It was created to "draw together and mobilize key stakeholders engaged in global health to help countries improve the way they plan for, educate and employ health workers" (World Health Organization, 2006). Despite a decade of attention, worrying global shortages, migration, and recruitment challenges remain far from resolved in 2008, and, in many nations, demand for nursing services continues to far outpace an adequate supply of nurses to provide them.

ADVANCING NURSING PRACTICE

A key problem with global nurse regulation is the dearth of data about *what* constitutes nurses' work and *how* it is shaped by healthcare service payments. In response, in 1989, the ANA proposed a council resolution urging national nurses associations to develop nation-specific classification systems for nursing care. The initiative may have been triggered by a difficult situation with which the ANA was confronted when the American Medical Association proposed introducing a new healthcare worker in the United States. The ANA, which successfully lobbied against such a decision, argued that the nursing profession must name its distinct contribution to health care to be recognized in worldwide healthcare planning and financing. The ANA offered to collect, document, and share data on nursing practice across countries, clinical settings, and patient populations to assist national associations in planning types and amounts of nursing needed, in determining skill mixes for various care settings and patient groups, and in evaluating clinical efficacy and cost.

Responding to the ANA resolution in 1990, the ICN board of directors invited June Clark (United Kingdom) and Norma Lang (United States) to develop a feasibility study for an International classification for nursing practice (ICNP). Gretta Styles, who was chair of the Professional Services Committee, nurse consultant Fadwa Affara, and Denmark's Randi Mortenson and Gunnar Nelson completed the team. From 1990 to 1997, they consulted with nurses and classification experts to collect, group, and rank nursing phenomena, interventions, and outcomes, with the ultimate goal of creating a universal nursing language (Brush, 1999a). In 2000, the ICN made ICNP an official program and continued to update and revise the classification system (ICN, 2004d). In that same year, the ICN published an updated version of its "Code of Ethics for Nurses" to provide nurses with a continuous resource to help maintain ethical practices worldwide (Fry, 2002).

Another pertinent issue arising through the 1990s was advancing nursing practice to respond to expanding primary healthcare demands and changing conditions of specialty nursing care. The ICN established an International Nurse Practitioner/Advanced Practice Nursing Network with the view to provide international resources for nurses practicing in these roles and to alert policymakers and health planners to the essential function of these roles in enhancing healthcare services. Again, the ICN sees it as a major responsibility to provide relevant data and to support nurses and countries in the process of expanding nurses' roles (ICN, 2004e).

THE ICN IN THE 21ST CENTURY

During the 1990s, the ICN prepared various policy decisions and initiated planning to lead nursing into the 21st century. In 1993, at the Council of National Representatives meeting in Madrid, the ICN adopted toward the 21st Century: A Strategic Plan, 1994 to 1999. The plan addressed the issues the ICN considered crucial to health planning for the new century, including formulating health and social policy, establishing professional standardization and socioeconomic equity, collaborating with other international bodies, disseminating nursing knowledge, and developing frameworks for identifying and measuring nurses' work. The strategic plan clearly laid out the ICN's goals for the future, which realistically could be accomplished considering available resources.

Two years later, at the 1995 Council meeting in Harare, Zimbabwe, the ICN endorsed several key position statements, emphasizing its expansionist agenda. Revisiting its 1981 Resolution of Female Excision, Circumcision and Mutilation, the ICN resolved to work with local, national, and international groups opposed to the practice. Position statements related to psychiatric mental health nursing and to the costs and value of nursing were also endorsed. Other resolutions specifically addressed issues of nurse titling, health policy participation, nursing school accreditation, and nursing students' roles in national nursing associations (Brush, 1999a; ICN, 2004a).

In 1997, Canadian Judith Oulton, formerly executive director of the CNA, assumed the post of CEO of the ICN. She brought with her the belief that it is critical for nurses in all countries to participate in shaping health policy and to have their work backed up by accurate data demonstrating nursing's contributions to health outcomes. During that year, some 5,000 nurses from 120 countries convened in Vancouver, Canada, to "Share the Health Challenge" at the ICN's 21st Quadrennial Congress. It was the first time Canada had hosted an ICN congress since the 1929 meeting in Montreal. Enhancement of nurses' political influence was a persistent theme: "We must raise our social status as a profession to our level of social contribution and our influence to the level of our strength," said outgoing ICN President Gretta Styles. "We must raise the intensity of our politics to the intensity of our ethics" (Brush, 1999a, p. 155).

At the 1999 Centennial Conference in London, the white heart was adopted as a symbol to commemorate a century of ICN nurses caring for and contributing to world health and welfare. ICN President Kirsten Stallknecht (Denmark) addressed the audience at the opening ceremony of the conference, urging nurses to "forge a renewed vision for nurses and nursing" that emphasized "high-touch" over "high-tech." At the end of her speech, she unveiled the ICN's vision statement for the 21st century, which opens as follows: "United within ICN, the nurses of all nations speak with one voice. We speak as advocates for all those we serve and for all the unserved, insisting that prevention, care, and cure be the right of every human being" (Brush, 1999a, p. 155).

Reflecting the demands and priorities of the world around it in a new century, ICN's diverse activities include human rights (including a focus on the rights of women and girls), the issue of task-shifting and its impacts on nursing, patient safety, and disaster preparedness. In 2006, it established the International Centre for Human Resources in Nursing in partnership with the Florence Nightingale International Foundation. Billed as a unique online service serving anyone involved in nursing human resources, the Centre is dedicated to "strengthening the nursing workforce globally through the development, ongoing monitoring and dissemination of comprehensive information, standards and tools on nursing human resources policy, management, research and practice" (ICN Web site, 2012a). The companion International Centre on Nurse Migration serves as "a global resource for the development, promotion and dissemination of research, policy and information on nurse migration" (ICN Web site, 2012b). It occupies a key role in establishing effective global and national migration policies and practices to facilitate safe patient care and positive practice environments for nurse migrants. And in line with both of these initiatives, ICN also hosts the International Socio-Economic Workforce Forum where interested member nations meet to hammer out these vexing human resources issues. Partnering with the Canadian Federation of Nurses Unions, CNA is always a participant in the forum, both providing information to the forum and sharing in it.

Judith Oulton completed her term as CEO in the fall of 2008, turning over the reins to David Benton, formerly a senior consultant at ICN. In 2009 more than 5,000 nurses from some 130 member countries met in Durban, South Africa, for the 110th anniversary Congress of the ICN, taking yet another step forward in ICNs illustrious journey of international leadership of nurses and nursing.

SUMMARY

This chapter has reviewed the evolution and major roles, priorities, and challenges of the CNA and the ICN. In Canada, the CNA's role is to advocate for the public, speak on behalf of the profession, and contribute solutions to strengthen the healthcare system. As the national voice of nursing, it focuses on the power of representation and regulatory policy. CNA's regulatory policy work is reflected in the educational field and in the evolution of credentialing in nursing. Examples of the power of representation include the CNA's influence on the initial Canada Health Act, and in the rich tapestry of work now being carried out by its policy departments. For example, during this decade CNA has developed significant expertise and leadership in health and human resources planning, quality nursing practice environments, and international development. Current priorities for the CNA include responding to the system transformation recommendations of its inaugural National Expert Commission, leading the dialogue about the future of nursing and maintaining a strongly collaborative voice for nursing in efforts across the country to build a stronger, better system of health and illness care. Future challenges for CNA include maintaining strong and united voices and messages, with increased representation in Ontario, Quebec, and British Columbia; development of appropriate leadership models to promote nursing values across multidisciplinary healthcare networks and delivery models; and growth and influence in the areas of credentialing.

The ICN's vision for nursing in the 21st century reflects the organization's century-long involvement in the politics of health care. The new century will undoubtedly present many challenges and opportunities, including the internationalization of markets, which may create an unknown effect on the process of reworking and redefining nursing. Tensions between generations of nurses and philosophical differences among ICN member associations also may pose new challenges to the ICN in the 21st century.

Both organizations are confronted by the shifting realities and possibilities brought about by technology. Born in an era of steamships carrying hand-written paper letters, CNA and ICN will have to continue to define their positions and purposes in a world where isolated nomadic tribes in Africa communicate using cell phone text messaging—and where nearly instant email has all but replaced the need for verbal telephone calls, never mind postal mail. Inexpensive social media means that savvy and sophisticated individual nurse citizens can communicate effectively with one another and with their governments, and those simple online tools have been the backdrop to toppling entire governments. Given that pace of change (which is only accelerating), historic leadership organizations such as CNA and ICN surely will be challenged to continually define new points of value in their roles as beacons for communication and collaboration as we move through the 21st century.

Online

Add to your knowledge of this issue:

Canadian Resources

Canadian Nurses Association	**www.cna-aiic.ca**
Canadian Association of Schools of Nursing	**www.casn.ca**
Canadian Federation of Nurses Unions	**www.cfnu.ca**
Canadian Healthcare Association	**www.cha.ca**
Canadian Nursing Students' Association	**www.cnsa.ca**

International Resources

International Council of Nurses	**www.icn.ch**
Organization for Economic Cooperation and Development	**www.oecd.org**
United Nations	**www.un.org**
United Nations Educational, Scientific, and Cultural Organization	**www.unesco.org**
World Health Organization	**www.who.int**

R E F L E C T I O N S *on the Chapter...*

1 Describe a professional association you are familiar with and explain what role it fulfills in society.

2 Over the past 20 years, what issues have been affected by the power of representation of the CNA? Select one and describe how the influence of the CNA changed the course of action.

3 What are two current policy priorities for the CNA and ICN? Discuss one priority and its progress at both the national and international levels.

4 Having read this chapter, in what ways are CNA's Web site (http://www.cna-nurses.ca), nurseONE portal (http://www.nurseone.ca/), and ICN's Web site (http://www.icn.ch) useful to you as a student and a beginning practitioner? If you have suggestions, how would you communicate them to CNA and ICN?

5 Discuss the impact of organized international nursing on changing healthcare demands and world health. Identify three political strategies nurses developed to change health care and health.

6 Identify three important issues that the ICN has faced throughout its history and discuss strategies it developed in response.

7 What roles does the ICN play in issues of regulation of nursing practice? How do they interrelate with CNA's roles?

8 Select a position statement from CNA Web site (http://www.cna-aiic.ca) or ICN Web site (http://www.icn.ch) and discuss its potential impact on health policy. How could the position statement contribute to informing or resolving the issue at the local level or in your nursing practice?

Want to know more? Visit thePoint for additional helpful resources:

- Journal Articles
- Learning Objectives
- Nursing Professional Roles and Responsibilities
- Bonus chapters:
  - Health and Nursing Policy: A Matter of Politics, Power and Professionalism
  - The NP Movement: Recurring Issues
  - When Difference Matters: The Politics of Privilege and Marginality

References

Brush, B.L. (1999). Leading nurses to a new century: ICN during the 1990s. *International Nursing Review, 46*(5), 151–155.

Brush, B. L., Lynaugh, J. E., Boschma, G., Rafferty, A.M., Stuart, M., & Tomes, N.J. (1999). *Nurses of all nations: A history of the International Council of Nurses, 1899–1999.* Philadelphia, PA: Lippincott Williams & Wilkins.

Canadian Institute for Health Information. (2007). *Workforce trends of registered nurses in Canada 2006.* Ottawa, ON: Author.

———. (2011). *Registered nurses database.* Retrieved from http://www.secure.cihi.ca

Canadian Nurses Association. (1958). *The first fifty years.* Ottawa, ON: Author.

———. (1968). *The leaf and the lamp.* Ottawa, ON: Author.

———. (1980). *Putting "health" back into healthcare: Submission to the Health Services Review.* Ottawa, ON: Author.

———. (1998). *The quiet crisis in healthcare.* Ottawa, ON: Author.

———. (1999). *Repair, realign, and resource healthcare.* Ottawa, ON: Author.

———. (2000). *Rebuilding Canada's health system starts with renewing the nursing workforce.* Ottawa, ON: Author.

———. (2001). *Revitalizing the nursing workforce and strengthening Medicare.* Ottawa, ON: Author.

———. (2010). *The Next Decade: CNA's Vision for Nursing and Health.* Ottawa, ON: Author.

———. (2012). Web site accessed Sept. 29, 2012 from www.cna-aiic/en.

Canadian Nurses Association & Canadian Medical Association. (2011). *Principles to Guide Health Care Transformation in Canada.* Accessed Sept. 29, 2012 from www2.cna-aiic.ca/CNA/documents/pdf/... Guiding_Principles_HC_e.pdf.

Fry, S. (2002). Guest editorial: Defining nurses' ethical practices in the 21st century. *International Nursing Review, 49*(1), 1–3.

Government of Canada. (1984). *Canada Health Act of 1984—Bill C-3.* Ottawa, ON: House of Commons, Government of Canada.

Health Action Lobby. (2012). Accessed Sept. 29, 2012 from www.healthaction lobby.ca/images/stories/ publication

Howard-Jones, N. (1981). The World Health Organization in historical perspective. *Perspectives in Biology and Medicine, 24*(3), 467–482.

International Council of Nurses. (1973). *ICN code for nurses: Ethical concepts applied to nursing.* Geneva: Author.

———. (2001a). *From vision to action: ICN in the 21st century* (revised February 2001). Geneva: Author.

———. (2001b). *The ICN credentialing framework.* Unpublished manuscript. Geneva: Author.

———. (2001c). *The ICN credentialing research registry—Draft 1.* Unpublished manuscript. Geneva: Author.

———. (2004a). *ICN position statements* [Online]. Retrieved on from http://www.icn.ch/policy.htm

———. (2004b). *Regulation: Regulation programme area overview* [Online]. Retrieved on from http://www.icn.ch/regulation.htm

———. (2004c). *About the International Council of Nurses' registry of credentialing research.* [Online]. Retrieved from http://www.icn.ch/rcrhome.htm

———. (2004d). *International classification for nursing practice (ICNP).* [Online]. Retrieved from http://www.icn.ch/icnp.htm

———. (2004e). *Nurse practitioner/advanced practice network* [Online]. Retrieved from http://icn-apnetwork.org/

———. (2012a). International Centre for Human Resources in Nursing. Retrieved Sept. 29, 2012 from www.icn.ch/pillarsprograms/international-centre-for-human-resources-in-nursing-ichrn/

———. (2012b). International Centre on Nurse Migration. Retrieved Sept. 29, 2012 from www.icn.ch/projects/international-centre-on-nurse-migration

Lemire Rodger, G. (1999). Intraorganizational politics. In J.M. Hibberd & D.L. Smith (Eds.), *Nursing management in Canada* (2nd ed., pp. 279–295). Toronto, ON: Saunders.

MacPhail, J. (1996). The role of the Canadian Nurses Association in the development of nursing in Canada. In J. Ross Kerr & J. MacPhail (Eds.), *Canadian nursing issues and perspectives* (3rd ed., pp. 31–54). St. Louis, MO: Mosby.

Malone, B. (2003). Guest editorial: Promoting the value of nursing in the context of a global nursing shortage. *International Nursing Review, 50*(3), 129–130.

Meilicke, D., & Larsen, J. (1988). Leadership and the leaders of the Canadian Nurses Association. In A.J. Baumgart & J. Larsen (Eds.), *Canadian nursing faces the future* (pp. 421–459). St. Louis, MO: Mosby.

Mhatre, S.L. & Deber, R. (1992). From equal access to healthcare to equitable access to health: Review of Canadian provincial commissions and reports. *International Journal of Health Services, 22*(4), 645–668.

Rafferty, A.M., & Brush, B.L. (1995). Conflict and consensus: The International Council of Nurses and international nursing. *International History of Nursing Journal, 1*, 4–16.

Ryten, E. (1997). *A statistical picture of the past, present, and future of registered nurses in Canada.* Ottawa, ON: Canadian Nurses Association.

Ryten, E. (2002). *Planning for the future: Nursing human resource projections.* Ottawa, ON: Canadian Nurses Association.

Villeneuve, M., & MacDonald, J. (2006). *Toward 2020: Visions for nursing.* Ottawa, ON: Canadian Nurses Association.

World Health Organization. (1978). *Primary healthcare: Report on the International Conference on Primary Healthcare,* Alma Ata, USSR, September 6–12, 1978. Geneva: Author.

World Health Organization. (2006). *New global alliance seeks to address worldwide shortage of doctors, nurses and other health workers.* Retrieved from http://www.who.int/mediacentre/news/releases/2006/pr26/en/index.html

Chapter

8

Canadian Provincial and Territorial Professional Associations and Colleges

Laurel Brunke

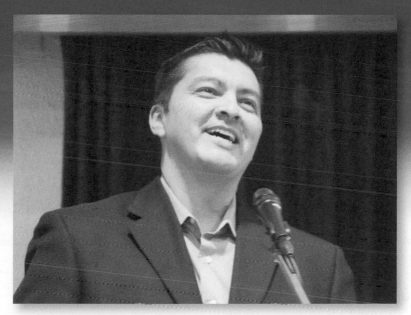

Hon. Jackson Lafferty, Minister of Education, Culture and Employment North West Territories speaks to nurse educators at a conference Aurora College, Yellowknife. (Used with permission. Photographer Anne-Mieke Cameron.)

Critical Questions

As a way of engaging with the ideas in this chapter, consider the following:

1. Are you aware of which groups of workers in the healthcare system are regulated and which are not? Who do you imagine is responsible for the regulation of healthcare workers?

2. In reflecting on what you know about the structure of the Canadian healthcare system and the tensions between national and

territorial and provincial political priorities, what would you anticipate as tensions arising in the regulation of registered nurses (RNs)?

3. Given the mandate of the International Council of Nurses (ICN) and the Canadian Nurses Association (CNA), what role do you imagine they might play in the regulation of RNs?

Chapter Objectives

After completing this chapter, you will be able to:

1. Describe the evolution of nursing regulation in Canada.

2. Recognize how differences in legislation have resulted in different approaches to nursing regulation.

(continued on page 144)

This chapter will assist the reader in understanding and appreciating the value of nursing self-regulation. To achieve this end, the evolution of nursing regulation in Canada is described, as are differences in regulatory approaches across jurisdictions, issues associated with these differences, and considerations for the future of the regulation of nursing by provincial and territorial nursing associations and colleges.

REGULATION

The purpose of regulating the nursing profession is straightforward: To protect the public, which makes regulation itself a most complex issue.

The What and Why of Regulation

What is regulation? Simply, regulation is the "forms and processes whereby order, consistency, and control are brought to an occupation and its practices" (International Council of Nurses [ICN], 1985, p. 7). The ICN states the following goals of regulation:

- Define the profession and its members.
- Determine the scope of practice.
- Set standards of education and competent and ethical practice.
- Establish systems of accountability and credentialing processes (Styles & Affara, 1997).

Finocchio et al. with the Taskforce on Healthcare Workforce Regulation (1995), take a broader view of regulation. They believe that regulation of the healthcare workforce best serves the public's interest if it promotes effective health outcomes and protects the public from harm; ensures accountability to the public; respects consumers' rights to choose their healthcare providers from a range of safe options; encourages a healthcare system that is flexible, rational, and cost effective and that facilitates effective working relationships among healthcare providers; and provides for professional and geographic mobility of competent providers.

Evolution of Regulation

Regulation of professions really began with the formation of crafts and guilds. There was, and always has been, competition among tradespeople in relation to the goods they sold and the services they provided. The crafts and guilds were made up of the people who were known to provide quality products and services, in part because they developed standards for these products and services. Of course, with increased quality came increased costs and, in some circumstances, a monopoly on the products and services the guilds were providing. From these guilds and crafts arose licensing laws intended to protect the public and ensure that only members of the crafts or guilds could provide the specified services and products (Cutshall, 1998). These traditional licensing laws provided for exclusive scope of practice, or what is sometimes referred to as *turf protection*. Today, there is a shift away from this approach to regulation, a topic discussed later in the chapter.

The nature of regulation has changed in other ways over the years. Historically, professional regulation focused essentially on gatekeeping, that is, setting the requirements for those who can enter the profession and disciplining those who fail to meet the standards of the profession. Finocchio, et al. (1995, p. vii) have said, in relation to healthcare workforce regulation in the United States, "Though it has served us well in the past, healthcare regulation is out of step with today's healthcare needs and expectations." However, nursing regulatory bodies in Canada have for some time embraced a more contemporary approach to regulation. This approach recognizes that there is more to regulation than gatekeeping.

The Canadian Nurses Association [CNA] (2007a, p. 1) believes that:

> Public protection is promoted when regulatory frameworks strengthen nursing practice and leadership in all domains of practice, including clinical practice, administration, education and research; when they provide supports to correct and improve practice; and when they focus not only on individual nurses but also on practice environments that support nurses in providing safe, competent and ethical care.

Some nursing regulatory bodies in Canada have adopted a regulatory framework of promoting good practice, preventing poor practice, and intervening when practice is unacceptable. The benefits of promotion and prevention strategies—the quality improvement approach—mean that intervention with unacceptable practice can be kept at a minimum.

REGULATION OF NURSING

Many nurses take it for granted that nursing is a profession and that, like other professions, nurses are entitled to collective professional autonomy, that is, the self-regulation of the profession as a whole. Professional autonomy means that, with appropriate public input, professional groups govern themselves. Canada has a tradition that communities of people within society take responsibility for meeting their obligations, both to themselves and the community at large. They do this by managing their affairs in a way that respects and furthers the good of society while recognizing the legitimate interests of their members. This is the essence of self-regulation (Registered Nurses Association of British Columbia [RNABC], 2000). However, self-regulation is a privilege of a profession, not a right. In Canada, self-regulation of nursing is less than a century old.

History of Nursing Regulation in Canada

The move to obtain registration for nurses began in 1893 with the formation of the American Society of Superintendents of Training Schools for Nurses of the United States and Canada. This was followed by the development of the Associated Alumnae of the United States and Canada in 1896. Securing legislation to "differentiate the trained from the untrained" (CNA, 1968, p. 35) was the purpose of the Associated Alumnae. When it was recognized that the fight for the nursing legislation had to be fought separately in each country, the Canadian and American groups separated. Consequently, the Canadian Society of Superintendents of Training Schools for Nurses was formed in 1907, with formation of the Provisional Society of the Canadian Nurses Association of Trained Nurses following in 1908 (CNA, 1968).

The development of provincial graduate nurses associations was due in large part to the increase in the number of nursing personnel that occurred at the end of the 19th century. Competition between trained professional nurses and nurses with little or no professional training was evident in the areas of wages and status. Moreover, no mechanisms for ensuring uniformity in nursing service standards were in place (CNA, 1968). Kerr (1996) identified two powerful social forces that affected the pursuit of legislation for the registration of nurses: First, consciousness raising regarding women's rights that was part of the effort to obtain the vote for women, and second, the increased valuing of nurses and nurses' services that occurred during World War I. Kerr speculated that these factors, as well as a general recognition that a mechanism was needed to ensure that nurses were qualified, led to the passage of legislation in all provinces over a 12-year period—a relatively brief time.

In 1910, the nurses of Nova Scotia became the first to have nursing legislation. Registration was voluntary, and nongraduate nurses could still practice. The Registered Nurses Act, which incorporated the Graduate Nurses Association of Nova Scotia, set out, among other things, the powers of the association and the duty of officers, admission of nurses as members, discipline of members, and appointment of examiners. Legislation proclaimed in Manitoba in 1913 was more in keeping with current legislation, as it set out minimum standards for admission, curriculum in schools of nursing, and the registration and discipline of practicing nurses. By 1914, all provinces except Prince Edward Island had a provincial nurses association.

Work to achieve legislation was not easy, as can be seen in the following example from British Columbia, where efforts to achieve legislation began in 1912. In 1914, the government decided that the nurses' bill could not be accepted as a government measure, and the association was advised to have the bill presented as a public measure introduced by a private member.

When the bill was reintroduced in 1916, it was suggested that the president and secretary of the College of Physicians and Surgeons should be members of the council of the nurses association and that the orders, regulations, fees, and bylaws should be subject to the approval of the College of Physicians and Surgeons. The nurses association decided to withdraw the bill rather than include these amendments. A letter was sent to the College of Physicians and Surgeons asking if these amendments met with their approval and if they wished to have graduate nurses under their control. This suggestion was unanimously opposed by the college. A revised bill was passed in 1918, and, interestingly enough, the first council was named by the College of Physicians and Surgeons (Kerr, 1944).

Ontario was the last province to achieve legislation for nursing because of objections from nurses who believed they could not meet the qualifications and because some hospital administrators feared that they could not meet education standards. However, by 1922, all nine provinces had some form of nurse registration.

The first act concerning nursing in Newfoundland came into effect in 1931, and the Newfoundland Graduate Nurses Association was incorporated in 1935. Newfoundland formed as a province in 1949 and enacted legislation for nurses, with mandatory registration, in 1953. Legislation regulating nurses in the Northwest Territories and the Yukon was enacted in 1988 and 1994, respectively. Membership in the Northwest Territories Registered Nurses Association, formed in 1975, was initially voluntary. Before the legislation enacted in 1994 in the Yukon, RNs working there had to be registered in another Canadian jurisdiction.

In 2010, the regulatory bodies in Alberta, British Columbia, Manitoba, Ontario, and Quebec announced their intention to form the Canadian Council of Registered Nurse Regulators (CCRNR). In 2011, the remaining provincial/territorial regulatory bodies indicated their intent to join CCRNR. CCRNR's purpose is to promote excellence in regulatory practice and serve as a national forum and voice regarding interprovincial/territorial, national, and global regulatory matters for nursing regulation.

Mandatory Registration

Initial legislation for nursing varied across provinces, and, in some instances, aspects of the legislation were inconsistent with the primary purpose of the regulation of the profession (i.e., protection of the public). Initially, not all nurses had to be registered to practice nursing. In some jurisdictions, these unregistered individuals were permitted to use the title "registered nurse" even if they did not meet the requirements for entry to the profession or uphold the profession's standards. In 1922, the Nova Scotia Act was amended to the effect that a register be kept "in which shall be entered the name of every member of the Association" and "only those persons whose names are entered in the register shall be deemed qualified to hold themselves out to the public as registered nurses" (S. Farouse, personal communication, 2002). Although not the same as mandatory registration, it was a first step toward this important mechanism for public protection.

Quebec was the first province to have mandatory licensing with the passing of the Quebec Nurses' Act in 1946 (CNA, 1968). The achievement of mandatory registration took considerably longer in other provinces, with British Columbia and Saskatchewan being the last to make this change to existing legislation. Mandatory registration was a requirement in the first acts for nursing enacted in the Yukon and Northwest Territories.

Authority of Nursing Regulatory Bodies

In Canada, authority to regulate the profession comes from legislation enacted by provincial and territorial governments. The nature of the legislation varies across Canada, although there is increasing interest from governments in enacting uniform legislation for all professions in a province or territory. Regardless of the form of the legislation, nursing regulatory bodies in Canada generally have authority for the following:

- Standards of education and qualifications for registrants
- Standards of practice and professional ethics
- Use of title
- Scope of practice
- Professional discipline
- Approval or recognition of education programs for entry to the profession
- Continuing competence requirements for registrants.

Responsibility for regulation of registered nursing rests with a provincial and territorial professional association or college. In Ontario, this authority rests with the College of Nurses of Ontario (CNO), which also has responsibility for regulating registered practical nurses. In other provinces, this group of professionals, also known as licensed practical nurses (LPNs) or certified nursing assistants, is regulated by separate organizations. Until recently, Ontario was the only jurisdiction in Canada to have both a regulatory organization and professional association, the Registered Nurses Association of Ontario (RNAO). The RNAO's mission is to pursue healthy public policy and to promote the full participation of RNs in shaping and delivering health services now and in the future. Contrast this with the mission of the CNO to protect the public's right to quality nursing services by providing leadership to the nursing profession in self-regulation. Risk (1992, p. 368) identifies that the uniqueness in Ontario "is based on the philosophical premise that there is an inherent conflict (real or perceived) between professional self-interest and public interest, and that regulatory decisions must be separate from professional advancement." At the heart of this issue is the question of whether an association that has as one of its goals the promotion of the profession can do this in a way that does not interfere with meeting its public interest mandate. The College and Association of Registered Nurses of Alberta (CARNA), has, as can be seen by its name, both a regulatory and association mandate.

In British Columbia, it is clear in how the Health Professions Act (HPA) is structured that it was not intended that health profession colleges in B.C. have a dual regulatory/association role. When it became apparent that the regulation of registered nursing would come under the HPA, RNABC made significant efforts to achieve amendments to the HPA to provide for the College to continue its past involvement in professional issues as provided for in the now repealed Nurses (Registered) Act. These efforts were unsuccessful.

When the College of Registered Nurses of British Columbia (CRNBC) replaced the Registered Nurses Association of British Columbia (RNABC) in 2005 as the regulatory college for registered nurses and nurse practitioners in B.C., it continued with RNABC's membership in CNA. There are conflicts, though, in the roles and purposes of the two entities. Unlike RNABC, CRNBC does not have a dual mandate as a professional association and a regulatory body. CRNBC's role is regulatory only and it does not carry out activities that RNABC was able to undertake as an association, such as advocacy on health and social policy issues, one of CNA's primary roles. In 2009 to 2010, a policy and legal review and analysis of the relationship between CRNBC and CNA was done to address how the College could sustain its membership in CNA given its regulatory mandate under the HPA. This evaluation concluded that the CNA function of lobbying government creates a perceived, if not an actual, conflict for CRNBC, given the College's public protection mandate under Section 16 of the HPA. In consideration of this, in April 2010 the CRNBC board decided to initiate a measured and managed withdrawal from CNA as a jurisdictional member.

CRNBC recognized that there was an opportunity for a new professional organization to establish itself to meet the professional needs and interests of B.C.'s registered nurses that were not being met in the province. To this end, the CRNBC board provided one-time funding to the RN Network of B.C. to build a business case to inform this need.

The Association of Registered Nurses of British Columbia (ARNBC) was incorporated in July 2010 and evolved out of the RN Network. ARNBC describes itself as "a professional organization that provides a forum for registered nurses to consider existing and emerging healthcare and professional issues" (Association of Registered Nurses of British Columbia, 2011).

Other differences between jurisdictional authorities relate to approval of nursing education programs, requirements for continuing competence for registration renewal, requirements for re-entry into practice, language requirements for registration, and approaches to regulation of nurse practitioners (NPs).

Approval of Nursing Education Programs

Of particular interest is the authority for approval or recognition of nursing education programs for entry to the profession. This authority typically includes establishing the criteria for approval of the nursing education program as well as actually approving the program. Essentially, this gives the profession the authority to establish the education, that is, the competency requirements for entry to the profession. In most instances, approval is limited to education programs for entry to the profession. However, CRNBC and the Association of Registered Nurses of Newfoundland and Labrador have authority to approve and recognize education programs for NPs. Until recently, the responsibility and authority for approving nursing education programs resided with the nursing regulatory body, except in Ontario and Quebec.

Until 2005 in Ontario, under the Nursing Act, 1991, authority for approval and monitoring of university programs was vested in the Council of Ontario University Programs in Nursing and the individual university's senate or governing council. Effective from January 1, 2005, changes to the Nursing Act provided for nursing education programs to be approved by a body or bodies designated by the council or by the council itself. This is a very significant change because formal responsibility for program approval now resides directly with CNO Council. The CNO designated the Canadian Association of Schools of Nursing as the agency to conduct the approval process. In Quebec, the Ministère de l'Éducation, du Loisor et du Sport has responsibility for nursing programs. In 2001, the Ordre des infirmières et infirmiers du Quebec was invited to participate in the consultation process for nursing curriculum for the first time. This consultation resulted in a revised nursing education program. In British Columbia, with the transition to regulating RNs under the HPA, the British Columbia cabinet must approve any changes to the schedule listing education programs recognized by the CRNBC. Many consider this requirement to be an erosion of the profession's authority to self-regulate.

Regulation of Nurse Practitioners

Another area of notable difference among jurisdictions is in the current or intended approaches to the regulation of NPs. RNs have been working in extended or expanded roles, predominantly in rural or remote settings, for many years. Although these roles are considered by some to parallel those of the NP, authority to carry out functions such as diagnosing, prescribing, and managing labor and delivery comes through delegated medical acts rather than legislation that authorizes RNs to carry out these functions autonomously. Pressures related to physician shortages, particularly in underserviced areas, and increasing pressures on health budgets have resulted in renewed interest in implementing the NP role. The use of NPs varies considerably across the country, as does the way in which the role is enacted. In some jurisdictions, collaborative relationships with physicians are mandated; in others, they are not. In some jurisdictions, such as Newfoundland, the title "nurse practitioner" is, or will be, protected; in others, there are no plans to protect the title. In some provinces, these nurses are identified in different ways; in Ontario, for example, they are registered as RN/Extended Class.

This variation raises questions as to how the public can be easily informed about which RNs have authority for some of the functions commonly associated with the NP role. Another significant difference is that, in some jurisdictions, the NP has authority for a "package" of functions, such as in Ontario and Newfoundland, whereas in others, such as Manitoba, authority will be given for each individual function.

The evolution of the regulation of NPs provides a good example of how differences in regulatory approaches can have implications for the consumer of health care. Consider how much easier it would be for consumers and other healthcare providers to understand the role and the responsibilities of NPs if the regulatory framework was the same in all jurisdictions. It also provides an example of how differing approaches to regulation can affect the mobility of nurses across the country because the requirements for recognition as an NP are beginning to vary across jurisdictions.

ISSUES IN REGULATION

As demonstrated in earlier sections of this chapter, there is a need for regulation to evolve to respond to the changing world and the needs of the healthcare system. Emerging issues in regulation are related to a variety of factors.

Impact of Globalization

Globalization of the economy presents significant challenges to countries to remain competitive in world markets. In this context, policies are being adopted that favor deregulation, decentralization, and, in some instances, a reduced role for government. Advances in technology are already affecting how health care is delivered, with increasing use of video and data communications. At the same time, trade agreements, such as the General Agreement on Trade in Services, the North American Free Trade Agreement, and the Treaty on European Union, are facilitating the movement of goods, people, and services across national boundaries. These agreements have significant implications for regulated professions because they promote uniform standards and reduce bureaucratic and regulatory barriers to mobility.

Mobility in Canada

In Canada, the Agreement on Internal Trade (AIT) requires governments to recognize mutually the occupational qualifications of workers who are qualified in any other province or territory and to reconcile differences in occupational standards. Effective from April 1, 2009, new labor mobility provisions required people with a specific professional or occupational certification in one province or territory to be recognized as qualified to practice their profession in all provinces and territories where their profession or occupation is regulated. In other words, a registered nurse in one Canadian jurisdiction must be granted registration on the basis of having been registered in another Canadian province or territory, without having to retrain, retest, or have his or her qualifications reassessed provided that the nurse's registration is in good standing and the nurse has met the requirements regarding current practice in the province or territory in which she or he is making application.

Similar trade agreements have been negotiated between provinces. In April 2006, the British Columbia and Alberta governments signed the British Columbia–Alberta Trade, Investment, and Labour Mobility Agreement (TILMA). One of the requirements of the agreement was that, by April 2009, workers certified for an occupation would have their qualifications recognized in both provinces. The New West Partnership Trade Agreement between British Columbia, Alberta, and Saskatchewan came into effect on July 1, 2010. Its obligations are consistent with those in TILMA.

Under these agreements, full mobility has been achieved for registered nurses within Canada. The same is not true for nurse practitioners due to differences in conceptualization of the streams of NP practice as well as entry-level education, examination, and continuing competence and quality assurance requirements; prior learning assessment; and lapsed practice and re-entry processes. Exceptions under AIT may be approved when there is a significant difference in occupational standards and the exception is based on a legitimate objective such as the protection of public security, health, and safety. Alberta has posted an exception related to primary care nurse practitioners from Quebec, and British Columbia has provided an exemption, under the B.C. Labour Mobility Act, related to nurse practitioners from all other Canadian jurisdictions. As a result, nurse practitioners affected by these exemptions/exceptions may be required to be reassessed, retested, or complete additional education.

Competencies or Credentials as the Basis for Registration

Government agreements about trade and mobility, such as AIT, have led to increasing emphasis on competencies rather than credentials as the basis for registration. The challenge is two-fold: First, how to achieve consensus across Canada regarding the competencies required for RNs' practice and second, how to develop an efficient, affordable approach to competence assessment.

Consensus on the competencies required for entry-level practice in 1996 and projected for 2001 for RNs, registered psychiatric nurses, and licensed/registered practical nurses was reached in 1997 through the National Nursing Competency Project (CNA, 1997). In addition, the project identified contexts for entry-level practice in 1996 and 2001 for these three nursing groups as well as entry-level competencies that are shared and those that are unique. The competency statements developed were intended to provide information for decision making regarding registration of new graduates, equivalence of out-of-province graduates, requirements for entry examinations, and curricula for basic nursing education programs. It was cautioned that the competency statements would need to be considered in the context of a healthcare system characterized by constant and rapid change. The report further cautioned that the competency statements are not at a level of specificity that would be required for measurement or assessment, and further work would be required to refine the results (CNA, 1997).

In 2004, a joint project was initiated by several regulatory bodies to revise the entry-level competencies with the aim of enhancing their consistency among the participating jurisdictions.

The goal is, overtime, to develop one set of competencies that are used at the jurisdictional level. By 2007, all RN regulatory bodies in Canada, with the exception of Quebec, had used the revised competency document (Jurisdictional Collaborative Project for Entry-level Competencies, Black, 2008). Work is now underway to revise these competencies with the goal of having them used by all RN regulatory bodies in Canada. The competencies for the Canadian Registered Nurse Examination (CRNE) draw on these entry-level competencies. The CRNE is a significant means of reducing barriers to mobility of the nursing workforce across Canada as required by the AIT.

Development of an efficient, affordable approach to competence assessment presents considerable challenge. The reality is that affordable assessment technology is not readily available. If competence assessment is to substitute for credentials as a mechanism for ensuring assessment for practice, the tools must be valid and reliable, and development of these takes both time and money. For example, estimates of the individual cost for assessment of competencies required for certification as an NP range as high as $4,000, not including developmental costs for the process. The question is who should pay—the practitioner, the profession through the regulatory body, or the governments driving this change? This is a significant question because competence-assessment processes must evolve as practice evolves and therefore do not represent a one-time cost.

Mount Royal College (MRC) in Calgary received funding from Health Canada to develop a competence-assessment process. The College now hosts the Internationally Educated Nurse (IEN) Assessment Centre, which is dedicated to assisting nurses educated in other countries to prepare for the RN credentialing process. MRC assesses the professional knowledge, judgment, and skills of IENs and supports them in completing their registration requirements in Alberta. The Western and Northern Health Human Resource Forum, with funding from Health Canada's Internationally Educated Health Professional Initiative, implemented, in collaboration with MRC and the nursing regulatory bodies, the Capacity Building for IEN Assessment Project in the Western and Northern provinces. Nova Scotia is also working with MRC, creating the possibility that, overtime, a consistent pan-Canadian approach to the assessment of IENs will be possible.

Registration Across Borders

As technology increases, the geographic borders of practice begin to disappear. RNs working in call centers, as well as those providing consultation or education services over the Internet, may be providing services to patients in other provinces, territories, or even countries. Canadian nursing regulatory bodies have agreed in principle that, when the nurse and the patient are in two different jurisdictions, the nurse is considered to be practicing in the jurisdiction in which he or she is located. As such, the expectation is that RNs provide these services in a manner consistent with the code of ethics, standards for nursing practice, practice guidelines, and relevant legal authority of the province or territory in which they are registered and practicing. Under this model, RNs must ensure that patients are aware of the nurse's name, professional designation, provincial or territorial regulatory body, and place of work to ensure that the patient has the information required to follow up with the nurse if needed or make a complaint regarding the nurse's practice, if needed (CNA, 2007b).

This approach differs from that being implemented in the United States, where the National Council of State Boards of Nursing agreed to establish a model for multistate recognition of the basic entry-level nursing license for RNs, LPNs, vocational nurses (VNs), and advanced practice nurses. The model, based on the driver's license model, provides for one license only to be issued by the state of the nurse's residence and allows the nurse to practice in other states (remote states) under the authority of the state of residence but the practice requirements of the remote states. Individual states are required to enter into interstate compacts that supersede state laws and may be amended by all party states agreeing and then changing individual state laws. As of May 2011, 24 states had enacted the RN and LPN/VN Licensure Compact with six others pending. To date, only Utah, Iowa, and Texas have passed the Advanced Practice Registered Nurse (APRN) Compact legislation. The rule writing between participating states has not yet begun, no date has been set for the implementation of the APRN Compact, and therefore no nurses are yet participating in this APRN Compact.

Advantages of the one-license concept include reducing barriers to interstate practice, improving tracking for professional conduct purposes, and facilitating interstate commerce (National Council of State Boards of Nursing, 1996–2001). Nurses will be held accountable to the nursing practice laws and other regulations in the state in which the patient is located at the time care is given.

In Australia, in March 2008, the Council of Australian Governments decided to establish a single National Registration and Accreditation Scheme for 10 health professions including nursing and midwifery. This came into effect on July 1, 2010. The Nursing and Midwifery Board of Australia has established state and territory boards to support the work of the national board in the national scheme. The national board will set policy and professional standards, and the state and territory boards will continue to make registration decisions affecting individual nurses and midwives. The new scheme is intended to "help health professionals move around the country more easily, reduce red tape, provide greater safeguards for the public and promote a more flexible, responsive, and sustainable health workforce." For example, the new scheme will maintain a public national register for each health profession that will ensure that a professional who has been banned from practicing in one place is unable to practice elsewhere in Australia (Australia's Health Workforce Online, 2010). Remaining to be seen are what differences, if any, emerge in implementing these different models to facilitate mobility. Of more relevance is that these models signal that regulation must continue to evolve in response to globalization and increased use of technology in health care. In 2001 a large Canadian newspaper printed an editorial titled, "End provincial lock on provincial licenses." Its author maintained that national licensing is the only way to ensure that skilled professionals do not have to "jump through hoops" when they wish to practice their profession in another province or territory. It further suggested that provincial licensing is a waste of time and money. The system of provincial licensing evolved because health, under the Canadian constitution, is a provincial and territorial responsibility, and we continue to see the federal, provincial, and territorial governments struggle with this issue. Is it likely that registered nursing in Canada will move to a national registration system? Perhaps. Is it also likely that the day will come when there will be agreement for nurses to move between countries with licensure or registration only from their home countries? Certainly, there is increasing pressure from the federal government to streamline the process of registration for out-of-country applicants. Significant funds are being directed by the federal government to this issue. If the day does come when nurses move between countries with licensure only from their home countries, as is happening in the European Union, care must be taken to ensure that regulatory responsibilities for activities such as monitoring the competence and conduct of members are not diluted.

Changing Approaches to Regulation

Governments across Canada have been exploring and, in some jurisdictions, implementing new approaches to the regulation of health professions. Driving these changes to legislative frameworks are concerns regarding accountability of professions to the public, turf protection, creation of economic monopolies by self-interested occupational groups, and lack of uniformity in legislation regulating health professions causing confusion for consumers.

Scope of Practice Legislation

Traditional licensing laws provide for exclusive scope of practice or turf protection. As identified earlier in the chapter, governments are beginning to move away from this approach to regulation and toward a model that is the same for all regulated health professions in the jurisdiction. This model includes a broad, nonexclusive scope of practice statement describing what the profession does, the list of reserved acts (also called *controlled acts* or *restricted actions*) that practitioners are authorized to carry out, and protected titles.

Use of broad, nonexclusive scope of practice statements is intended to break down unnecessary practice monopolies that limit a consumer's right to choose a health provider, inhibit access to health care through limiting consumer choice, and increase the cost of health care. Although some may consider that this approach serves the interests of powerful groups such as physicians, employers, and government because of the overlapping roles and the potential to use health professionals differently, others argue that this approach will result in new and exciting roles for RNs.

An example of a nonexclusive scope statement comes from the Ontario Nursing Act (2004) in which the practice of nursing is established as "the promotion of health and the assessment of, the provision of care for and the treatment of health conditions by supportive, preventive, therapeutic, palliative and rehabilitative means in order to attain or maintain optimal function" (p. 3).

The Ontario Nursing Act does not differentiate the scope of practice of RNs and registered practical nurses (known as LPNs in other Canadian jurisdictions) (College of Nurses of Ontario, 2004). In other jurisdictions, the scope of practice of these two nursing groups differs significantly, which poses the following question: Is there one scope of practice for the profession of nursing or is the scope different for each of the three nursing groups?

Within the new regulatory framework being implemented, differentiation of practice occurs primarily through the reserved acts that practitioners are authorized to carry out. Reserved acts are tasks or services performed by a health professional that carry such a significant risk for harm to the health, safety, or well-being of the public that they should be reserved to a particular profession or shared among qualified professions (Health Professions Council, 2001). The intended outcome of reserving only those acts that present a significant risk for harm is to ensure that the focus of professional regulation remains public protection and not the enhancement of professional status or control. The Manitoba Law Reform Commission (1994) identified three factors to evaluate in considering the seriousness of a threatened harm:

- Likelihood of its occurrence
- Significance of its consequences on individual victims
- Number of people it threatens.

Examples of controlled acts that RNs in Ontario are authorized to carry out include performing a prescribed procedure below the dermis or a mucous membrane; administering a substance by injection or inhalation; and putting an instrument, hand, or finger beyond the external ear canal, beyond the point in the nasal passages where they normally narrow, and beyond the larynx.

Procedures below the dermis include cleaning, soaking, irrigating, probing, debriding, packing, dressing, and performing venipuncture to establish peripheral intravenous access and maintain patency of the vessel using a solution of normal saline (0.9%), in circumstances in which the individual requires medical attention and delaying venipuncture is likely to be harmful to the individual.

Regulations under the Ontario Nursing Act set out the conditions under which RNs may initiate and carry out these acts. Legislation in British Columbia and Alberta is similar in its specificity. Important questions for consideration are: What impact will this specificity have on the ability of RNs to practice to the full scope of their competence? Can regulations be revised with sufficient frequency to reflect changes in practice? Does legislation such as this reduce nursing to a list of tasks and procedures? Will this approach to regulation ensure public safety while enhancing consumer choice? These questions remain unanswered.

Umbrella Legislation

The changing regulatory approach brings with it a changing legislative framework. Historically, every profession has had its own act that developed overtime in response to the needs of the profession and the public it served. The British Columbia Royal Commission on Healthcare and Costs (1991) concluded that, in British Columbia, lack of consistency in professional acts contributes to insufficient accountability to the public and that lack of uniformity in the structure, organization, and language of statutes results in confusion for the public. The same conclusions can be drawn from a review of health professions legislation across Canada. For example, in some jurisdictions, some regulatory bodies are called colleges while others are called associations. In Alberta, Alberta Association of Registered Nurses, coming under the HPA, became CARNA. Processes related to managing complaints from the public vary among professions, as do the legislated responsibilities of regulatory bodies.

Umbrella legislation, seen by some as a mechanism to address these issues, has been implemented in Ontario, Alberta, and British Columbia and has received royal assent in Manitoba. Different approaches to umbrella legislation range from one act for all professions to individual acts for each profession with parallel legislative language. The Ontario model relies on the Regulated Health Professions Act to set out the overall guidelines for the health professions, with each profession having its own satellite act. In British Columbia and Alberta, there is no provision for satellite acts. Instead, the requirements unique to each profession are set out in regulations under the act. It remains to be seen what differences in regulatory outcomes, if any, emerge from these differing models. On one hand, there may be more consistency in public policy as it relates to governance of health professions, and the public may be better able to understand how to get assistance with problems. On the other hand, the one-size-fits-all approach may be ineffective in addressing the differing issues of new and established professions and considering how differences in clinical practice should be reflected in regulation of the professions.

Public Participation in Regulation

It should come as no surprise that the public wants to play an increasingly active role in the regulation of health professions. Consumers believe that their complaints about the healthcare system are not heard, and the increased focus on "customers" in the private sector is beginning to spill over into the government and not-for-profit sector. In the 1970s, the Registered Nurses Association of British Columbia became one of the first to appoint public representatives to its board of directors. Today, most nursing regulatory bodies have, on their boards or councils, public representatives appointed by the government. In Ontario, public representatives make up just fewer than 50% of board members.

Public representation on the boards of regulatory bodies is an important public accountability mechanism as well as a means of ensuring that the public interest is served by the boards' decisions. For a profession to be truly self-regulating, public representatives should not exceed 50% of the membership of the board of directors. Even in this situation, an issue that polarizes the nurse representatives on the board can result in the public representatives being the decision makers on a significant nursing practice policy issue. In March 2001, the Ontario Health Professions Regulatory Advisory Committee (HPRAC) completed a review of the Regulated Health Professions Act and concluded that self-governance should be maintained by keeping professional members on boards in the majority. The HPRAC maintained that increased accountability for governing professions in the public interest "can be achieved through methods other than changing the mix of elected and appointed members and moving away from self-regulation" (Health Professions Regulatory Advisory Committee [HPRAC], 2001, p. 45). Contrast this with the view from the United Kingdom that "The Government is convinced that in order to establish and sustain confidence in the independence of regulators, all councils should be constituted to ensure that professionals do not form a majority" (The Secretary of State for Health, 2007). In

2008, changes to the governing legislation for the Nursing and Midwifery Council for England, Wales, Scotland, Northern Ireland, and the Islands changed the composition of the council to include seven registrant members and seven lay members, all appointed by government.

Essential to the success of public representation is that public representatives can meaningfully articulate the public perspective. Of concern is the practice noted in some jurisdictions of board appointments being based on political affiliation rather than on criteria, such as knowledge, abilities, and commitment to fulfill the public role as well as criteria that will ensure geographic, cultural, and demographic diversity. Also of concern is the orientation received by public representatives. Typically, the regulatory bodies assume responsibility for orientation. Although the regulatory bodies are best positioned to do this in relation to regulatory and profession specific issues, government must play a role in ensuring that public representatives are knowledgeable about their roles on boards and have access to information and other supports.

Challenges to Regulatory Authority

Challenges to the authority of regulatory bodies come from many sources. At the time of labor strife, governments and the public may question whether leaving decisions regarding the standards for entry to the profession has implications for the potential size of the labor pool and hence the wages that can be demanded. Others suggest that allowing regulatory bodies to establish education requirements can result in "credential creep," or increasing the academic credentials required for entry to a profession, which serves only to improve the status of the profession and has no direct impact on the outcome of care service provided by the profession. In 2003, the Conference of Federal/Provincial/Territorial Deputy Ministers of Health put in place a process to establish principles and policies to assist government to determine whether a change for a request in an entry to practice education credentials is based on a comprehensive, impartial process that would serve the interest of patient care and the effectiveness of healthcare delivery in the jurisdiction.

Some suggest that regulatory bodies entrench barriers to registration to ensure the required need for the regulatory body itself. The truth is that regulation does pose barriers—barriers that are intended to protect the public served by the regulatory body. The question that must always be asked is whether the regulatory body has achieved the appropriate balance in safeguarding the interests of the public and those of the profession. This is likely, in part, why the Ontario and Manitoba governments have appointed fairness commissioners with a mandate of ensuring that regulatory bodies' registration processes are transparent, objective, impartial, and fair. Similarly, the Nova Scotia government passed the *Fair Registration Practices Act* in 2008. Also established by government, in British Columbia and Ontario respectively, are the Health Professions Review Board and the Health Professions Appeal and Review Board, which have the authority to review registration and inquiry/complaints decisions. While regulatory bodies may have concerns related to the human and financial resources required to respond to these external bodies, most welcome the opportunity to review and improve their processes. Increasingly, regulators must be seen as transparent, flexible, and responsive and a benefit to the public in fulfilling their public protection mandate. If they are not, they risk becoming irrelevant and jeopardizing the future of nursing self-regulation.

SUMMARY

This chapter addresses the purpose of and issues associated with the regulation of nursing in Canada. Nursing regulation has evolved significantly since first set in motion in the early 1900s. The impact of globalization, evolving regulatory frameworks, and new roles for RNs will ensure that regulation in nursing is dynamic in meeting the healthcare needs of Canadians. The great unknown is how regulation will evolve and whether in its evolution it will serve to not only protect the public interest but also contribute to the advancement of the profession.

Add to your knowledge of this issue: *Online*

The Canadian Nurses Association	**www.cna-nurses.ca**
The International Council of Nurses	**www.icn.ch**
Provincial and Territorial Organizations	
Association of Registered Nurses of Prince Edward Island	**www.arnpei.ca**
Association of Registered Nurses of Newfoundland and Labrador	**www.arnnl.nf.ca**
College and Association of Registered Nurses of Alberta	**www.nurses.ab.ca**
College of Nurses of Ontario	**www.cno.org**
College of Registered Nurses of British Columbia	**www.crnbc.ca**
College of Registered Nurses of Manitoba	**www.crnm.mb.ca**
College of Registered Nurses of Nova Scotia	**www.crnns.ca**
Nurses Association of New Brunswick	**www.nanb.nb.ca**
Ordre des Infirmières et Infirmiers du Québec	**www.oiiq.org**
Registered Nurses Association of the Northwest Territories and Nunavut	**www.rnantnu.ca**
Registered Nurses Association of Ontario	**www.rnao.org**
Saskatchewan Registered Nurses Association	**www.srna.org**
Yukon Registered Nurses Association	**www.yrna.ca**

R E F L E C T I O N S *on the Chapter...*

1 Examine the legislation that regulates nursing practice and education in your province or territory and highlight the similarities and differences you note with other provinces and territories

2 Identify at least one issue in nursing practice that you would describe as a regulatory issue. What strategies would you formulate to address this issue?

3 What are some of the viewpoints you have heard from practicing nurses regarding regulation? What is your analysis of the differences in opinions?

4 What are the advantages and disadvantages of regulation of nursing practice and the registration of nurses?

5 How does the regulation of nursing practice compare to the regulation of healthcare professionals and other professionals?

6 Formulate and support a stance regarding the use of umbrella legislation to regulate health professions.

Want to know more? Visit thePoint for additional helpful resources:

- Journal Articles
- Learning Objectives
- Nursing Professional Roles and Responsibilities
- Bonus chapters:
  - Health and Nursing Policy: A Matter of Politics, Power and Professionalism
  - The NP Movement: Recurring Issues
  - When Difference Matters: The Politics of Privilege and Marginality

References

Association of Registered Nurses of British Columbia. (2011). [Online]. Retrieved from http://www.arnbc.ca/index.aspx

Australia's Health Workforce Online. (2010). [Online]. *National registration and accreditation.* Retrieved from http://www.ahwo.gov.au/natreg.asp

British Columbia Royal Commission on Healthcare and Costs. (1991). *Closer to home.* Victoria, BC: Province of British Columbia.

Canadian Nurses Association (CNA). (1968). *The leaf and the lamp.* Ottawa, ON: Author.

———. (1997). *National nursing competency project.* Ottawa, ON: Author.

———. (2007a). *Position statement: Canadian regulatory framework for registered nurses.* Ottawa, ON: Author.

———. (2007b). *Position statement: Telehealth: The role of the nurse.* Ottawa, ON: Author.

College of Nurses of Ontario. (2004). *Legislation and regulation. RHPA: Scope of practice, controlled acts model.* Toronto, ON: Author.

Cutshall, P. (1998). Regulating nursing: A new chapter begins. *Nursing BC, 30*(3), 35–38.

End provincial lock on professional licenses. (2001, January 18). *The Vancouver Sun,* p. A14.

Finocchio, L.J., Dower, C.M., McMahon, T., Gragnola, C.M., & The Task Force On Health Care Workforce Regulation. (1995). *Reforming healthcare workforce regulation: Policy considerations for the 21st century.* San Francisco, CA: Pew Health Professions Commission.

Health Professions Council. (2001). *Shared scope of practice working paper* [Online]. Retrieved from http://www.hlth.gov.bc.ca/leg/hpc/review/shascope.html

Health Professions Regulatory Advisory Committee. (2001). *Adjusting the balance: A review of the Regulated Health Professions Act* [Online]. Retrieved from http://www.hprac.org/downloads/fyr/RHPAReport.pdf

International Council of Nurses. (1985). *Report on the regulation of nursing: A report on the present, a position for the future.* Geneva: Author.

Jurisdictional Collaborative Project for Entry-level Competencies, Black, et al. (2008). Competencies in the context of entry-level registered nurse practice: A collaborative project in Canada. *International Nursing Review, 55*(2), 171–178.

Kerr, J.R. (1996). Credentialing in nursing. In J.R. Kerr & J. MacPhail (Eds.), *Canadian nursing: Issues and perspectives* (3rd ed., pp. 363–372). New York: Mosby.

Kerr, M. (1944). *Brief history of the Registered Nurses' Association of British Columbia.* Vancouver, BC: Author.

Manitoba Law Reform Commission. (1994). *Regulating professions and occupations.* Winnipeg, MB: Author.

National Council of State Boards of Nursing. (2011) *Nurse licensure compact. Fact sheet for licensees and nursing students* [Online]. Retrieved from https://www.ncsbn.org/2011_NLCA_factsheet_students_Rev_Jan_2011.pdf

Registered Nurses Association of British Columbia. (2000). *The regulation of nursing: Statement of principles.* Vancouver, BC: Author.

———. (2001). *Canadian registered nurse endorsement document.* Vancouver, BC: Author.

Risk, M. (1992). Regulatory issues. In A.J. Baumgart & J. Larsen (Eds.), *Canadian nursing faces the future* (2nd ed., pp. 365–379). Toronto, ON: Mosby.

Styles, M.M., & Affara, A.A. (1997). *ICN on regulation: Towards 21st century models.* Geneva: International Council of Nurses.

Secretary of State for Health. (2007). *Trust, assurance and safety—The regulation of health professionals in the 21st century.* London: The Stationary Office.

Nurses' Unions: Where Knowledge Meets Know-How

Pat Armstrong and Linda Silas

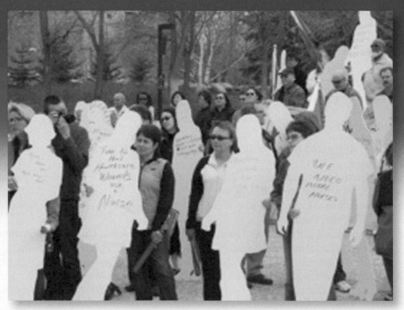

"Where are all the nurses?" Nurses at a 2008 rally in Alberta for National Nursing Week hold cardboard cutouts of nurses representing cut and unfilled nursing positions. (Used with permission of the Canadian Federation of Nurses Unions. Photographer Keith Wiley.)

Critical Questions

As a way of engaging with the ideas in this chapter, consider the following:

1. How do you understand the difference between the mandate for collective bargaining organizations and professional associations and colleges?

2. What assumptions do you hold about the relationships between nursing as a profession and nurses as members of collective bargaining units or unions?

3. Attitudes toward collective bargaining vary significantly from province to province and territory to territory in Canada. What do you already know about the nature of your province or territory that might influence these attitudes?

4. Consider what changes within society and in the nursing profession, as you understand it, might contribute to the changing face of unions and collective bargaining.

Chapter Objectives

After completing this chapter, you will be able to:

1. Understand the historical background of nursing and nurses' unions in Canada.

2. Understand the role of collective bargaining and of nurses' unions.

(continued on page 159)

Chapter Objectives (continued)

3. Articulate and analyze issues that arise in nurses' workplaces.

4. State past and current barriers to workplace representation.

5. Formulate strategies to resolve nurses' workplace issues.

For well over a century, nurses in Canada have worked together to improve conditions not only for themselves but also for those in their care. It has not been a smooth or uncontentious ride. Today, the overwhelming majority of nurses belong to a union and many also participate in other collective organizations. New issues are continually emerging and old ones linger. This chapter is about why nurses are highly unionized and what unionization means in nursing today.

The chapter begins by tracing the historical developments that have shaped collective organization among nurses. The direction and content of this chapter are based on the assumption that in order to fully understand nursing and its organizations today, we have to understand forces that operate at global, national, and local levels. In addition, it is important to understand forces within medicine that have influenced the demographics of nursing, how nursing is done, and why nurses formed unions. Politics and economics have played a role in shaping this understanding. So have physicians and ideas about both gender and healthcare. It is no accident that the overwhelming majority of nurses are women; nor is it accidental that nurses have turned to unions to protect themselves and their conditions for providing care.

After setting the stage, this chapter then moves on to look at nursing today. Given that over 80% of nurses belong to unions, it is important to understand the structure and organization of these unions. It is equally important to understand the current context for healthcare services, because this context influences not only how unions operate but also the issues they need to address on behalf of nurses and those in their care. While there are some new political and economic forces at work, there are also many old ideas and pressures that continue to structure healthcare, nursing, and nursing unions today.

HISTORICAL INFLUENCES

The nursing schools established in the late 19th-century Canada can themselves be understood as a form of collective action and resistance by women. Florence Nightingale was undoubtedly the single most important woman in that struggle, although she was certainly not alone. In mid 19th-century England, a woman of her class was expected to seek marriage and, in that marriage, to be obedient and passive. Nightingale used her class position to initiate the first nursing schools, after she had refused marriage, opposed her family, and exposed herself to the conditions of the Crimean War.

Of course, women were nursing in Canada long before nursing schools in the Nightingale tradition were established. Aboriginal women practiced midwifery and provided most of the care, commonly saving the lives of the white men who came from abroad to exploit the natural resources (Van Kirk, 1980). Jeanne Mance is recognized as being the first lay nurse to practice in North America. She is also known as one of the founders of Montreal and the founder of its first hospital, the Hôtel-Dieu de Montréal, built in 1645 (Library and Archives Canada [LAC], 2005). She served as a hospital administrator until her death in 1673. There were also nuns who worked in hospitals from the time the French settled in Canada. Indeed, the training systems they developed became models for care before Nightingale (Nelson, 2001).

The St. Catherines, nursing school, Ontario, established in 1874 by a physician and two Nightingale nurses, marked a significant change (Coburn, 1987, p. 447). It sought to meet "the desperate need of nursing services in Canada as well as of establishing nursing as a respectable profession for women," based on formal education in nursing skills (Coburn, 1987, p. 448). This successful school coincided with rapid industrialization and new developments in healthcare that contributed both to the expansion of hospital care and its effectiveness. "The emergence of the 'trained' nurse followed dramatic changes such as surgery, new diagnostic tools, and other medical techniques successfully undertaken in the hospital setting" (Keddy & Dodd, 2005, p. 440). The development of nursing schools also coincided with increasing activism among women in the prosperous classes who had lots of time to do good work, including the promotion of skilled care by women. At the same time, governments became more active in delivering care; thus, public hospitals became increasingly involved in educating nurses who provided labor in return for education.

One of the most notable examples of developments in nursing was the founding of the Victorian Order of Nurses (VON) by Lady Ishbel Aberdeen, wife of Canada's then governor-general, Lord Aberdeen. At a meeting for the National Council for Women in Halifax, Nova Scotia, Lady Aberdeen was asked to create an order of visiting nurses in Canada to respond to the desperate need for medical care for families in rural areas and rapidly developing cities and towns (Victorian Order of Nurses [VON], 2004). The services provided by the VON have helped Canada through many historical events, including both World Wars and the Halifax Explosion. VON nurses, who are represented by provincial and territorial nurses' unions, continue to be well known for their dedication to community building and homecare. Due to its charitable status, the VON's work relies on a large number of volunteers in addition to staff, and they remain dedicated to providing universal, not-for-profit healthcare.

Although the work of activists improved the skills and reputations of nurses, and even some of their working conditions, most nurses were working up to 14 hours a day in return for room, board, a small allowance, and education (Keddy & Dodd, 2005). In Montreal in 1889, the few graduate nurses employed were paid less than the hospital's rat catcher (Coburn, 1987). Some graduate nurses worked as supervisors if they were single or widowed, typically living in the hospital where their life was their work and their pay suggested religious devotion rather than reward for a day's work. Other graduate nurses were employed in private homes, although these women were single or widowed as well. Married women were not likely to be hired, and there was nothing preventing employers from refusing to hire them.

Hospitals were organized along hierarchical lines—not surprising given the tradition established by military and religious organizations. The male physicians were in charge. Indeed, they significantly outnumbered the nurses. In 1901, the census recorded 208 student and graduate nurses, compared to 5,000 physicians (Coburn, 1987). The training emphasis was on establishing nurses' respectability as well as their skills, reflecting both the influence of the upper class women reformers and women's subordinate status in the larger society. Given that students became the primary hospital nursing labor force after only 3 years of training, that graduate nurses often worked in private homes, that male physicians were in charge, and that ideas about female respectability dominated, it is not surprising that nurses were unable to join together to rebel.

ORGANIZING PRACTICES OF PROFESSIONAL NURSES

As their numbers and jobs grew, however, nurses started to work together for more than recognized training schools. The first recorded collective opposition was in 1878, when a group of Nightingale nurses threatened to return to England unless the Montreal General Hospital improved their working conditions (Canadian Federation of Nurses Unions [CFNU], n.d.). Such action was rare, however. Not surprisingly, their primary model for organizing was based on the model used by physicians. Long before most of their techniques were effective, physicians had started organizing to defend their interests and to establish standards for education (Naylor, 1986). By the beginning of the 20th century, the allopathic physicians had been largely successful in controlling who became a physician, by establishing their power within health services, and by requiring university education. They were also successful in convincing others that their organizations were about public interests rather than personal ones. Abraham Flexner, writing a report on North American medical schools that was profoundly influential in 20th-century health services, claimed that professions are intellectual disciplines, taught in educational institutions, based on a body of knowledge that is practical rather than theoretical, organized internationally, and perhaps most importantly, motivated by altruism. However, Flexner made it clear that nurses did not meet the criteria (Kerr, 1988); they were less esteemed than physicians.

One important leader in organizing nurses was Mary Agnes Snively, a Toronto nursing superintendent who worked regularly with physicians. She was primarily concerned with achieving legitimacy, power, and autonomy along the lines the physicians had already established (Mansell & Dodd, 2005). Snively held the position of Lady Superintendent of Nurses at the Toronto General Hospital's School of Nursing from 1884 to 1910. She began by working with others of her rank to organize alumnae associations, providing the basis for later formation of the Graduate Nurses Association of Ontario. Each province but Prince Edward Island had formed provincial associations by 1914 (Mansell & Dodd, 2005). The 1907 Canadian Society of Training Schools for Nurses became the Canadian Association of Nursing Education, which, in turn, created the Canadian National Association of Trained Nurses [CNATN] (1908) and, in 1924, the Canadian Nurses Association (CNA). The CNA, then, was organized primarily by nursing managers and teachers, although the structure allowed for representation of nurses in private duty, in public health, and in hospitals (Mansell & Dodd, 2005). While the CNATN sought "mutual understanding and unity among nurses in Canada" (Mussallem, 1988, p. 401), it also wanted to create a high standard of education and professional honor (Jensen, 1992). The CNA worked to control who could practice and what they would learn. They also wanted schools devoted to "the education of the nurse, and not as under the present system, to lessening the cost of nursing in the hospitals" (Mussallem, 1988, p. 403).

Just as the Crimean War had helped legitimate Nightingale and the other nurses who provided care there, so too did Canadian nurses gain leverage based on their work in World Wars I and II (WWI and WWII). Wars made the contributions of nursing visible, contributed to shortages at home, and enhanced women's sense of their own power. In WWI, military nurses "received the rank of lieutenant, along with all the advantages of rank: Salary, leaves, retirement plan" (Allard, 2005, p. 157), and the recognition of their work was a factor in the success of nursing organizations in the period immediately after the war. Similar patterns are evident during and after WWII.

This is not to argue for war as a strategy for improving the reputation of and conditions for nursing. Rather, it is to stress the importance of taking context into account in understanding strategies for change. In spite of their enhanced reputations, nurses found it very hard to find employment after the 1929 stock market crash that marked the beginning of the Great Depression. One report estimated that "40 percent of the private duty nurses in Canada were almost continuously unemployed and another 20 percent were only employed intermittently" (Toman, 2005, p. 176). Until the end of WWII, 60% of nurses were in private duty, usually working in private homes, making collective organization difficult (Richardson, 2005, p. 213).

It is important to note that nurses' associations were not nearly as successful as physicians' associations in their search for control over admission to their profession. Although their lobbying was successful in getting registration and the recognition of the title "registered nurse" (RN) in all provinces by 1922, the first mandatory registration was not introduced until the 1950s (Kerr, 1988). After years of effort, they only had a small degree of self-regulation and did not have the power to police their own (Mansell & Dodd, 2005, p. 202). It took just as long to end the dependence on student labor and develop schools that did not involve free labor. Even when employing strategies similar to those used by physicians, efforts did not bring the power and prestige nurses sought. This was likely because physicians' power did not result primarily from their skills, their education, or the nature of their work. Rather, it mainly followed from their effective organization, their class, their position in the health hierarchy, and their gender. Even though nurses managed to meet all Flexner's criteria for professionalization when they officially adopted the International Council of Nurses' (ICN) code of ethics in 1955, they still did not have nearly the pay, prestige, autonomy, or power that physicians had (Mansell & Dodd, 2005). Nursing was characterized by long or split shifts. It was still a low paid, insecure profession, with few vacations and benefits, no job security, and little protection from the whims of employers and supervisors.

In short, nurses were busy doing more than caring for patients in the century from the 1850s to the 1950s. They worked together to establish nursing schools and the regulation of nursing, which in turn helped ensure standards of care and enhance the reputation of nursing. They were supported in their efforts by the growing demand for skilled nurses in the wake of industrial expansion, urbanization, and new techniques in medical care. However, they were limited by physicians' power, the organization of hospitals, and the extensive use of private care, as well as by ideas about women and the lack of legal or other protections for their paid work. It was mainly the women superintending the nursing students and those teaching them, along with those working in public health, who organized in professional associations that followed the model set by physicians. These associations were eventually successful in reaching most of the criteria said to define a profession, but they were much less successful in achieving the power, prestige, pay, and autonomy that other professions enjoyed. Clearly, these criteria were not the only critical factors. Indeed, war was almost as important as the nursing schools and associations in enhancing nurses' power and pay.

EMERGENCE OF UNION PRACTICES

WWII, in particular, marked a major turning point for Canada, for women, for our healthcare system, and for the nurses who worked in it. The war ended the Great Depression and Canadians emerged from it to jobs, with a new faith in government and demands for more public services and more human rights. One of those demands was for public health services. They sought access to the medical advances developed during the war that made hospitals safer places that could provide effective care (Armstrong & Armstrong, 2003). Women joined the labor force and the military in large numbers during the war, earning significantly better wages than they had before and gaining experiences that made many unwilling to return to prewar inequities (Armstrong & Armstrong, 2001). Nurses, too, wanted better conditions and more equitable treatment. A number of factors contributed to both their increasing demands and their move to achieve them through unionization.

TRANSFORMATIONS IN HEALTH CARE

First, hospitals expanded and the demand for nurses grew. When after the war, the federal government failed to get provinces to agree on a national healthcare plan, it instead invested in hospital construction and training for physicians and nurses. In 1941, the census recorded 26,626 graduate nurses. By 1961, when public hospital insurance was in place, there were 61,553 of them. The number of nurses-in-training also doubled during this 20-year period (Dominion Bureau of Statistics, 1961). Most of these graduate nurses were employed in hospitals rather than in private homes, and they now outnumbered the supervisors and teachers significantly. Working together allowed them to share their concerns, and working as general duty nurses gave them experiences that were different from most of the nurses who had formed the associations.

TRANSFORMATIONS IN UNIONS

Unions were growing rapidly and achieving considerable success. "Between 1939 and 1945, the number of organized workers doubled" (White, 1993, p. 49). Although unions had been organized in Canada since the 19th century, it was not until the war that unions won legal recognition and established the formal procedures for certification that indicated legal recognition. Labor shortages added to their strength. Employers were required to recognize a union that represented a majority of its employees and were required to bargain in good faith with the recognized union. Collective bargaining, the process of negotiating terms and conditions of work between an employer and a union, became entrenched in industrial relations. In 1944, the year that emergency Order-in-Council P.C. 1003 legislation was passed, the CNA approved collective bargaining in principle (McIntyre & McDonald, 2006) and recommended that the provincial associations be certified as bargaining agents.

Unions not only grew, but their composition changed significantly. Government employees, many of whom defined themselves as professionals and many of whom were women, started to demand real collective bargaining rights. Prohibited from negotiating contracts on the grounds that their work was essential, public sector employees became increasingly restless as they saw gains made by private sector unions for people in similar jobs. Public servants in Quebec led the way by striking illegally in the 1960s, winning the right to bargain and even strike. By 1975, those in other provinces gained the right to bargain collectively too, although the right to strike was not granted in all provinces (White, 1993). Half of the unionized workers were in the public sector and the majority of these were women. Perhaps surprisingly to those who think of unions as defending private interests, the union movement in Canada has long supported programs such as public education that would promote the general good. In the period after WWII, unions became particularly active in supporting public healthcare services.

Lay nurses in Quebec had formed a union as early as 1939. Following the 1946 Quebec Nurses' Act that provided for collective bargaining, they organized a union with assistance from the Quebec Federation of Labour (Richardson, 2005). They, like nurses who were part of government bargaining units, saw their wages rise and conditions improve as a result. But they did not win these improvements without a struggle. Although the threat of a strike was enough to gain concessions from one Montreal hospital in 1962, a year later, nurses in the same city went on strike for 30 days before winning not only better salaries and working conditions but also the right to negotiate workloads and to apply the Rand formula. (CFNU, 2003). This, now widely accepted formula, requires all non-management employees in a unionized environment to pay dues, regardless of their union status. Some part-time, casual, and term employees, for example, are not unionized, but since they stand to benefit from the union's efforts, they are also required to pay dues. Such funding strengthens the union by providing economic stability.

CNA INFLUENCES ON THE MOVE TO UNIONIZATION

The CNA did not initially support unionization, and in 1946 passed a resolution against "any nurse going on strike at any time for any cause" (Richardson, 2005, p. 215). The organization did recognize that the poor conditions of work and pay required some action. In jurisdictions that prohibited provincial associations from acting as legal bargaining agents when they included managers in their membership, the CNA suggested associations establish a group to serve as their certifiable bargaining committee and a labor relations committee. The CNA offered advice through its own committee and through a labor consultant. There were several reasons why this was not a very satisfactory solution.

Perhaps most importantly, these collective bargaining agents had nothing to back up their requests. As Joan Harte, former provincial vice president of the Newfoundland and Labrador Nurses' Union (NLNU) explained in an interview about her experiences before unionization, "We had no power because we were not organized to bargain...nurses were getting whatever government wanted to give us because we had no power; we weren't a union" (Andrews, 1993, p. 1). "When we became a staff association we negotiated and got some things on paper, but we had no power to enforce provisions" (Andrews, 1993, p. 3). The things they won on paper disappeared in practice. With voluntary dues and membership, the association also lacked a firm financial base and evidence of commitment to bargaining agent negotiations. In addition, there were disagreements within the associations between those who did managerial work and those who did general duty nursing. Such disagreements weakened their overall position. The fact that other bargaining units were getting more benefits was something else under scrutiny. As Christine Kavanaugh, former Employment Relations Officer in the Prince Edward Island Nurses' Union put it, "the real catalysts [*sic*] was that nurses who were unionized in the civil service a year or two earlier had gotten significant increases, better working conditions, and pensions" (Andrews, 1993, p. 13). In some case, as Madelaine Steeves, former President of the New Brunswick Nurses Union (NBNU) explained, RNs "actually found themselves behind in salary compared to co-workers they were responsible for...I was an operating nurse and I would be in a theatre with an OR [operating room] technician who make [*sic*] more per hour than I did and I was responsible for her, the patient, and the theatre" (Andrews, 1993, p. 20). The issues nurses faced were difficult to address in associations that represented both management and workers and that opposed action against employers. These issues went beyond pay and pensions. In hospitals, lack of protection for patients and reporting mechanisms for nurses who tried to stand up for patients were of significant concern. "Nurses were caught in some really difficult employment situations—threats, intimidation," and "there was no onus on the employer to follow standards" (Steeves in Andrews, 1993, p. 22).

The CNA support for collective bargaining helped introduce nurses to union-like activities while its opposition to action (e.g., strike or other methods) drove momentum toward unionization. Nurses' lack of success in trying to improve working conditions and wages with the help of CNA pushed nurses further toward unionization. Then the law relating to unions changed. In 1973, the Supreme Court ruled that the Saskatchewan Registered Nurses Association could not represent nurses in collective bargaining because nurse managers were members of the governing body of the association, creating an inherent conflict of interest (Richardson, 2005). Nurses in Ontario already had separate bodies, and nurses in other provinces had begun to act more like unions by taking various kinds of actions against their employers when the CNA personnel policy approach failed (Andrews, 1993). Thus, the Supreme Court decision reinforced a trend that had already begun. After the decision, many associations helped establish independent nurses' unions and within a decade (by 1978) all provinces except Prince Edward Island and Quebec had one. In that same year, CNA drafted a code of ethics that would imply nurses' strikes were unethical because they placed self-interest, high wages, and improved working conditions before the needs of patients (CFNU, n.d.). Nurses' unions across the country eventually won the right to strike after many long and arduous struggles.

Led by the Saskatchewan Union of Nurses (SUN), the NLNU, and the PEINU, a committee was formed to discuss the potential organizational structure, funding, and constitutional provisions that would be needed to create a national organization to represent the voice of unionized nurses. Discussions, which began in 1978, led to the founding convention of the CFNU in April 1981. The CFNU allows nurses to share their skills and experiences and to develop national strategies related to their work. For example, the CFNU has taken a leadership role in the Canadian Health Coalition, an organization that works to defend and expand public health services. The

> **BOX 9.1**   Canadian Federation of Nurses Unions Mission Statement
>
> The birth of the CFNU in 1981 marked a new era for interaction among nurses' unions in Canada and provided a united front for action on problems that directly or indirectly affected the unionized nurses and the quality of healthcare.
>
> The rebirth of CFNU in 1999 as the national affiliating body for nurses to the CLC marks another era for nursing unions in Canada. Through this formalized relationship we have deepened and expanded our involvement and influence on the national labor scene.
>
> The core purpose of CFNU is to be a proactive, unifying national voice for quality health care and the socioeconomic welfare of nurses and others.
>
> CFNU is driven by the core values of democracy, collectivity, action, social justice, inclusion, and advocacy.
>
> CFNU's vision of the future is to become both a truly strong national organization for unionized nurses, representing all nursing unions in Canada, and part of a world voice for unionized nurses. We will have both the capacity and the influence as the experts on quality health care and health care policy.
>
> The strategic focus of CFNU will be on building a strong, clear, unified, national voice for the role of nurses, the protection and preservation of public health care, the advocacy of social justice and equity, and the development of an international network and international solidarity.

CFNU has also worked internationally with unions in other countries to collaborate on strategies for health care change.

Beginning with a mission statement (Box 9.1), the CFNU's constitution outlines the structure of the organization, its members, and its officials. The constitution explains that CFNU shall be governed by a National Executive Board when the convention is not in session and that the board shall comprise a president and secretary treasurer who are elected by membership at convention and national officers who are the presidents and or vice presidents of provincial nurses' unions. Currently, the following provincial unions and their members hold membership with CFNU: The PEINU, the NLNU, the Nova Scotia Nurses' Union (NSNU), the NBNU, the Ontario Nurses' Association (ONA), the Manitoba Nurses Union (MNU), the SUN, the United Nurses of Alberta (UNA), and the British Columbia Nurses' Union (BCNU). A recent addition to the National Executive Board is the President of the Canadian Nursing Students' Association (CNSA). Provincial unions and the CFNU are entirely funded by dues-paying members. While CFNU has a broad mandate to protect the health of patients and the national health system, and to promote nurses and the nursing profession at the national level, provincial unions focus more on workplace administration of collective agreements, grievances and occupational health and safety, and, of course, collective bargaining.

CHANGES IN NURSES' THINKING ABOUT COLLECTIVE BARGAINING

Unionization of nurses both reflected and reinforced a major shift in ideas about the public sector, professions, nursing, and women's work. Until the 1960s, those employed in the public sector were called civil servants, in part because it was widely assumed that they were dedicated to the public good and guided by that commitment as well as protected by a benevolent government. Professionals maintained they were governed by ethical considerations that would preclude forming organizations to defend their interests and unions were often seen as instruments of self-interest. For nurses, the notion of commitment to patients was combined with ideas about women's submission to others and about the value linked to professions. These perceptions undermined progress in the profession as nurses were constantly associated as akin to mothers, saints, and servants.

THE GENDERED NATURE OF ISSUES SURROUNDING COLLECTIVE BARGAINING

As Christine Kavanaugh explained (Andrews, 1993, p. 12), "the idea of nurses unionizing was considered demeaning" and those who unionized were seen as "less compassionate." This idea partly reflected an association in their minds with violence, with ideas that unions "are nasty, they damage homes, they threaten people in their homes," as Joan Harte put it (in Andrews, 1993, p. 4). The idea reflected preconceptions of a "woman's place." Harte recalls "a lot of interference from husbands and boyfriends telling their wives and girlfriends what was good for them and what wasn't…There was a lot of patronizing attitudes from hospitals, employers, treasury boards, husbands—everybody" (Andrews, 1993, p. 12). Until the mid-1970s, nurses were discouraged from questioning their working conditions or salaries. There were neither laws prohibiting employers from firing women when they got married or pregnant nor laws requiring women to be paid on the same basis as men, in part because it was assumed women would be supported financially by men.

All of this had started to change right after WWII, but the big transitions took place in the 1960s and 1970s—especially during the height of the women's movement. The relationship between the women's movement and nursing is complex, and, from a historical perspective, it has often been characterized by contradiction and conflict (Bunting & Campbell, 1990). Although this chapter will not explore this relationship in depth, it is valuable to note that the two—nursing and the feminist movement—have impacted each other in significant ways, though not always positively. Despite the fact that some believe the relationship should have been mutually enhancing, thanks to so many shared understandings between the two groups, particularly their common belief in a holistic approach to women's healthcare (McBride, 1984), feminists have often criticized nursing for a lack of commitment to women's movements (Bunting & Campbell, 1990) and nurses have criticized the feminist movement for ignoring and devaluing their work. Hunt's (1998) review of nursing and feminism's "turbulent history" offers a possible explanation: "A fear of feminism related to negative stereotyping and discrimination against feminist nurses, and the fear of losing nursing's 'caring' aspects, are some reasons why nurses did not want to be labeled as feminists. Ironically, this 'caring' aspect is thought to be the reason feminists have often excluded nurses." This, along with differing experiences and reactions to patriarchy in medicine and society in general, provide us with a sense of where tensions lay during those formative years.

Meanwhile, in the workplaces, public sector employees began recognizing that they would have to become more assertive if they were to match conditions and pay with their private sector counterparts. Commitment did not pay the rent, and governments were not necessarily good employers. The character of unions changed as many more professionals became union members. During this period, women moved into the labor force in large numbers, primarily because they needed the pay but also because many wanted the other rewards of paid jobs (Armstrong & Armstrong, 2001). Women also began entering universities in large numbers, having won battles to gain more equity in access and in financial support. Nursing education was moved from hospitals, where nurses provided much of the free labor and where they were closely supervised in residences, to colleges and universities where they enjoyed more freedom and saw more challenges to old ideas. Experiences with discrimination in both education and paid work in turn contributed to their dissatisfaction with the old inequities in the workforce and in unions. Feminists in and out of unions successfully fought not only for the right to their jobs after marriage and pregnancy and for access to birth control but also for paid maternity leave. Within unions they fought for equality as well as for women's issues to be placed high on the agenda (White, 1993). As a result, nurses stayed much longer in their jobs. Employed in large hospitals, they could share their grievances and work together over time for real change. Meanwhile, the experience of involvement in union actions (such as mass resignations in New Brunswick in 1969) made nurses more militant and promoted their negotiating skills.

Just as they saw that it was possible to be mothers and employees, so too did nurses start to see that they could unionize to fight for better working conditions, job security, and pay while maintaining their commitment to care and their code of ethics. Strikes still seemed to go against what all nurses were committed to as nurses, even though some physicians had resorted to such action. What was often thought of as "professional conduct" had not won them many traditional union benefits. Asking nicely did not work for nurses or their patients. Indeed, it became increasingly clear that good conditions for work and job security were necessary for good care. Job security gave nurses the right to say no to practices that would harm patients without fear of reprisal, allowing them to fulfill their professional role as patient advocates. It gave them the right to say no to sexual harassment and other forms of discrimination that could undermine their capacity to fulfill their professional responsibilities. Contracts also helped equalize conditions among nurses by addressing favoritism. With job security, decent conditions, and appropriate pay, nurses can provide better care. A 2002 United States study demonstrates this idea by showing a positive relationship between outcomes and unionization. Patients were significantly less likely to die after a heart attack if they were treated at a unionized hospital (Seago & Ash, 2002). Although strike action is the last resort, an action taken when all other avenues fail, nurses also learned that the public continued to support them even when they went on strike.

Joyce Gleason, former Executive Director of the MNU, recalls that in their 1975 strike, the physicians supported the nurses and even helped look after the patients (Andrews, 1993, p. 31). The dramatically improved pay and conditions that followed union negotiations and actions helped many nurses change their ideas about unions. However, outside perceptions of what it means to be a unionized nurse often leaves a lot to be desired. In the media, unionization is often associated with negativity, anger, and aggression. This type of imagery, when linked with nursing, paints a picture of an oppressed profession, despite innumerable testimonies from nurses who report feeling a great sense of personal and professional satisfaction from their work.

Nurses' unions have had to take dramatic steps to achieve benefits and to protect rights. The most significant example of such steps was probably the UNA hospital strike of 1988. In the fall of 1987, UNA began hospital negotiations with two employers who tabled major regressions, takeaways, and rollbacks. UNA was not willing to be forced into concessions at the bargaining table, and when no Memorandum of Settlement could be ratified, all hospital nurses were called out on strike. Since the strike was deemed to be illegal, the employers went to the Labour Relations Board and charged UNA with causing a strike (United Nurses of Alberta [UNA], n.d.). A timeline highlighting important events during the strike is contained in Box 9.2.

At the end of the strike, UNA was charged almost $427,000 in fines, but cash donations of support helped with their payment. It was not until negotiations in 1990 that most of the benefits of the 1988 strike were realized. In this round of bargaining, hospital nurses received many additional benefits, including an additional day of rest every 4 weeks (8-hour shifts) or every 6 weeks (12-hour shifts); a 19% wage increase over 2 years; an additional 8th salary increment level worth 3%; a guarantee of two weekends off in four; language expressly prohibiting employers from making individual agreements that contravene the Collective Agreement; and many others as well (UNA, n.d.).

A number of strategies undertaken by nurses' unions had an impact on how nurses and others view nursing. Perhaps the clearest example is the case of pay equity in Ontario. The ONA was active in the Equal Pay Coalition, an organization that brought together unions and community groups to work for equal pay for work of equal value. Once their efforts were successful in achieving legislation, ONA then focused on making sure it worked for nurses. In two ground-breaking cases heard by the Ontario Pay Equity Tribunal (Ontario Nurses' Association vs. Haldimand-Norfolk, 1989; Ontario Nurses' Association vs. Women's College, 1990), ONA

> ### BOX 9.2   United Nurses of Alberta Hospital Strike, 1988
>
> - January 25th: The Labour Relations Board granted some employers the right to cease the collection of union dues for 6 months. In displays of support and solidarity with the UNA, unions from across Canada began sending telegrams and letters with funds to prevent the financial destruction of UNA.
> - January 26th: A permanent court injunction was granted to prevent picketing at three Crown hospitals, but over 1,000 nurses responded by picketing those hospitals nevertheless.
> - January 27th: Individual nurses began being served with civil contempt of court charges. Over 75 charges were laid and heard by the end of the strike. This same day, UNA was also charged with criminal contempt of court.
> - January 29th: UNA was served with a notice to appear at a hearing to be held February 1st. The government of Alberta requested a $1,000,000 fine and sequestrations of the union's funds and assets.
> - February 3rd: Civil contempt hearings for individual nurses proceeded in courthouses in Calgary and Edmonton.
> - February 4th: UNA was found guilty and fined $250,000.
> - February 9th: UNA paid the $250,000 fine at the courthouse and was served a notice of motion of a second criminal contempt charge.
> - February 10th: Termination notices were given to individual nurses as "punishment."
> - February 11th: Fines up to $1,000 each for criminal contempt started being imposed on individual nurses. This same day, employers tabled an improved offer.
> - February 12th: Hearings on the second criminal contempt charge began and UNA was fined $150,000. UNA members voted to accept the employers' latest improved offer and a settlement was reached.
> - February 13th: Striking nurses returned to work.

was successful not only in making sure the skills, effort, responsibility, and working conditions involved in nursing were made visible and valued, but also in establishing criteria for job evaluation that are used throughout the world. The result was more than higher pay; it was public and legal recognition of the valued work nurses do every day in their jobs.

NURSES' WORKPLACES

This chapter has provided some insight into conditions that both contribute to and detract from a positive work environment. Research shows that the quality of the work environment, retention and recruitment of nurses, and the nursing shortage can all be interrelated and, consequently, play a role in shaping our nursing workforce. Workplace challenges including excessive workload, high rates of overtime, injury, and stress are all detrimental to the health and safety of nurses. The Canadian Labour Code requires a number of measures be taken to protect the health and safety of workers in all workplaces. One mechanism by which this is accomplished is through the creation of a joint health and safety committee. The role of this committee is to ensure that workplace and legislative health and safety policies are applied in practice. Members of the committee generally include occupational health and safety (OH&S) experts as well as representatives from labor and management so that in-depth, practical knowledge of the work is brought together with company policies and procedures to enhance cooperation and the resolution of health and safety problems (Canadian Centre for Occupational Health and Safety [CCOHS], 2007).

Despite the many challenges that nurses face in the workplace, they continue to provide safe, competent care to patients, and are highly trusted and respected as healthcare professionals. Nurses are employed in hospitals, community health agencies, residential and long-term care settings and where unions have taken many steps to improve the conditions of the work environment

Table 9.1	Canadian Registered Nurse Workforce Distribution from 2005–2009	
	PERCENTAGE OF NURSES	
PLACE OF WORK	2005	2009
Hospital	63.4	62.6
Community health agency	13.5	14.2
Nursing home/long-term care facility	11.7	9.9
Other	11.4	13.3

From: Canadian Institute for Health Information (2010). *Regulated Nurses: Canadian Trends, 2005 to 2009.* Retrieved Sept. 22, 2012 from https://secure.cihi.ca/estore/productSeries.htm?pc=PCC449

for nurses (Table 9.1). There are many examples across Canada, but the BCNU is often a leader in advocating for improvements to workplace health and safety and patient care. BCNU encourages nurses across the province to use a professional responsibility reporting process—detailed in their collective agreement—to inform managers about workplace situations needing change (BCNU 2011). This initiative has resulted in documentation by emergency room (ER) nurses who have identified the need to increase the number of full-time RNs on ER staff to reduce waiting times for patients and improve the workload and safety of both nurses and patients. "RNs on regular medical and postsurgical wards have been using their professional responsibility report forms to ask for more electric beds and overhead lifts to reduce injuries. Younger nurses are documenting the need to keep older nurses in the workplace to serve as mentors and use their experience to provide support" (McPherson, 2004). This is just one example of how unions work to improve the workplace environments for nurses and also patient safety. Another method is to bring solutions—proven by research—into action in the workplace; CFNU is working to promote balance and satisfaction in the workplace through the development of pilot projects that promote continuing education, mentorship, and professional development. These will be explored in more detail later in the chapter.

COLLECTIVE BARGAINING

"Collective bargaining is a very broad concept that has the potential to involve and strengthen all nurses" (New Brunswick Nurses' Union, n.d.). As nurses work to provide safe and effective care to the public, it is the job of unions to support them in achieving this important task by protecting their health, safety, and well-being. The collective bargaining process now addresses issues that range far beyond wages and benefits, including workplace health and safety issues, and workload. These are addressed by articles on flexible staffing and scheduling measures, mentoring, professional training and development, and measures to reduce violence in the workplace. Nurses' unions in at least five provinces have brought workload issues into contract negotiations (CFNU, 2007). One means of addressing these concerns is the establishment of professional practice committees and joint management-union committees. Meetings are often initiated by working condition reports or issues raised in professional responsibility report forms. All committee procedures are outlined in collective agreements. These committees value the input of front-line nurses, and give them the opportunity to review care delivery and working conditions, make recommendations to management, and promote excellence in nursing.

It has been said that collective bargaining is more of an art than a science; it is a process in which creativity is more valuable than analysis, in order to come to an agreement that is mutually acceptable to both the employer and the employee (Teplitsky, 1992). Unions vary in their procedures and techniques to negotiate collective agreements, but this section highlights a series of steps that generally takes place throughout the course of the bargaining process. Negotiation teams often examine research, explore contract language, and develop goals and priorities to be reviewed at bargaining conferences where local presidents are in attendance. Following preparations, prenegotiations begin whereby proposals are exchanged between the union and the employer's negotiating committee. At this time, procedures and processes are established for future meetings. After both parties commence discussion and explore options for settlement, each negotiating team attempts to persuade the other side of its position. As both sides move toward reaching a tentative agreement, each offers a "final" or "minimum position" on the issues at hand. When an impasse is reached—the two parties cannot come close enough together to form an agreement—a Conciliation Officer or Commissioner (title and process may change for each province because these are based on provincial labor relations legislation) may be engaged to meet with both groups separately in an attempt to facilitate negotiations. Sometimes, as a last resort, a strike vote is taken by members of the union to put pressure on the employer to meet the collective bargaining demands. A strike vote does not automatically mean that a strike will occur, but it sends a strong message to the bargaining table that members support the demands brought forth by the negotiating committee. Finally, when the union's negotiation team receives a final position from the employer that they feel is the best possible settlement, it is considered to be a tentative agreement. Ratification occurs after the majority of voting union members vote in favor of the settlement. Despite the structure and tradition of the collective bargaining process, it is important to recognize that (1) collective bargaining processes may vary from union to union, and (2) a number of external factors influence the nature and context for negotiations as well. Public opinion and the current political environment are two major factors. The public's high regard for nurses is something that strengthens their position, while government policies, such as legislated wage freezes, negatively affect bargaining power. It should also be noted here that although not all provincial unions have the right to strike, all have the right and power to influence decision making by placing political pressure on employers and governments by raising public awareness of issues that are important to the healthcare work environment.

Bargaining power is further strengthened by numbers, cohesion, and commonality of objectives within membership. Although provincial nurses' unions negotiate individually, their collective membership with CFNU allows them to receive information and research that will strengthen their individual bargaining power. The chief negotiators of the provincial member unions collaborate to produce a policy statement and national strategy for their common, long-term bargaining goals. The strategy is then adopted at the CFNU biennial convention. Though each union retains bargaining autonomy, these strategies recognize the national nature of many problems affecting nurses, and the importance of collaborating for common ends. A further example of collaboration is the comparative contract shown in Table 9.2. By sharing information, provincial unions can use the successes of other provinces as a model for their own negotiations.

It is important to note that the focus of collective bargaining is not solely monetary. Improving working conditions, professional practice and patient safety, and ensuring safe staffing levels are also fundamental objectives.

By the 1980s, Canada had public hospitals, physician care, and a highly unionized public sector as well as more egalitarian ideas, laws, and practices in relation to women. More than 9 out of 10 nurses were women and three-quarters of the nurses were unionized. This suggests that women who are nurses no longer see commitment to care and professional conduct as incompatible with being a woman and being in a union. This is not to suggest that all issues have been resolved or the tensions have disappeared, but it is often the unions—who have great strength in numbers—that are fighting to protect workers from external influences that damage their working conditions.

Table 9.2 Canadian Federation of Nurses Unions Contract Comparison Document: Salary at Contract Expiry (As of January 2012)

| UNION | DOLLARS PER HOUR | | ANNUAL INCOME | | STEPS | CONTRACT EXPIRY | ANNUAL HOURS |
	Minimum	Maximum	Minimum	Maximum			
UNA	32.42	42.45	62,270.72	81,535.84	9	3/31/2010	1920.75
ONA	29.36	41.70	57,252.00	81,315.00	9	3/31/2011	1950.00
BCNU	29.89	39.24	56,163.31	73,731.96	9	3/31/2011	1879.00
MNU	31.02	36.57	62,507.32	73,692.58	6	9/30/2009	2015.00
NSNU	29.24	34.17	57,014.00	66,630.00	6	10/31/2009	1950.00
SUN	32.62	42.34	63,569.86	82,512.19	6	3/31/2011	1948.80
FIQ	21.40	31.89	40,497.01	60,319.94	12	3/31/2010	1891.50
NBNU	28.99	34.60	56,762.42	67,746.80	6	6/30/2010	1958.00
PEINU	27.18	33.12	53,001.00	64,584.00	6	3/31/2011	1950.00
NLNU	28.44	35.22	55,465.80	68,688.36	6	6/30/2010	1950.00

Note that not all contract expiry dates are updated because at the time this chapter was written, some member organizations were in the process of bargaining. It should also be noted that some organizations offer long-term recognition steps beyond the standard salary scales and signing bonuses. The Canadian Federation of Nurses Unions provides this and other wage comparison documents through their website: www.nursesunions.ca.

UNIONS TODAY AND TOMORROW

Beginning in the 1980s, global pressure developed to turn back the clock on the development of public services. International organizations such as the World Bank and the International Monetary Fund promoted dramatic reductions in both public services and government regulation of private services. In Canada, growing government debts and deficits were used as a justification for "devolving responsibilities to other levels of government and to the private and voluntary sectors; reducing transfer payments to provinces, individuals and businesses; applying private sector management techniques to those federal activities that remain" (Swimmer, 1996, p. 2). Provincial governments had little choice but to follow this lead, although several did so enthusiastically.

Healthcare was one of the hardest hit, because it was one of the largest areas of government expense and because the private sector wanted to expand in health services, not only in providing services but also in financing and managing care. Healthcare is primarily based on labor, and nurses are the largest single occupational group in health services. It is perhaps not surprising, then, that nurses were among the primary targets for cost cutting and new managerial techniques taken from the for-profit sector. It should be noted, however, that it has been widely recognized that the most rapidly rising costs in health services are technologies and pharmaceuticals, not labor—and certainly not nurses' labor.

Nurses' unions found it difficult to resist this rising tide of cutbacks. They did manage to ensure orderly, fair layoffs and to maintain wages for the jobs that remained. They also maintained the right to say no to unreasonable work demands and the right to expose discrimination. But many nurses no longer had full-time jobs and some lost work altogether. To counter the trend, nurses' unions worked with health coalitions and other unions throughout the country to convince Canadians that public healthcare is the most effective and efficient way to deliver health services

BOX 9.3   Employment Trends of the Registered Nurse Workforce in 2009

Since 2002 the number of RNs who submitted for registration in Canada grew by an average annual rate of 2.1% for a 2009 total of 266,341.

In 2009, 58.7% of RNs were employed full time, while the proportion employed part-time and on a casual basis was 30.6% and 10.7%, respectively.

In 2009, RNs represented 76.4% of the regulated nursing workforce, a proportion that has been relatively stable over the preceding 5 years.

In 2009, 89.3% of the RN workforce lived in urban areas of Canada.

In 2009, 6.2 % of the RN workforce was male.

In 2009, 3,898 RNs with Canadian registration lived and/or worked outside of Canada. Of these, 83% (3,235) were employed in the United States.

Compiled from Canadian Institute for Health Information (2010). *Regulated Nurses: Canadian Trends, 2005 to 2009.* Retrieved Sept. 22, 2012 from https://secure.cihi.ca/estore/productSeries.htm?pc=PCC449

and that nurses are critical to care provision. When deficits, and even debt, could no longer be used as a justification for cutbacks in nursing, the strategy of working with others to support public care started to bear fruit. Governments began to put money back into health services and into nursing. Indeed, nurses' unions have been working with governments to address the growing nursing shortage.

However, much work remains to be done. The Canadian Nurses Association (CNA, 2010) projected a shortfall of 78,000 RNs for 2011, a shortage that will grow to 113,000 by 2016. An aging workforce that is not being replenished helps explain these numbers. According to the Canadian Institute for Health Information (CIHI, 2010), in 2009 the average age of a Canadian RN was 45.2 years old, an increase of 0.5 year over 2005. In the same year, almost a quarter (24.5%) of the RN workforce was 55 years old and over and nearly 4 in 10 (39.9%) were over 50 years old. (For an overview of the Canadian nursing workforce; see Box 9.3.) Working conditions also contribute to the shortage. In 2005, 37% of nurses reported experiencing pain over the preceding year that was serious enough to prevent them from carrying out their normal daily activities (Statistics Canada, 2006). The amount of overtime nurses' work is a clear symptom of the shortage. According to a report by the Canadian Federation of Nurses Unions (CFNU, 2009), nurses worked 21,560,100 hours of overtime in 2008, the equivalent of 11,900 full-time jobs. Overtime increased by 10% over 2005 and costs $879 million per year. In addition, unpaid overtime accounted for 12.9% of the time nurses worked.

In addition to addressing conditions of work and relating these to conditions of care, nurses' unions have been struggling to promote fair treatment on a range of issues. In their early forms of existence, most of the nurses' unions focused on negotiating contracts, handling grievances, and other labor relations issues. However, annual general meetings revealed that a number of issues relating to the healthcare system and social justice were also very important for nurses. For example, in 1982, MNU brought a resolution to the special convention that CFNU join the Canadian Health Coalition to champion Medicare and other social justice issues. Partnering with the CNA, the CFNU also co-founded "Nurses for Medicare," an initiative that promotes sustainable, publicly funded, and not-for-profit healthcare delivery in Canada. Unions have developed contract language on both sexual harassment and discrimination against racialized groups at the same time as they have sought to educate their members and the public on these issues. They have successfully demanded changes on health and safety matters, such as needles and reporting medical errors—matters that are critical to safe and effective care. Unions have also increasingly been at the forefront of demands for healthcare reforms that both recognize nurses' skills and protect equitable access to high quality, public care.

Since 1998, the CFNU has been an active member of the Canadian Labour Congress (CLC), the largest democratic and popular organization in Canada. With over 3.5 million members, the

CLC joins national and international unions, the provincial and territorial federations of labor, and 136 district labor councils (Canadian Labour Congress [CLC], 2007). Included in this group of affiliates is the International Trade Union Confederation, the world's largest trade union organization, which represents 176 million workers in 151 countries and territories around the world (International Trade Union Confederation [ITUC], 2011). In Canada, the CLC works to adapt policy and influence political agendas on issues like health and safety, pensions, and employment insurance. In recent years their campaigning has focused on childcare, education, the development of a national pharmacare program, pay equity, and pension protection. Recently, for example, the CLC has been actively campaigning for a doubling of Canadian Pension Plan benefits in order to ensure better minimum pensions. As a member of the CLC Executive Council, the strong collaborative relationship that the CFNU shares with the CLC provides all member nurses' unions with support for collective bargaining in areas such as occupational health and safety, pensions, and benefits.

The CFNU's advocacy for nurses extends beyond national borders, and its expertise on nursing workplace issues brings it into cooperation with nursing unions and associations around the world. Along with the CNA, the CFNU is a member of the ICN Workforce Forum. The ICN is a federation of over 130 nursing organizations representing more than 13 million nurses worldwide. From a global perspective, the ICN advocates for both quality of nursing care and the rights of nurses worldwide.

The CFNU also promotes justice abroad via its International Solidarity Fund. At the CFNU's 2005 Biennial Convention, nurses voted to create the fund, which supports worker-to-worker exchanges, provides humanitarian assistance, and builds the capacity of health workers.

NURSES' UNIONS AND POLITICAL ACTION

CFNU's elected officials and National Executive Board members have met with premiers, developed and released peer-reviewed papers and position statements, and hosted discussion panels and press conferences to address national nursing and healthcare system issues. Advocacy and campaigning efforts often lead the CFNU to lobby politicians on Parliament Hill, or at events like meetings of the Council of the Federation, or meetings of the provincial and territorial Ministers of Health. Over the past several years, the CFNU has also submitted briefs to parliamentary standing committees, like the Standing Committee on Health and the Standing Committee on Finance, and has appeared before committees to make recommendations.

Since 2005, the CFNU has been hosting "MP Breakfasts" on Parliament Hill. The breakfasts are an opportunity for MPs, Senators, and other key healthcare and labor stakeholders to come together and discuss issues central to nursing and the Canadian healthcare system. Recent topics include long-term care, pandemic preparedness, a national pharmacare program, and aboriginal health. Summaries of the breakfasts are available on the CFNU's website.

Nurses' unions also work hard to educate their members on important nursing and healthcare issues, and these efforts are redoubled during federal and provincial elections. During the 2011 federal election campaign, the CFNU promoted four priorities: A new Health Accord between the federal and provincial/territorial governments, a national poverty strategy, a national strategy on continuum of care, and a comprehensive national drug plan. The CFNU's website offered an election pamphlet, a printable postcard to be sent to candidates, and a host of useful information and resources. In addition, the CFNU sent a list of questions to each party in order to discern their stance on several of the organization's priority issues, including pharmacare, poverty reduction, senior care, child care, and the renewal of the Health Accord. Party responses were posted to the Web for the benefit of voters.

Nurses' unions believe that knowledge is power, and that the spread of knowledge can help effect positive change. Helping to educate the public is thus a high priority on the union action list. The

CFNU's research and publications have helped it become a recognized leader in several areas. Examples include policies on personal protective equipment, a report on how changes in nursing practices can improve the Canadian healthcare system (*Experts and Evidence: Opportunities in Nursing*), and books on the importance of rebuilding the Canadian long-term healthcare system (*Long-Term Care in Canada: Status Quo No Option*) and on the sustainability of the Canadian healthcare system as a whole (*The Sustainability of Medicare*). These documents are available online.

Provincial nurses' unions have implemented a number of successful action campaigns over the past several years. Some of these campaigns are described below: Further information is available on the respective union websites.

In 2010, ONA launched an innovative advertisement campaign aimed at highlighting the value of nurses. In the same year the Prince Edward Island Nurses' Union (PEINU) campaigned against the government's new Model of Care strategy that would have lead to the deletion of over 40 RN positions, arguing that without enough RNs, new models of care would be unsustainable.

In 2006, the Alberta government once again introduced plans for private insurance and for-profit healthcare in the province. Fearing these reforms would come at the expense of lower income Albertans, UNA and other Medicare advocates responded by launching the Third Way Campaign. Under the pressure, the Alberta government eventually backed down from introducing the legislation.

The BCNU workshop known as *Building Union Strength,* teaches participants about their workplace rights and responsibilities and how union tools and resources can help improve the workplace. NSNU has made effective use of television advertisements to promote its health and social priorities. NSNU has also partnered with the Nova Scotia Teachers Union to produce commercials in support of the *Read to Me* initiative, a program that promotes literacy by providing a bag of books to newborn and adopted babies in Nova Scotia.

Both the NLNU and the MNU have undertaken campaigns for the improvement of long-term care (LTC) in their provinces, a health sector that is often neglected. In 2010, Newfoundland and Labrador's provincial Minister of Health agreed to an NLNU request to undertake a new review into the skill mix and scope of practice of health workers in the province's LTC homes. A previous review in 2006 had excluded union participation and recommended reducing the proportion of RNs in LTC homes from 20% to 12%. For the new review the government promised the active participation of NLNU and other unions.

In 2009, the Saskatchewan government produced its "Patients First Review" that advocated for more patient-centered care. In response, SUN created their "Patients and Families First Initiative." Similarly, in 2011, NBNU launched a challenge called the "Wellness First Challenge" designed to generate ideas to help promote wellness, a goal that complements the efforts of front-line nurses.

These are just some of the tactics that nurses' unions employ to influence the collective bargaining environment and to generate political and public support for better workplace conditions and patient care.

BRINGING RESEARCH TO ACTION

Nurses' unions do not simply wait for change; they create change by applying creative, positive, research-based solutions to workplace problems. Research shows that nurse retention and high-quality patient care require a committed and engaged nursing workforce, and work settings that empower nurses to provide the care they are educated to provide (Cho et al., 2006). Recognizing this, nurses' unions have undertaken a variety of projects that promote nurse autonomy and leadership at all levels of nursing. Examples range from increased in-house education opportunities to the creation of mentorship programs and strategies to prevent the practice of hallway nursing.

In Nova Scotia and Saskatchewan, two pilot projects were implemented with funding from Human Resources and Skills Development Canada's Workplace Skills Initiative to improve the retention and recruitment of nurses. These projects have allowed nurses in two health regions to participate in continuing education or mentorship programs. Building on the success of these pilot projects, the CFNU partnered with the CNA, the Canadian Healthcare Association and the Dietitians of Canada to implement a Health Canada funded project known as *Research to Action: Applied Workplace Solutions for Nurses* (RTA). RTA ran from October 2008 to March 2011 and comprised 10 pilot projects across the country designed to increase the retention and recruitment of nurses. The pilots were all workplace-based and involved innovative strategies that brought research to action, including programs that address staffing ratios to enhance the quality of patient care, systems to offer support to new nursing graduates and opportunities for education and professional development. Each project was developed based on local needs and in partnership with employers, governments, unions, and other healthcare stakeholders in each jurisdiction. The results of the RTA project were impressive, including a 10% decrease in the categories of nurse turnover, overtime, and absenteeism. Nursing research has repeatedly shown that such results will translate into important health, social, and financial benefits. Further information on the 10 pilots can be found at www.thinknursing.ca/rta.

The CFNU and its member unions have been involved in several initiatives of this sort over the past years. For example, the SUN partnered with the government of Saskatchewan in 2008 to help stabilize and rebuild Saskatchewan's dwindling nursing workforce and ensure that their province can deliver high quality, timely, and accessible care to residents. In recognition of the need to retain a large number of experienced and skilled nurses, while also planning aggressive recruitment initiatives to increase the numbers of practicing nurses, several concrete strategies were put in place. Examples include the establishment of quarterly retention and recruitment targets, the recruitment of internationally educated nurses, and the provision of incentives for senior nurses to remain in the workforce longer by recognizing long-term service and providing opportunities to mentor new graduates and immigrant nurses (Saskatchewan Union of Nurses [SUN], 2008).

Another mechanism by which nurses' unions aim to address issues of retention and recruitment is by remaining current and informed about the changing needs of the workforce. By inviting the CNSA to sit on the National Executive Board, CFNU now represents over 176,000 members and associate members, making it the largest nursing organization in Canada. By working with the CNSA it is hoped that the future of nursing is well represented in current union activities and priorities.

Nurses' unions have been adept at making use of social media to further their workplace and social aims. Several unions and union presidents have active Facebook pages, Twitter accounts, and YouTube channels. All of Canada's major nursing unions, including the CFNU, have developed effective websites that help nurses stay informed about union activities, including bargaining and social justice campaigns. Many sites also offer nurses useful educational resources. In 2009, the CFNU launched a new site entitled *Think Nursing: Towards a Better Workplace*. Think Nursing provides research on positive practices designed to improve workplaces and patient care. It also offers a portal for nurses to connect with each other in order to promote collaboration and the sharing of best practices.

S U M M A R Y

In short, there are very good reasons why over 80% of nurses in Canada today belong to a union, and why unions have joined together to promote nurses' rights. Despite historical tensions between the notion of professionalism and unionization, nurses today experience support brought by union values and activities that bring continuous learning, challenges, and many rewards to their profession. Without unions, but with other forms of collective action, nurses were able to obtain registration and some control over the process of getting and retaining the right to be called an RN. However, until they formed unions, they were unable to significantly improve their conditions of work and, thus, the conditions for care.

Today, these unions work not only to promote the prestige and power of nurses but also to maintain a safe, accessible healthcare system that offers high-quality care. The CFNU is a founding member of the Quality Worklife Quality Health Care Collaborative (QWQHC, 2006), a national interprofessional coalition of healthcare leaders who are working together to develop an integrated action-oriented strategy to transform the quality of worklife for Canada's healthcare providers in order to improve patient care and system outcomes. The QWQHC (2006) maintains that "a fundamental way to better healthcare is through healthier healthcare workplaces; and it is unacceptable to work in, receive care in, govern, manage and fund unhealthy health care workplaces." A similar vision underlies the work of the Quality Work Life and Attendance Management Committee in New Brunswick, a partnership of NBNU, the Department of Health, the Regional Health Authorities, and the Office of Human Resources. Apart from improving patient care, the committee seeks ways to increase the retention and recruitment of nurses by providing them with the means to improve their own work environment, build their careers, and improve the satisfaction they derive from work.

Although a primary focus of nurses' unions is to ensure that nurses receive the same attention and care that they give to their patients, when nurses' unions work in collaboration with local employers, governments, and nursing stakeholders, the overall result can be seen in improvements not only in the quality worklife of nurses but also in increased quality healthcare and better patient safety.

Add to your knowledge of this issue:

Online

International Council of Nurses	**www.icn.ch**
Canadian Federation of Nurses Unions	**www.nursesunions.ca**
Canadian Nurses Association	**www.cna-nurses.ca**
British Columbia Nurses' Union	**www.bcnu.org**
United Nurses of Alberta	**www.una.ab.ca**
Manitoba Nurses Union	**www.nursesunion.mb.ca**
Saskatchewan Union of Nurses	**www.sun-nurses.sk.ca**
Ontario Nurses' Association	**www.ona.org**
Fédération Interprofessionnelle de la Santé du Québec	**www.fiqsante.qc.ca**
New Brunswick Nurses Union	**www.nbnu.ca**
Prince Edward Island Nurses' Union	**www.peinu.com**
Nova Scotia Nurses' Union	**www.nsnu.ns.ca**
Newfoundland and Labrador Nurses' Union	**www.nlnu.nf.ca**

REFLECTIONS *on the Chapter...*

1 How would you describe the transformation of nurses' unions in Canada?
2 Identify the appropriate documents that provide direction for nurses and their employers in the provision of professional practice environments.

3 What are the barriers in your practice environment to nurses providing safe and ethical care? How could you resolve these?

4 What are your views on the strengths and limitations of the strategies presented in the chapter or that you have seen utilized in the practice setting?

5 Identify at least one issue for nurses in the provision of a safe professional practice environment for their work.

6 What are the benefits and challenges associated with collective bargaining processes?

7 What other strategies can you suggest for the resolution of these issues?

8 How would you describe the stand of your provincial nurses' union on issues? How would you account for this stand?

Want to know more? Visit thePoint for additional helpful resources:

- Journal Articles
- Learning Objectives
- Nursing Professional Roles and Responsibilities
- Bonus chapters:
  - Health and Nursing Policy: A Matter of Politics, Power and Professionalism
  - The NP Movement: Recurring Issues
  - When Difference Matters: The Politics of Privilege and Marginality

References

Allard, G. (2005). Caregiving on the front: The experience of Canadian military nurses during World War I. In C. Bates, D. Dodd & N. Rousseau (Eds.), *On all frontiers: Four centuries of Canadian nursing* (pp. 153–168). Toronto, ON: University of Toronto Press.

Andrews, J. (1993). *Notes on the history of collective bargaining in current members of the CFNU: Interviews with key informants.* Ottawa, ON: Canadian Federation of Nurses Unions, May 1993.

Armstrong, P., & Armstrong, H. (2001). *The double ghetto: Canadian women and their segregated work* (3rd ed.). Toronto, ON: Oxford University Press.

———. (2003). *Wasting away: The undermining of Canadian health care* (2nd ed.). Toronto, ON: Oxford University Press.

British Columbia Nurses' Union (BCNU) (2011). *Professional responsibility form process.* Retrieved Sept. 22 from www.bcnu.org/ProfessionalPractice/ProfessionalPractice.aspx?page=Professional Responsibility Form (PRF).

Bunting, S., & Campbell, J. (1990). Feminism and nursing: Historical perspectives. *Advances in Nursing Science, 12*(4), 11–24.

Campbell, A. (2006). *Final report of the SARS Commission.* The SARS Commission, p. 254.

Canadian Centre for Occupational Health and Safety. (2007). *What is a joint health and safety committee?* Retrieved from http://www.ccohs.ca/oshanswers/hsprograms/hscommittees/whatisa.html

Canadian Federation of Nurses Unions. (n.d.). *Defending nurses and health care.* Ottawa, ON: Author.

———. (2003). Nursing unionism in Quebec. A bit of history (n.d.). *The Story of Canadian Labour.* Workshop handouts. Ottawa, ON: Author.

———. (2007). *Creating positive solutions at the workplace: Time to work together.* Presented in Geneva, Switzerland, March 23, 2007.

————. (2009). *Trends in own illness or disability-related absenteeism and overtime among publicly-employed registered nurses.* Ottawa, ON: CFNU, written by Lasota, M.

————. (2011). *CFNU contract comparison document.* Retrieved Sept. 22, 2012 from http://www. nursesunions.ca/news/2011-overview-key-nursing-contract-provisions

Canadian Institute for Health Information. (2010). *Regulated nurses: Canadian trends, 2005 to 2009.* Retrieved from http://secure.cihi.ca/

Canadian Labour Congress. (2007). *Welcome.* Retrieved from http://www.cihi.ca/cihi-ext-portal/internet/ en/document/spending+and+health+workforce/workforce/nurses/bul_30jun11

————. (2010). *2008 Workforce Profiles of Registered Nurses in Canada.* Retrieved from www.cna-aiic. ca/

Cho, J., Laschinger, H.K.S., & Wong, C. (2006). Workplace empowerment, work engagement and organization commitment to new graduate nurses. *Nursing Leadership, 19*(3), 43–60.

Coburn, J. (1987). I see and am silent: A short history of nursing in Ontario, 1850–1930. In D. Coburn, C. D'Arcy, GM. Torrance & P. Newman (Eds.), *Health and Canadian society* (2nd ed.). Toronto, ON: Fitzhenry and Whiteside.

Dominion Bureau of Statistics. (1961). *Census of Canada labour force occupation and industry trends.* Ottawa, ON: Minister of Trade and Commerce.

Hunt, J. (1998). Feminism and Nursing. *Nursing Monograph, 8,* 17–22.

————. (2011). *About Us (International Trade Union Federation).* Retrieved from http://www.ituc-csi.org/

Jensen, P. (1992). The changing role of nurses unions. In A. Baumgart & J. Larsen (Eds.), *Canadian nursing faces the future.* St. Louis, MO: Mosby.

Keddy, B., & Dodd, D. (2005). The trained nurse: Private duty and VON home nursing (late 1800s to 1940s). In C. Bates, D. Dodd & N. Rousseau (Eds.), *On all frontiers: Four centuries of Canadian nursing* (pp. 43–56). Toronto, ON: University of Toronto Press.

Kerr, J. (1988). Professionalization in Canadian nursing. In J. Kerr & J. McPhail (Eds.), *Canadian nursing issues and perspective* (pp. 23–30). Toronto, ON: McGraw-Hill Ryerson.

Library and Archives Canada. (2005). *Celebrating women's achievements: Women in science: Jeanne Mance.* Retrieved from http://www.collectionscanada.gc.ca/women/002026-410-e.html

MacDonald, P. (2006). Bullying in the workplace. *Practice Nurse, 32*(10), 1–4.

Mansell, D., & Dodd, D. (2005). Professionalism and Canadian nursing. In C. Bates, D. Dodd & N. Rousseau (Eds.), *On all frontiers: Four centuries of Canadian nursing* (pp. 197–212). Toronto, ON: University of Toronto Press.

McBride, A. (1984). Nursing and the women's movement. *Journal of Nursing Scholarship, 16*(3), 285–302.

McIntyre, M. & McDonald, C. (2006). Unionization: Collective bargaining in nursing. In M. McIntyre, E. Thomlinson & C. McDonald (Eds.), *Realities of Canadian nursing: Professional, practice and power issues* (pp. 303–316). Philadelphia, PA: Lippincott Williams & Wilkins.

Mussallem, H. (1988). The changing role of the Canadian nurses' association in the development of nursing in Canada. In J. Kerr & J. McPhail (Eds.), *Canadian nursing issues and perspectives* (pp. 35–46). Toronto, ON: McGraw-Hill Ryerson.

Naylor, D. (1986). *Private practice. Public payment.* Montreal: McGill-Queen's University Press.

Nelson, S. (2001). *Say little. Do much: Nurses, nuns and hospitals in the nineteenth century.* Philadelphia, PA: University of Pennsylvania Press.

New Brunswick Nurses' Union. (n.d.). *How the NBNU negotiates your contract.* Retrieved from http:// www.nbnu-siinb.nb.ca/pdf/negotiates.pdf

Ontario Nurses' Association vs. Women's College Hospital, Ontario Pay Equity Tribunal, 1990.

Ontario Nurses' Association vs. Haldimand Norfolk, Ontario Pay Equity Tribunal, 1989.

Quality Worklife Quality Health Care Collaborative. (2006). *Overview.* Retrieved from http://www2.cchsa. ca/qwqhc/

Richardson, S. (2005). Unionization of Canadian Nursing. In C. Bates, D. Dodd & N. Rousseau (Eds.), *On all frontiers: Four centuries of Canadian nursing* (pp. 213–224). Toronto, ON: University of Toronto Press.

Saskatchewan Union of Nurses. (2008). *Partnership between the government of Saskatchewan and the Saskatchewan union of nurses.* Retrieved Sept. 22, 2012 from www.sun-nurses.sk.ca/government-relations/government-sun-rha-agreement

Seago, J.A., & Ash, M. (2002). Registered nurse union and patient outcomes. *Journal of Nursing Administration, 32*(3), 143–151.

Statistics Canada. (2006). *2005 National Survey of the Work and Health of Nurses.* Catalogue no-83-003-XIE.

Swimmer, G. (1996). An introduction to life under the knife. In Gene Swimmer (Ed.), *How Ottawa spends: Life under the knife.* Ottawa, ON: Carleton University Press.

Teplitsky, M. (1992). *Making a deal: The art of negotiation.* Toronto, ON: Lancaster House.

Toman, C. (2005). Ready, aye ready: Canadian military nurses as an expandable and expendable workforce (1920–2000). In C. Bates, D. Dodd & N. Rousseau (Eds.), *On all frontiers: Four centuries of Canadian nursing.* Toronto, ON: University of Toronto Press.

United Nurses of Alberta. (n.d.). *1988 hospital strike.* Retrieved Sept, 22, 2012 from www.una.ab.ca/about/history pages/UNA History - 1988

Van Kirk, S. (1980). *Many tender ties: Women in fur trade society in Western Canada, 1670–1830.* Winnipeg: Watson and Dyer.

Victorian Order of Nurses. (2004). *A century of caring.* Retrieved Sept, 22, 2012 from www.von.ca/en/about/history.aspx

White, J. (1993). *Sisters & solidarity: Women and unions in Canada.* Toronto, ON: Thompson Educational Publishing.

Issues Related to Knowledge Generation and Dissemination

Part 2

Issues Related to Knowledge Generation and Dissemination

10 Challenges and Change in Undergraduate Nursing Education

Margaret Scaia and Kathryn McPherson

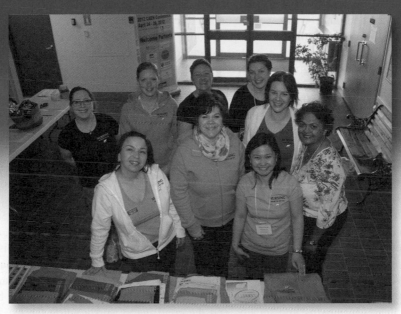

Undergraduate students and their instructor at Aurora College, Yellowknife, NWT. (Used with permission. Photographer Anne-Mieke Cameron.)

Critical Questions

As a way of engaging with the ideas in this chapter, consider the following:

1. What do you know about the history of undergraduate nursing education in Canada and how does that history inform current issues in nursing education?

2. How do issues in undergraduate nursing education affect you, nursing as a profession, health care in Canada, and Canadian society?

3. How does the current context of Canadian society, politics, and economics as seen through the lens of race, class, gender, and culture shape how you understand current issues in undergraduate nursing education?

Chapter Objectives

After completing this chapter, you will be able to:

1. Understand and identify significant events and issues in the history of undergraduate nursing education in Canada.

2. Situate current issues in undergraduate nursing education within past and present social, political, and economic contexts and describe how race, class, gender, and culture intersect to shape particular understandings of these issues.

3. Articulate and describe issues in undergraduate education in terms of the barriers, resources, and strategies available to nursing and nursing education to address areas of concern.

FRAMING THE TOPIC

Busy Busy Busy..........Rush Rush Rush............Organize, Prioritize, Be Efficient…

You see it, you hear it, and you live it. It seems like today it's more important to be efficient and be effective than to be human! Being human includes taking time to reflect, relax, think, converse, play, rest, and—yes—work. You are told about the importance of relationship building, about the nurse as the therapeutic agent, about the need to practice ethically, morally, legally, and with intention. You are expected to develop your own philosophy of nursing throughout your undergraduate program, reinforced through assignments that stress the value of self-reflection and the wise and considered acquisition of relevant disciplinary knowledge.

And so…is this what your life as an undergraduate student looks like? Do you have time to carefully prepare, thoughtfully act, and critically reflect, or, do you identify with the first imperative: Busy busy busy…rush rush rush…organize, prioritize, and be efficient! Keeping pace with present demands probably feels like enough of a challenge, but now you are expected to understand how the whole healthcare system works and how that system shapes and is shaped by the social, political, and economic context in which it takes place. In this chapter we will describe and articulate three issues that influence undergraduate nursing education today and analyze those issues from a historical, social, political, and economic perspective. Interwoven in the analysis are the ways dominant values, beliefs, and assumptions about race, class, and gender (feminist and postcolonial perspectives) intersect and influence how these issues are taken up by nursing and presented in the nursing literature in reference to undergraduate education.

While there are many issues in undergraduate nursing education, this chapter will focus on three: The stress of being an undergraduate student, the influence of racially based practices of exclusion in nursing and society, and the controversy surrounding the use of information technology in nursing and nursing education. The purpose of this chapter is to facilitate your understanding of how and why issues in undergraduate nursing education are significant for the recruitment and retention of nurses and for the growth of the discipline. How you perceive issues in nursing and nursing education count—nursing needs you! As you learned in the introduction to this text, nursing is a political act. Problem solving and decision making have shaped what nursing is about from the beginning of its modern history and so understanding issues that are sometimes framed as problems can lead to generating ideas that lead to decision making and resolution of those problems. Advocacy is also the mandate of nursing and a knowledgeable and informed perspective about issues that impact nursing is essential in understanding and addressing inequities, not just in nursing and nursing education, but in society as well.

Overview

The first section of this chapter situates the topic, that is, issues in undergraduate nursing education. I will present information about the issues of concern, review some of the literature that supports various ways of thinking about them, and talk about some of the values, beliefs, and assumptions that have shaped the particular debates that have arisen around them. In the next section, we will articulate some of the broader historical, social, political, and economic events that have shaped the direction of nursing and health care in Canada. Then we will take a closer look at each of the three issues; specifically, we will explore how students experience and respond to stress, issues around diversity, and finally debates about the use of information technology. The middle section of the chapter will analyze each of these issues using the lenses of history, politics, economics, society, and feminism. The final section will present ways of looking at barriers and strategies that might lead to the resolution of these issues, but here we will resist the inclination of assuming that barriers and strategies act as opposing forces. Instead, we will consider how barriers and strategies act along a continuum of possible actions and ways of seeing and understanding this topic and these particular issues.

Situating the Topic

Anticipating the next "need" for consumer goods and being excited about the next evolution/revolution in digital technology means that you are probably a member of the "NET" generation. For the NET generation, change has cachet. By now, however, you may not feel quite so positive about how change affects you as a nursing student. You may also have picked up on a theme that is popular in much that has been written about nursing and that is that nursing is a subservient and oppressed profession practiced at the mercy of its medical masters, unable to define its scope or purpose, and unable to regulate standards of educational preparation. This is an interpretation of history that matters in considering current issues in undergraduate education because it is the one that needs to be challenged. As D'Antonio et al. (2010) argues, there are many histories of nursing. In the face of rapid change students need to become aware of "the richness, complexity, and power in nursing's history" (p. 207). Appreciating the history of nursing as the history of a profession that has been at the forefront of social change facilitates an attitude of empowerment that will in fact change your thinking about issues in undergraduate education and hopefully inspire you to feel you can become an important change agent yourself. As D'Antonio has argued, nursing "is a history of how a small group of individuals transformed the most traditional of gendered expectations—that of caring for the sick—into respected and respectable work" (pp. 207–208). Let us look now at where some of the core values inherent in nursing come from.

For more than 100 years, the topic of undergraduate education has been a major focus of the political and policy initiatives of organized nursing in Canada. Preparation of the next generation of registered nurses (RNs) determines the viability of the profession and its ability to influence and respond to national and global health concerns. In advocating for change in undergraduate education, leaders in nursing have struggled to come to terms with tensions around the nature of nurses' work within the rapidly changing context of Canadian health care, society, politics, and economics. Previous assumptions about how best to address these tensions do not seem to be working. The stress of change and the expectation of instant solutions to historically entrenched issues create stress for nursing students and faculty and can be felt in most clinical settings (Gibbons, 2010). In this chapter, we will explore those historical tensions in relation to the issues that arise because of rapid change. The impact of rapid change in society and health care is an important consideration because while change has provided benefits to society, and technological changes, for example, digital technology, have made some aspects of life more exciting, convenient, and accessible, the practice and education of nurses is embedded within very large and complex systems such as political and economic systems that do not respond quickly. This lack of synchronicity means that when change happens, it is not always easy for nursing, nursing education, or health care to keep pace.

Articulating the Issues

What are some of the larger social, political, and economic systems in which change occurs? Let's go back in time a couple of decades. Probably the majority of nurses, nursing students, and Canadian citizens assume that the Canada Health Act, established in 1984, provides all Canadians with equal access to health care regardless of age, gender, race, class, or culture. In less than 20 years the influence of the neo-liberal approach to health care in Canada—that is, the market-driven approach to economic and social policy and other organizational pressures—has radically changed the way health care is provided in this country and indeed has transformed the ideology that every citizen deserves access to the basic entitlements of economic citizenship. Although the political will to provide equitable and accessible health care to all Canadians is embedded in the Canada Health Act and has been confirmed in each federal election, there is increasing criticism about that cost of health care. The cost of nursing care is one of the major costs of health care and nurses form the largest group of healthcare providers. This attention to the cost of health care, and consequently to the cost of nursing care, has at times led to lay-offs of nursing staff, cuts in educational programs, and more recently a shift in the ratio of Registered Nurses to patient care. Nursing has responded with research that validates and articulates the value registered nursing care brings to patient outcomes, but the constant shifts in staffing, short staffing, uncertain employment status, lack of adequate resources of time, and materials to provide nursing care at a standard demanded by the profession and other budgetary considerations have increased tensions in the workplace for most nurses. Students, as members of the nursing team, are exposed to these negative influences resulting in considerable stress. Students from minority populations are under additional stress due to embedded racism, gender bias, and classism in the broader society, including nursing.

Stress and Coping

How nursing students respond to stress and develop ways of coping is important because while nurses are generally well thought of and "a positive image of nursing attracts applicants" (Bolan & Grainger, 2009, p. 776), it is the quality of the educational and clinical experience that is a critical factor in retaining nursing students (Jackson et al., 2011). It is, therefore, essential that nurse educators and clinical nurses role-model relationships between students and themselves that not only make students feel welcome in nursing, but also role model the kinds of relationships that students can enact between themselves and their patients and clients. This positive mentoring is critical to the professionalization process. Through positive mentoring "we provide an alternative, and more productive image of nursing socialisation than the alternative model of oppressed group behaviour" (Jacksonet al., 2011, p. 107). According to Price (2009), professional socialization is "an essential process of learning skills attitudes and behaviours necessary to fulfil professional roles" (p. 12). Learning how to respond to change thoughtfully and critically as a professional nurse is thus part of the learning process of becoming a nurse. The assumption in this chapter is that nursing students' experiences are important in recruiting and retaining future nurses who are essential to the health of Canadians. This means that it is important for the growth of the discipline to understand, validate, and address issues in undergraduate nursing education including how students experience stress in their academic and clinical settings. The diversity of the nursing student body means that stress is experienced differently for each student, but there are some markers of difference that perhaps have a compounding influence on that experience.

Diversity

Race, class, gender, culture, as well as religion, geographical location, and sexual orientation are markers of difference that shape the individual's experience of health and illness and also shape how health care is provided. Students who have English as an additional language, students who need additional academic support to enter nursing programs, Aboriginal students, and students who come from non-white, non-Christian, and non-European heritages may differ in their assumptions about the meaning of health and illness, learning, and nursing. Although a 2009 CNA policy document promoting the value of embracing diversity in Canadian nursing explains that diversity is a benefit to the profession and to society (Sustaining the Workforce by Embracing Diversity, CNA, 2009), the traditions of nursing and nursing education continue to reflect the heritage of the white, Christian, gendered roots of the Nightingale model. These traditions have come down to nursing and continue to influence who is a nurse and how students perceive nursing education. How students perceive their place in nursing is important in recruiting and retaining nurses for the future and so the quality of the workplace for all students and nurses is an issue of concern. As Jackson et al. (2011) explain, "among nurses, workplace hostility is acknowledged as a leading cause of stress, illness…and depression" (p. 102).

As Choiniere et al. (2010) reveal, the majority of Canadian nurses experience "work-related illness, injury, disability, and /or violence" (p. 317). Nursing students, as vulnerable members of the healthcare team, are in a lesser position to mediate the impact of workplace hostility and are thus at greater risk for harm. In fact, according to Choiniere et al. (2010), nurses and nursing students are exposed to greater risk and injury in the workplace than other healthcare workers. This is even more so for students identified as members of a minority group. In a female dominated profession like nursing, violence against nurses has been attributed to biology—that women are less able to defend themselves than are men. However, this assumption ignores how gender is more than biology; it represents the (changing) way that society creates certain expectations of what it means to be male, female, or other. Particular ways of dressing, talking, walking, and even thinking are thought to be fixed through gender and in fact determined through gender, which is linked to biology. However, what is not acknowledged is the way that dominant (and changing) beliefs about race, class, and gender also create and then enforce what is considered "normal" human behavior. In Canada, and in nursing, these beliefs are shaped by white, Christian European traditions whereby whiteness and maleness are privileged. The experience of feeling inferior, including "feeling ignored or unwelcome…undervalued… invisible [and]…experiencing verbal abuse (Jackson et al., 2011, p. 103) is compounded by being singled out as not only a student, but a member of a recognizable minority (Gibbons et al., 2011).

Information Technology

A third issue impacting nursing and nursing education is the information technology. According to Fetter (2009), "improving information technology (IT) outcomes is a top nursing priority" (p. 78). Bembridge et al. (2010) explain that information technology is a term that "refers to any technology that has the capacity to accumulate, retrieve, control, convey or accept information by electronic means" (p. 18). The pervasiveness of Internet technology seems to create the expectation that if nurses just had the right information (which seems to be so readily available), they could produce "measurable outcomes" more quickly, efficiently, and cheaply. In health care, the information that nurses and nursing students are exposed to include (high-fidelity) patient simulation, electronic patient health records, tele-health, i-health, e-health, and related forms of patient charting and tracking. Not all nurses and nursing instructors embrace newer forms of information technology. Most nurses and members of the public feel that nursing is the profession most responsible for direct patient care and, for some, new technologies are antagonistic to what they perceive has historically defined the role of the nurse: The nurses' relationship to the patient, unmediated through technology, including health information technology (HIT).

ANALYZING THE ISSUES

An analysis of issues concerning undergraduate education includes an analysis of the changing historical, social, political, and economic landscape of Canada. In this chapter, we use an approach described as "feminist intersectionality." According to Van Herk, Smith, and Andrew (2011), a feminist intersectional approach "help[s] debunk the hegemony of the 'White, middle class' perspective that governs nursing research, practice, and education" (p. 30). Bilge (2010) explains that intersectionality is more than the analysis of race, class, and gender. Instead, a feminist intersectional approach acknowledges that more than one category of difference is involved in complex problems and political processes. Bilge argues that relationships between all categories of difference, including race, class, and gender, vary from person to person, across time, and between geographic, political, social, and historical locations. For example, not all women have the same experience of being labeled "woman." In the same way, not all nurses are caring just because they are nurses. Nurses must guard against making assumptions about difference or sameness in others based on personal experience. Therefore, in analyzing issues in undergraduate nursing education, we must be aware that there are multiple ways to describe and understand those issues, multiple barriers of resistance, and multiple strategies for resolution.

Analyzing Issues from a Historical Perspective

So far we have introduced four key issues in undergraduate nursing education: Students' experience of stress, diversity, the influence of information technology, and the challenge of interprofessional models of patient care. I have suggested an overall approach of feminist intersectionality as a way of understanding the historical, social, political, and economic contexts that have shaped those issues. The history of nursing education is one of those contexts.

In a profession like nursing, historical knowledge shapes everyday work life in a variety of ways. Individual practitioners, for example, accumulate experiences over the course of their careers. Those personal histories inform how nurses see their profession and respond to workplace issues, sometimes causing conflict or misunderstanding between nurses of different ages, with different experiences, and different personal histories. History is also reflected in nursing's legislative and regulatory frameworks: Laws determining who should be considered a nurse and what constitutes nursing continue to exert powerful influences on the profession long after they are passed. Nursing organizations and institutions, including schools of nursing, are invested in knowing about their pasts. They collect and preserve information about their own histories because they see how specific events and decisions in the past explain current practices. Nursing's past is also represented in popular culture and public opinion, where traditional images of nurses—however old-fashioned and outdated—are reproduced in film, television, and mass media. Throughout work life, then, nurses will encounter a range of ways that history is used—personal, legal, institutional, and popular. In these contexts, scholarly histories of nursing written by nurse-historians can offer some benchmarks from which to evaluate these sometimes competing versions of nursing's past, while also offering perspective on current issues and challenges for the future.

Over the past two centuries, the ways in which nurses were educated has fundamentally shaped the work nurses performed, the conditions in which nurses worked, and even who was considered a nurse. Indeed, nursing education has changed significantly since the early 19th century and examining some of those shifts helps illuminate how the definition of nursing is produced socially and historically. A historical overview of these shifts reveals that although the term "nurse" seems to represent a singular category of work and practitioners, it has contained over time a range of practitioners with a range of training and experience. Since at least 1800, when the British colonies of North America were expanding geographically and politically, there have been many paths to nursing, many routes to claim status as a nurse.

Diversity and Difference in the Early 19th Century

In the early 19th century, the particular combination of education, experience, and personal attributes varied widely among kinds of attendants and kinds of nursing care. Some, like the nuns of Catholic orders, acquired substantial expertise as healers by apprenticing under the senior members of the order and then working with the European-trained physicians and surgeons who returned to British North America to practice. In an era when physical health was directly linked to spiritual health and salvation, nuns combined religious ministry with more material services like bedside care, preparing pharmaceuticals, assisting with—and sometimes performing—surgery, and even midwifery. Because religious orders were responsible for Catholic institutions, many nuns were also skilled healthcare administrators, running large hospitals like Hotel Dieu in Montreal. Aboriginal societies, too, relied on midwives and female caregivers who were sanctioned by the community and might have been selected at early ages to apprentice as midwives.

Lay nurses rarely boasted such extensive formal instruction and sanctioned status. True, lay midwives—whose practice was not made illegal until later in the 19th century—might have well trained at one of the many lying-in hospitals in England, Scotland, and Ireland. Of course, many midwives gained their experience at a more personal level, giving birth to their own children and perhaps helping family members before becoming known in their community as "grannies" or "aunties" who could be relied upon for their experience, if not their formal education. These practitioners would have sought to distinguish themselves from domestic servants, nannies, or even governesses, all of whom would have been hired by middle-class and upper-class families.

Caregivers working in 19th-century hospitals would have had a harder time distinguishing themselves from the servant class. Lay hospitals inherited from the 18th century an uncomfortable alliance with poorhouses, and the women and men who staffed 19th-century hospitals were understood to provide custodial and domestic cleaning functions as much as any direct patient care. With the growth of hospitals in the later 19th century, what was expected of hospital staff began to expand, especially with respect to treating children and to performing surgeries. Hospitals thus began to mobilize to recruit a more respectable class of women to work as nurses and to retain those nurses who acquired specific skills as a result of working directly with staff doctors. These skilled staff nurses coexisted with older style nurses.

Nineteenth-century nurses claimed personal experience, informal apprenticeship with a doctor or pharmacist, structured apprenticeship with a religious order, formal midwifery certification, or knowledge derived from published manuals as the basis of their expertise. As a result, those who might call themselves nurses were also varied: Every ethnic or racialized community contributed to its local nursing workforce, though the degree to which nurses of one ethnic group could work in another depended very much on the specific politics of ethnocentrism and the prevailing economies of need.

Uniformed and Unified, 1880 to 1950

Changes in the nature of scientific medicine and the structure of Canadian society changed all this variability. By the 1880s, hospitals were becoming increasingly important sites of new medical procedures, and local medical associations started to more carefully control not only their own memberships but also which allied healthcare providers could practice and on what terms. Midwifery was made illegal, as was homeopathy and chiropractics. Medical authorities saw hospital nurses as particularly in need of reform, and, in 1874, a St. Catherines, Ontario, hospital instituted what would become the first of a long line of hospital-based nursing schools. Over the next 50 years, more than 70 hospital schools of nursing had opened across Canada. Initially organized around a 2-year curriculum, the 3-year program soon became the norm. Young, single women, between the ages of 18 and 35, with at least 1 year of high school to their credit, lived and worked in their institution, learning through some direct instruction and through extensive "on-the-ward" experience. When they graduated, they could call themselves "graduate nurses" and advertise their services on the private healthcare market, attending patients in their own homes or in private hospital wards and charging the family directly for services rendered.

The advent of the hospital-prepared nurse did not immediately eradicate the presence of the older style informally trained nurse of the 19th century. Indeed, nursing registries, established in urban centers to help families locate and hire nurses, continued to list "graduate nurses" alongside "other nurses" throughout the first decades of the 20th century. Nevertheless, a clear hierarchy was being produced, and, by the 1920s, graduates of hospital schools held significant prestige in the healthcare market. Meeting the entry requirements of hospital programs demanded that prospective students had completed at least some high school, a firm command over either English or French, and enough family resources such that their families could afford to live without their daughters' incomes for the 3 years of the nursing education program. Whatever their education, language, or financial status, nonwhite women and men of all ancestries were denied entry to most hospital schools of nursing. Thus, although early 20th-century graduate nurses hailed from rural and urban households and from a range of occupational backgrounds (including farming communities, working-class communities, and middle-class communities), the graduate nursing workforce was predominantly single, female, white, English-speaking (or French-speaking in parts of Quebec and New Brunswick), and had completed some high school. Graduate nurses thus held significant social prestige, even if they had to work to earn their living. Nursing was, then, a popular and prestigious occupational choice for young women seeking respectable work that would permit them economic independence and the ability to move across Canada and the world.

Working in hospitals with scientifically trained physicians and surgeons, student nurses gained valuable skills performing a range of procedures. This skill set included a solid theoretical knowledge of the germ theory and of disease and infection, including the symptoms of the most prevalent diseases of the day, such as diphtheria and tuberculosis, as well as sophisticated applied knowledge of how to maintain aseptic conditions, create a sterile field, assist in often-complicated surgical and medical procedures, and prepare and administer medications, including intramuscular injections. This skilled workforce was instrumental in making hospitals safe and efficient institutions for the delivery of scientific medicine.

In spite of the skills student nurses acquired, nursing leaders and educators grew increasingly frustrated with what they saw as flaws in this system. Hospitals were so reliant on student labor that too much learning was being done "on the job" and not enough time was set aside for classroom instruction and theoretical preparation. Classes were often held before and after students worked 12-hour shifts on the ward. As a result, nursing was not, in the eyes of some educators, attracting a "better class" of student: Too many applicants to nursing programs held the bare minimum of educational requirements. All nursing educators agreed that the proliferation of hospital nursing programs had resulted in an overproduction of graduate nurses, many of who were having trouble finding employment in private duty work.

With these concerns in mind, the CNA commissioned a study to investigate the crisis of employment. The 1932 "Weir Report on Nursing Education" recommended a significant increase in educational standards and a dramatic decrease in the number of hospital schools. The report also endorsed the efforts of dynamic nursing leaders like Kathleen Russell who were working to establish university nursing programs. By the end of World War II (WWII), new scientific and technological advances in health care combined with new state funding programs for hospital construction and growth resulted in significant changes in nursing education.

Specialization and the Emergence of the Canadian Welfare State, 1950 to 2000

The 1950s ushered in a very different set of educational structures and the definition of who was a nurse again changed. Between 1950 and 2000, the internal coherence and homogeneity of nursing was again transformed as new programs for educating nurses, new interest in recruiting a wider range of women and men from Canada and internationally, and the need to introduce new levels of subsidiary attendants combined to create a more heterogeneous workforce of nurses.

Many of these changes were sparked by the continued growth in hospitals after WWII and by new biomedical knowledge that accelerated Canadians' demand for scientific medicine. Put bluntly, during the second half of the 20th century, Canadians wanted and needed more health services, and the Canadian healthcare system wanted and needed more front-line attendants. The combination of new scientific knowledge and a constant shortage of nurses facilitated three kinds of changes to occur within nursing education. First, hospital administrators began to hire RNs to staff the wards: Student nurses didn't always have the advanced skills needed for some of the new procedures and many of the new procedures simply couldn't be learned "on the ward." As a result, hospital-based nursing programs began to devote more resources to classroom-based learning but still could not meet the constant demand for more graduates. In this context, community colleges initiated 2-year diploma courses in nursing. Meanwhile, the struggle to establish university-based baccalaureate programs in nursing had been won. By 1950, 10 Canadian universities offered Bachelor of Nursing or Bachelor of Science in Nursing degrees, and another dozen were established in the 1960s to 1980s. Some universities offered 4-year "integrated" degree programs, whereby students combined their basic sciences, liberal arts courses, and nursing-specific curriculum throughout the 4 years. Other universities offered 2-year "post RN" degrees that had to be completed once students had graduated from a hospital or community college diploma program. In 1982, CNA endorsed the position that the entry to practice for nurses should be a bachelor's degree and set the year 2000 to reach that goal, but the reality for the 1950 to 2000 era was that the nursing workforce boasted a range of educational credentials.

Back to the Present

If the postwar nursing workforce was characterized by the diversity of educational background, it was equally diverse in terms of the ethnic, racial, and national origin of its members. Few non-white women had been admitted to Canadian nursing schools before WWII. In 1944 and again in 1947, CNA passed resolutions advocating non-discrimination in student admission policies, but breaking racist barriers was a slow process. African-Canadian women and First Nations women were first admitted to Canadian nursing schools in the late 1940s, joining the small number of Chinese and Japanese-Canadian women who were enrolled. Despite the eradication of formal racist barriers, and reflecting the ethnic make-up of Canada at mid-century, nursing remained dominated by women of European ancestry until well into the 1960s and 1970s when immigration laws and patterns changed (Flynn, 2009). In those decades, foreign-born and foreign-trained nurses began to hold a greater presence in Canadian health care, reaching 13% of the RNs employed in 1971. The integration of male nurses was a slower process, with men representing less than 10% of the nursing workforce throughout the postwar era. In fact, the most pronounced change in the demographic composition of Canada's nursing workforce in this era was the marked increase in the presence of married women and of women with children—and, as a result, the age profile of nurses has grown older as nurses remain active longer throughout their life course.

Older, more ethnically diverse, including a larger number of men, and boasting a wide range of educational backgrounds: The workforce of RNs changed dramatically after 1950. Yet, in spite of these efforts to widen the pool of recruits, shortages within Canadian hospitals continued throughout the postwar era. Hospitals responded by introducing new levels of subsidiary workers to take up particular duties that had once been the domain of RNs or student nurses. Some, like LPNs, received formal training and certification; others were trained on the job. In some provinces, RPNs received distinctive education and licensing. In all provinces, university schools began graduating nurses with masters and doctorates in nursing or in related disciplines (such as education or administrative studies). The homogeneity that had once characterized the largest workforce in the Canadian healthcare system—the "nurse"—was gone. As in the 19th century, there were many paths to working at the bedside and many ways to become a nurse.

The particular critical feminist view of nursing history presented here examines nursing within the intersecting relationships of power, class, gender, and culture that have shaped how we understand nursing, nursing education, and health care and Canadian society in the 21st century.

Analyzing Issues from a Political Perspective

Our starting place is the idea that nursing is always already political whether we acknowledge these conditions or not. Not only are nurses' practices shaped by the formal "politics" of the day, which work to establish the specific economic and social contexts of healthcare, but there is a sense in which health is always a political issue having to do with judgments that instantiate values, create conditions of access, assign worth—and of course, reveal power.

(Cameron et al., 2011, p. 153)

A second way of contextualizing issues in undergraduate education is from a political perspective. As explained in the introduction to this text, most issues benefit from more than one type of analysis, but some will benefit from an emphasis on one particular aspect of analysis. Earlier, we explained that it is not possible to separate out particular aspects of identity such as race, class, gender, or culture because they intersect and change in meaning depending on a particular social and historical location. It is nonetheless important for you to be able to identify, articulate, and critique how issues in nursing education are influenced and shaped by particular historical, social, political, and social contexts and how these in turn are influenced by dominant beliefs about race, class, and gender.

One concept that links each aspect of our analysis together is the concept of power. Michel Foucault explains that power is not confined to a particular place, person, or thing. It is not something we are born with, but rather it is a word we give to a very complex set of relationships and attributes that are expressed at all levels of personal, societal, political, and economic organization. Petitt (2009) describes power in terms of the influence of race and gender—two axes of identity that are particularly relevant for nursing. Petitt's research focuses on the experience of nonwhite women in academia where "Whiteness is a critical issue in organizational culture and power. Because White individuals define, control, and shape organizational realities, policies, and practices" (p. 633). Thus, an analysis of how the "politics of power" is invested in systems such as health care, education, and government is a good place to understand how power has an impact on undergraduate education.

Analyzing Issues from an Economic Perspective

The Costs of Education and Diversity

In healthcare financing in many industrialized countries today, it is becoming increasingly important that every activity that goes on in a hospital, clinic, or nursing home be justified as cost effective. Skilled nurses are being challenged to prove that what they do cannot be sped up (so that fewer skilled nurses could be hired) or deskilled (so that hospitals could shift the work to lower-paid aides).

(Adams & Nelson, 2009, p. 3)

Our third perspective in analyzing issues in undergraduate education is from an economic perspective. Throughout the 20th century, nurse leaders fought to establish nursing as a discipline within institutions of higher learning and to eliminate the apprenticeship model that was popular even into the 1990s in Canada. Some have argued that the baccalaureate degree enhances nursing's status and profile in relation to other health professions; however, a recent editorial in the *Canadian Medical Association Journal,* (Dec. 22, 2009) comments that "the ongoing cost and stressors of a degree program not only prevent some people from entering but also weed out others along the way" (p. E132). In particular, the editor comments that the degree as entry to practice presents barriers and additional sources of stress to Aboriginal people and others who may need additional language or foundational courses to qualify for entry to a university degree program; thus the degree requirement increases the cost and length of the program.

The Costs of Technology

Another cost consideration in undergraduate education is the cost of providing opportunities for students to learn how to use HIT. These costs include the purchase of high-priced information technology simulators, and the cost of human resources to bring educators and technicians up to speed and ahead of the tidal wave of new technologies. According to Alexander and Staggers (2009), "having usable technology is imperative for contemporary nurses. Less optimal technology designs affect error generation and productivity, [and] create extreme frustration" (p. 252). Skiba (2010) argues that all nurses need to be HIT literate in order to be effective in today's healthcare system. For this to become a reality she claims, "informatics knowledge, skills, and attitudes must be integrated throughout the nursing curriculum. This is not optional" (p. 390). One particularly contentious topic is the use of Standardized Nursing Languages (SNL), now becoming common in the United States. The use of SNL is a part of what Farren (2010) describes as an effort to bring quality care in line with current professional knowledge. A review of the literature linked SNL to "improved accuracy, competency, and critical thinking" (p. 4) in nursing assessment, diagnosis, and intervention. The use of SNL or terminology is thought to be a way to document nursing's unique contribution to patient care as part of the increasing use of the patient Electronic Health Record (EHR) (Schwiran & Thede, 2011). Farren summarized the support for the use of SNL in patient charting as being related to the need for accurate nursing diagnosis and appropriate nursing interventions, the need for education and experience in using SNL for nursing students, and the efficacy of using SNL to enhance clinical reasoning. On the other hand, some nurse scholars argue that standardizing the language of nursing care strips away the heart of nursing practice—the relationship of the nurse to the patient—leaving only a shorthand notation dominated by medical terminology. For some nurses and nurse scholars, the use of standardized language threatens rather than enhances the autonomy of the profession by submerging non-quantifiable actions by nurses. As Cleveland (2011) explains

> The paradigm shifts and trends in health care and health information and the changes of information technologies demand crossing boundaries, creating much larger bodies of knowledge and skills for our professionals. This can bring extensive and radical ramifications for institutions of higher education (p. 66).

Despite these diverse views, Bembridge et al. (2010) argue that an investment in the cost of teaching students how to use HIT and other forms of information technology is justified because it is important that students learn the knowledge and skills that actually reflect the reality of the workplace. Learning how to use information technologies such as the electronic patient chart, which includes the use of SNL, helps to mitigate the effects of that reality shock. The authors cite studies going back to the 1930s that claim graduate nurse attrition can be related to "'reality shock,' a term which portrays the gap between undergraduate programs and the realities of the workplace...[and further] of particular interest is the role that information and communication technology (ICT) plays in the 'reality shock'" (p. 19).

Analyzing Issues from a Societal Perspective: Race, Class, and Gender

> *Critical educator Paulo Freire (2001) writes of education as "a form of intervention in the world" (p. 91). He reminds us that as an intervention, education can serve two ends, the continuation of prevailing ideologies and their unmasking.*
> *(Cameron et al., 2011, p. 155)*

A third perspective in analyzing issues in undergraduate education is from a societal perspective. Membership in the culture of nursing has historically included a process of "proving" oneself as a nurse in terms of what one knows about providing patient care and how one performs the act of nursing. Taking on the identity of a nurse and being accepted as a member of the profession includes becoming aware of and accepting the values, beliefs, and assumptions that shape the culture of nursing (Bolan & Grainger, 2009; Jackson et al., 2011). As D'Antonio et al. (2010) claims, nurses have contributed to improving society in numerous ways, particularly health care, but not only health care. D'Antonio points to nursings' contribution to "battling some of the deadliest diseases of the 20th century, and our place in making the academy a somewhat more hospitable place for women" (p. 113). Despite these successes, nursing, even today a predominantly female profession, still struggles for legitimation in a society that sees caring as women's work, and even the "natural" role of women. Being a good woman and being a good nurse are often linked within a gendered view of women as subservient to men, and nursing as subservient to medicine. As Levett-Jones and Lathlean (2009) explain, in the 19th century Florence Nightingale, "described the qualities of a 'good nurse' as restraint, discipline and obedience" (p. 343). These authors ask whether becoming accepted and acculturated into the hierarchy of the healthcare system still calls on nurses and nursing students to accept a subordinate role. In fact, Levett-Jones and Lathlean discuss a cross-national study of nursing students in Australia that looked at students' experience of nursing education and found "nursing students frequently engaged in strategies such as conformity and compliance, believing that to do so would improve their likelihood of acceptance by the nursing staff they worked with during clinical placements" (p. 343). Nursing students also reported a high degree of stress in their subordinate role as junior nurses. Goff (2011) used Gadzella's Student-life Stress Inventory (SSI) and Rosenbaum's Self-Control Scale (SCS) to examine the impact of stress on nursing students and found "high stress levels in nursing students may affect memory, concentration, and problem-solving ability, and may lead to decreased learning, coping, academic performance, and retention" (Goff, 2011, Abstract). Similarly, Galbraith and Brown (2011) identified significant stress levels in nursing students and claimed that the impact of stress contributed to sickness, absence, and attrition (p. 709). The authors of this systematic review suggest a number of interventions for reducing stress and highlight the importance of promoting such strategies in order to reduce attrition rates from schools of nursing and retain graduate nurses. A number of these strategies are presented later in this chapter.

The shifting demographics and greater diversity of society in Canada have been recognized as issues in nursing and nursing education. While each person is unique and thus diverse in many apparent and not so apparent ways, it is markers of race, class, and gender that are most often discussed as markers of social difference. As Munoz et al. (2009) explain, there is evidence that minorities, those people who stand out as different from the social norm, "experience a higher incidence of disability, disease, and death compared with the mainstream population"(p. 495). Students who exhibit markers of difference also experience the effect of society's attitudes toward minority groups. In addition to the background level of stress experienced by students who represent the mainstream demographic, Aboriginal students, foreign-born students, students with English as an additional language, and students with other markers of social difference face additional stress. Junious et al. (2010) identify "language issues, stereotyping, discrimination, cultural incompetence, financial issues, and lack of accommodation" (p. 261) as experiences that result in health-impacting stress for minority students and contribute to greater levels of student attrition and leaving nursing.

Analyzing Issues from an Ethical Perspective

Our fourth approach in analyzing issues in undergraduate education takes an ethical perspective. Obtaining the appropriate credentials is only one step in the process of assuming the role and identity of a Registered Nurse. This process includes coming to know the ethics, skills, relational practice, politics, history, and the culture of nursing practice. For some students, entering the workplace may present challenges and dilemmas about how to enact those standards of practice when they come into conflict with the culture of the paid working environment. Allen (2006) emphasizes that nurse educators strive to inculcate students with high ethical standards of practice but fail to recognize that in some settings these standards become eroded by pressures to work faster with fewer hands to provide high-quality nursing care. Despite these pressures, Van Herk et al. (2010) claim that it is an ethical imperative for nurses to consider how their position of power, afforded through their association with the dominant biomedical model, impacts their relationships with students. This critical self-examination is necessary in order to "practice as safe and caring professionals" (p. 30).

Critical Analysis of the Issues: Feminist and Postcolonial Perspectives

Our final lens of analysis employs a feminist and postcolonial perspective. Feminist intersectionality, introduced earlier in this chapter, is linked to a broader framework of analysis referred to as critical feminism or postcolonial feminism. Like feminist intersectionality, a postcolonial feminist analysis examines who is included and who is excluded from nursing and provides a way of understanding exclusionary practices in nursing. Postcolonial feminism seeks to understand how gender, class, and race identities are produced and reproduced within the context of local, national, and global relations of power. For example, postcolonial feminism critiques any characterization of women in the global south as passive victims in need of rescue—the "Third-World woman"—and insists that instead we need to listen carefully to what women in the global south say about their day-to-day struggles with economic and political instability. Postcolonial feminism also challenges women living in the global north to interrogate how colonialism also defines their societies and their lives. In Canada, this means acknowledging the ongoing effects of colonialism on Aboriginal Canadians. It means seeing how divisions of race, ethnicity, class, and sexuality have been created through state policies such as immigration regulations and through processes such as admission criteria for nursing schools. In addition, it means recognizing the racially produced privilege that white Canadians enjoy.

BARRIERS AND STRATEGIES: ISSUES IN PERSPECTIVE

According to Risjord (2010), the profession and discipline of nursing is notoriously fond of framing issues in terms of opposites and binaries. You are probably familiar with the binaries of the "theory/practice" debate, the "diploma/degree" debate, and the "profession/occupation" debate. The term "debate" already implies you are on one side or the other (opposing/binary) side of the "argument." Van Herk et al. (2011) suggest that a positivist paradigm, in which the medical model is legitimated, privileges binary and dualistic thinking. By binary and dualistic thinking I mean the assumption that through particular methods of scientific investigation, "the truth" can be found. The assumption that there is one truth that is to be found underpins the values, beliefs, and assumptions of the medical model and much of empirical scientific research. Van Herk et al. (2011) claim that this dualistic or binary thinking has invaded nursing and must be challenged. They claim that nurses must consider the contextualization of knowledge and the individuality of each nurse/patient encounter. If not:

> A divide is created between provider and patient which results in patients' receiving poor care that is unresponsive to who [sic] they are as human beings. This divide is the result of the dominance/subordination and privilege/oppression binaries associated with the biomedical model of health and the associated white, middle class perspective that often separates health-care providers from the context of the lives of marginalized individuals to whom they provide care (p. 29).

So, let's take this opportunity to go beyond "good issue/bad issue," "problem/solution," "conflict/resolution," and even "barrier/strategy" thinking in our consideration of barriers and strategies in relation to issues in undergraduate nursing education. As Gibbons et al. (2011) research demonstrates, we need to think differently about the complexity of issues and experiences, not whether they are right or wrong. A feminist intersectoral approach challenges binaries and artificial divisions such as race, class, and gender. Instead, an intersectoral approach would look at how issues might be addressed from a "both/and" rather than an "either/or," "barriers/strategies" approach. From this perspective, you might conclude that barriers are sometimes strategies, and sometimes strategies are the barriers we need to challenge. Let's start with stress.

Stress: The Good, the Bad, and the Possibilities

Gibbons et al. measured the impact of learning environment stress on nursing students' health related to "three factors: Learning and teaching, Placement-related and Course organization" (p. 623). The researchers found that students at greater risk for "stress-related illness, did not report sources of stress as more distressing than those [who did not] but did rate those sources of stress as providing far fewer opportunities to achieve" (p. 623). In other words, stressful events *can* present opportunities for growth and change—both personal and organizational. For instance, although students experience stress because of assignment deadlines and uncertainty in clinical settings, they also learn organizational and communication skills.

According to Gibbons (2010), research into stress in nursing students usually uses the term stress to mean psychological stress. Gibbon's research is one of the only studies to examine how stress can in fact "enhance well-being and, by implication, learning" (p. 1299). Gibbon's research examines how stress is moderated by coping measures, which can produce "eustress" or "good stress." Therefore, although nursing students experience stress, their adaptation to that stress or coping measures may in fact result in enhanced learning and enjoyment, depending on what style of coping mechanisms they employ.

A type of stress most often reported by students is the negative attitude toward students in clinical settings. The expectations that nursing students have of their profession can be shattered by negative clinical experiences; these stresses are compounded by the stresses and pressures of their academic program and competing demands at home. "Organisational aggression," (Jackson et al., 2011, p. 106) whereby students report that staff and instructor facilitators "sought to intimidate them through use of insult or, alternatively, they were 'belittled' by those more senior who wanted 'to pick a fight' with students" (p. 106), present serious barriers for recruitment and retention of nursing students. According to some research, however, some students used situations where they felt stressed and oppressed to develop skills to resist oppression and stress such as resistance, collaboration, and confrontation (Jackson et al., 2011). Students learned to support each other, primarily in the clinical setting where most students reported feeling most oppressed, but also in academic settings where similar types of oppression arose. Students explained practices such as joint advocacy and "backing each other up, reporting mistreatment, countering allegations of incompetence or blame and developing shared plans of action to address their repression. Through these acts of resistance, students (re)created for themselves a sense of respect, dignity and control" (p. 106). What about the classroom setting?

Gibbons (2010) and Gibbons et al. (2011) identified three coping strategies that instructors can encourage in students to decrease stress: Self-efficacy, control, support. In addition, reasonable workloads, the inclusion of students in deciding about topics, assignments, due dates, and learning activities promote self-efficacy and control. A learning environment that includes peer interaction and problem-based learning as well as the availability of additional learning support for language, writing, and study skills demonstrates that the instructor is taking a role in supporting student learning as an expectation of her/his professional role. Students on the other hand must be proactive in taking up opportunities for engagement and seeking out additional supports provided outside the classroom.

Diversity: Making It Work

In addition to stress created in the learning and teaching, placement, and course-related environments identified by Gibbons et al. (2010), students with English as an additional language, Aboriginal students, students who are immigrants to Canada, or students with other markers of difference experience additional stress. That students who have markers of difference have a high rate of failure and attrition from nursing programs is the result of a much larger issue in nursing and has to do with discrimination based on gender, class, and culture historically embedded in nursing's history. According to Ackerman-Barger (2010), recruitment and retention of students from diverse backgrounds is important within the Canadian healthcare system and supports the tenets of the Canada Health Act. Ackerman-Barger claims that this is particularly true in nursing because "nursing is based on human relationships and meeting patients' needs based on who they are and what is happening in their lives" (p. 677).

Canadian Nurses Association (CNA) supports the role of nursing within the Canada Health Act and has issued a policy brief claiming by 2016 there will be a shortage of 113,000 registered nurses (Sustaining the Workforce by Embracing Diversity, CNA, 2009). Our population is growing mainly through immigration and as a result it is estimated that by 2017, 20% of Canadians (up from 16.2 % in 2006) will be from a visible minority group. CNA looks to recruitment and retention of members of diverse groups to fill the ranks of nursing. Their rationale is not just to fill nursing positions, but reflects the more ideological position that, "innovative strategies are needed to transform the health workforce into a workforce of inclusiveness" (Sustaining the Workforce by Embracing Diversity, CNA, 2009, p. 1). The development of nursing courses such as those offered at the University of British Columbia (UBC) are examples of how nursing is responding to current issues such as cultural diversity. UBC has launched the Aboriginal Health Human Resources Initiative to increase the Aboriginal healthcare workforce. Dalhousie University's School of Nursing has a Recruitment and Retention of Students of African Descent Program to address issues that prevent students from African descent from being successful in nursing. Finally, the University of Victoria's School of Nursing partnered with Tsawout First Nation in Saanich, British Columbia, on the Reciprocal Partnership Model in Nursing Education Project, funded by the British Columbia Ministry of Advanced Education, Aboriginal Special Projects. Programs like the Integrated Nursing Access Program (INAP) in Northern Canada for Aboriginal students ladders students into mainstream programs through a 3-year process of university-level activities that are essential (Orchard, Didham, Jong, & Fry, 2010).

Ackerman-Barger (2010) recommends that teaching strategies are also essential to address barriers to ethnically diverse students. The first step to creating a positive learning environment for minority students is for educators to "acknowledge the multiple barriers that exist for traditionally underrepresented students and how nursing faculty contribute to those barriers. Self-reflection should lead to identifying "instrumentation bias" (p. 678) and to the creation of assessment instruments that reduce racial testing bias and promote a classroom environment "that is empowering for all students" (p. 678).

HIT: Complexity and Choice

According to Fetter (2009), the use of information technology "has vast potential to reduce health errors and improve care quality, access, and cost effectiveness" (p. 78). Many nurse scholars are calling for the integration of HIT competencies at all levels of the educational process. Despite this call, some nursing faculty are resistant to the use of technology and this is a major barrier to moving forward on integrating IT into nursing education. This resistance has been noted by Cleveland (2011) who argues that the nursing workforce is aging and that the average age of nurses is over 50. Many of these nurses did not grow up with information technology and are nearing retirement. For some, investment in new learning, despite the research that demonstrates positive patient care outcomes, is not worth their while. What are some of the directions that nursing needs to take to meet these challenges of the new IT age?

Bembridge et al. (2010) suggest that more research is needed to determine if information technology skills learned at the undergraduate level are applicable in the practice setting. There is also a perceived conflict between technological and humanized health care and this has not been adequately theorized. If information technology literacy is to become a nursing competency, then at this time there is no standard against which to measure those competencies in Canada. This lack of articulation with other countries that are already using information literacy competencies like the United States will limit student's mobility in the job market.

Another area of concern or potential growth related to the use of IT is shortage of clinical practice opportunities. Baxter et al. (2009) claim there are decreasing numbers of clinical settings available to nursing students and clinical time is severely limited. The level of patient acuity has also increased, and for this reason Baxter et al. suggest "one strategy [to address this issue] is the use of simulation" (p. 313).

How does simulation fit for a practice profession? If we accept that patient scenario simulation is useful in nursing education, then according to Baxter et al. (2009), simulation cannot replace "real-life" clinical learning. Research on faculty attitudes toward simulation range from enthusiastic to resistant. Generally, it is acknowledged that extra time and resources for faculty education is required to make simulation a positive experience for students. Time and training are resource intensive, and more work needs to be done on the efficacy of simulation as a teaching tool (Baxter et al., 2009). In addition to faculty education, students need access and time to become comfortable and familiar with simulation technology so that they do not feel threatened by its complexity. Not all students embrace technology equally and some find the experience "uncomfortable and stressful" (p. 865). Pairing students who are enthusiastic about simulation experiences with students who are fearful is suggested as one approach to easing students' anxiety. Debriefing and video-taping simulation exercises are also suggested in a review of the literature related to the use of high-fidelity patient simulation. Despite these challenges, research focused on third-year students' perceptions of high-fidelity simulation indicates that while students claimed that they learned best by interaction with real patients, more than 90% of students working in three scenarios with SimMan enjoyed their experience and found it worthwhile. In addition, 95% of students reported that knowledge gained was transferable to the clinical setting (Wotton et al., 2010; Wotton & Neill, 2011). The authors cautioned, however, that "high-fidelity simulation must be incorporated into the curriculum and not seen as a stand-alone educational tool" (p. 638). They also warned that more research is needed to validate the "relationship between the use of high-fidelity simulation and the development of students' clinical reasoning skills, to examine the relationship between confusion (i.e., 'feeling lost') and student learning, and to further explore the benefits of debriefing" (p. 638).

Information technology skills take time to develop and include faculty development and other resources such as simulation labs. A review of the literature also reveals that more research is needed in all areas of HIT in undergraduate education in order to justify claims of enhanced patient care at the bedside through the use of IT. Nonetheless, it appears that in Canada, as in the United States, the age of "information literacy competencies mapped to direct outcomes evaluation, curriculum mapping, and model module and documentation development" (Fetter, 2009, p. 78) is on its way. Not only nurses use information technologies. Nurses are part of a team of healthcare providers who are on a steep learning curve.

SUMMARY

This chapter has described and articulated three issues in undergraduate nursing education: The impact of stress on nursing students, diversity in nursing and undergraduate education, and the use of information technology. We have analyzed these issues from historical, political, economic, and societal positions using a feminist intersectoral approach that looks at the intersection of race, class, and gender in shaping meaning and experience. This is not an exhaustive list of issues but it suggests topics for further discussion that you perhaps had not previously thought of. These issues are your issues as you continue in your journey to become a politically active agent of change in your role as a professional nurse. Understanding the nature and implication of these issues will help you become that agent, not only in your student role, but also in leadership and advocacy roles to come.

Add to your knowledge of these issues:

		Online
Canadian Association of Schools of Nursing	**http://www.casn.ca**	
The Canadian Nursing Students Association	**http://www.cnsa.ca**	

REFLECTIONS *on the Chapter...*

1 What is the key point you take away from this chapter about the influence of change on undergraduate nursing education?
2 What points of view in this chapter do you not agree with?
3 What is the major cause of stress for undergraduate students?
4 Where does Information Technology fit in your nursing practice?
5 Do you agree that interdisciplinary models of practice should be integrated into undergraduate nursing education?

Want to know more? Visit the Point for additional helpful resources:

- Journal Articles
- Learning Objectives
- Nursing Professional Roles and Responsibilities
- Bonus chapters:
  - Health and Nursing Policy: A Matter of Politics, Power and Professionalism
  - The NP Movement: Recurring Issues
  - When Difference Matters: The Politics of Privilege and Marginality

References

Ackerman-Barger, P.W. (2010). Embracing multiculturalism in nursing learning environments. *The Journal of Nursing Education, 49*(12), 677–682. doi:10.3928/01484834-20100630-03

Adams, V., & Nelson, J. (2009). The economics of nursing: Articulating care. *Feminist Economics, 15*(4), 3–29. doi:10.1080/13545700903153971

Alexander, G., & Staggers, N. (2009). A systematic review of the designs of clinical technology: Findings and recommendations for future research. *ANS. Advances in Nursing Science, 32*(3), 252–279.

Allen, D.G. (2006). Whiteness and difference in nursing. *Nursing Philosophy, 7*, 65–78.

Baxter, P., Akhtar-Danesh, N., Valaitis, R., Stanyon, W., & Sproul, S. (2009). Simulated experiences: Nursing students share their perspectives. *Nurse Education Today, 29*(8), 859–866. doi:10.1016/j.nedt.2009.05.003

Bembridge, E., Levett-Jones, T., & Jeong, S.Y. (2010). The preparation of technologically literate graduates for professional practice. *Contemporary Nurse: A Journal for the Australian Nursing Profession, 35*(1), 18–25.

Bilge, S. (2010). Recent feminist outlooks on intersectionality. *Diogenes, 57*(1), 58–72. doi:10.1177/0392192110374245

Bolan, C., & Grainger, P. (2009). Students in the BN program—do their perceptions change? *Nurse Education Today, 29*(7), 775–779. doi:10.1016/j.nedt.2009.03.016

Cameron, B., Ceci, C., & Salas, A.S. (2011). Nursing and the Political. *Nursing Philosophy 12*(3), 153–155.

Canadian Nurses Association. (2009). *Sustaining the workforce by embracing diversity.* Retrieved September 7, 2012 from www.2.cna-aiic.ca/CNA/documents/...hhr_policy_Brief5_2009_e.p

Choiniere, J.A., MacDonnell, J., & Shamonda, H. (2010). Walking the talk: Insights into dynamics of race and gender for nurses. *Policy, Politics & Nursing Practice, 11*(4), 317–325. doi:10.1177/1527154410396222

Cleveland, A.D. (2011). Miles to go before we sleep: Education, technology, and the changing paradigms in health information. *Journal of the Medical Library Association: JMLA, 99*(1), 61–69. doi:10.3163/1536-5050.99.1.011

D'Antonio, P., Connolly, C., Wall, B., Whelan, J., & Fairman, J. (2010). Histories of nursing: The power and the possibilities. *Nursing Outlook, 58*(4), 207–213. doi:10.1016/j.outlook.2010.04.005

Farren, A.T. (2010). An educational strategy for teaching standardized nursing languages. *International Journal of Nursing Terminologies and Classifications: The Official Journal of NANDA International, 21*(1), 3–13. doi:10.1111/j.1744-618X.2009.01139.x

Fetter, M.S. (2009). Curriculum strategies to improve baccalaureate nursing information technology outcomes. *The Journal of Nursing Education, 48*(2), 78–85.

Flynn, K. (2009). Beyond the glass wall: Black Canadian nurses, 1940-1970. *Nursing History Review, 17*, 129–152.

Galbraith, N.D., & Brown, K.E. (2011). Assessing intervention effectiveness for reducing stress in student nurses: Quantitative systematic review. *Journal of Advanced Nursing, 67*(4), 709–721. doi:10.1111/j.1365-2648.2010.05549.x

Gibbons, C. (2010). Stress, coping and burn-out in nursing students. *International Journal of Nursing Studies, 47*(10), 1299–1309. doi:10.1016/j.ijnurstu.2010.02.015

Gibbons, C., Dempster, M., & Moutray, M. (2011). Stress, coping and satisfaction in nursing students. *Journal of Advanced Nursing, 67*(3), 621–632. doi:10.1111/j.1365-2648.2010.05495.x

Goff, A. (2011). Stressors, academic performance, and learned resourcefulness in baccalaureate nursing students. *International Journal of Nursing Education Scholarship, 8*(1), 1–5.

Jackson, D., Hutchinson, M., Everett, B., et al. (2011). Struggling for legitimacy: Nursing students' stories of organisational aggression, resilience and resistance. *Nursing Inquiry, 18*(2), 102–110. doi:10.1111/j.1440-1800.2011.00536.x

Junious, D.L., Malecha, A., Tart, K., & Young, A. (2010). Stress and perceived faculty support among foreign-born baccalaureate nursing students. *The Journal of Nursing Education, 49*(5), 261–270. doi: 10.3928/01484834-20100217-02

Levett-Jones, T., & Lathlean, J. (2009). 'Don't rock the boat': Nursing students' experiences of conformity and compliance. *Nurse Education Today, 29*(3), 342–349. doi:10.1016/j.nedt.2008.10.009

Munoz, C.C., DoBroka, C.C., & Mohammad, S. (2009). Development of a multidisciplinary course in cultural competence for nursing and human service professions. *The Journal of Nursing Education, 48*(9), 495–503. doi:10.3928/01484834-20090610-03

Orchard, C., Didham, P., Jong, C., & Fry, J. (2010). Integrated Nursing Access Program: An Approach to Prepare Aboriginal Students for Nursing Careers. *International Journal of Nursing Education Scholarship, 7*(1), 1–21.

Petitt, B. (2009). Borrowed power. *Advances in Developing Human Resources, 11*(5), 633–645. doi:10.1177/1523422309352310

Price, S.L. (2009). Becoming a nurse: A meta-study of early professional socialization and career choice in nursing. *Journal of Advanced Nursing, 65*(1), 11–19. doi:10.1111/j.1365-2648.2008.04839.x

Risjord, M.W., 1960. (2010). *Nursing knowledge: Science, practice, and philosophy.* Ames, Iowa: Wiley-Blackwell Pub.

Schwiran, P., & Thede, L. (2011). Informatics: The standardized nursing terminologies: A national survey of nurses' experiences and attitudes. *Online Journal of Issues in Nursing, 16*(2), 1F.

Skiba, D.J. (2010). The future of nursing and the informatics agenda. *Nursing Education Perspectives, 31*(6), 390–391.

Van Herk, K.A., Smith, D., & Andrew, C. (2011). Examining our privileges and oppressions: Incorporating an intersectionality paradigm into nursing. *Nursing Inquiry, 18*(1), 29–39. doi:10.1111/j.1440-1800.2011.00539.x

Wotton, K., Davis, J., Button, D., & Kelton, M. (2010). Third-year undergraduate nursing students' perceptions of high-fidelity simulation. *The Journal of Nursing Education, 49*(11), 632–639. doi:10.3928/01484834-20100831-01

Wotton, K., & Neill, M.A. (2011). High-fidelity simulation debriefing in nursing education: A literature review. *Clinical Simulation in Nursing, 49*(11), 632–639.

Graduate Education

Sally Thorne

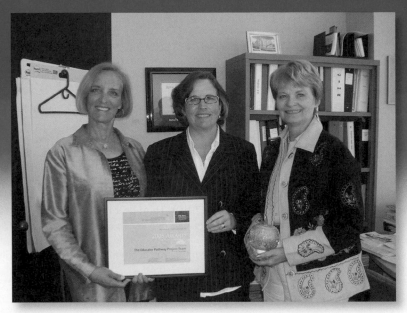

Nurse educators receive Golden Apple award for graduate nursing education. (Used with permission.)

Critical Questions

As a way of engaging with the ideas in this chapter, consider the following:

1. Have you ever considered graduate education in nursing as a possibility for yourself?

2. What would be important for you to consider in making a decision to pursue graduate education in nursing?

3. What difference might nurses prepared at the graduate level make to the study and practice of nursing?

4. What do you imagine is influencing the current proliferation of Canadian graduate programs in nursing?

Chapter Objectives

After completing this chapter, you will be able to:

1. Understand the implications of the historical context in which graduate nursing education in Canada has evolved.

2. Identify specific challenges faced in Canada by nurses with graduate preparation at various levels.

3. Recognize the impact of various social, economic, and political forces on the practice realities of Canadian nurses who have graduate degrees.

4. Interpret current issues and controversies associated with graduate nursing education in Canada.

(continued on page 203)

Chapter Objectives (continued)

5. Examine trends in society as they shape current graduate nursing education.

6. Identify opportunities for the nursing profession in Canada to direct its future through strategic advancement of graduate education.

This chapter focuses on the contributions made to the healthcare system by nurses educated at the graduate level. A special emphasis is placed on the contributions of nurses prepared at the master's level, whose focus is advanced practice, and those prepared at the doctoral and postdoctoral levels, whose focus is research.

Building on a historical overview of the evolution within graduate education in Canada, this chapter examines the impact of graduate education in general, as well as some of the specific contributions made by Canadian nurses with graduate-level preparation. Within this discussion, the reader will find a further exploration of some of the realities of graduate-prepared nurses in their places of work, the issues that arise for these nurses in practice, and the barriers that the profession needs addressed for the full potential of these nurses to be realized.

HISTORY OF GRADUATE NURSING EDUCATION IN CANADA

The second half of the 20th century brought graduate nursing education into the mainstream for the profession in Canada. In 1959, the first master's program in the country was launched at the University of Western Ontario, followed quickly by the inauguration of three more within the next decade, at McGill University, Université de Montréal, and the University of British Columbia (UBC). With a handful of new programs becoming available each decade, 27 universities were offering master's degrees in nursing by 2008 (Canadian Nurses' Association [CNA]) and Canadian Association of Schools of Nursing [CASN], 2010). The first doctoral program in the country, at the University of Alberta, admitted students in 1991, and over the next 2 decades, 13 doctoral programs in nursing were established across the country (Association of the Universities and Colleges of Canada (AUCC), 2011; CNA & CASN, 2010). The history of the evolution of graduate programs in Canada explains something of the shape that graduate nursing education has taken in comparison to that of other jurisdictions and provides a foundation for understanding some of the issues that nurses face with graduate preparation in the current academic, scientific, and social contexts.

Evolution of Master's Degree Programs

Although graduate degrees in other disciplines have been available to nurses for a much longer time, the history of master's programming in the country spans just over 60 years. As can be seen in Table 11.1, there has been a relatively stable proliferation of new master's degree programs in nursing every decade. Although many employers now specify a preference for graduate education in the discipline, master's programs designated as *nursing* degree programs still compete with a range of other disciplinary and interdisciplinary options open to nurses in Canada.

Before master's nursing programs were locally available in Canada, many nurses obtained their graduate preparation in other countries, particularly in the United States. Others undertook graduate work at Canadian universities in such fields as public health, education, medical science, social science, or business administration (Field et al., 1992). Although some of these

Table 11.1 Proliferation of Nursing Master's and Doctoral Programs in Canada

UNIVERSITY	MASTER'S PROGRAM	DOCTORAL PROGRAM
Athabasca University	2003	
Dalhousie University	1975	2003
Laurentian University	2004	
McGill University	1961	1993
McMaster University	1994	1994
Memorial University	1982	
Queens University	1994	2008
Ryerson University	2006	
Université du Québec	2001	
Université Laval	1991	
Université de Moncton	1997	
Université de Montréal	1965	1993
University of Alberta	1975	1991
University of British Columbia	1968	1991
University of British Columbia-Okanagan	2006	
University of Calgary	1981	1999
University of Lethbridge	2004	
University of Manitoba	1979	
University of New Brunswick	1995	
University of Northern British Columbia	2005	
University of Ottawa	1993	2004
University of Saskatchewan	1986	2007
University of Toronto	1970	1993
University of Victoria	2003	2006
University of Western Ontario	1959	2003
University of Windsor	1994	
York University	2005	

Note: Data compiled from most recent Canadian statistics.

From: Association of the Universities and Colleges of Canada (AUCC). (2011). *Directory of Canadian universities searchable database.* Retrieved from http://www.aucc.ca/ and, Canadian Nurses Association (CNA) and Canadian Association of Schools of Nursing (CASN). (2010). *Nursing Education in Canada Statistics 2008–2009.* Retrieved from http://www.casn.ca/vm/newvisual/attachments/856/Media/40605NursingEducationinCanadaStatistics20082009ENGFINAL.pdf Not listed above are collaborative sites without degree granting status, graduate programs leading to a degree other than nursing (such as the Master of Health Sciences, Master of Public Health, Maîtrise en sciences cliniques, interdisciplinary Ph.D., Doctorat en sciences cliniques) or degrees occurring outside of an approved nursing degree program, such as doctoral degrees by special arrangement.

degree programs drew nurses away from the main focus of their discipline for much of their academic development, others were quite sensitive to the special needs of nurse leaders and produced graduates with specialization in the study of problems directly relevant to their profession. In some instances, nursing faculty members with cross-appointments augmented the learning opportunities for nurses in those disciplines. In other instances, some nurses managed to retain their disciplinary focus within academic environments that were not entirely supportive.

For reasons of proximity and preference, some Canadian nurses continue to seek graduate education outside of the discipline, and, for the most part, the profession has enjoyed the healthy intellectual mix that can derive from an interdisciplinary perspective. In the early years, however, nurses tended to be less confident that their discipline would produce the highest quality graduate-level preparation for their advancement within such fields as nursing education and health administration (Beaton, 1990; Field et al., 1992; Ford & Wertenberger, 1993); hence, consciousness raising about the relevance of graduate preparation within nursing was a challenge throughout the early decades.

A continuing complication has been the availability of graduate programs designed specifically with nurses in mind but located somewhat outside of the disciplinary core, such as Master of Health Science or Public Health programs. In some universities, these programs have evolved collaboratively with the involvement of other disciplines as an evolutionary step toward more comprehensive nursing master's degree offerings (McBride, 1995). Thus it is not always self-evident to potential students which programs constitute *nursing* master's degrees.

In recognition of the urgent need for augmented graduate educational opportunities for nurses to advance the general academic level of professional nursing in Canada (Mussalem, 1965), nursing leaders creatively pursued a variety of strategies and mechanisms in developing master's programs. Among the strongest supporters of this initiative was the Kellogg Foundation. This foundation was a major presence in Canadian nursing education from 1949 to 1981 (Wood & Ross-Kerr, 2011). The foundation's fellowships to individual nurses helped Canadians obtain graduate degrees elsewhere, and its development grants supported initial programs in many Canadian universities in their early phases. Approvals to deliver graduate programs were accomplished individually by each university's senate and, in most instances, were explicitly built on a foundational history of high-quality undergraduate programming (McBride, 1995).

Within the Canadian nursing master's programs, the initial focus was primarily on filling the articulated needs within nursing education or nursing administration (McBride, 1995). Since the mid-1970s, that focus has shifted from those functional areas toward clinical specialization and leadership (Allen, 1986; McBride, 1995). Although nursing theory and science are still integral to the curriculum, the primary role of a master's degree program in preparing nurse researchers has gradually shifted since the 1980s as more Canadian nurses gain access to doctoral programs. Although rigorous research preparation was the standard within Canadian nursing master's programs until the advent of doctoral programs in 1991 (Kerr & McPhail, 1996), the appropriate placement for this level of training was a matter of controversy thereafter. Some master's programs in nursing continued to require a research-based thesis or include a thesis option; others no longer provided direct research training at this level (Gein, 1994; Kerr & McPhail, 1996; McBride, 1995).

Over its history, master's education in Canadian nursing has also experienced the effects of other trends and innovations. Although the dominant language of master's instruction in the country has remained English, the University of Ottawa was the first to offer a bilingual program, in 1993 (Kerr & McPhail, 1996). Because Canada's geography makes proximity to learning experiences a significant barrier for many nurses, and because the dominantly female constitution of the profession implies multiple demands upon learners, accessibility and flexibility of graduate education were consistently raised as important aspects of the ongoing discussion (Broughton & Hoot, 1995; Kerr, 1988). Over the years, with the rapid uptake of information and education technology innovations, many of the existing programs have some or all components available through web-based platforms or alternative delivery approaches. Two early innovations in the formatting of master's degree programs were the clinical training master's program available at the Family Nursing Unit in Calgary (Wright et al., 1985) and the generic master's program at McGill (Ezer et al., 1991).

Another major development in master's education in Canadian nursing in recent years has been the development of graduate-level nurse practitioner (NP) programs. Although the introduction of NPs into the health workforce in this country has taken a long and tortuous route, we now have a legislation to permit NP practice in one form or another across all provincial jurisdictions, and many provinces have launched educational programs. Despite the profession's strong consensus that the appropriate level of education for these programs is the specialized master's degree in nursing, this has not yet been achieved in all jurisdictions, and some provinces deliver NP education in the form of postbaccalaureate or postmaster's certificate programs. Although doing justice to the fascinating story of the evolution of educational programming for NP and other advanced practice roles is beyond the scope of this chapter, the issue has been extensively documented by leading thinkers in the discipline (Bryant-Lukosius et al., 2010; MacDonald-Rencz & Bard, 2010; Martin-Misener et al., 2010).

Although master's programs have rapidly proliferated and produced a generation of leaders for nursing practice, administration, education, and research, this evolution has not resolved the leadership shortage, let alone addressed the projected future demand at this point in our history (Mass et al., 2006). It is well recognized that, in the early 21st century, Canada has insufficient numbers of adequately prepared nurse educators and that a significant percentage of the current cadre of nurse educators is within sight of retirement (Canadian Institute for Health Information [CIHI], 2010; Hall, 2009). Thus, more than 3 decades after Beaton (1990) raised the alarm about the issue, consensus remains elusive as to what graduate education in nursing should constitute, how it ought to be funded and delivered, and whether academic or professional jurisdictions ought to take the lead in shaping the direction of future developments in master's education for Canadian nurses.

Evolution of Doctoral Degree Programs

The evolutionary process for doctoral nursing education in Canada has been much more recent and strategic than the development of master's degree programs. In 1978, the CNA sponsored a national seminar in which nursing leaders endorsed the value of working toward making doctoral nursing education possible in Canada (Zilm et al., 1979). From that, the Canadian Nurses Foundation (CNF) and the Canadian Association of University Schools of Nursing (from which today's CASN evolved) developed a proposal dubbed "Operation Bootstrap" to obtain funding for the infrastructure on which doctoral programs in nursing might be established (Kerr & McPhail, 1996). Although that proposal was never funded, the cooperative efforts involved in its development stimulated nursing educational leaders across the country to engage in sufficient strategic dialogue to create the basis on which explicit program proposals became successful a decade later. Through this process, Canadian nursing leaders developed a consensus with regard to the general conditions under which doctoral programs ought to be established, including the following:

- Universities with a successful track record in undergraduate and master's programming in nursing
- Close proximity to a full range of interdisciplinary doctoral and medical degree programs
- Sufficient numbers of doctorally prepared faculty members
- Explicit research development resources (such as programs of research or research units)
- Sufficient levels of research funding and a high degree of scholarly productivity shared among a range of faculty members (Field et al., 1992).

Although the first known Canadian nurse to obtain a doctoral degree was Sister Denise Lefebvre, SQM, Ph.D. (Docteur de Pédagogie) from Université de Montréal in 1955, the first to graduate with a doctoral degree in nursing on a special-case basis was Francine Ducharme from McGill in 1990 (Banning, 1990). Such special arrangement programs, allowing nurses to obtain doctoral degrees with a substantial nursing component, developed in a number of universities before the launching of formal nursing doctoral programs (Field et al., 1992; Wood & Ross-Kerr, 2011) and in some universities this model continues today. These programs differ from interdisciplinary doctoral degrees or degrees taken in another discipline by virtue of their explicit nursing focus, but they lack the programmatic core disciplinary component that the established nursing programs offer (Kerr & McPhail, 1996).

In 1991, the University of Alberta was the first in the country to launch a fully funded doctoral program in nursing, and its first official graduate was Joan Bottorff in 1992, who had been active in the program development process during her years as a special-case doctoral student there. The political negotiating involved in obtaining funding for that program and admitting the first group of students attracted considerable excitement across the country and was recognized as a landmark achievement (Brink, 1991; Field et al., 1992; Godkin & Bottorff, 1991; Rodger, 1991; Trojan et al., 1996). A second program, at UBC, admitted its first students later that same year (1991), and, in rapid succession, programs were launched at the University of Toronto and, by collaborative arrangement, at McGill University and Université de Montréal in 1993, and at McMaster University a year later (Kerr & McPhail, 1996).

Because of the commitment to dialogue and strategic planning throughout the developmental phase of advancing graduate education for the country, the character and shape of the Canadian doctoral nursing programs evolved in a somewhat distinct manner from those in other parts of the globe. A forum on doctoral education in Canada, held in late 1990 in Edmonton just before the country launched its first programs, contrasted the history of doctoral nursing education in the United Kingdom, the United States, and Europe and took advice from such international leaders as Rozella Schlotfeldt and Lisbeth Hockey. By unanimous agreement, the Canadian leaders who were present concluded that doctoral preparation in Canada should lead to a doctorate of philosophy in nursing, rather than a professional doctorate (Jeans, 1990).

A second invitational conference, held in Toronto in April 1995, brought together student and faculty representatives from the five doctoral programs in existence at that time, as well as from universities in which special-case opportunities were available for doctoral degrees in nursing, to examine the substantive context of Canadian Ph.D. nursing programs as they were evolving and developing (Wood, 1997). It was noted that the Canadian programs all had a rather similar structure, requiring an average of four or five core courses in foundational disciplinary knowledge and research, upon which both coursework and research training were individualized in conjunction with faculty supervision carefully matched to each student's substantive field over 3 or more years of study. Led by Ada Sue Hinshaw, who drew on American examples to point out the quality and resource challenges that a rapid proliferation of doctoral programs could create, participants at that meeting also grappled with such complex questions as how many doctoral programs Canada ought to support.

As doctoral programs took hold within the profession's national consciousness, it became apparent that they provided nursing not only with high-quality research training but also, and perhaps more importantly, with the capacity to study the clinical phenomena pertinent to the discipline, the conceptual leadership to direct the development of scholarly practice, and the grounded analytic skills to design systems of nursing practice and healthcare delivery (Field et al., 1992). In doing so, these programs began to create a cadre of future leaders with expertise in both the art and science of nursing.

The evolution of doctoral nursing education in Canada continues to be fraught with challenges. Among the most pressing concerns has been the difficulty in obtaining funding for student support (CASN, 2010b). In contrast to the academic trajectory in nonclinical disciplines in which doctoral degrees are pursued before the establishment of family and professional respon-sibilities, a majority of Canadian nursing doctoral students are still mid-career professionals, still primarily women, for whom full-time study is both expensive and logistically problematic. Financial support exclusive to nursing has been scarce, with the CNF able to provide only small numbers of graduate fellowships (Wood & Ross-Kerr, 2011). Further, many of the substantive problems associated with delivery and evaluation of nursing care and its outcomes that nurses wish to investigate, such as the experiential aspects of health and illness, and the socio-cultural complexities of interventional contexts, do not fit neatly into clinical (medical), health service, or social science priorities for competitive funding. Although many creative nurse researchers became highly successful in competing for funding within this difficult context, the CNA (2003) called on partners within government, healthcare agencies, universities, and nursing associations to plan cooperatively and share resources to support doctoral education for nurses.

With the advent of the Canadian Institutes of Health Research (CIHR), now the major fed-eral agency responsible for funding health research in Canada, in 2000, nursing leaders played an active role in shifting the traditionally narrow vision of health research in Canada beyond basic and biomedical science to include issues such as ethics, equity, and knowledge transfer. Although funding issues remain an ongoing challenge, there is room for optimism for the profes-sion's continued progress in doctoral preparation, and the exceptional caliber and productivity of Canada's early generations of nursing doctoral program graduates bodes well for the profession's continuing success in this regard.

PRACTICE REALITIES AND CHALLENGES FOR GRADUATE-PREPARED NURSES

In the early years of graduate nursing education in Canada, advanced preparation was generally understood to be a route away from the bedside and into teaching or administration. However, as the proportion of Canadian nurses prepared at the master's level has risen (as of 2009 it was 3.2% nationally [CIHI, 2010]), it has become increasingly apparent that a significant proportion of nursing's professional leadership and scholarship ought to be in the clinical practice arena. Although all aspects of nursing scholarship play a significant role in advancing nursing knowl-edge and influence, the unique contribution of the discipline to the Canadian healthcare system inherently depends on the application of knowledge in the practice arena.

Thus, since the early 1980s, many nursing master's programs have explicitly shifted their emphasis to professional and clinical leadership as a primary objective. Moreover, they have expanded the opportunities for a range of clinical leadership learning options. Similarly, when doctoral programs came on board in the 1990s, most nurses assumed that their primary goal would be to produce the next generation of academic nurse researchers. Although many gradu-ates have gone on to faculty positions, the potential for developing clinical scientists at that level has also been recognized (Mackay, 2009). Thus, the practice reality for nurses with graduate preparation in the discipline is a moving target, in keeping with the rapid changes in the popula-tion, the healthcare system, and knowledge proliferation within the society.

Among the more subtle but challenging practice realities for nurses at the graduate level has been the general level of skepticism and distrust within the mainstream nursing population for the value that advanced education brings to the profession (Donner & Waddell, 2011). In preparing this chapter, a wide range of students and recent graduates were interviewed for the purpose of clarifying the issues that might be included in the discussion. Many of them pointed out that, although attitudes are slowly shifting, it is not uncommon for nurses "coming back to do their master's work" to report the absence of endorsement or support from their colleagues. Even those who remain active in their clinical roles for the duration of their studies may find it an ongoing challenge to convince their practice colleagues that the university has anything relevant to provide to the practice setting.

Expertise and professional leadership within the practice setting are often attributed to the special qualities of an individual nurse, rather than to knowledge and skills that graduate education can bring to the effectiveness of nursing practice.* Perhaps because nurses have had long-standing debates about entry-to-practice levels and scope of responsibility, some remain reluctant to recognize the value of diversifying to achieve collective aims. Pressures from union ideologies, an inherent democratizing ideal, and a reluctance for self-promotion have made nurses more comfortable with the general notion that "a nurse is a nurse is a nurse" than with the ramifications of advanced practice levels and specializing nursing contributions.

Sadly, however, nurses have not always provided one another with a mechanism for understanding how their practice reality is shaped by the prominent forces of the day. Many simply fail to appreciate that the profession is advantaged, not disadvantaged, by an increasingly educated majority. Thus, nurses as a group have not always been supportive of the continuing educational advancement of their peers and may interpret "going back to school" as abandonment rather than as adding ammunition for their collective battles. Certainly, an emphasis on increasing social awareness and political analysis among the mainstream of practicing nurses will continue to be an important element in the general experience of graduate education and the practice reality of nurses prepared with graduate degrees.

A somewhat similar climate of misunderstanding can occur for doctorally prepared nurses with primary appointments in a clinical practice setting. Although the profession has had a generally high level of collective comfort with the traditional model of the academic researcher–educator, it seems much less comfortable with how to apply the skills of doctorally prepared nurses in the clinical context. Nurses in clinical leadership and scholar positions may find, for example, that the research component of their role is less valued than is the administrative aspect. As a result, although nursing has made great strides in cultivating a generation of accomplished researchers, this may have been at the expense of other critically important leadership roles. For example, many of the recent dean and director searches for Canadian nursing schools have been long and protracted, and it is generally understood that the available applicant pool has been diminished by other opportunities in research and scholarship as well as by an extended period of time in which nursing administrative scholarship was relatively unsupported (Laframboise, 2011). Thus, in contrast to the situation that faces the master's prepared nurse attempting to reenter the practice domain, doctorally prepared nurses graduate into a professional culture characterized by an inordinate valuing of specialized research training and acquiring protected time away from distractions to attain the highest level of research funding possible. In its own way, this attitudinal climate is as problematic and counterproductive as that of the academically resistant mainstream.

ISSUES AND CONTROVERSIES IN GRADUATE EDUCATION

In contrast to the career paths typical of many other professions, nurses still perceive the option to take their graduate education in nursing or consider advanced study in other disciplines. Although the proliferation of programs at the graduate level across the country and the availability of an array of distance offerings have made higher degrees in nursing a viable option for all Canadian nurses, many still decide to look elsewhere for their academic advancement. Certainly,

---

*As a teacher of graduate students, I have been fascinated by how prominent and resistant to change these negative attitudes can be within nursing. Increasingly, graduate students take seriously the "ambassador" role that they can play in showing their colleagues the value of their graduate education. New learning is made manifest not simply in the wearing of a new degree but, more importantly, in the new levels of confidence, critical thinking skills, and "big-picture" thinking that they begin to apply to their practice–Sally Thorne.

the history of the nursing profession in Canada has been well served by many noted leaders who returned to the fold after completing their master's or doctoral degrees in such fields as education, psychology, business administration, public health, anthropology, medical sciences, or sociology. From those disciplines, we have derived benefits in theoretical diversity, methodology, and analytic processes. We also recognize that the world in which nursing is practiced is inherently interdisciplinary and, therefore, that nurses have a natural affinity for the models, methods, and substantive knowledge of a range of disciplines.

At the same time, despite individual exceptions, leaders who lack an in-depth understanding of the complex theoretical, historical, and philosophical grounding of the nursing discipline can be considerably disadvantaged when they attempt to articulate a nursing perspective. Even more problematic may be a lack of awareness of the importance of this understanding. Nursing is sufficiently complex and multifaceted that it has proven impossible to delineate a singular and coherent definition that effectively captures the essence of its nature, scope, and boundaries (Thorne, 2011). Canada needs a cadre of leaders who have a strong conceptual grasp of the philosophical underpinnings of nursing's disciplinary knowledge and can effectively articulate the distinctive contributions of the profession within an ever-changing scientific and interprofessional context. Thus, although graduate preparation in nursing will remain a high priority for the discipline's development in this country, there are many opinions on how best to achieve it.

Theoretical Debates

An explicit concern for issues of a theoretical nature evolved in the second half of the 20th century in response to the explosion of new knowledge in the physical and social sciences and the availability of new theoretical challenges arising from the core projects of a variety of academic disciplines. Nursing theory emerged as a mechanism for organizing and making sense of "this infinitely dynamic and complex body of information" so that nurses could use knowledge in a "professional, accountable, and defensible manner" (Beckstrand, 1978).

As the influence of physicians and the medical model on healthcare delivery systems expanded, new species of healthcare professionals and technicians proliferated and nursing curricula evolved away from the more traditional medical science and apprenticeship structure. As such, nurses began to recognize an urgent need to articulate the uniqueness and distinctiveness of their profession among others in the healthcare system (Chinn & Kramer, 1999; Engebretson, 1997). To do this, they began to create conceptual maps that would depict the manner in which nursing informational and decisional processes might relate to a theoretically infinite range of clinical situations (Ellis, 1968; Johnson, 1974; McKay, 1969; Wald & Leonard, 1964). In calling such conceptual frameworks "nursing theory," they located nursing thought within the rather rigid academic and scientific communities of the era and, thereby, created a context within which nursing science could begin to acquire external legitimacy (Cull-Wilby & Peppin, 1987; Jones, 1997).

The conceptual model-building era that lasted from the mid-1960s through the mid-1980s was remarkable in its optimism and enthusiasm for extending the boundaries of existing scientific and philosophical thinking. In a context in which theory development in science was understood to follow a reductionist linear causation model, the nursing theorists were essentially attempting to capture complexity and infinite variation within a rigorous and systematic scientific matrix.

Considering some of the philosophical and scientific innovations in thinking with which we can now critically reflect on that project, some aspects of their efforts may seem naïve in retrospect. However, it can also be said that their efforts to develop a science accounting for both the generalities of substantive knowledge and theory as well as the particularities of an infinite range of new applications was impressive in its capacity to recognize the complexities inherent in excellent clinical nursing reasoning and to respect the diversities of expanding knowledge within which nursing operates (Barnum, 1994; Benner et al., 1996; Meleis, 1987; Raudonis & Acton, 1997; Thorne & Perry, 2001).

However, the model-building enterprise was not well understood within the dominant mainstream of nursing and, for the most part, remained a distinct enterprise from the research scholarship that developed through the latter decades of the century. As the theorists themselves became embroiled in debates about whose conceptual structure should dominate the discipline, mainstream academic nursing tired of the discourse and began to consider the theoretical debates a minor embarrassment in nursing's history (Engebretson, 1997). Indeed, where comparative analysis of the theoretical models had once been a prominent aspect of graduate education in nursing, many programs eliminated the issue from their curricula entirely in favor of a shift toward what Meleis (1987) termed the *substance* of nursing theory.

Because mainstream nursing was evolving away from traditional science and toward embracing aspects of a more humanistic orientation anyway, the "revolution" in nursing theorizing became something of a turf war in which ideologic claims about the underlying intent of those holding various theoretical positions began to take the form of abject generalizations about the beliefs and motives of those who did and did not sit on the same side of the paradigm fence (Thorne et al., 1999). Perhaps one fortunate consequence of this disciplinary infighting is that it brought the relevance of theoretical thinking back into the forefront of academic nursing and stimulated many nurse scholars to pay attention to the theoretical debates. Because of this, critical analysis of the implications of theoretical positioning has come back into favor in graduate nursing education as a relevant and entirely necessary component of nursing's scholarship. Further, that explosive era of unsettling misunderstanding and accusation among the discipline's theorists has forced academic nursing to recognize the imperative of understanding more fully its philosophical underpinnings.

Philosophical Challenges

Among the most overt and easily recognized philosophical challenges facing nursing scholarship from the 1980s to the present has been the qualitative–quantitative methodologic debate. Although research methodology has technical aspects, much of this debate underscores a number of much deeper and more complex philosophical schisms within the scientific and academic communities of which nursing is a member. Although overt attention to the philosophy of science was at one time rare in nursing curricula at any level, it is now well recognized as a hallmark of a credible graduate program in the discipline, and this recognition has crept downward into most undergraduate curricula as well. As a consequence, an appreciation for the philosophical positioning of the ideas of the discipline has emerged as a critically important element in professional leadership.

As a result of the popularization of the idea of paradigmatic thinking as the origin of revolutions within science following the publication of a seminal treatise by Kuhn (1962), academic discourse tends no longer to be characterized by indisputable facts and truths, but rather by claims and positions. A climate of *postmodern* thinking, which favors a more fluid and socially moderated interpretation of realities, permeates society. In this context, knowledge previously considered immutable by virtue of its scientific grounding has become fodder for deconstruction, or looking beneath the surface meaning of a term or concept to illuminate the multiplicity of ideas that tradition may have inscribed upon it (Haack, 1998; Hacking, 1999). The evolution of scientific knowledge is no longer understood as linear and rational, but rather as an entirely human enterprise, subject to ideational and political pressures over time (Van Doren, 1991). What we knew to be true yesterday is disputable today and may be considered reactionary tomorrow. For a discipline such as nursing, the dramatic shift from a realistic ontologic orientation, in which factual truths exist, toward consideration of knowledge as including social construction, in which there may be different ways of understanding truth, has had tremendous appeal. For example, nurses know that every practice principle must have its legitimate variations and that every theoretical claim one might make about human health and illness experience will break down in the face of individual human uniqueness. To some degree, one might argue that theoretical relativism and critical realism have always been philosophically consistent with the kind of curiosity, flexibility, and adaptability that are the hallmarks of excellent nursing practice. Because of this, nursing scholarship has enthusiastically embraced qualitative methods, subjective knowledge, and critical-emancipatory inquiry as consistent with its general moral foundation.

In a climate in which theoretical truths are no longer as comfortably solid as they once seemed, however, many nurse scholars now find themselves struggling to locate themselves on an increasingly slippery platform of disciplinary knowledge. For the profession to have a social mandate, certain basic philosophical truths or positions seem to be prerequisites. For example, although it might be interesting to philosophize about whether human pain and suffering exist apart from our ability to apprehend them subjectively, nursing is unequivocally bound to assume that they do and that nurses have a moral mandate to ameliorate them when possible, despite the individual variations they might manifest and the possibilities that they might simply be profound subjective constructions within the minds of those afflicted. Thus, in reaction to the notion that qualitative methods were more "true" to human subjective experience and, therefore, more relevant to the knowledge required for nursing practice, many scholars now recognize the inherent limits of any singular methodologic approach for generating knowledge suitable to a practice science. To develop useful knowledge in relation to a substantive field, for example, nursing might require population-based surveys, linear-regression modeling, phenomenologic interpretation, and emancipatory-action research. Thus, members of the nursing academy have scrambled in recent years to expand beyond their traditional methodologic expertise and develop the more rounded philosophical and methodologic buttressing that scholars of the future will require. For doctoral programs in nursing, this means that skill within a range of inquiry methods, including qualitative research, quantitative research, and philosophical analysis, will be foundational to producing a new generation of excellent scholars.

Although traditional doctoral training has relied heavily on mentorship models, the scholarship of the future will inevitably require a shift in student and supervisor relationships. The postmodern challenge within academia has raised awareness that traditional science recreates itself, such that genuine innovation must inevitably resist and react against the dictates of older models and authorities. Of course, in the extreme version, the notion of expertise is rejected entirely (Thorne, 1999). However, although that extreme version clearly exists within the academic community in Canada (Good, 2001), nursing's professional practice mandates seem to have kept it somewhat more grounded in a perspective in which the ideas one hold have meaningful implications for the society we live in and the individuals who constitute it. However, it seems also quite appropriate for Canadian nursing graduate students, especially those at the doctoral level, to view the scholarship forms of their mentors with a critical lens, to envision combinations of methodologic and philosophical approaches that extend beyond the specific expertise of their supervisors, and to chafe under academic regulations that create barriers to building their own programs of scholarship in a less rigid and bounded science than did their predecessors.

Practical Challenges

Although many of these debates underscore the challenge of understanding the theoretical and philosophical nature of the discipline, there are also a number of somewhat technical and practical issues that relate centrally to the question of core disciplinary knowledge. Historically and currently, Canada has few dedicated sources of funding for the development of nursing knowledge (the relatively minor amounts available from the CNF notwithstanding). The issue of a separate nursing fund was hotly debated during the developmental phase of transforming Canada's research infrastructure into CIHR. Although nurses have clearly demonstrated the capacity to successfully compete with other health disciplines for research dollars within the mandates of the specific institutes, the career opportunities within the more fundable substantive fields may have been at the expense of sustained inquiry into the core knowledge of the discipline.

For those whose graduate preparation was outside the discipline, the problems associated with core nursing knowledge may seem tangential to the larger enterprise. Given the contentious nature of the nursing theoretical debates, reluctance to engage in these issues is understandable. However, this tension between allegiance to "substantive" knowledge (such as children's health or family health) and "disciplinary" knowledge (such as the nature of nursing or the dynamics of clinical nursing reasoning) has played itself out in graduate nursing curricula, with some nursing scholars advocating immersion in the substance and others pressing for the disciplinary competence within which to ground it. Ongoing debates with regard to the optimal balance between such topics as the nature of nursing knowledge and interdisciplinary knowledge associated with distinct fields of nursing specialization are likely to continue and to complicate curricular planning for the foreseeable future.

A related practical challenge derives from the applied and practical nature of the science of nursing. Although graduate education has not always been understood as an inherent adjunct to the practice of nursing, increasing numbers of master's and doctoral students seek advanced degrees for the explicit purpose of enhancing and strengthening their practice effectiveness. Although it has been natural for the discipline to consider the conduct and dissemination of research as a scholarly enterprise, the notion of practice scholarship has been much more difficult to articulate. Although many Canadian universities continue to support and encourage advancement of practice knowledge using a variety of strategies, the continuous pressure to evaluate the quality of academic units and their faculty on the basis of the research dollars they attract and the publications they produce is unavoidable. Thus, particularly at the doctoral level, there has generally been less overt support for scholarship in the practice tradition than for more conventional health research scholarship, and students seeking to create clinical scientist careers may find themselves seduced by the apparent credibility afforded the more usual career track strategies.

These theoretical, philosophical, and practical challenges will continue to evolve as increasing numbers of nurses seek preparation at the graduate level, and as a broader range of higher education institutions try to make inroads into graduate programming. It will be important for the profession to find ways to come together to discuss and debate the social, political, and economic pressures affecting change, and to create consensus on the foundational principles it will retain through an inevitable period of dynamic change.

CHALLENGES FOR GRADUATE-PREPARED NURSES

Nurses prepared at the graduate level are the current and future leaders of the profession in Canada. In that capacity, they are vulnerable to the effects of the current healthcare climate. Various health reforms in Canada since the 1990s have reflected attempts to control health spending by shifting resources from the acute-care sector to the community sector, mechanisms to rationalize resource allocation decision making, and efforts to bring healthcare system decision making closer to home within national regions (CNA, 2000). The strongly held principles articulated in the Canada Health Act, and traditionally embraced by nurses, have been challenged as never before in the context of this conflictual health reform climate (Villeneuve, 2011). Nursing shortages and the "graying" of the profession occur in a climate in which nursing leadership is increasingly scarce (Laframboise, 2011; Mass et al., 2006).

The weight of navigating the discipline's journey through the health reform process over the next several decades will undoubtedly sit squarely on the shoulders of practice leaders, many of them prepared at the master's level. Clearly, their capacity to make nimble adjustments in health, human resource planning, economic accountability, health policy processes, and professional practice leadership will determine the shape of professional nursing for the next generation. Because these fields of inquiry have not been dominant within nursing's disciplinary scholarship over the most recent decades, there is a recognized shortage in scholarship related to nursing work, nursing service, and the delivery of nursing care. Because formal research scholarship has eclipsed academic and administrative leadership as a priority since the 1980s, it will take some time before graduate nursing programs can take a sufficient shift in course to cultivate a new generation ready to take up professional leadership. Meanwhile, collaborative partnerships between practice settings and universities will be essential to resolve the challenges inherent in the shortage of nursing personnel at all levels and in the conditions of nursing work. Thus, we can expect issues of the workplace to take an increasingly prominent position among the scholarship arenas of graduate education, such that issues traditionally considered the domain of the functional specialization of nursing administration will become mainstream and foundational expectations of nursing in any leadership role.

Although the number of nurses entering graduate programs continues to increase at all levels, the pressures on nurses to extend their academic commitment have also exponentially increased. First-rate graduates of master's programs are quickly seduced into doctoral programs, doctoral graduates are encouraged to shift immediately into postdoctoral training, and postdocs are expected to seek career award funding to protect their research investment. Although each of these progressions is laudable and necessary, it is also important for the profession to remain vigilant to the continuing need for nursing scholarship and leadership throughout the system (Cummings, 2010). University and college programs will increasingly be hungry for new faculty members to teach the next generation of nursing students, and clinical agencies will be desperate for nurses capable of combining practice knowledge with policy work, administrative strength, evidence-based practice development, and corporate leadership. As the current generation of faculty and administrators retires from the active roster, the demand for the next generation to fill the gaps will clearly exceed the current capacity of the profession to train and groom appropriate numbers (Hall, 2009; Mass et al., 2006). Thus, we can anticipate that the impact of nursing's global shortage across our workforce in Canada has only just begun (CIHI, 2010).

In the current climate, the healthcare community will more urgently demand that the university plays a strong role in resolving the critical human and material resource challenges that Canada will face in its development and delivery of health services to an increasingly diverse and complex population. Pressure to meet the emergent needs of the system will take the form of new professional practice roles, increasingly specialized training expectations, and greater numbers of excellently prepared graduates. Without dialogue and debate to create a national consensus on our shared beliefs, role definitions, and disciplinary core values, nursing may well experience discord and organizational disarray. Also, with the urgent demands on the system insinuating themselves on our education and practice contexts as well as on our research, it may be difficult in the next few decades to take the time we require to reflect on our past and direct our future.

STRATEGIES FOR ADVANCING GRADUATE EDUCATION

Canadian nurses have been strong advocates for the principles embedded in the Canada Health Act, and they have also been consistently proud of a national tradition of high-quality professional education and service delivery. As the pressures to increase the number of graduates inevitably lead to more programs and more diverse program delivery modes, it will be increasingly imperative for Canadian nursing to attend to the quality of the educational opportunities on which its leaders build their professional careers (Box 11.1).

Canadian nursing has no quality-monitoring mechanism at the graduate level. Programs preparatory to professional licensure are all regulated by provincial statute and professional

BOX 11.1	**Canadian Association of Schools of Nursing (CASN) Position Statements on Graduate Education (2006)**

CASN Position Statement on Master's Level of Nursing

Background

The purposes and nature of master's education are based on the following assumptions:

- Nursing practice is an inclusive term that incorporates care of individuals, families, and communities as well as involvement in nursing education, administration, research, and policy development.
- Many nursing practices are founded on rationales that have not been critically validated or critically examined.
- Nursing practice is enhanced by nursing-related research, scholarship, and theory.
- The Canadian healthcare system needs advanced practice nurses with the knowledge and skills necessary for appraising the "state of nursing science" in areas relevant to nursing practice, and transferring this to the practice setting.
- Master's level education is the minimum requirement for advanced nursing practice, leadership positions, and faculty positions in nursing education programs.

Position

At the master's level, students build upon the knowledge and skills acquired at the baccalaureate level. Emphasis is placed on developing the ability to analyze, critique, and use research and theory to further nursing practice. Provision should also be made for examination of current issues in healthcare and the ethical values that influence decision making. The master's curriculum should include a definitive component designed to enable students to synthesize research, theory, and practice at an advanced level. The focus of master's study may include the preparation of nurses with advanced skills in the practice of nursing (e.g., nurse practitioner). Master's programs encompass a *program continuum* that includes programs that require a master's thesis, programs that require a major project or practicum, and programs that are course based. Individual master's programs may include both required and elective courses designed to prepare graduates to assume positions in advanced nursing practice, teaching, administration, and policy development and to provide a foundation for Ph.D. study.

Doctoral Education in Nursing in Canada

Background

Canada will require significant increases in the number of nurses with doctoral preparation in order to:

- Build the faculty base necessary to educate sufficient numbers of new graduates to meet the healthcare system workforce needs.
- Generate the evidence required to address the health problems of Canadians, and
- Advance the knowledge base within which the practice of nursing is grounded.

Since 1991, a small number of Canadian universities have produced excellent graduates from nursing doctoral programs characterized by research, core disciplinary knowledge, and expertise within a substantive field. However, the production of new graduates has not kept pace with the country's requirements.

Position
Quality Standards
Because the traditional on-site, full-time Ph.D. training program model fails to reach some groups of talented and qualified potential students, CASN anticipates that innovative and creative delivery models will emerge and new programs will be developed. In order to ensure that this process occurs in an effective and constructive manner, explicit articulation of the quality criteria to which Canadian programs should be held is an imperative.

Among the criteria required for effective Ph.D. programs in nursing are the following:

- Research-intensive academic nursing units housed within universities with well-established graduate program infrastructure and access to high-quality interdisciplinary interactions.
- A critical mass of active faculty researchers capable of supporting the mentorship, research training, and socialization required to engage in the full complement of roles associated with success in the competitive Canadian health research context.
- Learning experiences related to at least three core components: (1) Research training, (2) core disciplinary knowledge related to the history, context, and theoretical underpinnings of nursing, and (3) knowledge of the current state of science and scholarship within a substantive field within the discipline.
- A combination of a modest amount of coursework, comprehensive examinations, and completion of a dissertation.

(continued on page 216)

BOX 11.1   **Canadian Association of Schools of Nursing (CASN) Position Statements on Graduate Education (2006)** (continued)

- Opportunities for active engagement in a scholarly learning environment.
- Evidence of a rigorous external evaluation benchmarking research effectiveness and productivity, infrastructure and resources, and outcomes.

The critical attributes of graduates of Canadian programs include the capacity for:

- Obtaining competitive research funding
- Conducting research that is both rigorous and original to address a problem of concern to the discipline
- Articulating and establishing a program of research
- Communicating effectively through peer-reviewed journal publication, presentation at scholarly meetings, and in professional and scientific interactions.

CASN proposes to undertake further work to more fully articulate necessary and expected attributes of Ph.D. in Nursing programs in Canada and implement processes whereby high-level quality standards can be assured.

Professional or Practice Doctorates
The Ph.D. in Nursing in Canada is a research-focused degree program. CASN does not support, at this time, the concept of the professional or practice doctorate, such as has been adopted in some other jurisdictions, and remains the subject of considerable controversy as an appropriate focus for Canadian universities at this time.

Accessibility
Strategies to increase accessibility to appropriate doctoral education must be multiple and creative. Recognizing that there are legitimate geographic and demographic barriers to access, creative strategies are required by which Canada's research-intensive programs can be made more accessible to the target audience, and thoughtful articulation of quality standards will assist with this process. In addition, CASN recognizes that some nurses who seek doctoral-level education will not be ideally served by a research-intensive Ph.D. in Nursing model. However, to address the particular needs of nurses who do not select to do research-intensive Ph.D.s, CASN encourages creative and collaborative mechanisms whereby these nurses may be appropriately accommodated through such means as interdisciplinary doctoral programs, special-case doctoral initiatives, or collaborative distance delivery mechanisms by which potential mentors from universities not currently delivering Ph.D. programs may become involved. CASN believes that active support of such creative options is an appropriate mechanism whereby researchers and scholars in the discipline can indirectly assist with this aspect of capacity building.

CASN believes that the future needs of Canada will be appropriately served by placing the current emphasis on the research-intensive Ph.D. in Nursing, and anticipates that this degree will become the expected basis for leadership roles across a variety of settings over the course of time. In this context, CASN recognizes the need for a clear and coherent communication mechanism whereby the explicit outcome criteria associated with the Ph.D. in Nursing are clearly articulated to potential students, potential employers, and others.

Students
In order to address the future needs of the Canadian healthcare system, ensure the development of an adequate professoriate to prepare the next generation of nurses, and to sustain the momentum that has been established within the nursing research community. Canadian nursing doctoral programs must target potential students at earlier points in their academic programs and in their careers and actively support their continuing development through to senior research and academic leadership roles. This focus requires efforts to actively engage students in research at an undergraduate level, to ensure the development of a strong base of master's prepared nurses, and to create the context in which excellent nurses anticipate and plan for doctoral education as a natural progression at an early stage within their career development.

Targets
In order to meet the needs of the Canadian healthcare system, explicit predictions are needed of the number of doctorally prepared nurses that will be required so that coherent strategies to meet those targets can be established.

Funding
In order to reach these goals, significant increases in funding will be required for doctoral students, for nursing research infrastructure, and for the infrastructures for graduate programs within schools of nursing. Because CASN recognizes that this will require concerted effort at all levels, including institutional, regional, and provincial, it strongly supports the development and implementation of a unified nursing voice to address this challenge at a national level.

Approved November, 2004, **Revised** June, 2006.

From: Canadian Association of Schools of Nursing. (2008). Retrieved from http://www.casn.ca/media.php?mid=205&xwm=true

organizations, and there is a voluntary accreditation system by which the quality of baccalaureate nursing programs is well supported. Although CASN has articulated strong position statements on master's and doctoral-level education to guide institutions in ensuring that essential quality criteria are in place (CASN, 2010a, 2011), graduate-program approval tends to be entirely within the authority of the individual university senate. In some jurisdictions, graduate program approval is at the mercy of each institution's interpretation of its own market demand and willingness to reconcile conventional academic quality criteria with its particular strategic objectives. Because university administrators tend to assume that graduate programs, especially at the doctoral level, attract fellowship dollars, increase the rate of faculty publication, and expand the research capacity of the organizational unit, some may be unconcerned that there is insufficient support within a nursing department for core disciplinary knowledge, research training, or scholarly mentorship when they seek to expand into graduate programming. Thus, preserving the quality of graduate education in Canada within an environment of pressure for rapid program proliferation has been recognized as an urgent priority (Wood et al., 2004).

Similarly, there is continuing pressure to expand the flexibility and accessibility of graduate programs (CNA, 2004). A review of program websites suggests that most Canadian nursing master's programs have some courses available in an alternative setting or online format, and many are offering full programs in this manner. Although there is no doubt that these fulfill an identified need, the implications of responding to the pressure *en masse* should be an important agenda for national discussion and deliberation. Some of the less objective characteristics of a high-quality master's program, such as developing the skills of collegial networking, challenging one's own concepts and core values, and being directly mentored by knowledge brokers and generators within the discipline, become experiences of a somewhat different nature when enacted asynchronously and/or in a virtual community (Bruce et al., 2008; Lindsay et al., 2009). Thus, it seems more important than ever for Canadian nurses to remain vigilant to the challenge of quality monitoring in graduate education and to take ownership of the standards by which excellence (and mediocrity) can be judged.

Because the financial imperatives of universities will undoubtedly continue to set the conditions within which scholarship is evaluated in the external world, research and academic leaders will have to find strategies by which a balance between lucrative and meaningful inquiry can be supported. In recent years, there has been an expansion of opportunity within the Canadian health research sector for funding projects, programs, and training centers in keeping with the national agenda of health system and health service demands. To the extent that nurses can align their scholarship with those national agendas as they unfold, they will be increasingly successful in attracting additional resources to their academic units. Unfettered adherence to these funding priority agendas, however, would have predictable and unacceptable effects on the culture and nature of nursing academic departments. Within any department offering graduate degree programs, it will remain important to have faculty who teach as well as do research, who engage in practice scholarship as well as traditional research, and who examine the philosophical and theoretical problems of the discipline as well as respond to the immediate expressed needs of the society around them.

Among the more complex challenges for academic nursing will be enacting strategies and processes that reward a range of professional leadership and scholarship (Boyer, 1990; Glassick et al., 1997) and creating the kinds of graduate learning environments that are both grounded strongly within the discipline and credible within the larger community. The nursing profession will require the capacity for healthy dialogue and consensus-building on matters relevant to a national strategy for graduate education if it is to remain the exemplar of world-class quality that we enjoy today. In the coming years, we will undoubtedly have to wrestle with new challenges, such as pressure toward the practice doctorate that has rapidly proliferated in the United States despite contentious debate (Acorn et al., 2009; Brar et al., 2010; Martin-Misener et al., 2010; Nelson, 2008), and a campaign toward a separate and distinct graduate degree option in psychiatric nursing on the part of registered psychiatric nurses in Western Canada (Ryan-Nicholls, 2004).

Nurses in Canada have made great strides toward developing professional scholarship and academic credibility during an era in which the pressing problems of society have demanded unprecedented attention. They have attempted to stay true to a vision of professional integrity as they flow with the changing tides of acceptable inquiry methods and theoretical locations. In an increasingly interdisciplinary world in which truth is never static and credibility is always open for discussion, nurses have collectively assumed a rightful place in the academy, in the healthcare delivery and policy arenas, and in society. And, as Florence Nightingale might have reminded us, the worth of a society can be measured by the quality of its nursing.

SUMMARY

Graduate education in nursing has advanced rapidly in Canada over the past half century. Today it serves to advance leadership within the profession in two distinct ways: Professional scholarship at the master's level and research-intensive training at the doctoral and postdoctoral levels.

Canada needs a cadre of nursing leaders who are adept at conceptualizing the discipline and its contributions in an ever-changing context of diverse theories and structures. A vibrant infrastructure of graduate education in nursing will serve to ensure that Canada sustains a knowledgeable nursing workforce in the years to come and that our discipline has the capacity to retain its ownership of the standards by which its excellence can be judged. Graduate education serves as the primary vehicle through which the nursing discipline maintains a philosophical grounding within its social mandate and its science, ensuring that a nursing angle of vision is brought to bear upon the challenges that confront the Canadian healthcare system of the future.

Add to your knowledge of this issue:		Online
Association of Universities and Colleges of Canada	**http://www.aucc.ca**	
Canadian Association of Nursing Research	**www.canr.ca**	
Canadian Association of Schools of Nursing	**www.casn.ca**	
Canadian Health Services Research Foundation	**www.chsrf.ca**	
Canadian Institute for Health Information	**www.cihi.ca**	
Canadian Nurses Association	**http://www.cna-nurses.ca**	

REFLECTIONS *on the Chapter...*

1 What priorities and trends have most influenced the changes in Canadian master's and doctoral nursing degree curricula since the 1960s?

2 Attitudes toward graduate education within the mainstream practicing nurse population may not have consistently supported nurses in their efforts to obtain master's or doctoral nursing education. Why do such attitudes exist? What social, political, and economic forces within nursing might contribute to their continuation?

3 It can be argued that many nurses with graduate degrees in the discipline are ambivalent about the value of studying "nursing theory" or the theoretical debates within the discipline. What characteristics of the theories or the understanding of them may have created this climate of misunderstanding?

4 As academic nursing evolves over the coming years, how can it appropriately attend to a balance between core disciplinary knowledge and the substantive knowledge that will drive advances in clinical practice?

5 Is a formal dialogue about the future direction of graduate education needed in this country? If so, what should be the primary objectives, and who should lead that discussion?

Want to know more? Visit the Point for additional helpful resources:

- Journal Articles
- Learning Objectives
- Nursing Professional Roles and Responsibilities
- Bonus chapters:
  - ○ Health and Nursing Policy: A Matter of Politics, Power and Professionalism
  - ○ The NP Movement: Recurring Issues
  - ○ When Difference Matters: The Politics of Privilege and Marginality

References

Acorn, S., Lamarche, K., & Edwards, M. (2009). Practice doctorates in nursing: Developing nursing leaders. *Nursing Leadership, 22*(2), 85–91.

Allen, M. (1986). The relationship between graduate teaching and research in nursing. In S.M. Stinson & J.C. Kerr (Eds.), *International issues in nursing research* (pp. 151–167). London: Croom Helm.

Association of the Universities and Colleges of Canada (AUCC). (2011). *Directory of Canadian universities searchable database.* Retrieved from http://www.aucc.ca/

Banning, J.A. (1990). Nursing PhD comes to Canada [Editorial]. *The Canadian Nurse, 86*(11), 3.

Barnum, B.J.S. (1994). *Nursing theory: Analysis, application, evaluation* (4th ed.). Philadelphia, PA: J.B. Lippincott.

Beaton, J. (1990). Crises in graduate nursing education. *The Canadian Nurse, 86*(1), 29–32.

Beckstrand, J. (1978). The notion of a practice theory and the relationship of scientific and ethical knowledge to practice. *Research in Nursing & Health, 1*(3), 131–136.

Benner, P., Tanner, C.A., & Chesla, C.A. (1996). *Expertise in nursing practice: Caring, clinical judgement, and ethics.* New York: Springer.

Boyer, E. (1990). *Scholarship reconsidered: Priorities of the professoriate.* Princeton, NJ: Carnegie Foundation for the Advancement of Teaching.

Brink, P.J. (1991). Editorial: The first Canadian Ph.D. in nursing. *Western Journal of Nursing Research, 13*(4), 432–433.

Broughton, K., & Hoot, T. (1995). Commentary: Canada needs accessible masters' programs. *The Canadian Nurse, 91*(10), 55.

Bruce, A., Stajduhar, K., Molzahn, A., MacDonald, M., Starzomski, R., & Brown, M. (2008). Nursing graduate supervision of theses and projects at a distance: Issues and challenges. *International Journal of Nursing Education Scholarship, 5*(1), art. 43. doi: 10.2202/1548-923X.1587.

Bryant-Lukosius, D., Carter, N., Kilpatrick, K., et al. (2010). The clinical nurse specialist role in Canada. *Nursing Leadership, 23*(special issue), 140–166.

Canadian Association of Schools of Nursing (CASN). (2010a). *CASN position statement on master's level of nursing.* Retrieved from http://www.casn.ca/vm/newvisual/attachments/856/Media/Masterslevelof-Nursing.pdf

———. (2010b). *Environmental scan on doctoral programs: Summary report.* Ottawa, ON: Author.

———. (2011). *CASN position statement on doctoral education in nursing in Canada.* Retrieved from http://www.casn.ca/vm/newvisual/attachments/856/Media/DoctoralEducation2011.pdf

Canadian Institute for Health Information (CIHI). (2010). *Regulated nurses: Canadian trends, 2005–2009.* Retrieved from http://publications.gc.ca/collections/collection_2011/icis-cihi/H115-48-2009-eng.pdf

Canadian Nurses Association (CNA) and Canadian Association of Schools of Nursing (CASN). (2010). *Nursing Education in Canada Statistics 2008–2009.* Retrieved from http://www.casn.ca/vm/newvisual/attachments/856/Media/40605NursingEducationinCanadaStatistics20082009ENGFINAL.pdf

Canadian Nurses Association. (2000). *Framework for Canada's health system.* Ottawa, ON: Author.

_____. (2003). *Joint Canadian Nurses Association and Canadian Association of Schools of Nursing position statement on doctoral preparation in nursing.* Retrieved from http://www.cna-nurses.ca/CNA/documents/pdf/publications/PS75_doctoral_preparation_e.pdf

_____. (2004). *Joint Canadian Nurses Association and Canadian Association of Schools of Nursing position statement on flexible delivery of nursing education programs.* Retrieved from http://www.cna-nurses.ca/CNA/documents/pdf/publications/PS74_flexible_delivery_e.pdf

Chinn, P.L., & Kramer, M.K. (1999). *Theory and nursing: Integrated knowledge development* (5th ed.). St. Louis, MO: Mosby.

Cody, W.K. (2000). Paradigm shift or paradigm drift? A meditation on commitment and transcendence. *Nursing Science Quarterly, 13*(2), 93–102.

Cull-Wilby, B.L., & Peppin, J.C. (1987). Toward a coexistence of paradigms in nursing knowledge development. *Journal of Advanced Nursing, 12*(4), 515–521.

Cummings, G. (2010). New knowledge and evidence for better leadership. *Nursing Leadership, 23*(3), 18–20.

Donner, G.J., & Waddell, J. (2011). Are we paying enough attention to clarifying our vision for master's-prepared nurses and ensuring that educational programs and workplaces are prepared to help achieve that vision? An invitation to engage in an important conversation. *Nursing Leadership, 24*(2), 26–30.

Ellis, R. (1968). Characteristics of significant theories. *Nursing Research, 17*(3), 217–222.

Engebretson, J. (1997). A multiparadigm approach to nursing. *Advances in Nursing Science, 20*(1), 21–33.

Ezer, H., MacDonald, J., & Gros, C.P. (1991). Follow-up of generic master's graduates: Viability of a model of nursing in practice. *Canadian Journal of Nursing Research, 23*(3), 9–20.

Field, P.A., Stinson, S.M., & Thibaudeau, M.F. (1992). Graduate education in nursing in Canada. In A.J. Baumgart & J. Larsen (Eds.), *Canadian nursing faces the future* (2nd ed., pp. 421–445). St. Louis, MO: Mosby.

Ford, J.S., & Wertenberger, D.H. (1993). Nursing education content in master's in nursing programs. *Canadian Journal of Nursing Research, 25*(2), 53–61.

Gein, L. (1994). Defending the master's thesis in nursing graduate programs: The Canadian context. *Journal of Nursing Education, 33*(7), 330–332.

Glassick, C., Huber, M., & Maeroff, G. (1997). *Scholarship assessed: Evaluation on the professoriate.* San Francisco, CA: Jossey-Bass.

Godkin, M.D., & Bottorff, J.L. (1991). Doctorate in nursing: Idea to reality. *The Canadian Nurse, 87*(11), 31–34.

Good, G. (2001). *Humanism betrayed: Theory, ideology, and culture in the contemporary university.* Montreal & Kingston: McGill & Queens University Press.

Haack, S. (1998). *Manifesto of a passionate moderate.* Chicago, IL: University of Chicago Press.

Hacking, I. (1999). *The social construction of what?* Cambridge, MA: Harvard University Press.

Hall, W.A. (2009). Whither nursing education? Possibilities, panaceas, and problems. *Nurse Education Today, 29*(3), 268–275.

Jeans, M.E. (1990). Advancing doctoral preparation for nurses. *Canadian Journal of Nursing Research, 22*(2), 1–2.

Johnson, D.E. (1974). Development of theory: A requisite for nursing as a primary health profession. *Nursing Research, 23*(5), 372–377.

Jones, M. (1997). Thinking nursing. In S.E. Thorne & V.E. Hayes (Eds.), *Nursing praxis: Knowledge and action* (pp. 125–139). Thousand Oaks, CA: Sage.

Kerr, J.R., & McPhail, J. (1996). *Concepts in Canadian nursing.* St. Louis, MO: Mosby.

Kerr, J.R. (1988). Nursing education at a distance: Using technology to advantage in undergraduate and graduate degree programs in Alberta, Canada. *International Journal of Nursing Studies, 25*(4), 301–306.

Kuhn, T.S. (1962). *The structure of scientific revolutions.* Chicago, IL: University of Chicago Press.

Laframboise, L.E. (2011). Making the case for succession planning: Who's on deck in your organization? *Nursing Leadership, 24*(2), 68–79.

Lindsay, G.M., Jeffrey, J., & Singh, M. (2009). Paradox of a graduate human science curriculum experienced online: A faculty perspective. *The Journal of Continuing Education in Nursing, 40*(4), 181–186.

MacDonald-Rencz, S., & Bard, R. (2010). The role for advanced practice nursing in Canada. *Nursing Leadership*, 23(special issue), 8–11.

Mackay, M. (2009). Why nursing has not embraced the clinician-scientist role. *Nursing Philosophy, 10*(4), 287–296.

Martin Misener, R., Bryant-Lukosius, D., Harbman, P., et al. (2010). Education of advanced practice nurses in Canada. *Nursing Leadership, 23*(special issue), 61–84.

Mass, H., Brunke, L., Thorne, S., Parslow, H.G. (2006). Preparing the next generation of senior nursing leaders in Canada: Perceptions of role competencies and barriers from the perspectives of inhabitants and aspirants. *Canadian Journal of Nursing Leadership, 19*(2), 75–91.

McBride, W. (1995). *State of the art and trends in graduate nursing programs in Canada.* Converging Educational Perspectives: An Anthology from the Pan American Conference on Graduate Nursing Education (pp. 255–257). Bogatá, Colombia: NLN Pub. No.19-6894.

McKay, R. (1969). Theories, models, and systems for nursing. *Nursing Research, 18*(5), 393–399.

Meleis, A.I. (1987). ReVisions in knowledge development: A passion for substance. *Scholarly Inquiry for Nursing Practice, 1*(1), 5–19.

Mussalem, H.K. (1965). *Nursing education in Canada.* Ottawa, ON: Queens University Printer.

Nelson, S. (2008). Yet another fork in the road? Nursing doctoral education in Canada. *Nursing Leadership, 21*(4). 52–55.

Parse, R.R. (1998). The art of criticism. *Nursing Science Quarterly, 11*(2), 43.

Pilkington, F.B., & Mitchell, G.J. (2003). Mistakes across paradigms. *Nursing Science Quarterly, 16*(2), 102–108.

Raudonis, B.M., & Acton, G.J. (1997). Theory-based nursing practice. *Journal of Advanced Nursing, 26*(2/1), 138–145.

Rodger, G.L. (1991). Canadian nurses succeed again! The launch of Canada's first doctoral degree in nursing. *Journal of Advanced Nursing, 16*(12), 1395–1396.

Ryan-Nicholls, K.D. (2004). Impact of health reform on registered psychiatric nursing practice. *Journal of Psychiatric and Mental Health Nursing, 11*(6), 644–653.

Thorne, S.E. (1999). Are egalitarian relationships a desirable ideal for nursing? *Western Journal of Nursing Research, 21*(1), 16–29.

Thorne, S. (2011). Theoretical issues in nursing. In J.C. Ross-Kerr & M.J. Woods (Eds.), *Canadian nursing: Issues and perspectives* (5th ed., pp. 85–104). Toronto, ON: Elsevier.

Thorne, S.E., & Perry, J.A. (2001). Theoretical foundations of nursing. In P.A. Potter, A.J. Perry, J.C. Ross-Kerr, et al. (Eds.). *Canadian fundamentals of nursing* (2nd ed., pp. 86–100). Toronto, ON: Mosby.

Thorne, S.E., Reimer Kirkham, S., & Henderson, A. (1999). Ideological implications of paradigm discourse. *Nursing Inquiry, 6*(2), 123–131.

Trojan, L., Marck, P., Gray, C., & Rodger, G.L. (1996). A framework for planned change: Achieving a funded PhD program in nursing. *Canadian Journal of Nursing Administration, 9*(1), 71–86.

Van Doren, C. (1991). *A history of knowledge: Past, present, and future.* New York: Ballantine.

Villeneuve, M. (2011). Policy is possible. *Nursing Leadership, 24*(1), 30–32.

Wald, F.S., & Leonard, R.C. (1964). Toward development of nursing practice theory. *American Journal of Nursing, 13*(4), 309–313.

Wood, M.J., & Ross-Kerr, J.C. (2011). The growth of graduate education in nursing. In J.C. Ross-Kerr & M.J. Wood (Eds.), *Canadian nursing: Issues and perspectives* (5th ed., pp. 389–409). Toronto, ON: Elsevier.

Wood, M.J. (1997). Canadian Ph.D. in nursing programs: A new age. *Clinical Nursing Research, 6*(4), 307–309.

Wood, M.J., Giovanetti, P., & Ross-Kerr, J.C. (2004). *The Canadian PhD in nursing: A discussion paper.* Canadian Association of Schools of Nursing. Retrieved from http://www.casn.ca/media.php?mid=60

Wright, L.M., Watson, W.L., & Duhamel, F. (1985). The family nursing unit: Clinical preparation at the master's level. *The Canadian Nurse, 81*(5), 26–29.

Zilm, G., Larose, O., & Stinson, S. (1979). *PhD (nursing).* Ottawa, ON: Canadian Nurses Association.

12

The Political Nature of Knowledge Generation and Utilization: Nursing Research in Canada

Carol McDonald and Marjorie McIntyre

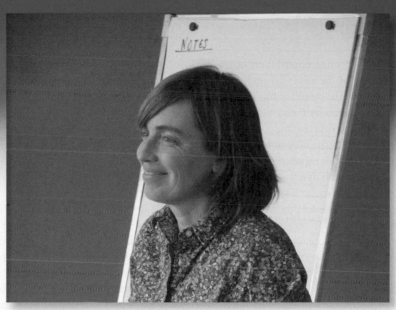

Coby Tschanz nurse educator, researcher, and practitioner in end of life issues and hospice care. (Used with permission. Photographer Anne-Mieke Cameron.)

Critical Questions

As a way of engaging with the ideas in this chapter, consider the following:

1. How do you understand the claim that research conducted by nurses is not necessarily "nursing research"?

2. What areas of research, apart from nursing research, do you imagine that nurses draw on in practice?

3. In your practice so far, what questions have come up for you that might benefit from research or inquiry?

Chapter Objectives

After completing this chapter, you will be able to:

1. Consider the history of nursing research in Canada.

2. Describe the obstacles nurses have had to overcome to develop research.

3. Identify challenges confronting the continued development of nursing research.

4. Describe obstacles to nurses and nursing using research in practice.

5. Discuss ways in which these challenges can be overcome.

Increasingly nurses' professional practice is informed by research-based evidence, often referred to as the best practice. In spite of this profile of nursing research in professional practice and nursing education, persistent questions point to the need for a deeper understanding of the issues surrounding nursing research. Questions such as: What constitutes *nursing* research, what counts as evidence in best practice and, who decides what research topics are worthy of funding, suggest the issue of nursing research benefits from exploration through political, economic, and social/cultural lens.

SITUATING THE TOPIC

Nursing research has contributed in many different ways to Canadians' health and healthcare, but the nature of the research undertaken by nurses does not usually result in products like the identification of the gene for muscular dystrophy, or the discovery of insulin—both the outcomes of *medical* research by Canadian scientists. Much of what nursing research has done to date is to inform clinicians (nurses and all healthcare professionals) of what patients are experiencing and what they prefer in the way of treatment, information, and approach. This knowledge positions the clinicians to work in more sensitive, helpful, and therapeutic ways with patients. Nurses have also contributed research that has improved the health of Canadians. An area in which Canadian nurse researchers in particular are making impressive contributions is in our understanding of how to staff and manage the healthcare system. This type of research, which relies heavily on databases that house information about patient case mix, lengths of stay, and mortality rather than on the collection of primary data, is increasingly important to our understanding of how to staff the healthcare system to achieve maximum efficiency and maximum patient outcomes. Nurses increasingly are undertaking experimental research, whether it be randomized controlled trials or theory-based experimental studies. In addition, nurses participate in research-based in other disciplines, as well as in interdisciplinary research with a focus beyond the scope of nurse's disciplinary knowledge.

This final point, of nurse's involvement in the research of other disciplines, leads to the topic of what the term *nursing research* refers to and where it fits alongside other research in healthcare. Nurses draw on research from many disciplines, such as psychology, pharmacology, medicine, and sociology, to inform their practice. One view of nursing research, the position taken in this chapter, is that nursing research is the generation of knowledge that contributes directly to nursing's disciplinary knowledge base. This disciplinary knowledge includes the knowledge that informs the work that nurses do, be that professional nursing practice, nursing education, or administration. It is also the case that nurses participate in research that contributes primarily to the knowledge of other disciplines, often as members of interdisciplinary research teams. In their professional nursing practice, nurses also use knowledge and thus research that has been generated from outside the discipline.

Nursing research is generated through diverse methodologies, which originate from various paradigms or worldviews. This means that research from various perspectives including empirical and interpretive approaches are valued in nursing. This topic will be discussed later in the chapter as we explore the question: What counts as evidence in evidence-based practice? (McIntyre & McDonald, 2013)

ARTICULATING THE TOPIC AS AN ISSUE

From a quantitative perspective, in which evidence is counted or measured, nursing research can be viewed as a successful endeavor of expansion over the past 5 decades. A focus on measurement of numbers demonstrates the growth of the preparation of nurse researchers, and publication of nursing research in Canada and elsewhere. From this same quantitative perspective, the chronic difficulties linked to the availability of funding for nursing research could be viewed as a problem to be solved, if simply more funds were made available, rather than as an issue to be explored and understood. In keeping with the intention of this book, however, we encourage you to critically consider the political nature of nursing research. In this instance, viewing the political nature of research raises questions that help us see research as more than the unproblematic or ideal-ized activity of knowledge generation. Closely connected to the topic of nursing research is the topic of nursing knowledge, which can be seen as the product of research. Issues arise from the political nature of nursing research/knowledge in asking the questions: Who decides what topics are worthy of research/research funding, and what knowledge is valued as evidence in evidence informed practice?

ANALYZING THE ISSUE: WAYS OF UNDERSTANDING

An analysis of the issues concerning nursing research helps us understand what lies beneath the issues, and what makes the issues significant for Canadian nurses. As you will see, the analysis moves beyond describing the current and historical situation, to raise questions that challenge some of the taken-for-granted assumptions that surround nursing research.

Understanding the Evolution of Nursing Research Historically

The current issues in nursing research can be elucidated in part by viewing the evolution of nursing research in Canada. This history not only recalls events as they unfolded but critically analyzes how the current situation has been constructed. As part of this analysis the evolution of nursing research in Canada is contrasted with that of the United States, one that has been more favorable to the development of discipline-specific knowledge.

It is significant that Canada, following the American model of nursing education, has located such education in universities. This does not mean that all or even most nursing educa-tion occurred in universities, but in Canada from 1919 onward when the University of British Columbia commenced a degree program to prepare nurses for public health, nursing was associ-ated with universities. This association was very important in the evolution of nursing research because universities and their affiliated teaching hospitals are where the vast majority of health-related research occurs. Furthermore, the usual academic progression of baccalaureate to mas-ter's to doctoral education was adopted in Canadian nursing (as it was in the United States), and this set the pattern for the preparation of nurse researchers in the same mold as other academic disciplines (Pringle, 2010).

Preparation of Nurse Researchers

The establishment of programs of research depends on having well-prepared researchers. This requires education programs of study and funds for students while they study. Preparation at the doctoral level is seen as necessary for most people to undertake the role of principal investigator, the person who takes major responsibility for designing and managing research studies. Canada was late to develop doctoral programs in nursing relative to other countries. Our first programs occurred in the early 1990s, whereas the United States already had four doctoral programs by 1975. By 2000 the United States had 75 doctoral programs (Wood, Giovannetti & Ross-Kerr, 2004), and Finland, Japan, Korea, and Thailand all had doctoral programs in nursing.

In the mid-1980s, McGill University, followed closely by the University of Alberta, began to plan in earnest for doctoral programs in nursing. In the case of McGill, the governing body of the Faculty of Medicine—in which the School of Nursing is located—challenged the plan. The

Faculty of Medicine did not think that nursing had demonstrated sufficient resources or a sufficient body of knowledge to justify a PhD degree in the discipline. The Faculty of Nursing at the University of Alberta saw their program approved at the university level, but the government was not prepared to provide funding for it. Here it can be seen that even the earliest plans for doctoral nursing programs were undermined by political issues such as funding availability and the authority of adjacent disciplines such as the Faculty of Medicine to challenge the establishment of a doctoral program in nursing.

Although it took a long time to initiate doctoral education in Canada, once started, five programs began within a 3-year period. In 2012 there are 12 PhD programs in nursing in universities across the country, delivered by both face-to-face and distributed, or distance, learning, so it is now possible for nurses who wish to pursue a PhD in nursing to choose from many excellent programs (CNA, 2012).

Like everything else in the establishment of the nursing research enterprise in Canada, the mounting establishment of doctoral programs did not come easily. Nursing had to prove itself as a legitimate academic field of study in several of the universities. Only a few faculties and schools actually received additional funding to support these programs, and the rest stretched their budgets to include this new resource-intensive activity. These programs do, however, provide the infrastructure for the continued production of researchers without which all the other elements of the conduct of research could not proceed. The establishment of doctoral programs without dedicated funding has not been without its challenges and can be seen to have contributed to ongoing limitations of what can be accomplished through nursing doctoral programs.

Funding to support nursing doctoral students has not proved as buoyant as the programs themselves. Few sources of funding are available to doctoral students in nursing. The absence of a specific source of funds for nurses is felt every time the Canadian Institute for Health Research (CIHR), currently the major funding body for doctoral students, releases the list of successful candidates for doctoral fellowships. There is an enormous demand for doctoral support, and the CIHR funds fewer than 20% of the applications it receives. Previous sources of funding of doctoral students, including the Social Sciences and Humanities Research Council (SSHRC), have altogether stopped funding research related to health (SSHRC, 2012). This decision excludes the vast majority of nursing students from SSHRC funding, a loss that further erodes the feasibility of doctoral studies for many nurses.

The limited access to funds means that many doctoral students work full-time or part-time throughout their programs. This necessity tends to slow their progress and creates a great burden on the individual, who may be raising a family at the same time. This is a continuing struggle and one that requires creative solutions by nursing agencies. When considering that only 0.2% of Canada's registered nurses have currently completed the doctoral level of education, the lack of funding available for this pursuit is an additional unfortunate barrier (Pringle, 2010).

Funding of Nursing Research

The funding of nursing research in Canada is no less challenging for nurses once they have completed their PhD education. Research takes time and resources: Time to undertake the review of the current state of knowledge in the area of interest; time to assemble a research team and to meet with them; time to determine the most appropriate design, data generation approach, and/or measurement instruments; time to figure out the data analysis and interpretation strategies; and time to write the grant for funding and receive ethics approval from institutional review boards. Because it is so time intensive, research commonly is relegated to second or third place behind other responsibilities. Nurses in academic settings find themselves with heavy teaching loads, a situation that requires them to fit research into weekends and evenings. Administrators and clinical nurse specialists, who have heavy demands on their time but are expected and encouraged to do research, face similar dilemmas.

Conducting research takes funds, and funds are often scarce to support the kinds of research that nurses undertake. The Medical Research Council (MRC) of Canada was launched in 1960 with a mandate to "promote, assist, and undertake basic, applied, and clinical research in Canada in the health sciences" (MRC Act), but because of the meager funding available, MRC decided to limit its support to *biomedical research*. This limitation did not change in any fundamental way until the mid-1990s and, as such, did not support research by nurses.

The alternative major national source of funding available to nurses (and other nonbio-medical researchers) was the National Health Research and Development Program (NHRDP) of Health Canada (previously Health and Welfare Canada). Unlike MRC, which operated in an arm's-length relationship with the government and could develop its own research priorities, NHRDP was a department of the government and was expected to support research that assisted the government to meet its objectives. This meant the research that received funding was research that aligned with government objectives rather than research that was seen to be important by nurse researchers themselves. This early situation of government-directed focus in research high-lights the way in which political agendas can take the lead in generating a research agenda that might be better served from leadership within the healthcare or, specifically, the nursing arena. In addition, the size of their budgets differed enormously: When MRC and NHRDP merged into the CIHR in 2000, MRC's budget was $350 million and NHRDP's was about one tenth of that. Furthermore, NHRDP's budget fluctuated every year depending on the government's largesse. Because NHRDP was the major general research fund (i.e., not limited to a specialty area) avail-able at the national level to nurses and several other nonbiomedical disciplines like epidemiology, occupational therapy, and family medicine, the competition was fierce and the size of the avail-able grants was limited. The highly competitive atmosphere for limited funds and a government-directed focus can be seen to account for nursing research grants being shaped by the political agenda. In other words, researchers in need of funding constructed their research grant applica-tions to align with government agendas. Doctoral students were encouraged to pursue research in fundable areas and the art of grant craftsmanship gained increased visibility in the pursuit of research funding.

Despite the constraints of both a limited budget and government-directed focus, NHRDP proved to be a great benefactor to nurses. Many nurses who pursued doctoral education from 1975 until 2000 received fellowships from NHRDP that supported them during their studies. Nurses won these fellowships in national interdisciplinary competitions that demonstrated their ability to compete head-on with the best candidates from other health disciplines. NHRDP was also a source of project grants required by nurses for research.

Charitable organizations with special interests in particular diseases, for example, the Heart and Stroke Foundation of Canada, the Canadian Diabetes Association, the Alzheimer Foundation of Canada, and the Canadian Cancer Society, raise money to support research in those diseases. Most began their funding programs favoring biomedical research because of an orientation to seek cures rather than to focus research on caring for individuals with the disease. Even under these circumstances, some nurses were successful in receiving grants from competitions held by these organizations and built important research programs based on this funding. Fortunately, the policies of these foundations have evolved over the years, and nursing research is now part of the range of studies they fund.

Because of the very limited funding available at the national level, the Canadian Nurses Foundation (CNF) was established by the Canadian Nurses Association (CNA) in 1962 initially to provide support for nurses studying at the master's and doctoral levels. In 1984, small grants for research were added. As with many nursing-based endeavors, the CNF has struggled since its inception to secure sufficient funds to keep itself in business. Much of its support has come from donations from nurse researchers themselves. In the days before NHRDP and MRC fund-ing, CNF was frequently the sole resource nurses could turn to. Even today, CNF will fund stud-ies that address topics unique to nursing that would not likely be successful in interdisciplinary competitions. In 2002, CNF entered into a partnership with the Canadian Health Services Research Foundation (CHSRF, described later) to increase their resources substantially.

The SSHRC has been an important source of funding for many nurse researchers. SSHRC is a national foundation established in 1977 on the same basis as MRC, that is, funded by but at arm's length from the federal government. (The third national body in Canada that makes up the research funding triumvirate is the Natural Sciences and Engineering Research Council.) SSHRC has always had a substantially smaller budget than MRC and its successor, CIHR. In 2007 to 2008, its budget was $312,700 million while CIHR had a budget of $700 million. As its name suggests, the SSHRC fund research that examines questions relevant to the social, cultural, economic, technologic, environmental, and wellness dimensions of life. For many qualitative nurse researchers and those interested in the ethical, historical, and psychosocial dimensions of nursing, SSHRC has been a major source of funding. The peer-review committees understand and value qualitative methods to address questions and have expertise in content areas relevant to nursing. Nurses also have received doctoral fellowship support from SSHRC. However, the size of the overall budget dictates that most SSHRC grants are relatively modest in comparison to those available from CIHR. Unfortunately, since 2011 it was decided that this federal agency would no longer fund health-related research. Thus, the task of obtaining funds to conduct research is further challenged when the agendas of national funding bodies shift, and researchers are compelled to construct grant applications that align with the goals of health research for one arm of the government (CIHR) and wellness research for another (SSHRC).

Some provincial granting bodies have had a tradition of providing funds to nursing research, for example, the Fonds de recherche scientifique du Québec, the Michael Smith Foundation for Health Research in British Columbia (MSFHR), and the Alberta Heritage Foundation for Medical Research (AHFMR). As with the national funding bodies, however, the historical portrait of these provincial organizations includes an original focus on biomedical research countered by a challenge from nursing organizations, often resulting in small accommodation of funds for nursing research that all too often disappear during the next round of decision making.

The CHSRF was established in 1997 with an initial endowment of $66.5 million that was increased by an additional $60 million in 1999. Its mandate is to fund research on health services management and policy. In 1999, $25 million was allocated to CHSRF for the funding of nursing research over a 10-year period. CHSRF was the recipient of the funds because the CNA argued that workplace difficulties and workforce shortages were at crisis levels in Canada and required serious research attention. The agreement between Health Canada and CHSRF specified that $500,000 per year was to be spent on clinical research; the rest was to go to health services and policy research relevant to nursing. CHSRF was a significant source of funding through open competitions for nurse researchers from 1999 to 2005. Since that time, however, CHSRF has not offered open competitions and has focused instead on commissioned research.

Almost simultaneously with the CHSRF developments, MRC undertook a national study that resulted in a reinterpretation of its mandate to embrace all types of research. New peer-review committees were developed, and nurses and researchers from other disciplines, such as occupational and physical therapy, epidemiology, and family medicine, were able to compete. This reinterpretation was followed quickly by a redevelopment of the entire health research enterprise. The CIHR was approved by the government of Canada in June 2000. MRC and NHRDP ceased to exist, and CIHR became the major source of health-research funding for the nation. As previously mentioned, in 2005, the CHSRF transferred the open grants competition to CIHR. This move, along with the SSHRC reconfiguration that has excluded health research means that currently, CIHR is the major source of funding for nursing research in the country.

Thirteen "virtual" interdisciplinary institutes were created within CIHR to represent such diverse areas of science as genetics, aging, cancer, aboriginal health, and gender and health. Each institute reflects four areas of research: Basic biomedical, clinical, health services, and population health. A target had been set to try to achieve $1 billion in funding annually by 2006 but clearly this target was not met. This shortfall is a problem for all health researchers and speaks to the limited commitment of the federal government to research relative to other countries, such as the United States, where the National Institutes of Health (NIH), the American equivalent of CIHR, had a budget of $28 billion in 2008.

In addition to the limited funds available, researchers face steep competition in the selections process. For example, between 2005–2006 and 2010–2011 CIHR experienced a 31% increase in funding applications. With increasing numbers of applications there is even less likelihood of funding for individual researchers. In 2001–2012 CIHR funded 5.6% of the applications submitted for operating grants (CIHR, 2012).

Nurses are an integral part of CIHR. There are nurses on most institute advisory boards, and nurses sit on all the appropriate peer-review committees. They chair some committees and serve as scientific officers on others. Nurse researchers now compete for the much larger grants available through the CIHR and take their places alongside scientists from all other disciplines. The structure of CIHR is not, however, what nursing had hoped for.

Given the frustration created by MRC's exclusion of nursing research for so many years and the tentative steps to include an applied research agenda in the 1990s, nursing had hoped that the new approach to research funding would include an institute for nursing research. However, very early in its development, the CIHR embraced a strictly interdisciplinary agenda and declared that no institute would be disciplinary based.

In the United States, nursing research has had a different history. After many years of concerted and well-coordinated lobbying by nurses, a National Center for Nursing Research was created in 1985 as part of the NIH. The center was elevated to the status of a National Institute of Nursing Research (NINR) in 1992. The American National Institutes of Health are organized very differently from their Canadian counterparts in that they have dedicated buildings, they conduct research within the institutes (intramural research), and they mount competitions for researchers to apply for funds (extramural research). The NINR's autonomy and resources (a budget of $148 million [USD] in 2012) mean that American nurses are able to identify areas of particular interest to nursing or areas that require special attention and establish directed competitions (in addition to their regular competitions) to drive research into them. Canadian nursing cannot do this under the CIHR structure and must seek other routes to gain attention for areas with special needs. This battle for the recognition of nursing research is not over. Nurses are well positioned within the CIHR, and there is no reason to believe that individual nurse researchers will not continue to do well in competitions for grant support, but nursing has yet to develop strategies within the unique funding opportunities in Canada that will allow it to focus on areas of unique or special interest to nurses (Pringle, 2010).

Publishing Nursing Research

The impetus for much early Canadian nursing research came from McGill University and the leadership of Dr. Moyra Allen. Dr. Allen completed her PhD at Stanford University and returned to Canada and to McGill. She saw the need for a nursing research journal to serve Canadian researchers, and *Nursing Papers* was launched in 1969 with just two editions per year. It was renamed the *Canadian Journal of Nursing Research/Revue Canadienne de Recherche en Sciences Infirmiéres* in 1988. Maintaining this journal represents one of the struggles in the development of nursing research in Canada. There was never enough money, manuscripts— particularly in the early days—were hard to come by, and circulation was low. However, it was crucial and remains so for Canadian nurse researchers to have a vehicle in which to publish their works, some of which address topics of particular interest to the Canadian scene. In addition, the editorials reflect issues in Canadian healthcare and nursing education and what research has to bring to these issues (Gagnon, 1999; Gottlieb, 1999). The journal remains at McGill, and four issues a year are published.

Other journals have been established in Canada since 1969, including journals that support specialty fields, for example, the *Canadian Journal of Cardiovascular Nursing,* the *Canadian Journal of Nursing Leadership,* the *Canadian Gerontological Nurse,* and the *Journal of the Canadian Gerontological Nurses Association.* Several of these journals began by publishing articles about clinical practice with very little research reflected in them. This lack of research has changed over the years. They all now publish reports of research on topics relevant to practitioners in their specialty areas. Of course Canadian researchers publish well beyond journals based in Canada and well beyond nursing journals.

Nearly all journals have introduced peer review, which means that people with expertise in the field review the reports submitted by the researchers to determine whether the research is sufficiently sound to warrant publication. The reviewers are not informed who the authors are; hence, the peer review is called a "blind" review. This prevents the reviewers from bringing positive or negative biases colored by any relationships they might have with the authors of the research. Despite the excellence of many journals and the filter of the peer-review process, the caveat "reader beware" still holds true. Consumers of research, including nurses considering the use of research findings in practice, must bring a critical perspective to reading all published research to determine whether the findings of the study can or should be applied to their own practice.

A review of the history of nursing research in Canada tells us that nursing research, particularly in the area of funding, has not been well served by the structures of government funding bodies. As we move to political analysis of nursing research the notion of inadequate funds and of the highly competitive nature of achieving funding for research accompanies the topic.

UNDERSTANDING THE RELEVANCE OF RESEARCH FOR NURSING PRACTICE POLITICALLY

Evidence-based practice, which is sometimes referred to as *best practice,* means that the type of care delivered (or in health promotion arenas, the health promotion strategy used) is based on the best research evidence about that practice and, ideally, is integrated with knowledge about the patient's preferences, culture, emotional status, information needs, and unique physiologic responses, among other things.

Research is now regarded as central to the determination of what constitutes best practice. Basing nursing practice on research evidence was not possible until recently because there was simply not enough research available in most areas of nursing practice to influence the decision. This is still the case in some areas of nursing practice. Nevertheless, the evidence is mounting, and increasingly nurses can turn to research studies to help them determine what is best for individual patients or classes of patients (e.g., patients being supported by mechanical ventilation or recovering from coronary artery bypass surgery). This ability represents a significant change in how nurses approach patient care and will change the view that nurses turn to each other rather than to research literature to answer questions about what is the most current thinking on the care of patients with specific problems. While this *ideal* of evidence-based practice is widely accepted, questions are raised about decision making to incorporate research knowledge, in particular the question of what counts as evidence in evidence-based practice.

It is a common misconception that systematic reviews can be undertaken only on experimental research and that the randomized controlled analysis is the gold standard for all research (Jennings, 2000; Petticrew, 2001). This misconception is closely connected to the politics of knowledge, in which some kinds of knowledge are seen as more valuable than others. In a 2011 article Earle-Foley, a Canadian doctoral student, presents what she calls the evidence-based hierarchy and questions "whether evidence-based practice is even a reasonable or attainable goal within the discipline of nursing" (p. 40). She goes on to explain, "While many agree that broad definitions of evidence are needed in nursing, when scholars take a more narrow view of evidence as meaning 'conclusive statements from randomized control trials' (Mitchell, 1999, p. 30), it becomes very problematic and rather impossible for a practice discipline such as nursing to achieve" (Earle-Foley, 2011, p. 40). In the historical review of funding for nursing research earlier in this chapter it was revealed time and time again that national and provincial bodies have shown preference for biomedical research over nursing research. When competing with other disciplines for research dollars, nurses sometimes focus on the quantitative approaches to research that could be seen as most competitive in this setting. Nursing research includes a number of randomized controlled trials, but much of nursing practice does not lend itself to experimental treatment where outcomes are counted or measured. A tension exists when the knowledge that is most valued as evidence does not align with disciplinary knowledge. Nursing relies heavily on qualitative research that generates understandings of the meaning of experiences rather than measurable outcomes; furthermore, interventions that include a strong interpersonal component, as much of nursing practice does, are best researched using qualitative methodologies. The relevance of the knowledge that is generated through research surely also affects whether or not the research is utilized at the point of care.

There is a huge gap between what is known as a result of research and its utilization in patient care. Research utilization, also called knowledge translation, is a developing area of science, and a Canadian nurse scientist, Dr. Carole Estabrooks, and her colleagues at the Knowledge Utilization Studies Program at the University of Alberta Faculty of Nursing have taken the lead in explicating the factors that influence health professionals to use research findings in their practice (Estabrooks et al., 2007; Cummings et al., 2007). It seems that simply knowing what works best does not usually lead to practicing on the basis of that knowledge. The reasons are complex and involve issues at the level of the individual nurse and the context in which the nurse practices. Estabrooks et al. (2007) have identified factors that contribute significantly to research utilization, which include nurses who use the Internet more and feel less emotionally exhausted at work; higher levels of nurse-to-nurse collaboration; someone available to facilitate the uptake of research; high levels of nursing autonomy; organizations that are innovative, responsive, and employ adequate staff and are supportive of them; and, finally, the presence of nursing leadership.

Nursing education has been profoundly affected by the development of research in terms of what is taught and who teaches it. Forty years ago, faculty members in university programs were educated at the baccalaureate or master's levels, and teachers in diploma programs themselves had only diplomas or baccalaureate degrees. Research had little presence in the programs by virtue of the fact that little existed. Textbooks were the cornerstone of course work. In the 21st century, that trend has changed dramatically. Most university professors of nursing now hold a PhD, and the minimum preparation found throughout nursing education programs is the master's degree. These are not just paper qualifications. They mean that the faculty in nursing programs consists of both educators and researchers, thus profoundly changing teaching.

In research-intensive university programs, opportunities are available to undergraduate students to work as research assistants on research projects throughout their education. These opportunities commonly serve as incentives for students to pursue graduate education immediately to acquire the research skills that will allow them to become principal investigators.

Nursing is still struggling with how to make research an attractive and attainable career goal for an increasing number of students entering the profession. Most students enter nursing to realize their desire to care for people who are ill. In the course of their studies, they find that many different career paths are available to them. If they are exposed to research and have the opportunity to participate actively in it, they might come to see research as a possible future.

In schools of nursing with master's and doctoral programs, undergraduate nursing students are exposed to graduate-level students in those programs. The students interact in their roles as teaching assistants or in social encounters. This interaction makes graduate education very real and attainable. If undergraduate students are not in a research-intensive environment, then faculty members have to use imaginative ways of making research alive for the students. It may mean attending research days at other universities; having days when faculty and graduate student research is presented; or having researchers or doctoral students come and meet with students, present their work in interactive seminars, and discuss the realities of research careers. Students need encouragement to see graduate school as a logical step in their career plans. They also need tangible financial support to be able to pursue their education. Students who are excited by the possibilities of research, who in the course of their studies raise questions that have been investigated or can be investigated using research methods, and who challenge current practice are excellent candidates for future research careers in nursing.

From a political perspective the question of who decides what topics are worthy of research/ funding is relevant and controversial for students considering graduate education. In other words, the politics of knowledge, suggesting that some types of knowledge are more valued than others, is also embedded in funding decisions. Decisions about what research topics are current and what populations, processes, or experiences are worthy of funding are typically made by national or provincial boards or organizations far removed from the point of care. A commonly repeated mantra that "funding begets funding" means that researchers who have been successful in receiving funding from a large agency such as CIHR are more likely to be funded again for the same research topic and the students are more likely to be funded if they work with supervisors who have broken into this competitive funding process. One might consider the serious shortcomings of this reality including the limitations for researchers whose interests fall outside of what could be seen as fundable topics.

STRATEGIES TO ADDRESS ISSUES OF NURSING RESEARCH

In this chapter we have discussed challenges that underlie the generation of nursing research and the production of nurse researchers as well as the limitations to the utilization of research in practice. To some extent the political influence on the generation of nursing researchers is beyond the reach of most individual nurses. While we must rely on the sound intentions of nurse leaders in academia and research agencies to implement some strategies there are always ways to participate through raising awareness and voicing your position on an issue. Individual nurses can actively and meaningfully influence research utilization in practice and educational settings, as we will discuss in the following section.

Strategies to Address Research Utilization

A critical issue facing nursing research is the need to accelerate the translation of research into practice. As discussed earlier, the uptake of research into best practice is at an early stage of development in nursing and in all the health disciplines. The rate of research production in nursing, however, means that if the transfer process does not accelerate, research knowledge will languish in journals years before it is used in patient care.

A force on the horizon for research utilization is an increasingly better-educated nursing workforce. Research will increasingly influence the way nurses practice as more nurses are educated to read research with understanding, to conduct systematic reviews, and to seek out research as their first resource when trying to answer practice questions. This utilization of research-informed knowledge extends beyond nursing research to research from other disciplines, relevant for nursing at the point of care. The increase in nurses with the technical literacy to access digital data bases will support this move toward the integration of research-informed knowledge in practice.

It bears repeating that nurses are likely to resonate with, and perhaps to utilize, research findings that have relevance for their daily practice. Such research that explicates understandings or meanings of patient experiences, or that generates theory from experience is as important to consider as randomized control trials in the development of evidence-based nursing practice (Aikin Murphy, 2011).

What is needed is an understanding by and commitment from all practicing nurses to attend to research findings and to seek opportunities to use the results of research in their practice, which means that nurses must be prepared in their initial education or through continuing education opportunities to read, comprehend, and critique research. It puts a special demand on nursing practice leaders, such as nurse managers, clinical nurse specialists, and nurse educators, to assist nurses in appreciating the value of research and in finding creative ways of bringing research into practice. Organizations that employ nurses have a special responsibility to provide the resources and the infrastructure supports that make it possible for nurses to access research, to have time to read it, and to have individuals available to them to assist them in understanding and in utilizing research informed knowledge.

The responsibility to facilitate the transfer of knowledge does not, however, rest only with nurses in the practice setting, be they leaders, managers, or educators. A critical analysis encourages a discerning look at all of those involved in research generation and dissemination, including nurse researchers themselves. In the academic setting, tenured and tenure-track faculty faces a strong imperative to engage in funded research and to publish the findings of their research. While the publication of research in peer-reviewed journals, or presentations at conferences, is from one perspective viewed as knowledge dissemination or knowledge transfer, it is often the case that this new knowledge does not reach practicing nurses directly. This critique raises the political question: Whose needs are being served by nursing research?

Strategies to Generate Nurse Researchers and Nursing Research

Canada entered the 21st century in the throes of a nursing shortage and with the probability that this shortage would intensify over the next decade. The shortage is distributed across all dimensions of the profession including researchers who will replace the cohort of researchers retiring during the next 10 to 15 years.

Canada needs more nurse researchers, not fewer. Medical science is making enormous progress in addressing the treatment of disease. For every development in medical care, nursing must respond by determining patients' responses and needs and by developing interventions that complement the medical treatment. For every advance in our understanding of what promotes health or prevents disease, nursing must develop programs at the individual and population levels that build on this new knowledge. Furthermore, there is much catching up to do. Because the undertaking of nursing research is so recent, much of what nurses do and most of what patients experience and need to understand about their health situations has not been studied.

Creating incentive programs to support nurses while they pursue graduate education and developing creative and stimulating opportunities to help undergraduate and graduate students see research as a viable and desirable career choice are desperately needed to ensure the future of nursing research.

As noted earlier, Canadian nursing does not have its own institute within the CIHR structure, which emphasizes interdisciplinary research. Although some nurses are well positioned within the CIHR institutes, the discipline has yet to develop strategies for working with the agency so nursing is heard when new initiatives are required to better understand issues that are either unique to nursing or in which nurses play a major role. Individual nurse researchers, graduate students directly from point of care, and nurses as members of interdisciplinary teams, to name a few, have the capacity to identify gaps in nursing knowledge that are worthy of research. It is this knowledge that will advance disciplinary knowledge and inform nursing practice. A critical strategy to support the expansion of knowledge means undertaking research that is needed, rather than research that is high on a "currently fundable" agenda of national or provincial agencies.

SUMMARY

Nursing research has been developing since the 1960s in Canada, and enormous strides were made in the 1990s. Doctoral programs in nursing were launched, and more nurses than ever before achieved doctoral preparation. The funding environment changed, new sources of funds became available to support nursing research, and a number of opportunities developed to allow nurses to devote more of their time to conducting research. Nursing research achieved an increasing share of the research dollars that are distributed annually. These changes did not come easily. Opposition both inside and outside universities had to be overcome before PhD programs became established, but nurses worked strategically to ensure that they gained access to the new sources of funding.

Research is now regarded as central to determining what constitutes best practice, that is, care delivered based on the best research evidence available *combined with* knowledge about the patient's unique circumstances. An understanding of how to bring about best practice and research utilization more broadly is in its infancy and research utilization at point of care is a challenge. Issues of the politics of knowledge, the value of some forms of knowledge over others, and the unquestioned relevance of all approaches to research for nursing practice may influence research utilization.

Nursing education has been profoundly influenced by research. As nurse educators are better prepared and bring knowledge about research into their teaching, students graduate with higher research literacy and interest in developing research careers themselves.

Despite its relative youth, nursing research has made major contributions to our understanding of what patients are experiencing and what they prefer in the way of treatment, information, or approach to their care; how to better care for patients experiencing a variety of health conditions; how to run the healthcare system more effectively and efficiently; and how to help people to live healthier lives. The potential for even more substantive contributions is immense.

Of the many issues facing nurses, a few stand out: The challenge to prepare sufficient researchers to replace those who will retire over the next 10 to 15 years and to meet future demand; the challenge of using the structure and resources of the new CIHR to meet the needs of nursing research; the challenge of increasing research utilization in practice; and the need to question and disrupt the politics of knowledge.

Add to your knowledge of this issue:		
Canada Association for Nursing Research (CANR)	**www.canr.ca**	
Canadian Association of Schools of Nursing (CASN)	**www.casn.ca**	
Canadian Health Services Research Foundation (CHSRF)	**www.chsrf.ca**	
Canadian Institutes of Health Research (CIHR)	**www.cihr-irsc.gc.ca**	
Canadian Nurses Association (CNA)	**www.cna-nurses.ca**	
Canadian Nurses Foundation (CNF)	**www.canadiannursesfoundation.com**	

Online

R E F L E C T I O N S *on the Chapter...*

1 Identify one or two nurse researchers whose work interests you. Trace their publications through electronic databases such as the Cumulative Index to Nursing and Allied Health Literature and MEDLINE. What journals are they publishing in? Are they working alone or with a consistent team of collaborators? How would you summarize their contributions?

2 Think about an area of practice that interests you (e.g., managing the symptoms of children being treated for cancer or helping mothers maintain a sense of control during labor) and then develop a nursing practice question. Go to the electronic databases and search for research that addresses that question. Has research been done on it? If there is research, who has done it, and how much of it has been done by nurses? If there is no research, are there opinion pieces, editorials, or descriptions of how various places manage? Describe the state of knowledge at this time on the practice. Would you recommend research or more research on the question?

3 Think of one practice setting you have been in. What strategies are in place to apply research findings to practice? How successful are they? If there are no obvious strategies, describe what could be done to bring research to practice.

4 Go to the CIHR website, http://www.cihr-irsc.gc.ca/. Visit the web pages of the 13 institutes. Review their mission statements and the types of research they are interested in. How many are focused on research that is relevant to nursing? Look at their staffing and the members of their advisory boards. How many have nurses on their boards? Is there a relationship between mission and research focus and the membership of their boards?

Want to know more? Visit thePoint for additional helpful resources:

- Journal Articles
- Learning Objectives
- Nursing Professional Roles and Responsibilities
- Bonus chapters:
  - Health and Nursing Policy: A Matter of Politics, Power and Professionalism
  - The NP Movement: Recurring Issues
  - When Difference Matters: The Politics of Privilege and Marginality

References

Aikin Murphy, P. (2011). Evidence-based practice: What evidence counts? *Journal of Midwifery and Women's Health, 56*(4), 323–324.

Canadian Institute of Health Research. (2012). *Frequently asked questions.* Retrieved from: www.CIHR-IRSC.gc.ca/e/4478.html

Canadian Nurses' Association. (2012). Graduate Programs. Retrieved from: www.cna-aiic.ca/en/professional/development/graduate-programs/

Cummings, G.G., Estabrooks, C.A., Midodzi, W.K.,Wallin, L., & Hayduk, L. (2007). Influence of organizational characteristics on research utilization. *Nursing Research, 56*(4S), S24–S39.

Earle-Foley, V. (2011). Evidence–based practice: Issues, paradigms and future pathways. *Nursing Forum, 46*(1), 38–44.

Estabrooks, C.A., Midodzi, W.K., Cummings, G.G., & Wallin, L. (2007). Predicting research use in nursing organizations. *Nursing Research, 56*(suppl. 4), S7–S23.

Gagnon, A.J. (1999). Do editors have anything to teach us? A review of 30 years of journal editorials. *Canadian Journal of Nursing Research, 30*(4), 23–26.

Gottlieb, L.N. (1999). From nursing papers to research journal: A 30-year odyssey [Editorial]. *Canadian Journal of Nursing Research, 30*(4), 9–14.

Jennings, B.M. (2000). Evidence-based practice: The road best traveled? [Editorial]. *Research in Nursing & Health, 23*, 343–345.

McIntyre, M., & McDonald, C. (2013). Nursing philosophies, theories, concepts, frameworks and models. In B. Kozier, G. Erb, A. Berman, S. R. Bouchal, S. Hurst, L. Yiu, L. S. Stamler, & M. Buck (eds.), *Fundamentals of nursing: Concepts process and practice.* Toronto, ON: Pearson.

Medical Research Council of Canada. [Online]. Retrieved from http://strategis.ic.gc.ca/epic/internet/inrti-rti.nsf/en/te01458e.html

Mitchell, G. (1999). Evidence-based practice: Critique and alternative view. *Nursing Science Quarterly, 12*(1), 30–35.

Petticrew, M. (2001). Systematic reviews from astronomy to zoology. *British Medical Journal, 322*, 98–101.

Pringle, D. (2010). The realities of Canadian nursing research. In M. McIntyre & C. McDonald (eds.), *Realities of Canadian Nursing: Professional, practice and power issues* (3rd ed.), pp. 259–280. Philadelphia: Lippincott, Williams and Wilkins.

Social Sciences Humanities Research Council (SSHRC). (2012). Guidelines for the eligibility of applications related to health. Retrieved from: www.sshrc-crsh.gc.ca/funding-financment

Wood, M., Giovannetti, P., & Ross-Kerr, J. (2004). *Canadian PhD in nursing: A discussion paper.* Retrieved from www.casn.ca/en/

Nursing, Technology, and Informatics: Understanding the Past and Embracing the Future

W. Dean Care, David Michael Gregory, and Wanda M. Chernomas

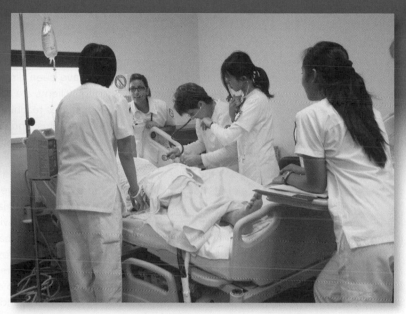

Students participate in a simulated learning experience. (Used with permission, University of Manitoba, Faculty of Nursing.)

Critical Questions

As a way of engaging with the ideas in this chapter, consider the following:

1. What is your comfort level with the use of technology?

2. What are your assumptions about the usefulness of technology in nursing education and professional nursing practice?

3. Can you identify what your learning needs are with respect to technology and nursing practice and how they can be addressed?

4. How do you think that nursing compares with other professional practice disciplines regarding the use of technology in practice and in education?

Chapter Objectives

After completing this chapter, you will be able to:

1. Discuss the relationship between nursing and technology.

2. Discern the technology and informatics foundations, theoretical and practical, expected in a baccalaureate nursing program.

3. Describe the role of technology and informatics in nursing.

4. Explore the possibilities of the use of technology and informatics in nursing.

(continued on page 238)

Chapter Objectives (continued)

5. Discuss the issues related to applying technology and informatics in education and practice.

6. Identify the barriers to technology in education and practice contexts.

7. Formulate strategies for resolving these barriers in practice settings.

It is the year 2015. You are a public health nurse with the regional health authority. Your primary responsibilities include following up on clients who have been discharged from the cardiac surgery program at the local tertiary care hospital. Clients are now being discharged 1 to 2 days after surgery. The care you provide includes teaching, wound care, symptom management, assessing and monitoring health status, and coordinating the interdisciplinary team. Most (90%) of the clients you serve have access to the Internet and personal computers (PCs) in their homes.

A typical day for you looks something like this: You arrive at work and log on to your desktop PC. You receive notice of the cardiac clients who were discharged yesterday. You call or e-mail five of these clients and set up appointments for the day. Having downloaded their electronic medical records onto your desktop computer, you review the files in preparation for home visits. You then transmit these files onto a wireless, handheld personal digital assistant (PDA), which accompanies you on all home visits. It provides access to your e-mail messages and Internet databases and it has an intranet feature that allows instant access to the other members of the healthcare team. This tool is also a cell phone, and it contains your appointment schedule, word processing documents, and address book; it is your personal organizer. It has 32 GB of memory and contains a voice recognition system that allows you to verbally record and store your "Nurse's Notes," which will be digitalized and downloaded to a permanent record when you get back to your office.

Most of your clients wear electrocardiogram (ECG) leads. You are able to monitor their cardiac rhythms and vital signs from both your desktop and PDA. Each client has an e-mail account from which they can send you messages and ask you questions. Before you leave the office, you receive a call from a 5-day postoperative client who is experiencing chest discomfort. You ask him to turn on his video Web cam, which is provided to each client upon discharge. It is mounted on the top of his desktop PC and allows you to view his appearance, assess his medical and emotional conditions, and speak with him "face to face." He attaches a Dynamap to his arm, and you receive instant blood pressure and pulse readings; an oxygen saturation reading is transmitted from the finger probe he is wearing. Using your desktop computer, you upload his ECG to get a "real-time" image of the client's cardiac rhythm. Next, you upload a visual image of his normal cardiac rhythm and compare it to his current ECG. You decide to make a home visit to assess this client's situation more thoroughly.

This brief vignette sets the stage for a discussion of the issues and trends arising from technology and informatics as they apply to nursing. Like the vignette, this chapter focuses on common uses and applications of technology in nursing practice and education. It also identifies issues arising from this technology and broaches the future of technology in nursing and healthcare. Relevant historical events are introduced, particularly as they relate to the significant shift in Western society from an industrial focus to an information ethos. Both rely heavily on technology but in vastly different ways.

The Industrial Age (late 19th and early 20th centuries) was characterized by an emphasis on productivity, efficiency, division of labor, and hierarchical organizations. In contrast, the Information Age (present era) is distinguished by a heavy dependence on telecommunications, knowledge and information explosion, global operations, decentralized organizations, and networked employees. The Information Age provides society with rapid access to and manipulation of information. In the area of healthcare, the Information Age fosters advances in health and telecommunications technology, which has had, and will continue to have, a profound effect on nurses and the organizations for which they work.

Historically, the relationship between technology and nursing has been marked by tension and unrest. Until recently, nursing and technology were framed as a dichotomy—nursing at one end and technology at the other—polar opposites, in a sense. Technology has been viewed as masculine, scientific, mechanistic, and reductionistic. In contrast, nursing in this dichotomous thinking has been conceptualized as feminine, nurturing, a soft science, humanistic, and holistic. Thus, technology has been identified as innately negative and dehumanizing to nursing— potentially obstructing or impeding nursing care (Gadow, 1988). The long-term utility of framing nursing and technology in this manner (i.e., masculine versus feminine, hard versus soft science, and reductionistic versus holistic caring) is questionable. Of course, the advent of new biomedical technologies can have ethical, moral, and philosophical implications for nursing and Canadian healthcare (e.g., genetic marker assessments, techno-treatments, diagnostic technology, etc.). Nurses are concerned with the resultant impact of technologies on the lives of patients and nursing practice.

In this regard, nurses do serve as "cultural brokers" between technology and patients. In this role, nurses translate technology for patients and provide explanations about the technology. On another plane of discussion, however, the development and adoption of information and communication technology (ICT) has the potential to optimize client and patient outcomes. ICT can permit nurses to readily access the knowledge they need to support their care (Mathieu, 2007). The Canadian Nurses Association ([CNA], 2006) recognizes the importance of nursing information and knowledge management.

> Competencies in information management and the use of communication technology are integral to nursing practice. Competencies in information management and the use of communication technology are no longer add-ons to traditional methods of health-care delivery. Rather, these competencies are an integral part of health care and nursing practice. CNA supports the Health Council of Canada's statements that health-care providers "need reliable and accurate patient health information at the point of care and the best evidence available to determine treatment options" and that electronic tools to manage this information are a necessity (p. 1).

RELATIONSHIP BETWEEN NURSING AND TECHNOLOGY

What exactly is the relationship between nursing and technology? To date, nurses have rarely been "at the table" in regard to developing much of the biomedical technology that affects their practice. As a profession, nursing most often inherits or receives technology developed by other disciplines. Medical technology is not nursing technology, and yet this technology is most often imposed on nursing (Purnell, 1998). In contrast to the importation of biomedical technology, there is the promising presence of nurses in the development and application of ICT. For example, nurses were involved in the development of an electronic information gathering and dissemination system to support both nursing-sensitive outcomes data collection and evidence-based decision making at the point of patient care (Doran et al., 2007). At the point of patient care, nurses can use technology to improve the quality of patient and client care and generate data about nursing outcomes. This and other related technologies are thus poised to provide freedom to nurses, the freedom to engage in holistic and humanistic care for patients and clients and their families.

Despite such recent developments, there are several factors that may be contributing to a *technology lag* within the profession itself. A closer look at these factors may help us to better understand why this technology lag exists.

- As Booth (2006) observes, nursing education programs "have yet to conquer the larger issues surrounding the necessary knowledge, skills, and practice competencies required for nurses to function in the future" (p. 3). Although there is growing movement in Canadian nursing curricula to address such shortcomings in undergraduate nursing education, there is a need for faculty development in the areas of e-Health (electronic health), including informatics, technology, and ICT. (See next section regarding e-Health.)
- Although new graduates from baccalaureate nursing programs may be lacking in literacy skills with respect to e-Health, the need for ongoing literacy education becomes clear when looking at the demographic profile of the profession. In 2009, more than 50% of practicing nurses had graduated 20 years ago and 37.3% of all registered nurses (RNs) in Canada were aged 50 or older. In 2009, Canada had more RNs employed in nursing at ages 50 to 59 (29.4%) compared to any other age group (Canadian Institute for Health Information [CIHI], 2009). This is not to suggest that older nurses lack the capacity or aptitude to embrace and master technology or informatics. Rather, they likely have had to become techno-literate through individualized continuing education and staff development efforts. And if we consider that formal and informal education and socialization processes may disadvantage women with respect to e-Health literacy, then there may also be a gender gap within the profession (i.e., 93.8% of RNs are women; 6.2% are men [CIHI, 2009]). Further research regarding the possibility of the gender–generation technology gap within nursing is required.

Recently, sectors within the Canadian healthcare system are implementing a range of e-Health–related technologies to improve patient care. Although the progress to date can be considered slow and ad hoc, the widescale adoption of new technologies will likely occur at a very fast pace over the next few years. This trend has significant—perhaps even dramatic—implications for the education of future RNs. Similarly, nurses currently working within the healthcare system in Canada will require adequate supports and education. For example, the Association Québécoise des Infirmières et Infirmiers en Systèmes et Technologies de l'Information is authoring a position paper on the need for the systemic training of nurses in the area of informatics (Mathieu, 2007). The need for nursing informaticists is clear as is the need for nurses to embrace technology and care. Thus, the stage is being set for future developments in the relationship between nursing and technology.

NURSING INFORMATICS

According to Simpson (1998, p. 22), "Part of the reason nursing informatics is so hard to define is because it is a moving target." Two decades later, there remains some confusion regarding the concepts of health information technology, health informatics, and e-Health (Loiselle & Cossette, 2007). Booth (2006) suggests that "e-Health" serves as the umbrella term for many of these concepts, including ICT. In its broadest sense, nursing informatics is understood as the integration of information technologies and communications into nursing practice (Mathieu, 2007).

Staggers and Bagley Thompson's (2002) definition is helpful in understanding the breadth and depth of nursing informatics:

> Nursing Informatics is a specialty that integrates nursing science, computer science and information science to manage and communicate data, information and knowledge in nursing practice. Nursing informatics facilitates the integration of data, information and knowledge to support patients, nurses and other providers in their decision making in all roles and settings. This support is accomplished through the use of information structures, information processes and information technology (p. 255).

Today's nurse is affected by an ever-changing healthcare system dominated by a focus on outcomes, evidence, performance measurement, and the use of technology to provide and support care delivery. Information is key to effective decision making and integral to quality nursing practice (CNA, 2007). In their evolving role as "knowledge workers," nurses are increasingly being called on to access information systems to facilitate evidence-based practice. In addition, as more patients become comfortable with information technology, expectations will be placed on nurses to have similar skills. "In fact, nurses may find that their patient education encounters will increasingly occur through distance technology" (Gassert, 1998, p. 266).

APPLICATIONS OF NURSING INFORMATICS AND TECHNOLOGY IN PRACTICE

The application of nursing informatics as an umbrella concept takes various forms in practice. More recently, the term "e-Health" is used to refer to "the application of information and communication technologies in the health sector" (Health Canada, 2007, p. 1) reflecting the integration of telehealth technologies with the Internet (Riva, 2000). The proliferation of terms relating to care practices using distance technology has created confusion and difficulty when exploring related issues. Terms such as *telemedicine, nursing telepractice,* and *tele-education* are used in the literature. Collectively, they refer to different components of healthcare delivery through technology and, in certain instances, as subsets of telehealth. This section will discuss telehealth, emphasizing nursing telepractice with the telephone, electronic mail, and Web-based information as the vehicles for knowledge dissemination, information exchange, communication, and electronic health records.

Telehealth and Nursing Telepractice

The term *telehealth* encompasses a broad range of healthcare and service delivery systems provided through distance or electronic technology (Gassert, 2000). "Nursing practice in telehealth includes all client-centered forms of nursing practice and the provision of information, and education for healthcare professionals occurring through, or facilitated by, the use of telecommunications or electronic means" (CNA, 2007, p. 1).

The geographically dispersed population of Canada provides an ideal opportunity for the application of telehealth to reduce barriers related to healthcare access. Telehealth has the potential to provide borderless, seamless, and accessible healthcare in all reaches of the country, delivering fast, accurate diagnoses and treatments in situations where face-to-face visits may not be possible. For example, Alberta's extensive telehealth network offers clinical services including specialist consults and follow-up care, rehabilitation services, and patient education sessions (Alberta Telehealth, 2007).

Nursing telepractice uses the nursing process, within the context of the nurse–client relationship, to assess, plan, and implement care through the provision of information, referral, education and support, evaluation, and documentation (CNA, 2007).

In real time, nurses can perform a wide variety of assessment, education, and intervention skills at varying frequencies. They can listen to heart and chest sounds, read and interpret ECG results, assess wound status, review downloaded blood glucose information, and observe and facilitate the patient's self-care (Russo, 2001). Mobile phones and PDA technology exist to communicate health information, such as ECG and blood pressure readings, to clinicians anywhere in the world from a mobile consumer (Rasid & Woodward, 2005). The opportunities for nursing within this area may be limited only by the technologic resources available and the knowledge and ability of nursing to advocate for our expanded role in implementation, care, and evaluation.

Within telehealth, the need remains for nurses to practice according to the established standards of practice, codes of ethics, legislation, and competencies of their regulatory bodies. Several related issues and challenges are apparent within the telehealth environment. There are guidelines for telephone practice in some jurisdictions but not all have such policies for their practitioners. (See, for example, "Practice Guideline: Telepractice," College of Nurses of Ontario, 2005.) These telepractice guidelines address many of the broad practice expectations within a telehealth environment. CNA's position is that the regulation of nurses' practice and accountability lies within the jurisdiction of their registration (CNA, 2007). However, policies on the provision of telehealth across provincial registering bodies have yet to be developed through coordinated efforts. In addition, educational standards or credentials have not been established for this area of practice. Issues related to maintaining privacy and confidentiality pose challenges that are still being understood. Without a comprehensive consideration of the aforementioned issues, liability issues, and employer responsibilities become unclear. The following question remains relevant: How do professional nursing organizations and regulatory bodies promote safe and competent practice, prevent substandard nursing practice, and intervene or investigate complaints as necessary when the RN and patient may be thousands of miles apart and their interactions are electronic (CNA, 2000)?

Care Delivery by Telephone

The earliest use of the telephone as a tool for providing public health or private duty nursing occurred in the early 1920s (Sandelowski, 2000). Nurses have long since been offering advice over the telephone, particularly from emergency rooms and public health areas. Today, eight provinces and one territory offer "24/7" access to nurses by telephone, thus ushering in a new era in nursing telephone practice (Goodwin, 2007).

In addition to the guidelines for telehealth practice noted above, a wide range of protocols also exists to support nurses' decision making and judgment. Questions and issues remain regarding the frequency of review of protocols, the qualifications and education required of the practitioner, and nurses' involvement in developing these standards.

Manitoba's Health Links is an example of telephone technology that provides 24-hour province-wide nursing access for health information and advice. Experienced RNs with a broad range of expertise and skills usually provide this service. Another example is British Columbia's HealthLink NurseLine, which makes 24-hour, toll-free, province-wide nursing access available. Nurses use software to assist in guiding patients' healthcare decision making. NurseLine is part of an expanded program endorsed by the College of Registered Nurses of British Columbia. The program consists of a printed HealthGuide handbook and an online health database. Commercially available software can be customized, at a cost, to meet needs for evaluation and monitoring of calls, including the number and type of calls and users, automated evaluation of disposition or outcome, patient satisfaction, and patient knowledge of services.

Whether the protocols are available online or on paper, telephone nursing can be compared with more traditional triage. Telephone nursing uses nursing assessment to guide or coach the decision making of the patient concurrently with an empowerment approach rather than directed decisions. The inability for nurses to incorporate nonverbal patient behaviors can be viewed as a limitation, or as a challenge, to their assessment skills. However, the advent of visual images may address this limitation.

The Aboriginal Nurses Association of Canada supports the use of telehealth practices to improve the health of First Nations, Métis, and Inuit communities. According to a discussion paper, "inequities exist in the health and the health care services of Aboriginal people compared to the general population of Canada" (Aboriginal Nurses Association of Canada, 2001, p. 9). The Manitoba Telehealth First Nations Expansion Project links 10 northern, remote First Nations communities. Videoconferencing can now be used to improve access to specialist care, health-related education, and visits with family members located in healthcare facilities elsewhere in the province (Manitoba Telehealth, 2007). However, patients from these communities and others without phones, computers, or computer skills are at a disadvantage. The introduction of advanced technology in some communities may inadvertently create a "digital divide" that further marginalizes people in remote communities who do not have access to that technology. (Refer to the Digital Divide Website for more information on this topic.)

Electronic Mail and the Internet

Electronic mail (e-mail) and the Internet are means of providing telehealth services in an e-Health world. As more patients become comfortable with and gain access to e-mail, this form of communication may be used increasingly as a means of contact and consultation with healthcare providers. Some patients may experience greater comfort using e-mail as a form of communicating, especially if their concerns are of a personal or sensitive nature. With e-mail, patients and nurses have some flexibility in regard to the timing of consultations, inquiries, and responses. However, the issues of privacy and confidentiality remain unresolved. In addition, it may not be possible to verify that the individual initiating communication is indeed the patient and that the question and the nurse's response will not be read by others. The nurse's e-mail response could also be circulated to other care providers, with the potential for the nurse's response to be misinterpreted or taken out of context. The lack of live communication may belie the complexity of the patient's situation, leading to tendencies for both the patient and the provider to inadvertently simplify or exaggerate their concerns, assessments, and responses. Liability for care practices and potential misdiagnoses or care provided through distance or electronic technology is issues warranting careful exploration.

Health-seeking Behaviors

Similarly, the Internet has provided the opportunity for health-seeking behavior by patients, often before contact with a health professional. Potentially, the Internet offers privacy, immediacy, breadth of information, different perspectives, and infinite repetition of information (Bischoff & Kelley, 1999). The proliferation of Web-based resources provides individuals with access to health information not easily obtained prior to the advent of the Internet. Conversely, the amount of information, quality of presentation, and often-conflicting information can create confusion. Patients and care providers may be unaware of how to evaluate the accuracy and credibility of Web-based information. Provider resources for such evaluation are growing, as exemplified by the inclusion of guidelines and standards for Web-based publishing on many Websites. The nurse may find her or his practice extending into patient education about how to evaluate Internet sites. Local public and academic libraries are beginning to provide information on how to evaluate the quality of Web-based information. An example of an interactive Internet service that promotes health-seeking behaviors with palliative care patients is the Canadian Virtual Hospice. This service represents a network of information and support for people dealing with life-threatening illness and loss. After registration, people can access this Website as a patient, friend or family member, healthcare provider, or volunteer. This is a credible and well-recognized health service offered by healthcare professionals. This site is in contrast to the myriad unregulated Internet sites that have been established and maintained by nonprofessional "experts" in various areas of healthcare. Consumers of health and those seeking healthcare information need to be aware of the potential for information that is not validated or credible being posted to authentic-looking Websites.

Online Support Groups

In addition to its use for patient self-education, the Internet is used for support groups through online synchronous chat rooms (real-time discussion) and asynchronous interaction (anytime discussion), which provide patients with the opportunity to seek support and to consult with others independently. The content of online healthcare and related discussions may vary according to the nature of the disorder and the composition of the group (White & Dorman, 2000). Topics may revolve around general themes, such as personal experience and opinion, encouragement and support, treatment, symptoms, alternative therapies, caregiver concerns, and coping strategies. As with e-mail, using technology may ease communication for those who feel inhibited by face-to-face support groups, who seek the company of those who are similarly affected, or who are geographically isolated. Future research will need to explore the role that nurses play in such online support groups, how effective groups are conducted, and the role of such groups in health promotion. Active participation or "listening" to online support groups also helps the nurse to understand patients' concerns. Nurses need to be familiar with the opportunities that online support groups provide.

Despite the challenges of this technology, e-mail, Internet, and telehealth practices have the potential to substantially decrease the indirect and social costs of healthcare. Costs associated with travel to healthcare facilities and absenteeism from family, school, or work may be reduced. This cost savings is particularly relevant to patients and families isolated by geography or care needs.

Electronic Health Records

Since 2001, Canada Health Infoway has been working with Canada's 14 federal, provincial, and territorial governments to improve the accessibility, safety, and efficiency of healthcare by developing private and secure *electronic health records* (EHRs). An EHR is the health record of a person that is accessible online from many separate, interoperable automated systems within an electronic network (Office of Health and the Information Highway [OHIH], 2001). This definition infers the complexity of the issues involving EHRs, such as the need for additional resources, infrastructure, and economic challenges related to accessing an integrated electronic network. Health Canada (2001 as cited in CNA, 2002) notes the following characteristics of EHRs:

- Electronic—voice, video, images, and data related to the client or patient are available electronically
- Longitudinal—data on the client or patient are collected and stored over time
- Accessible—authorized health professionals can access the record to support the delivery of care
- Comprehensive—the record includes service encounter data from various health professionals and across the continuum of health-service delivery.

Thus, the EHR is a secure and private lifetime record of an individual's health and healthcare history, available to authorized healthcare providers. It is designed to tie together the output of a number of information systems. Some of these systems are in use today, while others are in development. Canada Health Infoway (2009), an independent and nonprofit organization, is involved in a number of projects to develop systems that form the essential building blocks of an EHR, such as digital imaging, summaries of drug prescriptions, immunizations, and lab test results. Provinces and territories across Canada are working together with Infoway to accelerate the development of these systems. The move to EHRs has been stimulated by technologic development, increased social mobility, public and government demand for accountability, and care by a wider range of healthcare professionals—all of whom will require information (OHIH, 2001). Healthcare decision makers and policy analysts increasingly require access to data for the evaluation and support of appropriate healthcare programming. The electronic availability of a patient's record promotes accessibility of the information by a variety of healthcare providers— linked to the network—who are involved in the patient's care. EHRs could eliminate duplication of services, improve efficiency of the system, and provide accurate documentation over time. With access to complete records, physicians and nurses will have far better information for decision making. This information is especially critical when prescriptions and treatments are being provided by multiple care providers, or when a patient is in an emergency situation.

Limited patient access to health records also becomes a possibility with EHRs. Such access may support enhanced personal decision making in health behaviors. Potentially, patients can be more informed about their health status, which may facilitate discussions with healthcare providers. In this way, patients will be empowered to take a more active role in their health. Privacy and security are fundamental to EHRs. Health Canada Infoway (2009) is working with jurisdictions and privacy commissioners to implement an EHR information governance structure. The agency is also completing a conceptual EHR privacy impact assessment. In addition, it is planning to conduct (with the Office of the Privacy Commissioner of Canada and Health Canada) a comprehensive survey of public attitudes and concerns about privacy and electronic health. Ideally, only authorized healthcare providers will have access to confidential patient information.

The value of EHRs in relation to renal nurse practitioner care has been noted (Allen, 2007). Information technology in the form of the EHR "can profoundly affect clinical workflow, enhance and expand the NP's [nurse practitioner's] ability to work with client data and information. EHRs have the potential to greatly improve client safety by making it possible for clinicians to have information available to enable them to make informed decisions" (p. 44). Thus, EHRs can offer point-of-care information to clinicians.

ISSUES IN THE APPLICATION OF BIOMEDICAL TECHNOLOGY AND NURSING PRACTICE

In terms of biomedical technology, a study by Cooper and Powell (1998) revealed how such technology created extreme uncertainty and profound physical, emotional, psychological, and spiritual vulnerability among patients undergoing bone marrow transplantation. It was, however, nurses who attended to these vulnerabilities. The researchers observed the following about how nurses incorporated technology as part of their nursing care:

> It is no exaggeration to suggest that these nurses created a sacred space in this highly technologic enterprise for patients to do the work of making meaning of the experience...One extraordinary feature of this [nursing] care resides in the fact that it occurred in the context of a highly technical endeavor. Capturing the essence of this feat, one patient insightfully asked, "How can the nurses be at the end of technology [in a spectrum of technology and care] and thank goodness they are because I'm here today because of it—and then how can they be at this touch-feel end at the same time?" (p. 65).

Ethical Dilemmas

The nurse experiences firsthand the ethical dilemmas associated with new biomedical technology. Ethical and moral knowledge moves nurses to action in relation to technology. Reproductive technologies, for example, are a special concern of women, their families, and practitioners, and, within nursing, there is a substantial body of work related to the ethics of reproductive technology. Availability of genetic testing requires women to examine their personal situations and beliefs to determine whether they wish to access the technology. Nurses may need to provide counseling as a woman decides what is best for herself. In addition, society at large varies in its perception of the right or the need of government, resource availability, funding, and community values to influence the utilization and distribution of technologies.

Decision Making

Decision making regarding access to available biomedical technology has further ethical implications when technology is costly or in limited supply. Who should have access? What criteria should be used? Who should develop the criteria for access? These are some issues that emerge in the face of new technology. For example, at this time, not all people who need dialysis have locally available access to this technology. One mechanism to address determination of access under high-demand, limited-availability situations is to refer decision making to review boards. Such boards establish criteria in reviewing candidates for access to the technology. Nurses may be members of such boards or they may be called on to assess a patient's suitability for access to the technology. Then, too, nurses are in positions to provide information, advocacy, and emotional support to patients and families denied access to these services.

Decision-making criteria to purchase technology or make it accessible to units are also limited (Purnell, 1998). In most instances, incorporation of technology onto nursing units occurs as a consequence of criteria established by medical and, increasingly, non-nursing administrators. As nurses are left out of technology development, they are similarly distanced from decision making related to technology application in their workplaces.

ISSUES IN THE ALLOCATION OF TECHNOLOGY IN EDUCATION

Timothy, a nursing student, is about to graduate and thinks he is well prepared to face a workplace filled with technology. Computers are commonplace in his life as a student. Nursing informatics is a required course that he took at the beginning of his program. He uses a word processing program to construct and format papers. He finds that electronic mail and Internet access are helpful to search Websites, stay in touch with classmates, keep informed about university and faculty information, and take courses offered by Moodle. He is adept at locating electronic information and is skilled at critiquing the quality and credibility of the information.

Timothy is enjoying the high-fidelity simulation experiences that are part of the learning laboratory course. Because of the limited access to clinical practice sites, Timothy and his fellow students are now substituting a clinical day a week for a simulated learning experience. He is concerned that this reduced exposure to "real" patients in the clinical setting will reduce his ability to critically think and develop his competency as a practicing nurse.

Computer technology is a significant tool for nursing education and practice. However, according to Ehnfors and Grobe (2004), the largest dilemma facing nursing and health professional education is accurate identification of the future competencies that will be required to function in a technology-infused workplace. If nurse educators expect students to use technology in their practice as graduates, students must become proficient and comfortable with healthcare-related technology in their basic programs. The new generation of university students has been raised with an appreciation for and a working knowledge of technology. They bring with them thousands of hours of playing video games, text messaging, blogging, and social interaction on MySpace, YouTube, and Facebook. The challenge for educators involves taking these previously learned skills and adapting them to the world of healthcare informatics.

Extent of Computer Literacy

Computers are available in most schools of nursing but their use is neither systematically nor routinely included in programming, unlike the situation described in the previous vignette. Until recently, few programs in Canada had a required nursing informatics course. Postsecondary institutions may believe that incoming students possess the necessary computer skills because of their experience with computers in primary and secondary schools. However, empirical evidence shows that although nursing students had access to computers in primary and secondary schools, they had limited opportunity to use them for tasks other than word processing (Gassert, 1998) and social interaction.

The life experiences of today's students are vastly different from that of previous generations'. The new generation of postsecondary student, often called Generation X (comprising young adults in their late 20s to early 30s) and Generation Y (in their early to mid-20s), exhibits unique learning characteristics and needs (Hessler & Ritchie, 2006). These young learners function better in learning activities that are structured, involve teamwork and experiential activities, and include the use of technology (Collins & Tilson, 2001). This generation wants quick access to information; has little tolerance for delays; and prefers interactive, collaborative learning styles. Members of this generation represent a challenge for instructors who rely on a traditional teacher-centered lecture style of course delivery. Part of the tension that exists in higher education today is related to the differences between the experiences and preferences of students versus the capacity of our educational institutions and faculty to adapt to these changes.

Many institutions of higher learning are increasing their use of teaching innovations. In some cases, technology is being used to address the issue of increasing student numbers, multiple-site campuses, declining numbers of faculty, and limited financial resources. The potential exists for technology to become a means to address these complex administrative problems without due consideration for maintaining educational standards and quality programming. Educational facilities need to guard against the temptation of substituting quality of instruction for increased student access and financial gain.

Simulated Learning

Technology has always played an integral part in the learning laboratory experience. The era of using stationary models and filmstrips has evolved into the use of more high-fidelity simulated learning experiences. Nursing has followed high-risk professions like airline pilots and adopted simulated learning because of the concern for patient safety and quality care. Recently, increased enrollments in nursing programs, reduction in faculty numbers, and reduced access to clinical sites has caused a heightened interest in the use of simulated learning in nursing education. Early studies have shown that critical thinking, clinical judgment, and confidence levels can increase when nursing students are exposed to computer-based simulations in their programs of study (Lasater, 2007; Schoening et al., 2006). The recent movement toward substituting simulated learning experiences for clinical practice time requires further debate at the faculty level. In a systematic review of literature, Harder (2010) concluded that "institutions have adopted simulation to help educate their students and healthcare professionals; however, intervention effectiveness evaluation continues to be an area requiring research" (p. 23).

Options for Distance Learning

Nursing education is experiencing unprecedented changes in student characteristics. Students of the 21st century are more likely to be of diverse backgrounds and nontraditional in their learning styles. These characteristics are fueling the need for educational facilities to consider alternative approaches to teaching, such as distance-learning options. The same can be said for providing opportunities for practicing nurses who require enhanced job skills, such as physical assessment or leadership abilities.

Technology-based pedagogy enables us to conceive of education without the restrictions of the classroom; hence, the usual mechanisms and parameters around course delivery need to be rethought. For example, traditional lectures, which commonly are the foundation of knowledge delivery in higher education, become nonexistent in a learner-centered, Web-based environment. In this scenario, a faculty member and student may never see each other, despite having lengthy "discussions" that have the potential to shape a student's thinking for life. At the same time, nursing education values strategies that facilitate the learning of a wide range of skills. Nursing education also values knowledge that includes assessment skills, promotion of health in families, adoption of the ethical values of the profession, and communications skills. Jukes (2005) has suggested that engaging students in e-learning can make learning fun and relevant, can deliver learning faster, can encourage "just-in-time" learning, and can provide opportunities for multitasking, networking, and interactivity. However, two questions remain: How does e-learning address the affective domain; and how does e-learning influence socialization into the professional nursing role? Until these questions are answered, educators will remain skeptical of the merits of e-learning.

Learning Distribution Systems

There are four general categories of distributed learning systems that support instructional delivery and communication. These include (1) print, (2) audio conferencing, (3) videoconferencing, and (4) Web-based and blended delivery.

Print-based Delivery

Print-based and correspondence courses employ prepackaged courses and self-contained learning modules. Faculty–student interaction is limited to occasional telephone contact and written feedback on submitted assignments. In recent years, distance-education providers have incorporated technology, such as facsimile machines, e-mail, and assignment submissions through the Internet, to supplement print-based courses. This mode of course delivery requires maintaining an expensive and extensive infrastructure and is not a popular method of choice today.

Audioconference Delivery

Instructional delivery has been enhanced by advancements in digitalized audio capabilities. This medium includes two-way telephone interaction between the faculty member and groups of students gathered at remote sites. Courses can be offered anywhere in the world that has telephone lines. Audioconferencing provides for real-time delivery at a fairly reasonable cost. It is ideally suited to students who cannot attend courses offered on campus or who do not have easy access to computer technology. One drawback of this method is the lack of visual stimuli to enhance the teaching–learning experience. This drawback is especially evident for students who have been exposed to video games, television, virtual learning experiences, and other hi-tech classes with slide presentations and graphic illustrations of course materials.

Videoconference Delivery

Interactive video networks use compressed digital video technology to deliver two-way audio signals and visual images to distant sites. Although the initial investment in videoconferencing requires an expensive technologic infrastructure, ongoing costs are usually limited to long-distance telephone charges and technical support. Student participation is encouraged through the use of multimedia presentations and interactive capabilities. Recent innovations in technology include the development of desktop video applications and simulations.

This form of delivery best approximates a face-to-face learning experience by allowing students to join a class and a professor in a distant locale. It also permits students in remote locations to have access to faculty expertise that may not be available in their home community. However, the expectations of this technology are often exceeded by the realities of the technical difficulties that can occur. The more complex the technology, the more complex the problems; this is one reason that more technical support is needed before and during course delivery. Preparing for a videoconference course requires considerable preliminary planning, knowledge of the technology, and the ability to solve problems and use the available technology to its fullest. Another drawback is that students on the receiving end tend to feel isolated from the faculty member, which may result in a perception of substandard and unequal treatment. Extensive faculty development is needed to assist educators to use this method of teaching.

A study by Care et al. (2006) showed that Aboriginal nursing students located in a northern community were often intimidated by the videoconference experience. They often positioned themselves off camera so they could remain anonymous and invisible to the remotely located instructor and students. Aboriginal students were often uncomfortable speaking out in class when videoconferencing with their more verbal southern counterparts. The study found that the faculty who made the extra effort to personalize the video technology were more effective in fostering a positive teacher–student relationship.

Web-based and Blended Delivery

To participate fully in a Web-based course, students must have regular access to a computer with Internet capacity. Web-based delivery allows students to engage in online interaction with the teacher and other students in a virtual learning environment. The instructional medium is through such software programs as Moodle. Interaction occurs through online discussion forums, chat rooms, and e-mail. New hybrid learning technologies combine the use of audio, video, and computer applications, creating multidimensional course delivery options. Courses can be structured as synchronous (real time) and asynchronous (anytime) offerings. This delivery method virtually eliminates geographic and access barriers to education. Blended delivery, "the thoughtful fusion of face-to-face and online learning experiences" (Garrison & Vaughn, 2008, p. 5) is increasing in popularity. In this method, a portion of traditional classroom hours are restructured and replaced with appropriate online learning experiences.

The rapid advances in instructional technologies have created a need for a transformation in higher education. This transformation has resulted in the need to address a myriad of issues in nursing education.

ISSUES IN ADOPTING TECHNOLOGY IN NURSING EDUCATION

The adoption of advanced instructional technology, like Web-based and blended delivery, has become commonplace in continuing and higher education. It has been viewed as both an educational boon and a technologic "money pit." Using advanced instructional technology in higher education also challenges educators to rethink the teaching and learning enterprise.

Changing Models and Roles

In the traditional paradigm of education, the educator was the "sage on the stage," and lectures were the dominant teaching practice. Students were expected to listen passively and absorb large quantities of content in a single serving. This "tell 'em and test 'em" approach saw the teacher as the expert and provider of information. In a learner-centered paradigm, the principles of constructivism, that is, "learning is a process of meaning making or knowledge building in which learners integrate new knowledge into a pre-existing network of understanding" (Young & Maxwell, 2007, p. 9), can be applied in an online learning environment. In this constructivist paradigm, teachers facilitate the learning process and, as such, become "guides on the side" for students.

The adoption of technology in education requires a paradigm shift that has a dramatic impact on the roles of faculty and students. With online courses, faculty and students have limited or nonexistent face-to-face interactions. The instructor is less likely to be the primary source of content expertise or information for the student. The role of facilitator has been commonly used to characterize how an educator functions in the technology-based pedagogy (Care et al., 2007). Specific aspects of the faculty role have been defined as assisting with access and navigation, explaining expectations for students, clarifying the faculty role, stimulating critical thinking, sharing professional expertise, and providing encouragement to online students (VandeVusse & Hanson, 2000). These changing responsibilities and relationships can affect the receptivity of students and faculty to embark on Web-based teaching and learning.

Carryover to Curricula

Rapid advances in the use of technology in practice have put pressure on the faculty to integrate the types of technology used in healthcare and nursing into already "packed" undergraduate curricula. Educational programs need to make decisions about the extent of use of technology in the delivery of curricula. For example, the adoption of PDAs is becoming popular in nursing education. According to Martin (2007), PDAs help to reduce student anxiety in clinical practice by making readily available a large volume of information and evidence. In a rapidly changing healthcare system, current information about medications, policies and procedures, and laboratory tests and values are readily available on a PDA at the point of care. Access to empirical evidence and medical and nursing information has been shown to have a positive effect on reducing medication errors, delivery of more comprehensive care, improving the continuity of care, and reducing stress levels in healthcare practitioners (Martin, 2007). On the other hand, Koeniger-Donohue (2008) raises concerns that introducing handheld technology into clinical courses can be an additional cost to students, and raises issues about security of confidential patient information and concerns about students becoming dependent on a PDA "at the expense of development of critical thinking skills" (p. 77).

Demands on Time and Career Activities

A troublesome area for the faculty in adopting technology into their teaching is time. The use of technology may actually increase the amount of time needed for teaching. This increased amount of time takes the faculty away from other aspects of their academic roles and responsibilities such as scholarly and research activities. Bates and Poole (2003) suggest that online courses increase faculty workload in all aspects of course design and implementation. Halstead and Billings (2005) believe that "time management frequently becomes an issue for faculty teaching online courses because of the amount of student communication typically generated within the course through threaded discussion postings, e-mail, and phone calls" (p. 429). This additional time commitment can be offset by establishing policies about "capping" enrollment in online courses as well as allocating preparation time and reducing the teaching load for the faculty engaged in online teaching. One of the greatest barriers in implementing Web-based instruction in higher education is the lack of recognition it affords to the faculty. University environments, in particular, place a high value on research and scholarly achievements in the criteria for tenure and promotion. Faculty members who persist in incorporating advanced instructional technologies in their courses serve the curriculum in significant ways, but the time spent on this activity may be perceived as detracting from their other academic roles. If so, the faculty may be reluctant to take on this type of instruction. Faculties and schools of nursing need to make important decisions about the value placed on using advanced technologies in their programs. Sufficient resources and faculty development activities will help to reduce this significant barrier.

Gains and Losses

One of the benefits of Web-based, online instruction is increased access by students who live in remote locations. For example, education becomes a reality for underrepresented populations like the Aboriginal community. A concern with this instructional medium is the loss of face-to-face contact between teachers and students and among students themselves. What becomes of the high value placed on socialization, role modeling, and development of the student–teacher relationship? Can a chat session replace the level of dialogue and discourse that exists in a traditional classroom? It is only after these issues are resolved that the faculty will feel comfortable adopting this approach on a large scale.

Isolation

The inherent nature of distance education includes the geographic separation of students from the faculty and from other learners. This separation can often contribute to feelings of social and psychological isolation. Moore and Kearsley (1996) coined the phrase "transactional distance" to describe the psychological distance that occurs in learners. This transactional distance is often caused by miscommunication and psychological gaps occurring between learners and instructors. In a traditional classroom, students are in touch with the nuances of nonverbal communication. Their presence in class contributes to a sense of community with other students and the instructor. In a virtual classroom, the instructor must make a conscious effort to bridge the psychological distance experienced by learners. This bridge can be achieved by promoting the establishment of a community of learners among students.

Effect of Advanced Instructional Technology on Career Choices

There is a call for a critical examination of the use of and growing reliance on technology in education. Mallow and Gilje (1999) caution the faculty about the rapidity of adopting technology in nursing education without careful thought about its impact. They note that research to date supports the effectiveness of technology in conveying factual information, and they report student satisfaction. However, little evidence exists regarding "student progress in affective domain criteria such as outcomes related to humanism, moral knowledge development, ethical development, interdisciplinary communication, or caring attributes." Mallow and Gilje recommend that educators consider the core values and social processes of the profession before using technology in the curriculum. The faculty often struggles to balance the use of technology with the need to develop valuable working relationships with students.

In Canada, it is becoming clear that certain clinical areas within nursing practice are "passed over" by students in favor of more technologically challenging environments. Nursing students are drawn to the "power and prestige" of technology. This theory was substantiated in a longitudinal study by Australian researchers (Stevens & Crouch, 1998). Of note was how nurse educators and nurses in clinical settings championed high-technology areas of nursing practice (e.g., emergency room and intensive care nursing) and created favorable technologic bias in students. The 156 students who were studied responded accordingly and, after graduation, gravitated toward these high-technology nursing practice domains. Because of this socialization by educators and clinicians, students valued specialized training experiences (e.g., intensive care, spinal trauma, and pediatric and neonatal intensive care) over basic nursing. Students and graduate nurses in the Australian study perceived that high-technology activities attracted power, prestige, and the nod from the elite of the profession, whereas basic nursing had low status and no power and was marginalized from the profession (Stevens & Crouch, 1998, p. 14). At issue then, is how the new generation of computer-literate, technologically savvy nurses will be attracted to and retained in low-technology practice areas, such as long-term care, or in practice agencies that do not have the financial means to support the newest technologies.

Information and instructional technologies can enhance the quality of the educational experience if used for the right purpose. The adoption of advanced technology in education does not in and of itself guarantee a positive outcome. How can this technology contribute to the overall effectiveness of the educational process in a way that maximizes student learning? Until this question is adequately addressed, educators must be cautious of wading into the technologic sea.

FUTURE OF TECHNOLOGY IN EDUCATION AND PRACTICE

Although the future is unclear, one thing is certain: Technology will continue to evolve and advance. The computer has become to the Information Age what the automobile was to the Industrial Age. The Internet is accessed by millions of people daily. The explosion of a digital society has brought about significant transformations in the way people interact, access and process information, and solve problems. Healthcare professionals are only beginning to appreciate the impact this revolution will have on the ability to deliver comprehensive and safe care. These challenging times call for healthcare professionals who can think critically and adapt to change quickly.

Impact of Nursing Science on Practice Technology

The development of nursing science, that is, knowledge relevant for nursing practice, will have an impact on the development and use of technology in nursing practice. Clinical nursing information systems for data categorization and storage depend on the taxonomic structures developed to reflect the phenomena of the discipline (Graves & Corcoran-Perry, 1996). If nursing science continues to be reflected in numerous classification systems, those that are selected to frame data management programs will have their presence more strongly embedded in the discipline. Concerns develop when one considers whose interests are being met with the implementation of standardized language and taxonomies found in EHR systems. Issues raised by Petrovskaya et al. (2009) caution us that the EHR is a product of government and industry that may not serve the needs of patients and client-centered nursing practice. Will the voices of patients and nurses alike be lost in the movement toward standardized codes and categories?

Extent of Informatics in Curricula

At this point in nursing's history, it is not surprising that there is a need for more education, support, and research for optimal utilization of computer technology and information systems for practicing nurses, educators, and undergraduate and graduate students (Link & Scholtz, 2000; Smith et al., 1998). As the next decades unfold, improved understanding and skills among all these groups are likely, as is concurrent acceptance of advanced information technology as part of nursing.

The Canadian Nursing Informatics Association completed a national research study of undergraduate nursing education informatics in Canada (Clarke & Nagle, 2003). Among its recommendations, the study suggested a holistic approach to nursing informatics and that the use of ICT be required in education, healthcare, research, and policy development. Schools of nursing should also plan and implement a strategy for faculty development in the area of nursing informatics. Progress to date has been limited, and there is the risk that Canadian nursing students will graduate without the requisite knowledge and skills related to informatics (Nagle, 2007).

As a result, the extent of inclusion of nursing informatics within nursing undergraduate curricula is now being discussed in faculties across the country. Fostering this discussion is the position statement on baccalaureate education and baccalaureate programs offered by the Canadian Association of Schools of Nursing (CASN). CASN notes that baccalaureate programs are "characterized by the presence of information technologies and infrastructures" (Canadian Association of Schools of Nursing [CASN], 2006, p. 1). Existing and new curricula must demonstrate not only their commitment to ICT, but also the manner in which students are provided with the education and hands-on experience to make them e-Health literate. Research into the effectiveness of advanced technology in nursing education will provide valuable information in refining how we incorporate technology into delivering nursing knowledge in undergraduate programs.

Potential for Greater Learning Access

Technology has the potential to improve the availability of basic and continuing nursing education for those for whom geography or other barriers have prevented access, which is a particularly significant issue in Canada for nurses and students who live great distances from major cities where higher education or facility-based continuing education is more likely to be located. Today's public demands education that is convenient and flexible. Moreover, in the face of busy lives, the ability to access education from home is appealing. Developments in the kind of available distance-education modalities have expanded the options and increased the quality of communication that is now possible with students who prefer to obtain degrees from their living rooms.

Faculty and student roles will change as the means of communication between the faculty and students takes different forms. This can also be said about nursing practice as technology is further incorporated into the healthcare system. Although computer skills and knowledge will be important in the 21st century, interpersonal relations that rely on basic language and communication skills will remain significant in the provision of nursing care. Relationships with patients and their families can be facilitated through technologic advances, because it is the way nurses enact their knowing with patients that defines the practice. Technology facilitates and alters this but does not replace nursing knowledge about the work with patients.

Whatever technologic innovations emerge in the future, nursing must remember that technology offers the profession tools to use in its mandate to provide care to individuals and their families in illness and in health promotion. Technology is a means toward the goal of health and quality patient care. Thoughtful development and use can serve nursing and recipients of care well.

S U M M A R Y

Nursing informatics—the integration of information technologies and communications into nursing practice—has a profound effect on nurses and the organizations where they work. The relationship between technology and nursing is evolving and, literally, at a crossroads. The advent of nursing informatics presents challenges and opportunities. CNA recognizes that technology can improve healthcare, but technology without education and support may also negatively affect clients, families, healthcare professionals, and the health system in untoward ways.

Some applications of nursing informatics are telehealth (the use of advanced telecommunications technologies to exchange health information and provide healthcare from vast distances), videoconferencing, remote monitoring, and electronic health records.

Challenges associated with technology include "short-shifting," as real-time demands replace patient care with a litany of technical tasks and a focus on outcomes (evidence), performance measurement, and technical expertise that calls for acquiring related knowledge and competence in information technology.

Applied informatics will require nurses to adhere to standards of practice, codes of ethics, provincial legislation, and competencies established by regulatory bodies. To this end, nurses will need to develop or follow telephone standards of practice, policies on providing telehealth across provinces, educational standards and credentials, provisions for maintaining privacy and confidentiality, protocols to guide decision making and judgment, and advice on professional liability issues and employer responsibilities.

Additional challenges to nursing practice are the geographic invisibility of the client and liability for care practices—potential malpractice or misdiagnoses—delivered by distance or electronic technology. On the other hand, changes influenced by informatics will be incorporated into the healthcare system, offering nurses tools to use in promoting health and caring for the sick.

Benefits to practice include greater client involvement in health-seeking behaviors and health choices, possibly because electronic communication is perceived to offer privacy, immediacy, breadth of information, and different perspectives.

Additional benefits apply particularly to education. One of the benefits of Web-based, online instruction is increased access by students who live in remote locations. Information previously disseminated in classrooms and in textbooks and other print media is now available to students and faculty in remote locations at nontraditional times. The benefits are obvious, as are the challenges prompted by change. The faculty must clearly articulate the need for information technology in nursing curricula to ensure that all nurses have the skills needed to practice effectively. The faculty must acquire technical skills and adjust to altered roles as collaborators, facilitators, and guides of learning. Technology is fundamental to ensuring that nursing remains at the forefront of healthcare and continues to contribute to its natural evolution.

Add to your knowledge of this issue:		
Informatics Association	**www.cnia.ca**	*Online*
Canada's Health Information Informatics Association	**www.coachorg.com**	

R E F L E C T I O N S *on the Chapter...*

1 From your experience, consider the application of technology and informatics in your practice.

2 How would you describe the relationships among technology, informatics, and nursing practice in these examples?

3 Identify issues related to the use of technology in your practice or in practice situations you have observed.

4 What strategies have you used or observed being used to overcome barriers to the use of technology and informatics in practice?

5 What barriers have you experienced in using technology in your nursing studies?

6 What strategies have you used or could you use to overcome these barriers?

Want to know more? Visit thePoint for additional helpful resources:

- Journal Articles
- Learning Objectives
- Nursing Professional Roles and Responsibilities
- Bonus chapters:
  ◦ Health and Nursing Policy: A Matter of Politics, Power and Professionalism
  ◦ The NP Movement: Recurring Issues
  ◦ When Difference Matters: The Politics of Privilege and Marginality

References

Aboriginal Nurses Association of Canada. (2001). *Impact of technology on Aboriginal nursing: A discussion paper.* Retrieved from http://www.anac.on.ca/web/techinfo.html

Alberta Telehealth. (2007). *Telehealth services: Clinical telehealth services.* Retrieved from http://albertatelehealth.com/content.asp?category_id=5&root_id=2

Allen, S. (2007). Benefits of electronic health records to renal nurse practitioner care. *The CANNT Journal, 17*(3), 44.

Bates, A.W., & Poole, G. (2003). *Effective teaching with technology in higher education: Foundations for success.* San Francisco, CA: Jossey-Bass.

Bischoff, W.R., & Kelley, S.J. (1999). 21st century house call: The Internet and the World Wide Web. *Holistic Nursing Practice, 13*(4), 42–50.

Booth, R.G. (2006). Educating the future e-health professional nurse. *International Journal of Nursing Education Scholarship, 3*(1), 1–10. doi: 10.2202/1548-923X.1187

Canada Health Infoway. (2009). *Business plan.* Retrieved September 7 from www.infoway-inforoute.ca/BusinessPlan-2008-2009-en-final-1.pdf

Canadian Association of Schools of Nursing. (2006). *CASN position statement on baccalaureate education and baccalaureate programs.* Retrieved from http://www.casn.ca/content.php?doc=33

Canadian Institute for Health Information. (2009). *Workforce trends of registered nurses in Canada, 2009.* Retrieved from http://www.cihi.ca/CIHI-extortal/internet/en/document/spending+and+health+workforce/workforce/nurses/stats_nursing_2009

Canadian Nurses Association. (2000). Telehealth: Great potential or risky terrain? *Nursing Now: Issues and Trends in Canadian Nursing, 9,* 1–4. Retrieved from http://www.can-Nurses.ca/CNA/documents/pdf/publications/Telehealth_November2000_e.pdf

———. (2002). Demystifying the electronic health record. *Nursing Now: Issues and Trends in Canadian Nursing, 13,* 1–4. Retrieved from http://www.cna-nurses.ca/CNA/documents/pdf/publications/Demystifyinghealthrecord_April2002_e.pdf

———. (2007). *Position statement: Telehealth: The role of the nurse.* Retrieved from http://www.cna-nurses.ca/cna/documents/pdf/publications/ps89_telehealth_e.pdf

———. (2006). *Position statement: Nursing information and knowledge management.* Retrieved from http://www.cna-nurses.ca/CNA/documents/pdf/publications/PS87-Nursing-info-knowledge-e.pdf

Care, W.D., Gregory, D.M., Russell, C., & Hultin, D. (2006). Aboriginal students and faculty experiences with distance education. In R. Riewe & J. Oakes (Eds.), *Aboriginal connections to race, environment, and traditions* (pp. 101–109). Winnipeg, MB, University of Manitoba: Aboriginal Issues Press.

Care, W.D., Russell, C.K., Hartig, P., Murrell, V., & Gregory, D.M. (2007). Challenges, issues, and barriers to student-centered approaches in distance education. In L.E. Young & B.L. Paterson (Eds.), *Teaching nursing: Developing a student-centered learning environment* (pp. 484–502). Philadelphia, PA: Lippincott Williams & Wilkins.

Clarke, H., & Nagle, L. (2003). *OHIH research project: 2002–2003—Final report.* Retrieved from http://www.cnia.ca/OHIHfinaltoc.htm

College of Nurses of Ontario. (2005). *Practice guideline: Telepractice.* Retrieved from http://www.cno.org/docs/prac/41041_telephone.pdf

Collins, D.E., & Tilson, E.R. (2001). A new generation on the horizon. *Radiological Technology, 73,* 172–177.

Cooper, M.C., & Powell, E. (1998). Technology and care in a bone marrow transplant unit: Creating and assuaging vulnerability. *Holistic Nursing Practice, 12*(4), 57–68.

Doran, D.M., Mylopoulos, J., Kushniruk, A., et al. (2007). Evidence in the palm of your hand: Development of an outcomes-focused knowledge translation intervention. *Worldviews on Evidence-Based Nursing, Second Quarter,* 69–77. doi: 10.1111/j.1741-6787.2007.00084.x

Ehnfors, M., & Grobe, S.J. (2004). Nursing curriculum and continuing education: Future directions. *International Journal of Medical Informatics, 73,* 591–598. doi: 10.1016/j.ijmedinf.2004.04.005

Gadow, S. (1988). Covenant without cure: Letting go and holding on in chronic illness. In J. Watson & M. Ray (Eds.), *The ethics of care and the ethics of cure* (pp. 5–14). New York: National League for Nursing.

Garrison, D.R., & Vaughn, N.D. (2008). *Blended learning in higher education: Framework, principles, and guidelines.* San Francisco, CA: Jossey-Bass.

Gassert, C.A. (1998). The challenge of meeting patients' needs with a national nursing informatics agenda. *Journal of American Medical Informatics Association, 5*(3), 263–268.

Gassert, C.A. (2000). Telehealth and nursing. In B. Carty (Ed.), *Nursing informatics: Education for practice* (pp. 232–251). New York: Springer.

Goodwin, S. (2007). Telephone nursing: An emerging practice area. *Nursing Leadership, 20*(4), 37–45.

Graves, J.R., & Corcoran-Perry, S. (1996). The study of nursing informatics. *Holistic Nursing Practice, 11*(1), 15–24.

Halstead, J.A., & Billings, D.M. (2005). Teaching and learning in online learning communities. In D.M. Billings & J.A. Halstead (Eds), *Teaching in nursing: A guide for faculty* (pp. 423–439). St. Louis, MO: Elsevier Sanders.

Harder, B.N. (2010). Use of simulation in teaching and learning in health sciences: A systematic review. *Journal of Nursing Education, 49*(1), 23–28. doi: 10.3928/01484834-20090828-08

Health Canada. (2007). *eHealth.* Retrieved from http://www.hc-sc.gc.ca/hcs-sss/ehealth-esante/index_
e.html

Hessler, K., & Ritchie, H. (2006). Recruitment and retention of novice faculty. *Journal of Nursing Education,
45*(5), 150–154.

Jukes, I. (2005). *Understanding digital kids (DKs): Teaching & learning in the new digital landscape.*
Retrieved from http://www.ldcsb.on.ca/schools/cfe/internet_safety/documents/understanding%
20digital%20kids.pdf

Koeniger-Donohue, R. (2008). Handheld computers in nursing education: A PDA pilot project. *Journal of
Nursing Education, 47*(2), 74–77.

Lasater, K. (2007). High-fidelity simulation and clinical judgment: Students' experiences. *Journal of
Nursing Education, 46*(6), 269–276.

Link, D.G., & Scholtz, S.M. (2000). Educational technology and the faculty role: What you don't know
can hurt you. *Nurse Educator, 25*(6), 274–276.

Loiselle, C., & Cossette, S. (2007). Health information technology and nursing care. [Guest Editorial].
Canadian Journal of Nursing Research, 39(1), 11–14.

Mallow, G.E., & Gilje, F. (1999). Technology-based nursing education: Overview and call for further
dialogue. *Journal of Nursing Education, 38*(6), 248–251.

Manitoba Telehealth. (2007). *MBTelehealth innovation: Current project highlights.* Retrieved from
http://www.mbtelehealth.ca/innovation_research.php

Martin, R. (2007). Making a case for personal digital assistant use in baccalaureate nursing education.
Online Journal of Nursing Informatics (OJNI), 11(2) [Online]. Retrieved from http://eaa-knowledge.
com/ojni/ni/11_2/martin.htm

Mathieu, L. (2007). Nursing informatics: Developing knowledge for nursing practice. *Canadian Journal
of Nursing Research, 39*(1), 15–19.

Moore, M.G., & Kearsley, G. (1996). *Distance education: A systems view.* Belmont, CA: Wadsworth.

Nagle, L. (2007). Everything I know about informatics, I didn't learn in nursing school. *Canadian Journal
of Nursing Leadership, 20*(3), 22–25.

Office of Health and the Information Highway, Health Canada. (2001). *Toward electronic health records.*
Retrieved from http://www.hc-sc.gc.ca/hcs-sss/pubs/ehealth-esante/2001-towards-vers-ehr-dse/
index-eng.php

Petrovskaya, O., McIntyre, M., & McDonald, C. (2009). Dilemmas, tetralemmas, reimagining the
electronic health record. *Advances in Nursing Science, 32*(3), 241–251. doi: 10.1097ANS.
0b013e3181b1056e

Purnell, M. (1998). Who really makes the bed? Uncovering technologic dissonance in nursing. *Holistic
Nursing Practice, 12*(4), 12–22.

Rasid, M.F.A., & Woodward, B. (2005) Bluetooth telemedicine processor for multichannel biomedical
signal transmission via mobile cellular networks. *IEEE Transactions on Information Technology in
Biomedicine, 9*(1), 35–43. doi: 10.1109/TITB.2004.840070

Riva, G. (2000). From telehealth to e-health: Internet and distributed virtual reality in health care. *Cyber-
psychology & Behavior, 3*(6), 989–998. doi: 10.1089/109493100452255

Russo, H. (2001). Window of opportunity for home care nurses: Telehealth technologies. *Online Journal
of Issues in Nursing, 6*(3). Retrieved from http://www.nursingworld.org/ojin/topic16/tpc16_4.htm

Sandelowski, M. (2000). Thermometers and telephones: A century of nursing and technology. *American
Journal of Nursing, 100*(10), 82–85.

Schoening, A.M., Sittner, B.J., & Todd, M.J. (2006). Simulated learning experience: Nursing students'
perceptions and the educators' role. *Nurse Educator, 31*(6), 253–258.

Simpson, R.L. (1998). A few points about point-of-care technology. *Nursing Management, 29*(11),
19–22.

Smith, C.E., Young-Cureton, V., Hooper, C., & Deamer, P. (1998). A survey of computer technology utilization in school nursing. *Journal of School Nursing, 14*(2), 27–34.

Staggers, N., & Bagley Thompson, C. (2002). The evolution of definitions for nursing informatics: A critical
analysis and revised definition. *Journal of the American Medical Informatics Association, 9*(3), 255–262.
doi: 10.1197/jamia.M0946

Stevens, J., & Crouch, M. (1998). Frankenstein's nurse! What are schools of nursing creating? *Collegian,
5*(1), 10–15.

VandeVusse, L., & Hanson, L. (2000). Evaluation of online course discussions: Faculty facilitation of active student learning. *Computers in Nursing, 18*(4), 181–188.

White, M.H., & Dorman, S.M. (2000). Online support for caregivers: Analysis of an Internet Alzheimer mailgroup. *Computers in Nursing, 18*(4), 168–179.

Young, L.E., & Maxwell, B. (2007). Student-centered teaching in nursing: From rote to active learning. In L.E. Young & B.L. Paterson (Eds.), *Teaching nursing: Developing a student-centered learning environment* (pp. 3–25). Philadelphia, PA: Lippincott Williams & Wilkins.

14

Changing Picture: From "Medical Rounds" to Interprofessional Practice

Olga Petrovskaya

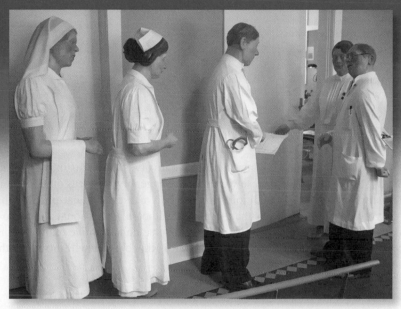

Medical (and nursing) rounds: Waxwork model. Museum of Nursing History, Kolding, Denmark. A former tuberculosis sanatorium for children, est. 1911. (Photograph by O. Petrovskaya.)

Critical Questions

As a way of engaging with the ideas in this chapter, consider the following:

1. From your observations as a nursing student in a hospital or community healthcare agency, how would you describe the relations among the healthcare professionals with whom you work?

2. Think of a situation that you identify as an example of effective collaboration among various health providers (including different groups of nurses such as NPs, RNs, and LPNs).

What made this collaboration effective? Who defines what *effective* means?

3. What personal qualities (e.g., knowledge, skills, and attitudes) and organizational factors are required to make collaborative work effective?

4. What challenges do you think can arise in interprofessional practice (IPP)?

Chapter Objectives

After completing this chapter, you will be able to:

1. Explain the expressions *inter-* and *intraprofessional healthcare practice, interdisciplinary research,* and *interprofessional education (IPE).*

2. Identify micro-, meso-, and macro-factors required for successful collaborative work in healthcare.

(continued on page 260)

Chapter Objectives (continued)

3. Articulate social, political, and economic aspects of interprofessional healthcare as well as historical changes that influence contemporary relations among various health providers.

4. Identify some of the international, national, and provincial documents (i.e., reports, legislations, and professional colleges' regulations) that shape interprofessional work.

5. Discuss moral dilemmas and issues of accountability arising from working with unregulated care providers.

6. Envision possibilities existing amidst the complexities and challenges of interprofessional work.

INTRODUCTION

Any discussion of contemporary nursing practice involves the terms interprofessional and interdisciplinary. Some authors use these words interchangeably, whereas other authors prefer to distinguish between the two. In addition, it is not only nurses' clinical practice that increasingly involves working alongside other-than-nursing healthcare professionals, but also nurses' education and research activities are taking place in diverse collaborative teams. Using a framework for analysis presented at the beginning of the book, this chapter will introduce the reader to the terminology of and issues related to IPP.

SIGNIFICANCE FOR NURSES AND FOR THE PROFESSION

The necessity for nurses to be aware of issues in IPP can be illustrated by two straightforward observations: Contemporary nursing practice happens in collaboration with other professionals and the topic of interprofessional collaboration has attracted the attention of Canadian policy makers on all levels of the healthcare arena as well as professional organizations, as reflected in several documents guiding the practice of nurses.

Who Do Nurses Work with?

Nurses work in collaboration with other people. In large urban healthcare settings, such as teaching hospitals or community care centers, collaborative teams may involve more than a dozen members, whereas in remote settings a nurse–client dyad and sometimes a few other providers may work together. Thus, IPP can be carried out by well-defined teams of individuals who work in close proximity. In contrast, IPP can also occur when geographically dispersed professionals work on the same patient case attending to different aspects of it asynchronously. This latter example of IPP goes beyond traditional team work to include a multilevel integration of services within complex healthcare systems.

Nursing practice involves interaction with regulated and unregulated health providers as well as informal caregivers and patients. As the term suggests, *regulated* health and social care providers are those whose practice is regulated by their respective provincial or territorial professional colleges, such as College of Nurses of Ontario or Physiotherapy Alberta College or College of Registered Psychiatric Nurses of British Columbia. Regulated health professions and their titles vary across Canadian jurisdictions. For example, in the province of Ontario, 23 self-regulated health professions include chiropractors, dental hygienists, dieticians, massage therapists, medical laboratory technologists, medical radiation technologists, midwives, nurses, occupational therapists, optometrists, pharmacists, physicians and surgeons, physiotherapists, psychologists, respiratory therapists, and speech–language pathologists (see the online resources box at the end of the chapter for the link to the OMHLTC website). As regulated professionals, Canadian nurses make up a heterogeneous group comprised, variably in different jurisdictions, of registered nurses (RNs), licensed practical nurses (LPNs; or registered practical nurses in Ontario), registered psychiatric nurses (RPNs), and nurse practitioners (NPs).

In contrast, *unregulated* health worker is an "umbrella term used to describe care providers or assistant personnel who provide some form of health service and who are not licensed or regulated by a professional or regulatory body" (CNA, 2009, p. 1). Personal support workers and care aides are examples of unregulated providers working alongside nurses in many settings. Collaboration in professional nursing practice also involves patients, patient families, and significant others. Ideally, healthcare collaborative practice not only regards the patient, or a service user, as a nominal figure on the team, but the provision of care is actually structured around the needs of this individual. The analysis in this chapter, however, will suggest that, despite the rhetoric of patient-centeredness, specific mechanisms ensuring that the patient's needs are given priority appear to be marginalized whereas other priorities take precedence in the climate of austerity characteristic of many aspects of today's health and social care provision.

Interprofessional Practice in National and Provincial Nursing Documents

With an increasing impetus on interprofessional collaboration observed in the healthcare sector across the country over the last 2 decades, the Canadian Nurses Association (CNA) engaged in a pan-Canadian committee called *EICP: Enhancing Interdisciplinary Collaboration in Primary Health Care*. The work of this committee "focused on how to create the conditions for health professionals to work together in the most effective and efficient way so that they can produce the best health outcomes for individuals and their families" (EICP, 2006, p. 1). Subsequently, based on the EICP report, the CNA issued a Position Statement (CNA, n.d.) titled *Interprofessional Collaboration* outlining principles of effective collaboration and structural support factors required to sustain collaboration among health professions and professionals.

Another national document, the *Code of Ethics for Registered Nurses* (CNA, 2008), stipulates that nurses have a responsibility to uphold ethical values when working with members of a healthcare team, where team is defined as "a number of healthcare providers from different disciplines (often including both regulated professionals and unregulated workers) working together to provide care for and with individuals, families, groups, populations, and communities" (p. 25).

Guidelines and standards of practice developed by provincial and territorial nursing regulatory bodies also reflect the importance of effective collaboration. For example, the College of Nurses of Ontario (CNO, 2002) professional standard *Relationships: Professional Relationships* outlines an expectation of each nurse to establish and maintain collegial relationships based on trust and respect with all members of healthcare team; to demonstrate an understanding of roles of other team members; to share knowledge appropriately; and to use communication, interpersonal, and conflict-resolution skills. In addition, beginning in the year 2011, the CNO annual Quality Assurance, or continuing competence, program includes a component on interprofessional care, requiring each nurse to reflect on this aspect of their practice (CNO, 2010).

SITUATING THE TOPIC AND FRAMING THE ISSUE

A Brief Note on Terminology

Even a brief review of the literature on the topic under discussion reveals a multiplicity of terms used to refer to what appears to be synonymous with *IPP:* Interprofessional collaboration, interdisciplinary or multidisciplinary practice, healthcare team work, or simply collaborative practice. In the United Kingdom, for example, a phrase *interprofessional working* is common (Pollard et al., 2010). In Canada, although many of the listed expressions, such as *collaborative practice,* have been in use for at least 2 decades, and still seem to be relevant, a preference in the official discourses of governments and professional regulatory colleges has clearly shifted, replacing *collaborative* with *interprofessional.* (Later in the analysis I will return to the significance of this shift.) As you read the chapter you may want to consider whether a change in language is simply a preference and caprice, or whether this linguistic shift both reflects and brings about other changes—in how people think and practice.

Box 14.1 explains terminology widely used in nursing. So far, the discussion in this chapter concerns IPP. However, health professionals collaborate not only for the purpose of providing direct services to patients, but also for the purpose of conducting research. Even when research is carried out in hospitals or community and involves clinical practitioners, research is usually associated with academic departments at universities (i.e., academic disciplines); hence the expression *interdisciplinary research.* Studying complex problems requires bringing together multiple perspectives, and interdisciplinary research has a potential to accomplish this goal. Another, newer term that usually refers to research and academic programs, is *transdisciplinarity.* This term is often explained as a collaboration that collapses disciplinary boundaries for the purpose of creating unified knowledge and generating new insights for an increasingly complex world. A growing body of literature suggests that professionals can be prepared for a process of interprofessional and interdisciplinary collaboration. *Interprofessional* or *interdisciplinary education* is proposed as an effective strategy to help students in health disciplines as well as practicing professionals to understand the roles and values of various healthcare team members and to be able to communicate and work collaboratively (Barnsteiner et al., 2007; Bilodeau et al., 2010; Mann et al., 2009; Takahashi et al., 2010).

BOX 14.1   Terminology at a Glance

● **Multiprofessional/Multidisciplinary** (from Latin *multus* much, many): People from different disciplines or professions are involved but this may or may not imply collaboration (adapted from Goodman & Clemow, 2008, p. 13).

● **Interprofessional/Interdisciplinary** (from Latin *inter* between, among): Professionals *collaborating* to work together more effectively to improve the quality of patient care (adapted from Goodman & Clemow, 2008, p. 13). Emphasizes professionals; may or may not include patients/ clients and unregulated providers.

● **Intraprofessional** (prefix *intra-* from Latin *intra* within, inside): Collaboration among various groups within one profession (e.g., NPs, RNs, and LPNs working together).

● **Collaboration:** Working together with one or more members of the healthcare team who each make a unique contribution to achieving a common goal. Each individual contributes from within the limits of her/his scope of practice (CNO, 2008). More inclusive; implies involvement of patients/clients and unregulated providers.

Interprofessional Education

A definition of IPE widely adopted in Canada was proposed by the UK-based Centre for the Advancement of Interprofessional Education (see the online resources box for the link to the CAIPE website). This definition states that IPE consists of two or more professionals from different disciplines learning with, about, and from each other. It is acknowledged that no single discipline or profession can address health and social care needs of patients/clients with complex conditions; therefore, a team approach where "a right professional provides right service at the right time" is recognized as a suitable model for healthcare delivery. Proponents of IPE state that it is no longer enough to narrowly educate specialists in their respective disciplines and then to expect that they will be able to practice collaboratively. The culture of "silos-education," write D'Amour and Oandasan (2005), needs to shift toward IPE. In a process of IPE beginning early in learners' educational programs, students from various health disciplines learn together and have collaborative practicum placements. With the adequate support from educational institutions and healthcare agencies, and appropriate guidance from their mentors, students are expected to develop an understanding of each profession's unique contribution to the team, acquire interpersonal skills, build collegial relations, and appreciate how the model of patient-centered interprofessional collaboration can meet the goals of quality care, positive patient outcomes, effective service provision, and efficient resource utilization (Barnsteiner et al., 2007; Bilodeau et al., 2010; Mann et al. 2009; Takahashi et al., 2010).

A number of initiatives in IPE were established in Canada in the last decade. A few examples follow (see the online resources box for the links):

- The Canadian Interprofessional Health Collaborative (CIHC)/Consortium pancanadien pour l'interprofessionnalisme en santé (CPIS)
  This national organization, funded by Health Canada, offers health providers, teams and organizations, and the resources and tools needed to apply an interprofessional, patient-centered, and collaborative approach to healthcare.
- Interprofessional Education for Collaborative Patient-Centred Practice (IECPCP)
  This multi-year initiative, funded by Health Canada, supports the development and implementation of various facets of IPE for collaborative patient-centered practice across all health sectors in Canada.
- The University of Manitoba Interprofessional Education Initiative (UofM IPE Initiative)
  This initiative creates collaborative opportunities for the health science students, including nursing. The Faculty of Nursing at the UofM incorporates interprofessional learning opportunities into its undergraduate program. For instance, a partnership among the Faculty of Nursing, the UofM IPE Initiative, and the Winnipeg Regional Health Authority enables the simultaneous clinical practicum placements of students from different health professions at the hospital and community settings (Ateah, 2011).
- The McGill Educational Initiative on Interprofessional Collaboration: Partnerships for Patient and Family-Centered Practice
  This initiative, funded by Health Canada, began in 2005 with the purpose of developing IPE and IPP. The schools of Medicine, Nursing, Physical and Occupational Therapy, and Educational Psychology are involved in this project between McGill University, the McGill University Health Centre, and the Sir Mortimer B. Davis-Jewish General Hospital.

Why Become Interprofessional?

A growing attention to IPP and IPE in health and social care in Canada, the United Kingdom, and other countries in recent years can be attributed to a number of factors and influences (Castro & Julia, 1994; Goodman & Clemow, 2008; Pollard et al., 2010). At the systemic and organizational level, IPP is seen as compatible with, and a vehicle for, the redesign of healthcare that seeks to utilize providers to a maximum of their capacity, eliminate duplication in services, enhance public access to services, and generate the best value for the cost (Buchda, 2008; Kearney-Nunnery, 2008; Pollard et al., 2010). The governments' goal of healthcare efficiency seems to be related to their attempts to regulate, through legislation, certain aspects of (self-) regulated health professions, which have multiplied significantly over the last decades (Field, 2011; King, n.d.; Lahey, 2011). Thus, professional regulatory colleges were asked by the governments to identify ways of possible collaboration among colleges and professionals, specifically to identify ways of streamlining some of the requirements for practice among health professions (CNO, 2008). Pointing to the difficulties with streamlining, professional colleges nevertheless actively promote the idea of interprofessional care among its practitioners through guidelines and a yearly Quality Assurance program (CNO, 2010).

On the other hand, at the level of individual healthcare organizations and community and social care services and across these sectors, concerns have been expressed about fragmentation of services. This fragmentation is seen as a result of the increased complexity of patients' conditions and a growing number of specialists required to attend to each complex case. Negative effects of such fragmentation transpire in the form of miscommunication, medication errors, client and provider dissatisfaction, and legal lawsuits in some instances. Motivated by a desire to avoid these negative consequences, organizations encourage collaborative team work among various providers.

Moreover, individual providers, or groups such as nurses on hospital units, appreciate the experience of truly effective collaboration. When a team of professionals works cohesively, considers the client's perspective, and builds satisfactory relations with unregulated staff, everyone benefits. Notions of quality care and positive patient outcome come alive in such examples. This ideal picture, however, might not be easily attainable. As will be discussed, issues arise in IPP. Some of these issues pertain to the assumption of "the common goal" made about IPP as reflected in the above discussion, specifically, that multiple stakeholders have their differing interests aligned in IPP (Pollard, 2010). A question that can be raised at this point, and which casts doubts on the optimistic tone of many commentators on IPP, is whether it is possible to satisfy all stakeholders' interests through IPP as if the needs and goals of the governments, professional regulatory colleges, healthcare organizations, individual providers, and patients were all aligned.

Interprofessional Practice: Principles and Factors for Successful Collaboration

Principles of successful IPP identified in the literature are drawn from both observations of well-functioning collaborative teams and reflections on and imaginings of possibilities of collaborative work in health and social care. These principles include: Understanding of one's own professional role, knowledge of the roles of other health professionals, effective communication, respectful and trusting relationships, goal of patient care at the center of team efforts, effective leadership on all levels, and organizational support for collaborative work (MacDonald et al., 2010; Orchard, 2010; Pollard & Harris, 2010).

These principles lead to a consideration of so-called micro-, meso-, and macro-factors contributing to IPP. Among micro-, or personal level, factors are knowledge, skills, and attitudes required from health providers for team work. Meso-factors may include the context and environment of health team's work such as geographical proximity of providers or organizational leadership. Finally, macro-level factors encompass, among other, healthcare system's priorities and governments' and professions' regulations.

There is general agreement in the reviewed literature that nurses (and other health professionals for that matter) should have a good knowledge of their professional role as stipulated by the scope of practice, professional standards, and expectations of a particular job.

Understanding one's profession, however, usually presupposes more than the practitioner's ability to perform specific skills and articulate practitioner's technical role (or controlled acts, as the Ontario *Nursing Act, 1991* calls it). This requirement to understand one's profession is typically thought of as including values of a profession, its philosophy, its preferred conceptual frames of reference, its specific modes of thought and action—in short, its *culture*. Introduction into the culture of the profession begins early in learner's educational experience, and is called a process of *socialization*. An outcome of this process is a formation of professional *identity*. This discussion uses concepts drawn from sociological analyses of professions (Miers, 2010a, 2010b; Pollard, 2010). If you reflect on your educational experiences in your nursing program, you will identify implicit or explicit instances of your socialization into the nursing profession and shaping of your identity as a nurse. As further analysis in this chapter will show, strong professional identity, paradoxically, can be both an asset and a deterrent for IPP.

Apart from understanding one's own professional responsibilities and obligations and performing one's role as a nurse, it is certainly a requirement for IPP to understand other team members' roles and contributions to the team, both unique and shared. Such knowledge eliminates duplication of services, utilizes each provider appropriately, contributes to seamless integration of services, better meets patient's/client's needs, and in some cases allows fewer providers to be involved in each client's case.

Clearly, to just *know* the roles of all team members is not sufficient; communication and interpersonal skills as well as particular attitudes are required for collaboration to thrive. In general, nursing undergraduate education across Canada prepares nurses well in this regard: Many course assignments promote collaborative group work, and practice experiences encourage effective communication with mentors, patients, and colleagues. Ability to advocate, negotiate, ask for assistance, question, challenge, and resolve conflicts are other desirable qualities for health professionals. Some examples follow: In situations of overlapping scopes of practice, team members negotiate their areas of responsibilities. When doubts arise about correctness of information, for instance, the doctor's order, a nurse is expected to clarify and, if needed, challenge the order. Considering that IPP sometimes involves practitioners located in different geographical locations, this might be not an easy endeavor—the doctor who wrote an order can be located in another hospital and contacting him or her may take additional time and effort (Duck, 2010). Further, it is a mistake to think that team work is always smooth sailing and that conflict should be avoided at all cost (Thomas, 2010). On the contrary, understanding the inevitability of conflict might serve team members well. Thus, assertiveness and the ability to disagree, along with skills to resolve conflict, are necessary for nurses and other health professionals. Sellman (2010) delineates three conditions for successful IPP: *Willingness* of providers to engage in team work, mutual trust and respect among them, and effective leadership. These conditions presuppose such personal qualities as being humble in recognizing one's own limitations in knowledge and skills, being open to peer's constructive feedback, willing to learn from others and to reconsider stereotypes one possibly holds of other professions, and being respectful of all people on the team and their diverse perspectives (Sellman, 2010).

It is useful for nurses to realize that not all health professionals are socialized into values of collaborative relations. Traditionally, medical education and on-the-job socialization emphasized the hierarchical nature of relationships among providers working alongside each other with physicians placed at the top of hierarchy (Miers, 2010a). Although this situation is changing, nurses might still encounter a "top-down chain of command" approach. Nurses, however, are usually well equipped to challenge and even transform such practices. What might also be important is that nurses pay attention to their own style of relations with other nurses (i.e., intraprofessional practice) and unregulated staff.

This section of the chapter sought to situate the topic of IPP by highlighting the most common themes elaborated in nursing and other literature. Concluding this section is a consideration of the role that patient/client/service user plays in IPP. You might have noticed in a process of your nursing education that the majority of published sources such as government documents, professional colleges' standards, and journal articles on the topic of IPP seem to unanimously emphasize the importance of the patient, around whose needs health and social services are supposedly structured. This rhetoric notwithstanding, a few analysts are more skeptical about such claims (Pollard, 2010). At the very least, in a situation of competing interests and agendas in the healthcare system, in order to benefit patients, health professionals need to make an effort to keep patient's priorities visible. Even the shift in terminology, which I mentioned earlier, is worth noticing. A phrase *collaborative practice* (Gottlieb & Feeley, 2005), which was more inclusive, is replaced by *IPP,* which signals a focus on professions and professionals as opposed to patients/clients (Payne, 2000, as cited in Thomas, 2010). In addition, Gask (2005) writes that phrases *seamless care* and *holistic approach,* often used as descriptors of IPP, gloss over complexities of and issues in interprofessional health work. It is to a more detailed analysis of some of the issues that we now turn.

(FURTHER) ANALYZING THE ISSUE

Historical Analysis

Until relatively recently, a context of nursing practice involved few groups of providers and was markedly hierarchical: From physicians to head nurses to nurses with some preparation to nurses with less preparation to care aides. This structure, however long-lasting and strong in some respects, has undoubtedly changed (Goodman & Clemow, 2008). Horizontal relationships, in which nurses engage in current practice, involve a multiplicity of providers and range from working in close proximity but independently, that is, side-by-side, or interdependently, with various degrees of integration that span even geographical distances.

Medicine–nursing Relations Reconsidered

Throughout the 20th century, and more intensely in the second half, the dominance of the medical profession in the healthcare arena has been continuously challenged (King, n.d.; Lahey, 2011; Miers, 2010a, 2010b). Arguably, five main forces can be recognized as contributing to lessening the traditional power of physicians in society in general: Emergence and growth of other health professions; women's rights movements as subverting the traditional dynamic of male physician/female nurse hierarchy; patient rights movements; government's current, growing involvements in re-regulation of certain domains considered a purview of self-regulated professions; and increasing alignment of healthcare provision with methods and strategies of industrial efficiency attained through new forms of management. The latter process is referred to as managerialism (Traynor, 1999) whereby managers, not physicians or other healthcare providers, exercise ultimate, albeit indirect, control over practice matters. However abstract these factors or forces may seem for a nurse in clinical practice, they all play out tangibly in how IPP unfolds on the ground level of provider–patient and provider–provider relationships. These historical forces and occurrences and the ways in which nurses encounter them in interprofessional work will be further discussed in the remaining sections of the chapter. Considering these historical forces, what can be said with certainty is that the picture of nursing practice is changing: Nurses' relations among themselves, with the patients, as well as with other health professionals are shifting. You can instantly identify some of the more visible shifts by reflecting on your practicum placements and on how "patient rounds," or case meetings, look now (e.g., who is involved, how participants behave, and so on) and comparing this picture with a photograph at the opening of the chapter that depicts medical (and nursing) rounds from a century ago.

From "Intersectoral Cooperation" to "Interprofessional Integration"

A 1978 WHO report outlining a new approach to healthcare delivery, namely Primary Health Care, was one of the first international reports widely embraced by the Canadian nursing and interpreted as emphasizing the importance of interdisciplinary collaboration for the provision of health and social services (Calnan & Lemire Rodger, 2002; CNA, 2005). Specifically, one of the five principles of Primary Health Care, namely intersectoral cooperation, was interpreted broadly in the following way: "Health and well-being are linked to both economic and social policy. Intersectoral means experts in the health sector working with experts in education, housing, employment, immigration, etc. It also means health professionals from various disciplines collaborate and function interdependently to meet the needs of Canadians" (Calnan & Lemire Rodger, 2002, p. 3).

In the wake of healthcare reforms called for by the federal government and elaborated upon, for example, in the 2002 Kirby Commission report, the CNA (2005) supported the vision of reforms as emphasizing the role of interdisciplinary teams.

Nurses are addressing the challenge of working more effectively as members of multidisciplinary primary care [PC] teams…PC teams, which include family physicians, nurses, and other health professionals working side-by-side as partners, produce better health outcomes, improved access to services, more efficient use of resources, and greater satisfaction for both patients and providers (p. 2).

The notion of simply working *side-by-side,* however, seems to be challenged most by the notion of IPP. Specifically, IPP emphasizes *integration* of services and skills, promotes blending of professions to the point of their interchangeability whereby fewer providers, and (in some instances) with less preparation, are proposed to be involved in each patient's case. An often unarticulated expectation of healthcare providers with such *integration* is to cross- and multi-task. At the level of discussions, integration of services in IPP has much appeal: It is profiled as advantageous both for patients in terms of greater continuity of and access to care and for providers as promising to free up their time currently spent on unnecessary duplication of or performance of un-skilled procedures. No doubt, this prospect is difficult to argue against. What remains to be seen, however, is how the rhetoric of service integration with blending of professionals' skills will unfold on the ground level and what implications such blending will have for individual health professions and patients.

Critical Feminist Analysis

A feminist critique is inevitably bound to recognize a gendered nature of nursing. A legacy of lasting and, until recently, deeply entrenched tradition of a male physician/female nurse hierarchy can still be observed in practice (Pollard, 2010). Several authors who write about how gender hierarchy plays out in nursing practice cite an observation that the psychiatrist Leonard Stein initially made in the 1960s of the "nurse–doctor game" (Stein, 1967). He argued that because of the subordinate status of nurses and women in general, nurses could not openly challenge the authority of the physician, but instead indirectly influenced his decisions through a form of communication that maintained the impression that it was the physician himself who made that decision. Two decades later, Stein et al. (1990) documented a change that they observed in relationships between nurses and physicians. No longer playing the "game," nurses acted assertively in situations of disagreement with physicians and other members of the healthcare team. There is evidence to suggest that relationships among nurses, physicians, and other health professionals are indeed more collegial and egalitarian (Goodman & Clemow, 2008). In some situations, medical residents are encouraged by their mentors to recognize nurses' expertise and consult nurses on patient-related matters.

As a description of the framework for analysis in Chapter 1 usefully suggests, the critical feminist lens does not privilege one gender over the other, but rather brings questions of inequality to our attention. Inequality can become visible on a health team along the lines of gender, ethnicity, seniority, or professional affiliation, as well as intersections among these and many other factors. From this vantage point, it becomes obvious that, for example, neither a "feminization of a medical profession" nor "bringing more men into nursing" will automatically guarantee equal status of team members (Pollard, 2010). Instead, an equal degree of actual (as opposed to tokenistic) participation of all health providers on a team in a decision-making process is perhaps a hallmark of egalitarian IPP. Although relations between physicians and nurses and other providers have changed in general, it is still not uncommon to encounter situations when the notion of "a common goal" for the team and an understanding of what constitutes a "good teamwork" become contentious issues. Specifically, nurses might want to examine power relationships that underpin teams and to question teamwork that camouflages power inequities.

Social and Cultural Analysis

This section draws on a number of sociological perspectives advanced by social scientists including nurse researchers (Allen, 1997; Dingwall, 1983; Miers, 2010a, 2010b; Pollard, 2010). Rather than focusing on a detailed discussion of those theories, the goal here is to deepen the reader's understanding of issues emerging in IPP through a presentation of summarized cultural and sociological theoretical insights. Specifically, a discussion will highlight tensions observed and theorized between the so-called *professionalization project* versus IPP as well as *identity work* versus *shifting boundary work*. In addition, a process of *skilling-up* in contemporary healthcare will be addressed. Although overlapping in practice, these processes will be partially disentangled for the purpose of discussion.

Professionalization Project or Interprofessional Practice?

In the last 5 decades in Canada many new health professions branched out and specialized in their respective fields. Initially carrying a designation as vocations, these new trades, ever-expanding in number and ever-narrowing in scope, emulated the model of the established medical profession to obtain professional status (Dingwall, 1983; King, n.d.; Miers, 2010a, 2010b). Health providers who claimed unique skills organized into groups, competed for influence through advancing providers' educational level and building a body of specialized knowledge, and developed regulations and codes of ethics, striving for government's recognition as self-regulated professions. Self-regulation means that the profession autonomously decides on its educational and practice standards, regulates licensure process, and assures quality practice of its members. You may recall from the beginning of the chapter that Ontario, for example, recognizes 23 self-regulated health professions. The processes of the rise of professions in society, their attempts to compete for influence, and their efforts to demarcate and protect their respective territories of expertise are termed *professionalization projects.* In other words, any profession pursuing a professionalization project strives to enhance its status and prestige in society, expand its territory, and create and strengthen professional identity of its members (Nettleton, 2006, as cited in Pollard, 2010; Witz, 1992, as cited in Miers, 2010b). Clearly, for self-regulated professions, their respective professionalization projects clash with the goal of IPP that calls for an abandonment of territorial claims and integration of skills and regulations. This clash is proposed as one of the factors contributing to resistance toward interprofessional collaboration from individual professions' and its members'.

Identity Work or Boundary Work?

According to Allen (1997) and Miers (2010b), traditional theorizing of professional identity suggested that members belonging to a specific profession, as a group, are struggling to build and maintain their identity, which then remains fixed. Current theorizing, however, emphasizes shifting boundaries between realms of various professions as well as evolving identities of its members (Allen, 1997; Miers, 2010b). For example, nurse practitioners are authorized to order certain tests, a function that only physicians could previously perform. To give another example, a physiotherapist, who assists a patient in a community setting with a range of motion exercises, can change a patient's wound dressing that was removed for the purpose of exercising, thus carrying out a task that is usually the responsibility of a nurse.

"Skilling Up"

With constantly shifting boundaries between professions' realms of expertise, the following parallel processes are observed in practice settings: Unregulated staff is increasingly assigned and delegated tasks that were the responsibility of regulated staff in the past; LPNs increasingly take on responsibilities of Registered Nurses (RNs); and nurses, especially a relatively new group of nurse practitioners (NPs), are performing procedures that physicians used to perform. This phenomenon, sometimes called skilling-up, is viewed in contradictory ways by different parties. For instance, an introduction of the role of the NP is usually discussed as an achievement for the nursing profession that allowed expanding nurses' domain of expertise. Some nurse scholars, however, raise concerns with the NP movement, as with the notion of interdisciplinarity, on the account that these developments serve to advance bio-medical goals of physicians rather than the goals unique to the discipline of nursing as presented by the nursing philosophies, theories, and conceptual frameworks (Cody, 2001). To clarify, this objection is not against interdisciplinary/ IPP *per se,* but about nurses' limited ability to formulate and convey their particular, discipline-specific, unique contributions to the team. "The risk of nursing being swallowed up and its unique nascent knowledge disappearing is very real," which results in nurses following others' agendas (Cody, 2001, p. 277).

Another aspect of the phenomenon of skilling up is that healthcare organizations perceive it as economically advantageous for their staffing decisions. In times of fiscal constraints, the tendency is to prefer unregulated providers, who are paid less, over costly professional staff. Next, as will be discussed in the political analysis below, the governments' umbrella regulations of health professions stimulate regulatory professional colleges to collaborate and, in turn, to promote interprofessional collaboration in practice. On a ground level, however, these intentions sometimes transpire in a form of "turf wars": Some physicians perceive NPs and RNs as usurping their responsibilities (Oliver & Keeping, 2010), and, in turn, RNs might feel that LPNs and unregulated care providers (UCPs) are taking over their jobs, which is (or is perceived as) threatening RNs' employment (Miers, 2010b; Pollard, 2010).

These challenges emerging in inter- and intraprofessional work and related, at least to some degree, to shifting boundaries between various professions in contemporary healthcare, can understandably contribute to nurses' apprehension about attempts to merge services and integrate skills.

However, rather than discounting nurses' concerns about IPP as simply being about their professional identities or motivated by their self-interests, nurses should be listened by nursing and organizational management and leaders. Nurses' resistances to align their voices with a dominant voice on a team be it a voice of a manager or a physician or another player often result from their observations that patients' concerns are pushed aside in an environment of cost containment.

Political Analysis

Political analysis usually involves questions of power. Ways in which power is exercised in society are changing, and also changing are theories in sociology, philosophy, political science, and nursing about the phenomenon of power. In the past, nurses' position as a group in our society has often been described as powerless and oppressed. The status of nurses as subordinate to physicians and an unpaid or underpaid workforce for the hospitals contributed to an image of nurses as lacking power. In this view, historical steps that nurses have undertaken to build a profession and a discipline are viewed as instances of seizing power and successfully wielding it.

Another conceptualization of power, developed by French intellectual Michel Foucault in the 1970s and early 1980s, suggests that power in contemporary society should be viewed in terms of micropolitics, as being exercised everywhere, as not (only) negative, seeking to oppress, but as productive, shaping our personalities, behaviors, and determining what is considered true (the truth) in particular periods in history (Smart, 1983). From this perspective, ethical issues that arise in IPP or issues addressed in a critical feminist analysis and even a question of why the topic of IPP is included in this current edition of the text but not in the previous ones—all these issues and questions are instances of power relations in a Foucauldian sense.

The following section uses an example from Ontario to highlight one aspect of healthcare politics—healthcare legislation influencing IPP. Specifically, certain Ontario government's steps potentially mean significant changes in the status of self-regulated health professions. As mentioned before, this re-regulation enacted in a few provinces is one of the factors contributing to a decrease of power of a medical profession in Canada in the last decades and is also affecting all other self-regulated health professions (Lahey, 2011).

Governments' Re-Regulation of Self-Regulated Professions

The key government legislation, *Regulated Health Professions Act (RHPA), 1991,* sought to bring a unifying approach to all self-regulated health professions in Ontario. Called "umbrella health professions legislation," this approach is based on "controlled acts model" (Field LLP, 2011, p. 3). Controlled acts, defined as actions that health professionals are authorized to perform when providing healthcare services to a patient/client, are listed in the *RHPA, 1991.* Based on this key document, health professional colleges have issued their respective Acts, such as the *Nursing Act, 1991,* by the College of Nurses of Ontario (CNO), which stipulates nurses' scope of practice in terms of selected controlled acts. It is obvious that more than one group of health professionals are authorized to perform certain controlled acts. This overlap in scope may be interpreted as suggesting a certain interchangeability among members of the healthcare team (CNO, 2008 May). For example, both nurses and physicians are authorized to put "an instrument, hand or finger... beyond the external ear canal" (see links to the *RHPA, 1991* & *Nursing Act, 1991,* in the online resources at the end of the chapter).

After Quebec, the province of Ontario was the first one in English-speaking Canada to introduce in 1991 this umbrella legislation for regulated health professionals (King, n.d.). British Columbia, Alberta, Yukon, Manitoba, and Newfoundland followed suit, albeit with some variations (Field, 2011).

In light of the *RHPA, 1991,* the CNO engaged in consultations with other health professions' regulatory colleges to identify strategies for collaboration (CNO, 2008, 2009b). A recent amendment to the *RHPA* and *Nursing Act* is Bill 179, which was passed by the Ontario government in 2009. When approved, this Bill introduced changes into the practice of nurses in Ontario, notably prescribing authority of NPs and dispensing authority of RNs, and mandates all nurses to carry legal liability protection, which was optional before (CNO, 2009c).

Although various groups of professionals have worked more or less collaboratively for many years, there appears to be a new dimension to this collaboration brought about by the *RHPA, 1991.* Arguably, the notion of IPP conveys more than just working side-by-side; it infers integration of services so that fewer providers can be involved in each case, skills can be mixed and matched, and more can be required from each provider through mechanisms of individual accountability. Potential implications of governments' steps to re-regulate health professions can be inferred from the CNO (2009c) reply:

> Some... recommendations appear to emphasize the performance of individual controlled
> act procedures over the collective competencies and knowledge base of the profession.

Nursing practice is more than a collection of discrete controlled acts. Regulatory processes must reflect the full scope of practice and support the application of nursing knowledge, skill, and judgment that includes, but is not limited to, the performance of controlled acts (p. 2).

Ethical Analysis

A professional responsibility of nurses to work collaboratively with other members of healthcare team is stipulated in the *Codes of Ethics* (CNA, 2008) and provincial practice standards (CNO, 2002). Issues that arise in everyday practice, however, are not necessarily easily solved by citing what nurses ought to do or abstain from doing. Uncertainty and complexity often characterize nursing practice, including work in teams.

In collaborative practice, dilemmas can be experienced in relationships among nurses and other providers (interprofessionally) and among different groups of nurses (intraprofessionally). Some of the issues that create moral unrest for nurses have been pointed out throughout the chapter, for instance, witnessing patients' concerns being discounted; disagreeing with other health providers over the team goals; challenging the *status quo* on the "collaborative" teams; addressing gender inequalities; or feeling torn between competing priorities of the employer (e.g., health organizations and agencies), professional expectations, and patients' wishes (see also Benjamin & Curtis, 2010). This section will surface the issues around accountability for nurses when working with UCPs. An important point to remember is that "nurses are regulated and accountable to clients, the (regulatory college), and the employer; whereas UCPs are unregulated and accountable to the employer" (CNO, 2009a, p. 3). Although drawing on Ontario examples—mostly the CNO guidelines—the discussion below has a wider resonance to many nurses across Canada.

Working with Unregulated Care Providers

In the current organizational context of cost-containment, nurses may observe growing utilization of UCPs on a hospital unit, where the proportion of RNs and LPNs decreases and the proportion of care aides and other UCPs increases (Catalano, 2008). Another example is nursing homes, where the workforce is comprised primarily of UCPs. The role of UCPs is usually thought of as assisting clients with activities of daily living when the outcome of care is predictable and has been established over time, that is, in relatively uncomplicated cases, which do not require supervision from nurses. But in contemporary, busy health settings, nurses are faced with situations when they need to delegate more complex procedures or tasks (e.g., controlled acts identified in the *RHPA, 1991*) to the UCPs. In other words, dilemmas may arise for RNs in a situation where they believe that to fulfill an obligation of safe, competent, and ethical client care, they must *directly* provide a specific service to or perform a procedure for a patient. And yet, other competing demands on nurses' time do not afford such a possibility, that is, a necessity arises to assign or delegate a task to UCPs.

Assigning means "allocating responsibility for providing care," whereas delegating means "transferring the authority to perform a controlled act procedure to a person not authorized" (CNO, 2009d, p. 6). Both decisions, to assign and to delegate, require nurses to be knowledgeable about processes involved in making such decisions and about their accountability (including legal), and to understand the potential risks involved. Nursing regulatory colleges' guidelines are devised to assist nurses with thinking about whether and how to delegate to UCPs. It is worth quoting from the CNO Practice Guideline *Utilization of Unregulated Care Providers* (2009a):

The nurse is:

- Accountable for her/his actions and decisions when working with UCPs;
- Accountable for knowing and understanding the roles and responsibilities of UCPs and collaborating and consulting with UCPs when required. Collaboration includes appropriate

communication and sharing of information among caregivers, and taking action on client information when needed;

- Accountable for her/his decisions and actions when delegating, teaching, assigning, and supervising UCPs. UCPs are accountable to the employer for using the information appropriately;
- Responsible for taking action to ensure client safety. This includes informing the employer of concerns related to the conduct and/or actions of UCPs;
- Not accountable for decisions or actions of other care providers when there is no way of knowing about those actions (p. 6)

As can be seen, although nurses are not directly accountable for the actions of UCPs, they *are* accountable for their own decision to delegate (which might feel as a necessity rather than a choice on a busy unit, for instance), teaching the UCP, setting expectations around clear and regular communication, and ensuring continuing supervision. Considering the heated discussions around issues of working with UCPs that registered nurses from across Canada bring to the CNA annual general meetings (CNA, 2009), it is clear that issues arising in intraprofessional practice are more complicated than they may appear.

Economic Considerations

As discussions of various issues in this book demonstrate, it is quite difficult to separate an economic aspect of any contemporary issue in healthcare provision from other aspects of it. In fact, current financial priorities in health and social care are often *driving* the issues addressed in this and other chapters. Goals of cost containment and attempts to maximize efficiency, that is, to achieve greater measurable outcomes with less expenditure, are often behind governments' and organizations' imperatives to promote interprofessional collaboration and integration among services and providers (Kearney-Nunnery, 2008). It is likely that the emphasis on cost/benefit calculations will become even more prominent, influencing nurses' work and foregrounding questions of quality assurance through mechanisms of individual provider's accountability (Buchda, 2008).

RECOGNIZING BARRIERS, DEVISING STRATEGIES: CREATING POSSIBILITIES WITHIN CONSTRAINTS

IPP is an issue of interest for multiple stakeholders, whose visions of and goals for IPP can be divergent. It is anticipated that this form of collaborative work holds a potential to benefit patients/clients, providers, and the Canadian healthcare system. Considering the issues surrounding IPP, what does it take then to make IPP work well for nurses, patients, and others?

Effective IPP requires that nurses and other team members understand and are able to articulate and demonstrate the unique contributions that their respective professions, as well as other regulated and unregulated providers, make for the patient/family/community. In other words, it is important for nurses to possess a clear understanding of their roles and contributions within particular settings, and to exercise skills to competently, ethically, and safely perform these roles. However, considering that the roles and accountabilities of nurses and other providers are shifting as a result of government regulations and other historical and societal changes (e.g., emergence of new professions and implementation of managerial strategies directed at reducing costs of health provision), nurses are faced with a double necessity: On the one hand, to be knowledgeable of the current roles and responsibilities as reflected in professional standards, guidelines, legal requirements, and employer's regulations, and on the other hand, to recognize that these are continuously evolving, and that what might have been considered a familiar and fixed role or accountability of health providers (e.g., a physician, NP, LPN, or UCP) is changing too.

IPP depends on nurses' and other professionals' willingness and skills to communicate and negotiate effectively with others, while building and maintaining a climate of trust and respect among persons involved and rebutting stereotypes about other professions. Nurses in general are well prepared through their classroom education and practicum placements to meet the challenges of interpersonal communication on teams: To be able to ask questions, negotiate, disagree, and resolve conflicts. However, when teams are faced with competing goals and diverging priorities, it is sometimes difficult not to lose sight of what nurses' consider to be important and to advocate for it. For instance, keeping patients' perspectives in play might be quite challenging when acute care settings expect that patients are moved through the system faster (Campbell & Rankin, 2006). Moreover, questioning a *status quo* of a team player whose voice has been dominant requires courage, good understanding of a situation, and an ability to build alliances with those who are supportive. In addition, ethical dilemmas of delegating to UCPs when nurses are concerned about patient safety require that nurses possess the skills to navigate these dilemmas and to educate their employers about professional accountability.

IPE has the potential to assist student nurses to enter a world of interprofessional collaboration. To overcome challenges of IPE such as scheduling difficulties or lack of financial support the following is necessary: Allocating dedicated staff to coordinate student placements, willingness of health authorities and health organizations to accommodate student teams, and various forms of support from universities. In relation to the goals of IPE, however, it is not sufficient for learners to memorize what other providers do and to learn to communicate. What is also important is to nurture a sense of flexibility and curiosity, to recognize and be able to live with uncertainty, and acquire political acumen to see the bigger picture, that is, to understand how health organization or agency functions, what its priorities are, and how those shift with societal changes.

Insightful nursing leadership and organizational support are crucial factors for IPP. In the last 2 or 3 decades, nurses have witnessed, with a sense of dissatisfaction, powerlessness, and anger, that several patient services were terminated and funding of some programs stopped, and that organizational cost saving measures in acute care did not materialize in better funding for community and home care, despite stated intentions. Questions can be asked: Is there a danger that inter- and intraprofessional practice, despite its stated objectives of patient-centeredness and bridging fragmented services, will unfold on the ground in the form of "turf wars"? Will a call for integration of skills mean that each provider is expected to do more with fewer resources? It is important to have strong nursing leaders within healthcare settings and beyond, who will not only align with organizational goals, but will listen to nurses working in close proximity with patients and will bring their voices to the discussion table. Another aspect of nursing leadership in a context of IPP is that nurse leaders, both in formal leadership roles and on all organizational levels, should be able to see what is possible within the constrains, that is, creative approaches to service provision are needed and there might be opportunities for funding new, pilot programs. Healthcare organizations are in a search for new solutions, so teams of committed and politically astute professionals can actually lead a development of interprofessional services that will directly benefit patients.

SUMMARY

Nurses rarely work in isolation. Even when practicing in geographically remote settings, nurses are working not only with their patients/clients, but also with other health providers, through direct communication and consultation or through integration of service provision that occurs at the level of healthcare organizations and agencies. IPP is a relatively new phrase that seems to be gradually replacing other expressions such as collaborative practice or team work.

This change in terminology, as the chapter suggests, is reflective of complex processes taking place in the provision of healthcare.

Over the last 2 or 3 decades, in a time of significant changes in the healthcare system, provincial and territorial governments, nursing professional regulatory bodies (as well as other health professions' colleges), and the CNA have all placed increasing attention on IPP. In this context, educational institutions and other organizations are launching projects for IPE as a strategy to assist health professionals to acquire knowledge, skills, and attitudes to work together to maximize professionals' potential, overcome fragmentation of care, provide quality services to patients/clients, and meet organizational goals of effective and efficient outcomes.

A close look at a government's legislation and regulatory nursing college's documents of one of the Canadian provinces, Ontario, suggests that IPP is shaped by the government's agenda of re-regulation of (self-) regulated health professions and is taken up by the regulatory bodies as an attempt to preserve their respective areas of expertise while at the same time balancing shifting boundaries between health professions.

Transformations in healthcare as well as changes in a wider society resulted in "flattening" of hierarchical relationships among health professionals, most notably physicians and nurses, with nurses gaining confidence as knowledgeable team players. However, nurses may observe that IPP is sometimes understood by more powerful participants as their right to define the goals of service provision with which all other providers are expected to agree. A challenge for nurses is to confront the *status quo*. Nurses are also encouraged to keep concerns unique to the discipline and the profession of nursing in play, to highlight voices of nurses on a team, while hearing others and contributing to building cohesive groups.

Despite the rhetoric of patient-centeredness found in a vast literature on IPP, a close look at the topic identifies organizations' agenda of cost containment as driving changes in practice. These changes can affect nurses in various ways: Create opportunities for new practice models that promise improved, measurable outcomes, and enhance nurses' satisfaction with team work, or the opposite: Preclude professionals from benefiting their clients in a more meaningful way and contribute to animosity and "turf wars" among providers. In any case, nurses are increasingly required to balance multiple competing priorities—a situation in which patients' priorities get easily pushed aside. To work with this challenge, nurse leaders on all levels of practice are required to understand how the system works, see the bigger picture, and find opportunities to preserve and advance what is important for nursing, with the ultimate goal of benefiting patients.

Add to your knowledge of this issue: *Online*

The Ontario Ministry of Health and Long-Term Care (OMHLTC) website	**http://www.health.gov.on.ca**
Centre for the Advancement of Interprofessional Education (CAIPE)	**http://www.caipe.org.uk**
The Canadian Interprofessional Health Collaborative (CIHC)	**http://www.cihc.ca**
Interprofessional Education for Collaborative Patient-Centred Practice (IECPCP)	**http://www.hc-sc.gc.ca**
The University of Manitoba Interprofessional Education (IPE) Initiative	**http://umanitoba.ca**
The McGill Educational initiative on Interprofessional Collaboration	**http://www.interprofessionalcare.mcgill.ca**

R E F L E C T I O N S *on the Chapter...*

1 This chapter uses examples of legislation, professional standards, and guidelines from Ontario. In the province or territory where you attend the nursing program, what official documents regulate the intra- and interprofessional aspect of nursing practice? In what ways are they similar to or different from the ones implemented in Ontario?

2 How do you perceive a shift in terminology around collaborative practice that happened over the last 2 decades? Does language matter and in what ways? Why or why not? What might be the assumptions that underlie your answer?

3 Who are regulated and unregulated providers with whom you interact in your clinical practicum courses? What facilitates your interactions or impedes them?

4 Observe the work of an established team in a healthcare or community setting. How are decisions made? Is there a "dominant voice" on a team? What is nurses' role on this team? In what way, if any, is patient/client involved in teamwork?

5 How could your perspectives on the goals of IPP shift if you try on various metaphorical hats: That of the official on a provincial government, of an advisor on nursing policy at a nursing regulatory college, of a nurse practitioner on a transplant unit of a teaching hospital, of a nursing aide on the same unit, of a registered nurse doing home visits, of a senior manager in a hospital, of a patient, and so on? What are the assumptions and values that can underlie each of these diverse perspectives?

6 In your educational institution, are there initiatives promoting interdisciplinary/IPE? Have nursing students taken part in them? What do you perceive as advantages and disadvantages of such initiatives? What are the assumptions that underlie your perspective?

Want to know more? Visit thePoint* for additional helpful resources:

- Journal Articles
- Learning Objectives
- Nursing Professional Roles and Responsibilities
- Bonus chapters:
  - Health and Nursing Policy: A Matter of Politics, Power and Professionalism
  - The NP Movement: Recurring Issues
  - When Difference Matters: The Politics of Privilege and Marginality

References

Allen, D. (1997). The nursing-medical boundary: A negotiated order? *Sociology of Health and Illness, 19*(4), 498–520.

Ateah, C. (2011, January). *Interprofessional education (IPE) activity report.* Retrieved from University of Manitoba, Faculty of Nursing, IPE Information and Activities Web site: http://umanitoba.ca/faculties/nursing/current/media/jan_2011_report.pdf

Barnsteiner, J. H., Disch, J. M., Hall, L., Mayer, D., & Moore, S.M. (2007). Promoting interprofessional education. *Nursing Outlook, 55*(3), 144–150. doi:10.1016/j.outlook.2007.03.003

Benjamin, M., & Curtis, J. (2010). *Ethics in nursing: Cases, principles, and reasoning* (4th ed.). New York: Oxford University Press.

Bilodeau, A., Dumont, S., Hagan, L., et al. (2010). Interprofessional education at Laval University: Building an integrated curriculum for patient-centred practice. *Journal of Interprofessional Care, 24*(5), 524–535. doi: 10.3109/13561821003724026

Buchda, V. L. (2008). Managing and providing care. In R. Kearney-Nunnery (Ed.), *Advancing your career: Concepts of professional nursing* (4th ed., pp. 269–288). Philadelphia, PA: F. A. Davis.

Calnan, R., & Lemire Rodger, G. (2002). *Primary Health Care: A new approach to health care reform.* (Remarks to the Senate Standing Committee on Social Affairs, Science and Technology). Retrieved from CNA website: http://www.cna-nurses.ca/CNA/documents/pdf/publications/PHC_presentation_Kirby_6602_e.pdf

Campbell, M.L., & Rankin, J.M. (2006). *Managing to nurse: Inside Canada's health care reform.* Toronto, ON: University of Toronto Press.

Castro, R.M., & Julia, M. C. (1994). *Interprofessional care and collaborative practice. Commission on interprofessional education and practice.* Pacific Grove, CA: Brooks/Cole.

Catalano, J. T. (2008). Professional ethics. In R. Kearney-Nunnery (Ed.), *Advancing your career: Concepts of professional nursing* (4th ed., pp. 250–268). Philadelphia, PA: F. A. Davis.

CNA. (2005). *CNA backgrounder. Primary Health Care: A summary of the issues.* Retrieved from http://www.cna-nurses.ca/CNA/documents/pdf/publications/BG7_Primary_Health_Care_e.pdf

———. (2008). *Code of ethics for registered nurses.* Ottawa, ON: Author. Retrieved from http://www.cna-nurses.ca/CNA/documents/pdf/publications/Code_of_Ethics_2008_e.pdf

———. (2009). *Issues discussion at annual meeting: Increasing use of unregulated health workers.* Retrieved from http://www.cna-nurses.ca/CNA/documents/pdf/publications/Annual_Meeting_Issues_Disc_UHW_e.pdf

———. (n.d.) *Position statement: Interprofessional collaboration.* Retrieved from http://www.cna-nurses.ca/CNA/documents/pdf/publications/PS84_Interprofessional_Collaboration_e.pdf

———. (2002). *Professional standards.* Toronto, ON: Author. Retrieved from http://www.cno.org/Global/docs/prac/41006_ProfStds.pdf

———. (2008, May). *Interprofessional collaboration among health colleges and professions. (Submission to the Health Professions Regulatory Advisory Council).* Toronto, ON: Author. Retrieved from http://www.hprac.org/en/projects/resources/hprac-1433May28CollegeOfNurses.pdf

CNO. (2009a). *Practice guideline: Utilization of unregulated care providers.* Toronto, ON: Author. Retrieved from http://www.cno.org/Global/docs/prac/41055_UtilizeUCPs.pdf

———. (2009b, January). *The College of Nurses of Ontario's response to: An Interim Report to the Minister of Health and Long-Term Care on Mechanisms to Facilitate and Support Interprofessional Collaboration among Health Colleges and Regulated Health Professionals (March 2008).* Toronto, ON: Author. Retrieved from http://www.cno.org/Global/docs/policy/hprac_InterprofColl_and_NP_Response_Jan302009.pdf

———. (2009c, September). *The College of Nurses of Ontario submission to The Standing Committee on Social Policy: Bill 179, Regulated Health Professions Law Statute Amendment Act, 2009.* Toronto, ON: Author. Retrieved from http://www.cno.org/Global/docs/policy/Bill179SubmissionStanding Committee_Final_CouncilApproved.pdf

———. (2009d). *Practice guideline: Working with unregulated care providers.* Toronto, ON: Retrieved from http://www.cno.org/Global/docs/prac/41014_workingucp.pdf

———. (2010). *Self-assessment: A guide to developing your learning goals and learning plan 2011.* Toronto, ON: Author. Retrieved from http://www.cno.org/Global/docs/qa/44041_qaGuide2011.pdf

Cody, W.K. (2001). Interdisciplinarity and nursing: "Everything is everything," or is it? *Nursing Science Quarterly, 14,* 274–232. doi: 10.1177/08943180122108562

D'Amour, D., & Oandasan, I. (2005). Interprofessionality as the field of interprofessional practice and interprofessional education: An emerging concept. *Journal of Interprofessional Care, 19*(Suppl. 1), 8–20. doi: 10.1080/13561820500081604

Dingwall, R. (1983). 'In the beginning was the work...': reflections on the genesis of occupations. *Sociological Review, 31*(4), 605–624.

Duck, E. (2010). Accountability within interprofessional healthcare. In M. Standing (Ed.), *Clinical judgement and decision-making in nursing and interprofessional healthcare* (pp. 153–166). Berkshire: McGraw Hill & Open University Press.

Enhancing Interdisciplinary Collaboration in Primary Health Care. (2006). *The principles and framework for interdisciplinary collaboration in primary health care.* Ottawa, ON: Author. Retrieved from http://www.caslpa.ca/PDF/EICP_Principles_and_Framework_final.pdf

Field, L.L.P. (2011). *Appendix D. A primer on umbrella health professions legislation across Canada.* Presented to Steering Committee of the Health & Social Services Umbrella Legislation Project, Department of Health and Social Services, Government of the Northwest Territories. Retrieved from http://www.hlthss.gov.nt.ca/english/services/professional_licensing/pdf/hss_profession_legislation/appendix_d.pdf\

Gask, L. (2005). Overt and covert barriers to the integration of primary and specialist mental health care. *Social Science & Medicine, 61*(8), 1785–1794. doi:10.1016/j.socscimed.2005.03.038

Goodman, B., & Clemov, R. (2008). *Nursing and working with other people.* Exeter: Learning Matters.

Gottlieb, L. N., & Feeley, N. (2005). *The collaborative partnership approach to care: A delicate balance.* Toronto, ON: Elsevier Canada.

Kearney-Nunnery, R. (2008). Management in organizations. In R. Kearney-Nunnery (Ed.), *Advancing your career: Concepts of professional nursing* (4th ed., pp. 206–228). Philadelphia, PA: F. A. Davis.

King, M. C. (n.d.) An introduction to the *Health Professions Act.* Report for the Calgary Regional Health Authority. Retrieved from http://www.calgaryhealthregion.ca/clin/adultpsy/documents/king_hpa1.pdf

Lahey, W. (2011, May). Is self-regulation under threat? *Canadian Nurse.* Retrieved from http://www.canadian-nurse.com/index.php?option=com_content&view=article&id=451:is-self-regulation-under-threat&catid=4:perspectives&itemid=39&lang=en

MacDonald, M. B., Bally, J. M., Ferguson, L. M., Lee Murray, B., Fowler-Kerry, S.E., & Anonson, J.M.S. (2010). Knowledge of the professional role of others: A key interprofessional competency. *Nurse Education in Practice, 10*(4), 238–242. doi:10.1016/j.nepr.2009.11.012

Mann, K. V., McFetridge-Durdle, J., Martin-Misener, R., et al. (2009). Interprofessional education for students of the health professions: The "Seamless Care" model. *Journal of Interprofessional Care, 23*(3), 224–233. doi: 10.1080/13561820802697735

Miers, M. (2010a). Learning for new ways of working. In K. C. Pollard, J. Thomas, & M. Miers (Eds.), *Understanding interprofessional working in health and social care. Theory and practice* (pp. 74-89). Basingstoke: Palgrave Macmillan.

Miers, M. (2010b). Professional boundaries and interprofessional working. In K. C. Pollard, J. Thomas, & M. Miers (Eds.), *Understanding interprofessional working in health and social care: Theory and practice* (pp. 105–120). Basingstoke: Palgrave Macmillan.

Oliver, B., & Keeping, C. (2010). Individual and professional identity. In K. C. Pollard, J. Thomas, & M. Miers (Eds.), *Understanding interprofessional working in health and social care: Theory and practice* (pp. 90–104). Basingstoke: Palgrave Macmillan.

Orchard, C. A. (2010). Persistent isolationist or collaborator? The nurse's role in interprofessional collaborative practice. *Journal of Nursing Management, 18*(3), 248–257. doi:10.1111/j.1365-2834.2010.01072.x

Pollard, K. C. (2010). The medicalization thesis. In K. C. Pollard, J. Thomas, & M. Miers (Eds.), *Understanding interprofessional working in health and social care: Theory and practice* (pp. 121–155). Basingstoke, UK: Palgrave Macmillan.

Pollard, K. C., Thomas, J., & Miers, M. (Eds.). (2010). *Understanding interprofessional working in health and social care: Theory and practice.* Basingstoke: Palgrave Macmillan.

Pollard, K., & Harris, F. (2010). Interprofessional working. In D. Sellman & P. Snelling (Eds.), *Becoming a nurse: A textbook for professional practice* (pp. 138–166). Essex: Pearson.

Sellman, D. (2010). Values and ethics in interprofessional working. In K. C. Pollard, J. Thomas, & M. Miers (Eds.), *Understanding interprofessional working in health and social care: Theory and practice* (pp. 156–170). Basingstoke: Palgrave Macmillan.

Smart, B. (1983). *Foucault, Marxism and critique.* London: Routledge & Kegan Paul.

Stein, L. (1967). The doctor-nurse game. *Archives of General Psychiatry, 16*(6), 699–703.

Stein, L., Watts, D., & Howell, T. (1990). The doctor–nurse game revisited. *New England Journal of Medicine, 322,* 546–549.

Takahashi, S., Brissette, S., & Thorstad, K. (2010). Different roles, same goal: Students learn about interprofessional practice in a clinical setting. *Canadian Journal of Nursing Leadership, 23*(1), 32–39.

Thomas, J. (2010). Service users, carers and issues for collaborative practice. In K. C. Pollard, J Thomas, & M. Miers (Eds.), *Understanding interprofessional working in health and social care: Theory and practice* (pp. 171–185). Basingstoke: Palgrave Macmillan.

Traynor, M. (1999). Managers and measurement: Taking a literary approach to managerial discourse. In J. Robinson, M. Avis, J. Latimer & M. Traynor (Eds.), *Interdisciplinary perspectives on health policy and practice: Competing interests or complementary interpretations?* (pp. 119–139). London: Churchill Livingstone.

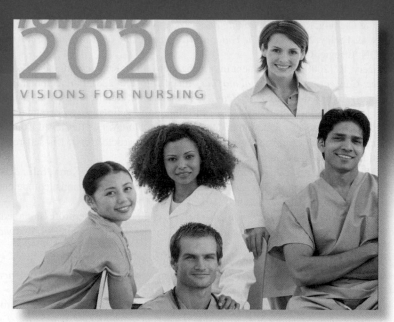

An image from the cover of the DVD "Toward 2020: Visions for Nursing," which challenges long-held stereotypes of gender in nursing. (Cover photo: Comstock. Used with permission of CNA and NurseONE.)

Critical Questions

As a way of engaging with the ideas in this chapter, consider the following:

1. How have you come to hold the views you hold of gender and gendered roles?

2. How is it that historically some work has been thought of as women's work?

3. How does value get assigned to particular work?

Chapter Objectives

After completing this chapter, you will be able to:

1. Understand the idea of gender as socially constructed and the ways that gender is bound by cultural, temporal, and social realities.

2. Recognize gender as attributed to both individuals as well as to larger realities, such as the profession of nursing.

3. Recognize gender as one of a number of intersecting identities, including race, class, age, ethnicity, and sexual orientation, through which we are uniquely constituted as individuals.

4. Articulate the nature of nurses' work, nurses' knowledge, and nurses' public representation as gendered, and discuss the historical social discourses of women's work and nurses' work that have contributed to this understanding.

(continued on page 279)

5. Discuss the barriers that interfere with the resolution of issues that arise from societal assumptions about gender and the significance attributed to nurses' work.

6. Identify strategies that will serve to interrupt the taken-for-granted notions of gendered work that underlie the undervaluing of nurses' work.

This chapter presents opportunities to consider the idea that societally derived concepts about gender are inherent in claims about the value of nurses' work and the importance of nursing knowledge. The chapter challenges readers to look beneath the taken-for-granted assumptions about what is called women's work in general and nurses' work in particular. Exploring the topic of the gendered nature of nurses' work relies on thinking of the idea of gender in two interrelated but different ways. The first is the idea of gender as an expression of the masculinity or feminin- ity of the individual person; in this case, the gender of the nurse. The second, and perhaps more important idea, is the gendered nature of the profession, meaning nursing itself is inscribed with meanings of gender. As we will discuss, both of these views of gender can be understood as socially constructed, that is, beliefs and assumptions about gender and therefore the way that gender is expressed are strongly shaped by societal norms and ideals.

Ideas about gender, in particular the value attributed to women's work and whether this work requires significant knowledge, responsibility, and skill contributes to the devaluing of nurses' work within the healthcare system and society at large. Using the framework for analysis from Chapter 1, this chapter examines the issues of the gendered nature of nurses' work from histori- cal, social, cultural, critical feminist, and legal perspectives. Ideas about care as central to nursing practice, and the topic of men in nursing, are discussed as well.

ARTICULATING THE ISSUE FOR NURSING

How does the topic of gender arise in a discussion of the issues currently affecting Canadian nurses in education and in practice? Gender is a concept in our society that is simultaneously taken for granted and poorly understood. In this chapter, *gender* refers to the ways in which a person lives a life that demonstrates or reflects masculinity and femininity. As the chapter explores, gender can be thought of as constructed through social influences outside of a particular individual. And although there is undoubtedly some interrelationship between biologic sex and gender, this chapter addresses gender as distinct from the categories of biologic sex.

In exploring the significance of gender in relation to nursing practice, nursing knowledge, and nurses themselves, we begin by acknowledging the complexity of gender per se. Then we need to explore ways of thinking about gender beyond distribution, beyond the numbers of nurses who are female or male. These ways of thinking about gender will anchor us in the world of social realities where nursing is practiced and where concepts of gender and gender practices are formed.

The Gender Binary

The commonly used binary genders are the taken-for-granted categories of boy/girl or man/ woman assumed by many to be closely linked to the biological sex categories of male and female. While we will later discuss the idea that all of these categories are socially constructed and in some sense "empty categories," the role played by this categorization of gender in society is very real. From the moment of birth the first identifying knowledge of a person is a categorization of

BOX 15.1   Glossary of Terms and Definitions

This list describes the way some terms are used in the content of this chapter. They should not be taken as absolute definitions of the words.

- **Complicity**—our own participation in, for example, supporting or reinforcing societal norms that undermine the value of women's work.
- **Essentializing**—seeing something as representative of all members of a particular group or category. For example, essentializing nurses' work in a woman's domain implies that there is something about nursing that could only be performed by women.
- **Discourses**—social practices, values, and cultural beliefs that prevail in a given culture or subculture at a specific historical moment and shape a collective sense of what is right, proper, worthwhile, or valuable (Thorne et al., 1997, p. 2).
- **Discourses of care**—the ways in which ideas about care have been represented in nursing, particularly the values and beliefs that have placed care central to nursing practice.
- **Discursive process**—how we learn to be and to behave in particular ways through the messages received in social discourses.
- **Gender**—the ways in which femininity and masculinity are reflected in the lived life. Gender is distinct from the biologic sex of a person. Culturally, there is value attached to particular genders and the way in which that gender is performed.
- **Ideologies**—not merely ideas, but a powerful and authoritative voice in society that tells us who we are and how we are to behave.
- **Location of gender**—gender is constructed through the interaction of the person with the social realities, values, and beliefs of a culture at a particular time in history. In this sense, gender resides both within and beyond the individual.
- **Naturalized**—when some quality is taken to be innately, or obviously "the way it is," without questioning the beliefs on which that assumption is formed. For example, the symbol of a "woman" (wearing a dress) and a "man" (wearing pants) have become naturalized in our culture to represent the washrooms in public places to be used by women or men. Although there is nothing innately natural about these symbols representing men or women, we have come to interpret them unquestioningly in this way (Fig. 15.1).
- **Reinscribing**—reinforcing or reproducing a concept or belief, at times without the thoughtful intention of doing so.
- **Social construction**—ideas, concepts, and roles that are understood to be formed or built up through the agreed-on ideologies of a society.
- **Transparency**—the ways in which we can see something clearly, or obviously (high transparency), or in which something is obscured from our view. For example, increasing our awareness of material and social realities that contribute to gendering of nurses' work will improve our ability to see, or make transparent to us, the manner in which nursing is undervalued because it is "women's work."

sex—"it's a girl"—announces to the world that this particular body will be read as female. While it can be argued that many of these early determinations into the binary choices are arbitrary, the focus of this discussion is with the presentation of gender that moves beyond biology to the presentation of the person in the social realm.

It is in childhood that we are acculturated to the social regulations that underpin our local world. Anyone who has spent time with early-school-aged children might recognize the dominance of gender in their language and questions as they struggle to master the reading of bodies as gendered. The limitation of the binary choices ring clearly in the repeated question: Is that a boy or a girl? And for some of us, are you a boy or a girl? There is almost an urgency to be able to place people as one—or the other. For children, the binary is clearly differentiated in the gendered nature of toys, clothing, and activities. And in case you consider this an outdated argument, reminiscent of the 1950s, take a look at the dominance of pink in what is referred to as the "girls side" of the children's wear shop, or the resurgence of Barbie and Barbie-like dolls on offer. The point here is that the maintenance of the gender division is alive and well, and that the continued reinscription of this division enforces the well-engrained although sometimes unconscious ideas that society holds about what is suitable, appropriate, or even "natural" for boys and girls, men and women.

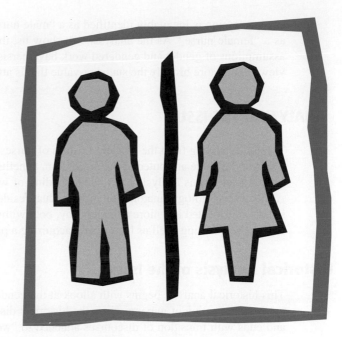

FIGURE 15.1 The symbols of a "woman" (wearing a dress) and a "man" (wearing pants) have become naturalized in our culture to represent the washrooms in public places to be used by women or men. Although there is nothing innately natural about these symbols representing men or women, we have come to interpret them unquestioningly in this way.

Gender as Socially Constructed

As concepts, gender, women's work, and nursing itself derive their meaning in society through social construction. Social construction means that ideas, concepts, and roles are understood as formed or built upon the shared assumptions and beliefs of a society. Over time these shared assumptions become discourses that develop the authority to tell us who we are, what we are to think, and how we are to behave. In other words, discourses are "social practices, values and cultural beliefs that prevail in a given culture or subculture at a specific historical moment and shape a collective sense of what is right, proper, worthwhile or valuable" (Thorne et al., 1997, p. 2).

In *Revisioning Gender*, Nakano Glenn (2000) notes that "feminist scholars adopted the term *gender* precisely to free our thinking from the constrictions of naturalness and biological inevitability attached to the concept of sex" (p. 4). In this sense, gender moves us to a broader understanding of what it is to live one's life in ways that reflect masculinity and femininity. Butler (1990), a prominent feminist thinker, discusses gender not as the expression of an internal identity but rather as a performance in which the person acts a script that is written in and through social discourses. Although the socially sanctioned scripts for gender that are currently provided and normalized through social discourses offer little alternative to the categories of man and woman, this idea of gender as socially constructed means that we are free to recognize the feminine and the masculine within each of us, and to live our lives in ways that comply with or disrupt normative ideas of gender.

The Gendered Nurse as Socially Constructed

Just as gender can be seen as constructed, rather than innate, the concept of a *nurse* is not a naturally occurring phenomenon. Rather, the concept of *nurse* has been constructed over time, through discourses of what constitutes or makes up the role of a nurse. Although we may acknowledge intellectually that there is no natural role or personality attributable to a *nurse*, we often, unthinkingly, act as if the opposite is so. It is not surprising, for example, when a man who chooses nursing as a profession is inevitably identified as a "male nurse," whereas a woman is rarely referred to as a "female nurse." As the analysis will show us, the historical influence of social norms and assumptions of gender and gendered work have persistently shaped the way in which nurses are viewed and more broadly the status or value that is attributed to the profession.

ANALYZING THE ISSUE

The issues arising from the gendered nature of nurses' work, in particular, the influences of this issue on the value attributed to the profession, benefits from various perspectives of analysis.

Crucial to this analysis is an understanding of what may be called the *location of gender*. Although the biologic anatomy of an individual resides with that person, gender as a social construction is located in a more complex way, both within and beyond the particular person. In this way we see nursing itself as historically acquiring a profoundly gendered profile.

Historical Analysis of the Issue

This historical analysis begins with a look at the gendered nature of knowledge that predates the professionalization of nursing, visits the historical discourses of nursing education and practice, and ends with transition of discourses attached to "women's work." Through time, nurses have been influenced by the discourses around several bodies of knowledge. Before the industrialization of nursing, women healers and caregivers were privileged to gynocentric (feminine-centered) knowledge, for example, midwifery and herbal pharmacology, as well as the knowledge necessary for the care of home and family (Ginzberg, 1999). These areas of knowledge have lost value in the foreground of Western science and scientific knowledge, which was produced with an androcentric (masculine-centered) focus. Critiques of science in the 20th century suggest that "knowledge produced by the sciences is part of the social and political tradition within which it is produced" (Welch, 1999, p. 423). Such critiques support the notion that particular "women's activities haven't been called 'science' for *political* reasons, even when those activities have been model examples of inquiry leading to knowledge of the natural world" (Ginzberg, 1999, p. 441).

Nursing practice has long been equated with "female virtues"—the virtues of care, nurturance, and altruism. In an exploration of classism, genderism, and racism in nursing, Turkoski (1992) notes that, historically, nursing has been "described in purely genderised terms as: 'women's mission, ministry, humanitarian service,' a 'service of womanly duty and conscience,' and 'the noblest and most womanly of professions'" and reminds us that these descriptions "reinforced the assumption that nursing is essentially related to one's biological makeup" (p. 162). In a fascinating and disturbing critique of nearly a century of nursing education, Walker and Holmes (2008) provide repeated examples, decade by decade, of anti-intellectual rhetoric that portrays the ideal nurse as the ideal woman of the Victorian era. The valorization of the feminine character of the nurse through a great deal of the 20th century includes the intellectual subservience of the profession to medical knowledge.

"Gentleness and quietness were required of Nightingale's nurses, and many nurses in today's work force that 'trained' in the 1960s and earlier can attest to the importance attached to those virtues" (Falk Rafael, 1996, p. 9). Some of those nurses, who are still in practice, were expected to demonstrate as their "professional" behavior, unquestioning deference to physicians, for example, standing when physicians entered the room, vacating chairs and opening doors for them, as well as obediently, even unthinkingly, carrying out physicians' orders. Abbott and Wallace (1990) argue that even though "nurses no longer see themselves as handmaidens to doctors, they have remained trapped in their status as subordinate to doctors" (p. 22). In support of this argument, Abbott and Wallace remind us of nurses being accountable for administering medication that they are not authorized to prescribe.

At any given point in time, there may be multiple discourses participating in the social construction of the nurse. "Just as the cosmetic and fashion industries created the 'ideal woman,' so nursing texts, be they in popular press, television, or textbook form, create images of the ideal nurse" (Cheek & Rudge, 1994, p. 589). These idealized images of nurses are by no means unified. Part of the complexity of attaining the ideal is that it comprises mixed and conflicting messages and changes over time.

Regardless of the variables that form this ideal—including race, ethnicity, age, and sexuality—"both the nurse and the work of nursing are firmly associated in the public mind with the female sex" (Davies, 1995, p. 2). As suggested by Davies (1995) in the introduction to her text *Gender and the Professional Predicament in Nursing,* "a closer acquaintance with nursing, however, shatters any cozy image of women doing work that is somehow *natural* to them and hence being entirely comfortable in and satisfied with the role they have chosen" (p. 2; emphasis added). A current American television portrayal of an emergency room nurse as an autonomous, independent, respected, and compassionate professional conveys a particular appeal to nurses entering the profession. The actual social and material realities of this nurse's professional world may, in fact, be as much of a fabrication as the professionally submissive representation of the fictional "Dr. Welby's nurse" of the 1960s. Although vastly different from one another, both of these media portrayals of the nurse reflect an idealized image of "woman" formed through the prominent social discourses of the day.

A feminist historical analysis connects the value attached to work ordinarily performed by women in the public sphere to the changing value attached to work performed by women in the private sphere (Bunting, 1992). In preindustrial times, before the advent of large-scale productivity and commercialization, the work ordinarily performed by women was associated with the maintenance and care of home and family and was more closely aligned, in worth, to the work ordinarily performed by men. The refocusing of modern society on a production- and wage-oriented economy resulted in a devaluation of the care work ordinarily performed by women in the private sphere. Women were placed in the "position of performing services and producing products for the family that have no recognised market value" (Bunting, 1992, p. 58). Along with Bunting, we might wonder about the "connections between the devaluing of women's care in the home and the difficulty of gaining recognition for *nurses'* contributions of care" (Bunting, 1992, p. 60). Bunting (1992) finds a relationship between the invisibility and taken-for-grantedness of caregiving in the private sphere, based on the absence of financial remuneration, and the low status of nursing as a profession.

Social–cultural Analysis of the Issue

This social–cultural analysis, which explores prevailing attitudes and assumptions, continues with a view of nurses' work through the lens of "women's work." As Walker (2009) and others (Brown, 2009; McGee, 2009; Walker & Holmes, 2008) describe nursing as a "profoundly gendered profession" (p. 163) where worldwide, women constitute over 90% of the membership, it is understandable that nursing falls within the category of women's work. While in itself the idea of women's work is unproblematic, the values ascribed to this work over time continue to be a challenge.

"The gendered division of labor in the home and in the work place is part of a negotiated order that is accomplished within the social context of a prevailing set of normative conceptions or ideologies, about what activities are appropriate for men and women" (Angus, 1994, p. 24).

In exploring the working lives of Canadian women, Angus (1994) notes that the "labour force is characterized by marked horizontal (occupational) and vertical (hierarchical) gender divisions" (p. 32). This means that women in preponderate numbers enter a limited subdivision of the workforce: A subdivision understood to be gender-typed as "women's work." Among these occupations is nursing, which composes part of about 80% of women workers who are "employed in labor-intensive occupations. . . . concentrated in the public sector. . . . where cost containment has produced additional burdens and frustration" (Angus, 1994, pp. 32, 38).

Angus' (1994) work also comments on the vertical division of labor by gender in certain occupations. This division refers to the socially created reality that occupations dominated by men are better rewarded than those dominated by women. According to Angus, this phenomenon is attributable to the dominant discourses in our society that support the valuing of technical skill over interpersonal skill. It is also evident that, within many occupational groups, women are less likely to be promoted to administrative positions or to be financially rewarded as generously as their male counterparts.

Although this argument within the nursing profession is open to debate, the challenges that women often negotiate as the primary caregivers in their personal or familial situations along with the demands of professional nursing practice are rigorous. The requirements of personal responsibilities may be experienced as incompatible with the additional demands of administrative work or participation in professional or union organizations, thus limiting the participation of nurses—in particular, women nurses—from positions of power and politics (Angus, 1994). This is not to suggest that men in nursing may rise to particular positions by virtue of being men, but it does open questions about the social landscape on which the realities of the demands of labor reside. Other questions may be raised as well. How do these social arrangements contribute to what some have called an "over-representation (of men) in top positions compared with their minority status in the profession" (Davies, 1995, p. 9)?

A feminist critique would suggest that we resist the temptation to assign responsibility for the work-life choices that women are forced to make to the individual nurse. Instead, we might examine the social conditions of nurses' lives, such as primary caregiving responsibilities, a lack of child-care resources, and the incompatibility of these social realities with the career demands of nursing.

Critical Feminist Analysis of the Issue

A critical feminist analysis questions the assumptions held about gender and often interrogates the intersection of gender with other discursive realities that form personal identity. In addition, this analysis of the gendered nature of nurse's work explores myths that underlie stereotypical gender roles, the meanings attached to *care* in nursing and some of the paradoxes for men in nursing.

Gender and the Intersectionality of Identity

In recognizing how dominant social discourses influence who we are to be, the production of identity becomes a discursive process (Scott, 1992). The term *discursive process* refers to how we learn to be, in particular ways, through the messages we receive in social discourses. Our concept of ourselves as gendered, the way we live as masculine and feminine, is one way in which we become people with particular identities. The gendered self is one of a number of the selves or identities through which we are uniquely formed as people. The gendered self intersects with other discursive processes such as race, class, age, ethnicity, and sexual orientation, in the constitution of each individual. It is not merely the "facts" of one's personal attributes that form this intersecting identity, but the relative value that is attributed to these identities in particular contexts. The experience of living one's life as a young, black, middle-class, heterosexual, male nursing student would be quite different from the experience of living as a white, middle-aged, working class, lesbian, single-mother nursing student. The difference of experience, although influenced by gender and what it means to be gendered in particular ways, is also constructed through material realities, such as economics and availability of social resources, as well as through the influence of dominant social discourses.

The idea of the intersecting identities of nurses is addressed in Reverby's (1987) historical critique of American nursing. In her exploration of some of the historical unrest in the discipline,

Reverby suggests that class differences among individual nurses and between groups of nurses with diverse training contributed to an internal hierarchy within nursing. Although the oppression of women was a reality for these nurses, they were also bound by their own participation in classist assumptions and ideologies. In this case, the "commonalities of the gendered experience could not become the basis for unity as long as hierarchical filial relations, not equal sisterhood, underlay nurses' lives" (Reverby, 1987, p. 201). Reverby describes a situation in which the class identities of these nurses held more influence than their shared gender identity.

The significance attributed to particular social positions and particular identities, including gender, is neither random nor benign. Collins (1997), a black feminist scholar, reminds us that "race, gender, social class, ethnicity, age and sexuality are not descriptive categories applied to individuals. Instead these elements of social structure emerge as fundamental devices that foster inequity in resulting groups" (p. 376). In other words, the meanings that are attached to these identities and social positions shape what is possible: The ways in which we live our lives and the ways that others see us. And while it is important to remember that not all of these differences matter in the same way, we are challenged to keep in our awareness the difference that the meanings attributed to gender makes.

Stereotypical Gender Attributes

In an article discussing the tensions between power and caring in the nursing profession, Falk Rafael (1996) itemizes the characteristics traditionally associated with femininity and masculinity as follows (p. 5):

FEMININITY	MASCULINITY
Submissiveness	Strength
Helplessness	Aggression
Dependency	Mastery
Tenderness	Independence
Nurturance	Logic
Altruism	Being unemotional
Competitiveness	
Ambition	

Falk Rafael (1996) notes that these traditional notions of femininity and masculinity have been constructed in a way that associates the masculine with power and the feminine with care.

Furthermore, we should note that these qualities are stereotypical, frequently inaccurate, and form the basis of unfounded assumptions about the abilities of men *and* women. In fact, "behavior that results from the underlying belief in sex role stereotypes" is named gender bias (Cushner et al., 2006, p.1 as cited in Crude & Winfrey, 2007). Nonetheless the prevalence of discourses supporting gender role stereotypes and the association of care with femininity play an active role in the construction of nursing as a feminized profession.

Discourses of Care

The association of nursing with *caring* is complicated by the social belief in care as an innately female quality. When viewed as a natural or essential quality—meaning care resides innately in all women—care is undervalued, as merely a "feminine virtue."

How is it that the value of care has been so compromised by society? Condon suggests we consider a feminist understanding that appreciates caring as a "positive dimension of our lives that has been socially devalued by a patriarchal and capitalistic order" (Condon, 1992, p. 73). In this way, the concept of care continues to be valued, and the effort is directed toward interrupting the social discourses that contribute to the devaluing of care. In contrast to duty and calling, which she calls "old masculine metaphors," Condon (1992) maintains that care provides an "infinitely more authentic metaphor grounded in the experience of women and capable of being practiced by anyone who chooses it as a social, as well as a professional, ethic" (p. 81).

A critical feminist analysis seeks to disrupt the notion of women as naturally caring. To say that women are naturally caring suggests that all women are caring, just by "nature" of being women. This also implies that men are not (as) caring as women. In reality, some women and some men in our culture are socialized to behave in caring ways. In addition, the "caring" that is involved in the caring relationship between a nurse and client is a "quality of relating" that is fully developed through nursing education, by nurses who are women and nurses who are men.

Men in Nursing

Although the commonly held history of nursing leads us to identify Nightingale as a lead figure in the development of nursing, another historical account of nursing places men at the center of nursing history (Cude & Winfrey, 2007). In this account, men, as members of the military and religious orders, formed the dominant gender of nurses during the Middle Ages. Male nurses provided care during plagues in Europe and during war time worldwide. According to Anthony (2004), Nightingale excluded men from nursing in her effort to construct a viable profession for women during Victorian times. Currently men are resuming their participation in the profession, although the percentage of male registered nurses in practice remains at 5.6% in Canada, with 41% of those men practicing in Quebec (2006 Workforce profile of Registered Nurses in Canada, retrieved from www.cna-aiic.ca).

Not surprisingly, men describe their experiences in nursing education and in practice as being treated differently by their female colleagues. More troubling, however, is that many men experience gender bias and discrimination in their nursing educational experience (Cude & Winfrey, 2007). While these authors suggest nurses and nurse educators may unwittingly participate in gender bias that is subconscious, it should go without saying that discrimination within the profession, based on any difference, be it gender, ethnicity or class, is unethical and undermines the integrity of the profession as a whole.

Walker (2009), a scholar and an academic in nursing in Australia, describes the situation of men in nursing as complex and puzzling. While acknowledging that men live with the experience of being a minority gender group in the profession, he further notes: "The paradox in this, as is well reported here and elsewhere, is that men enjoy enormous privilege and authority in nursing as they take up higher qualifications to advance their careers, rise up the ranks in education, management and clinical roles and take home more money; furthermore they achieve these goals in a shorter time than their female counterparts" (Walker, 2009, p.164). Similarly, Brian Brown (2009) concurs that men "appear to be well served by a career in nursing" (p. 120) and suggests that rather than focus on the individual difficulties that some men may experience in nursing, the profession would be better served by addressing the broader social inequities of gender and the sociopolitical context of the nursing.

Finally, in returning to the discussion of *caring* as central to nursing, it is worthwhile to note that men become nurses for the same reasons as women: Caring for others is identified as a principle reason for pursuing a career in nursing by both men and women (Cude & Winfrey, 2007; Kouta & Kaite, 2011).

BARRIERS TO AND STRATEGIES FOR ISSUE RESOLUTION

Several barriers to resolving the issues of the gendered nature of nursing need to be identified before strategies for change can be devised.

Identifying Barriers: Furthering Our Understandings

"The dilemma of nursing is too tied into the broader problems of gender and class in our society to be solved solely by the political efforts of one occupational group" (Reverby, 1987, p. 207). The barriers to the resolution of issues of gender in nursing are embedded in the society. As nurses, we require both the knowledge and the willingness to critique and to challenge these social discourses. In particular, we can consider the following barriers that impair movement toward understanding the issues:

1. The gendered nature of work in general, and nurses' work in particular, is concealed—or implicitly present—in nursing practice. Although the effects of gendering on nursing practice are part of our experience, there is a lack of discussion that identifies these experiences as the problematic effects of gender and power.
2. The effects of power and gender in nurses' work and nursing knowledge are taken for granted in nurses' practice and education. The lack of transparency regarding the gendered nature of nurses' work (see Barrier 1) contributes to our inability to question the embedded assumptions regarding gender and nurses' work.
3. Historically, nurses have lacked a critical feminist analysis that provides a framework to critique and question the taken-for-granted social discourses of gender, nurses' work, and the valuing of care in society.
4. Although the gendered divisions of labor have long been ingrained in society, only recently has the gendered nature of work been called into question in academic discourses that are accessible to nursing.
5. Understandings of the gendered nature of nurses' work are impaired by the lack of clarity and articulation of the nature of nurses' work in general. The inaccurate and limited public representations of the nurse and nurses' work contribute to the limited understanding and devaluing of nurses' work and nursing knowledge.
6. Individual efforts to disrupt the taken-for-granted ideas of gender require one to challenge social discourses and dominant views. This necessary strategy produces a barrier for the individual by placing her or him in tension with commonly held societal views.

Devising Strategies: Voice and Action

1. Several of the barriers to resolving issues of gender and power, and their impact on the significance attributed to nurses' work, can be broken down by providing knowledge regarding the gendered nature of nurses' work both historically and as it is currently embedded in nursing practice. The knowledge necessary for a thorough understanding of the gendered nature of nursing is complex and requires familiarity with a structure that can be used to critique and challenge the taken-for-granted assumptions embedded in these issues. Knowledge of the gendered nature of nurses' work may be supported by feminist analysis, which focuses on the idea of the formation of gendered subjects through social discourses and the disruption of those assumptions of gender conformity. This knowledge and the means to illuminate and question assumed truths belong in nursing curricula early in undergraduate nursing education. Much of the complexity of this knowledge lies in our lack of familiarity with concepts of gendering and social construction. As nurses become fluent in knowledge and language, the transparency regarding the gendered nature of nurses' work will improve.
2. As identified in the aforementioned barriers, there is a tension generated between the origin of social discourses of gender and the value of particular types of work in society, and the disruption of these discourses must begin at an individual level. Important strategies to interrupt discourses that undermine the significance attributed to nurses' work begin with increasing our own awareness of these taken-for-granted discourses in our daily lives. Influencing these discourses in ways that call into question the way things have always been or the way things have always been done requires confidence and courage for the individual nurse.

3. As members of society, nurses and women have been socialized to suppress difference. To challenge effectively what is taken for granted about the role of gender and its powerful influence on nurses' work, we must be willing to notice difference and to acknowledge the way that differences, such as gender, class, race, ethnicity, and sexual orientation, matter in the ways our identities are lived and viewed by the world. Nurse educators have a particular responsibility to bring to consciousness the experience of male student's experience as a member of the gender minority in the profession. As with other differences of identity we are ethically bound to develop a critical consciousness of gender bias in educational and professional practice settings.

4. Social discourses of gender are more than ideas. They are intimately connected to the social and material realities of our lives. Exerting influence that will change or disrupt discourses of gender necessitates action that will improve, in particular, the material realities of women's lives. This means, for example, advocating for changes in the workplace that support the lives of women as they negotiate family and work responsibilities and demands. Adequate resources for childcare and family responsibilities are gendered workplace issues. Attending to these needs influences the value and respect attributed to women's multiple roles, including the significance attributed to nurses' paid work.

S U M M A R Y

This chapter explores multiple issues associated with the gendered nature of nursing, of nurses' work, of nursing knowledge, and of the public representation of the nurse. Central to the issue are the social discourses about gender that are inherent in the value attributed to nurses' work and the importance attached to nurses' knowledge.

One question examined is: Is the value accorded to nurses' work representative of the societal devaluing of work that is ordinarily performed by women? The exploration extends our understanding of gender in nursing beyond the idea of the distribution of gender in the profession, that is, beyond the number of nurses who identify as women or men. The significance of nurses' work and the value accorded to this work are steeped in societal structures and discourses that surpass the particular gender of the nurse who is performing the work.

The gendered nature of nurses' work and education has been with us since the inception of nursing. The gendered division of labor has, according to the view of history, placed nursing in the realm of women's work, a division that was supported through the early educational program for nurses that focused on "womanly virtues" and "moral character." The legacy of this account of nursing has been the conceptualization of care as both an innately feminine virtue residing in all women and a discourse central to nursing practice. The significance of nurses' work parallels the devaluing of care in a society that has increasingly valued science and a production-focused economy.

Given the Victorian image of nursing as a natural extension of feminine virtues, we may be tempted to assign responsibility for "gendering" to the pioneering women of nursing practice and education. This chapter argues that the gendering of work occurs not with particular individuals but through society's discourses. The current and perhaps more difficult challenge is to recognize the less overt but no less present discourses of gender that structure current nursing practices. These discourses of gender—the nature of the work called "women's work" and the value that is afforded to caregiving in our society—underlie the significance of nurses' work.

In locating the discourses of gender in society, we need not look beyond ourselves. Our complicity is evident as we participate in the reinstatement of gendered discourses birthed in the societal ideologies from which we cannot extricate ourselves. The challenge, then, is to look for opportunities to recognize and to disrupt the taken-for-granted notions that define and constrain the possibilities for gendered people who are practicing and being nurses.

R E F L E C T I O N S *on the Chapter...*

1 How do you understand gender as socially constructed? What are the implications of your understanding for nurses, for nurses' work, and for nursing as a profession?

2 What does a feminist analysis of gender add to our understanding of the value and of nurses' work?

3 What are the benefits and limitations of placing gender in a central place in our analysis of nurses' work? How does gender intersect with other realities and conditions of nurses' lives?

4 How would you explain the social–political context that contributes to the paradox for men in nursing as both a minority gender and a group who are well served by a career in nursing?

5 From your own nursing experience, provide an example of your participation in a taken-for-granted, socially sanctioned norm regarding gender. In retrospect, how might you have acted to interrupt this particular social discourse around gender?

Want to know more? Visit the Point for additional helpful resources:

- Journal Articles
- Learning Objectives
- Nursing Professional Roles and Responsibilities
- Bonus chapters:
  - Health and Nursing Policy: A Matter of Politics, Power and Professionalism
  - The NP Movement: Recurring Issues
  - When Difference Matters: The Politics of Privilege and Marginality

References

Abbott, P., & Wallace, C. (Eds.). (1990). *The sociology of the caring professions.* London: Falmer Press.

Angus, J. (1994). Women's paid/unpaid work and health: Exploring the social context of everyday life. *Canadian Journal of Nursing Research, 26*(4), 23–42.

Anthony, AS. (2004). Gender bias and discrimination in nursing education: Can we change it? *Nurse Educator, 29*(3), 121–125.

Brown, B. (2009). Men in nursing: Re-evaluating masculinities, re-evaluating gender. *Contemporary Nurse, 33*(2), 120–129.

Bunting, S. (1992). Eve's legacy: An analysis of family caregiving from a feminist perspective. In J. Thompson, D. Allen, & L. Rodrigues-Fisher (Eds.), *Critique, resistance and action: Working papers in the politics of nursing* (pp. 53–68). New York: National League for Nursing Press.

Butler, J. (1990). Performative acts and gender constitution: An essay in phenomenology and feminist theory. In S. Case (Ed.), *Performing feminisms: Feminist critical theory and theatre* (pp. 270–282). Baltimore, MD: Johns Hopkins University Press.

Canadian Nurses Association (2006). *Workforce profile of Registered Nurses in Canada.* Retrieved from www.cna-aiic.ca

Cheek, J., & Rudge, T. (1994). The panopticon revisited? An exploration of the social and political dimensions of contemporary health care and nursing practice. *International Journal of Nursing Studies, 31*(6), 583–591.

Collins, P.H. (1997). Comment on Hekman's "Truth and method: Feminist standpoint theory revisited": Where's the power? *Signs: Journal of Women in Culture and Society, 22*(2), 375–381.

Condon, E. (1992). Nursing and the caring metaphor: Gender and political influences on an ethics of care. In J. Thompson, D. Allen, & L. Rodrigues-Fisher (Eds.), *Critique, resistance and action: Working papers in the politics of nursing* (pp. 69–84). New York: National League for Nursing Press.

Cude, G., & Winfrey, K. (2007). Hidden barrier gender bias: Fact or fiction. *AWHONN Nursing for Women's Health, 11*(3), 254–265.

Cushner, K., McClelland, A., & Safford, P. (2006). *Human diversity in education: An integrative approach.* Cited in Cude, G., & Winfrey, K. (2007). Hidden barrier gender bias: Fact or fiction. *AWHONN Nursing for Women's Health, 11*(3), 254–265.

Davies, C. (1995). *Gender and the professional predicament in nursing.* Philadelphia, PA: Open University Press.

Falk Rafael, A. (1996). Power and caring: A dialectic in nursing. *Advances in Nursing Science, 19*(1), 3–17.

Ginzberg, R. (1999). Uncovering gynocentric science. In E.C. Polifroni & M. Welch (Eds.), *Perspectives on philosophy of science in nursing: An historical and contemporary anthology* (pp. 440–450). Philadelphia, PA: Lippincott Williams & Wilkins.

Kouta, C., & Kaite, C. (2011). Gender discrimination and nursing: A literature review. *Journal of Professional Nursing, 27*(1), 59–63.

McGee, P. (2009). Who says we're all equal? Gender as an issue for nurses and nursing care. *Contemporary Nurse, 33*(2), 98–102.

Nakano Glenn E. (2000). The social construction and institutionalization of gender and race: An integrative framework. In M.M. Ferree, J. Lorber, & B. Hess (Eds.), *Revisioning gender* (pp. 3–43). New York: AltaMira Press.

Reverby, S. (1987). *Ordered to care: The dilemma of American nursing, 1850–1945.* Cambridge, UK: Cambridge University Press.

Scott, J. (1992). Experience. In J. Butler & J. Scott (Eds.), *Feminists theorize the political* (pp. 22–40). London: Routledge.

Thorne, S., McCormick, J., & Carty, E. (1997). Deconstructing the gender neutrality of chronic illness and disability. *Health Care for Women International, 18*(1), 1–16.

Turkoski, B. (1992). A critical analysis of professionalism in nursing. In J. Thompson, D. Allen, & L. Rodrigues-Fisher (Eds.), *Critique, resistance and action: Working papers in the politics of nursing* (pp. 149–166). New York: National League for Nursing Press.

Walker, K., & Holmes, C. (2008). The 'order of things': Tracing a history of the present through a re-reading of the past in nursing education. *Contemporary Nurse, 30*, 106–118.

Walker, K. (2009). Epilogue: Nursing, gender, aporia. *Contemporary Nurse, 33*(2), 163–165.

Welch, M. (1999). Science and gender. In E.C. Polifroni & M. Welch (Eds.), *Perspectives on philosophy of science in nursing: An historical and contemporary anthology* (pp. 423–426). Philadelphia, PA: Lippincott & Wilkins.

Workplace Realities

Chapter

16

Issues Arising from the Nature of Nurses' Work and Workplaces

Marjorie McIntyre and Carol McDonald

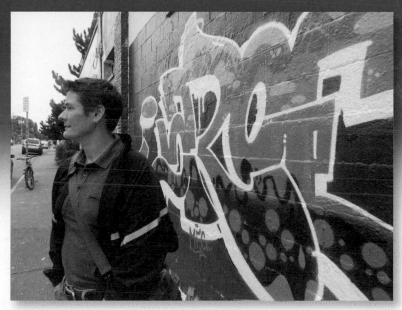

Nurses work in many environments and adapt to many conditions. The setting for this nurse is the inner city. (Used with permission. Photographer Andrea Monteiro.)

Critical Questions

As a way of engaging with the ideas in this chapter, consider the following:

1. Before beginning your nursing education, where did you imagine that nurses worked? How has that changed for you?

2. Before your first practicum experience, what work did you imagine nurses would do? How does this fit with the realities of your nursing experience?

3. What do you think nurses would identify as their major concerns around their work and their workplaces?

4. As a student, what, if any, concerns do you have about your future work and workplaces?

Chapter Objectives

After completing this chapter, you will be able to:

1. Articulate issues arising from the nature of nurses' work and their workplaces.

2. Frame and analyze issues arising from the nature of nurses' work and the places in which that work is carried out.

3. Identify barriers to resolving issues arising in nurses' work and workplaces.

4. Formulate strategies for resolving issues arising in nurses' work and workplaces.

5. Trace the links between nurses' work, nurses' health, and the health of Canadians.

6. Recognize the conflicting loyalties between the goals of organizations and nurses' professional goals.

This chapter highlights relevant issues arising from the nature of nurses' work and the significance of these issues for the health of nurses and the health of Canadians who need nursing care. Issues arising from the nature of nurses' work are closely related to and sometimes overlap the issues arising within the environments in which nurses' work takes place. However, there is increasing Canadian and international research substantiating the importance of understanding the nature of nurses' work as distinct from nurses' work environments. Thus, this chapter highlights some of the distinctions between the issues arising from the work that nurses do and the places in which this work takes place.

THE NATURE OF NURSES' WORK

Themes throughout the literature on the changing nature of nurses' work include confusion about what constitutes nurses' work, the increasing demands of nurses' work, the lack of control that nurses have over the work they do, and the incongruity between what nurses are prepared as professionals to do and what they are expected to do in practice.

The lack of clarity in defining nurses' work is due in part to the lack of clear boundaries between nurses' work and non-nurses' work and the increasing expectation that nurses perform work other than nursing care. Changes in administrative structures and in the way auxiliary workers are utilized means nurses take on work that has been traditionally performed by others. In other situations, nursing practices have been relinquished to auxiliary workers. In addition to the increasing demand to do more work, nurses are also faced with the increasing demands of the work itself. Patients in care are more acutely ill, and the care nurses provide is increasingly complex. There are demands on nurses for increasing technical competence.

In practice, nurses are often faced with a lack of control over the work they do. Decisions about what care will be provided, who will provide that care, and in what setting the care will be provided are made by someone other than the nurses expected to provide the care. Nurses' work often occurs in a climate of diminished resources without support to meet the demands of their work with competence and confidence. The increased demands of nurses' work and the lack of support provided to sustain the work may contribute to the disturbing reality that nurses are unable to nurse in the ways that they have come to expect they should. Nurses increasingly experience incongruities between the work that they are prepared to do, both educationally and philosophically, and the expectations that they encounter in practice.

THE NATURE OF NURSES' WORKPLACES

The nature of nurses' work and the workplaces themselves are interrelated; both contribute to nurses' experiences of job satisfaction, recruitment and retention, and well-being. For example, many writers and researchers have linked Canada's current nursing shortage to inadequate and inferior work environments (Ceci & McIntyre, 2001). Baumann et al. (2001) claim, "Canada's nursing shortage is at least in part due to a work environment that burns out the experienced and discourages new recruits. But that environment can be changed" (p. iii). Despite the seriousness of the real and potential shortcomings of nurses' work environments, there is evidence that governments, employers, and nurses are taking action to improve the situation. Further, there is an acknowledgment on the part of these groups that they must work together to create and maintain healthy nurse workplaces. Research suggests that recruitment and retention strategies will be successful only if this action is implemented on a large scale (Sochalski, 2001). More recently, Laschinger et al. (2009) suggest that despite our knowledge of what constitutes healthy workplaces for nurses, we have yet to act on this evidence.

Understanding what constitutes a healthy work environment and selecting those environments in which to work will positively affect not only the individual's work-life experience but also the quality of care that individual is able to deliver. As more desirable work environments are created, nurses already in practice will undoubtedly be attracted to those employment situations, promoting the continued production of healthy work environments. Some employers offer nurses and other employees onsite services that have been identified as indicative of a quality work environment, such as fitness centers, hot food services 24 hours a day, wellness programs, and provision of onsite childcare (Baumann et al., 2001).

THE SIGNIFICANCE OF NURSES' WORK ISSUES

Issues arising from the nature of nurses' work relate directly to the recruitment and retention of nurses, the health of the nursing workforce, and the quality of care that nurses are able to deliver. The belief that all we need to do to address the recurrent shortages of nurses is to produce more nurses overlooks the point that it is the issues arising from the nature of nurses' work that sustain and perpetuate nursing shortages. Unless these issues are addressed, it is unlikely that existing vacancies will be filled, that student enrollments will increase, or that nurses, given other opportunities, will stay in nursing. This chapter challenges the inevitability of healthcare systems doing more with less in the short term when downsizing and restructuring occur at the expense of nurses' health and well-being.

For the most part, nurses' work environments are and always have been complex, and barriers to providing quality professional practice environments are considerable. However, given the authority, adequate resources, and support of colleagues, it is assumed at the outset of writing this chapter that nurses can provide such quality practice environments as those envisioned by the Canadian Nurses Association (CNA).

According to the CNA position statement (2001, p. 1) on nurses' work environments, nurses have an obligation to their patients to "demand practice environments that have the organizational and human support allocations necessary for safe, competent and ethical nursing care." The CNA position states that a quality nursing practice environment for professional nurses is one in which "the needs and goals of the individual nurse are met at the same time the patient or client is assisted to reach his or her individual health goals, within the costs and quality framework mandated by the organization where the care is provided" (p. 1). The CNA holds that the development and support of quality practice environments for professional nurses are responsibilities shared by practitioners, employers, regulatory bodies, professional associations, educational institutions, unions, and the public.

In November 2006 the CNA Board of Directors approved a joint position statement titled "Practice Environments: Maximizing Client, Nurse and System Outcomes," jointly developed by the CNA and the Canadian Federation of Nursing Unions (CFNU). This document extends the earlier CNA position statement by identifying seven characteristics of quality practice environments (Box 16.1).

ISSUES ARISING IN NURSES' WORK AND WORKPLACES

In any discussion of nurses' work, one cannot overlook the nature of the work itself and the availability of nurses to do this work. Despite the positive initiatives of select groups of employers, for many Canadian nurses the realities of the workplace continue to be reflected in themes of professional and social isolation; disrupted workplaces, and acts of bullying that result in alienation from nurse leaders, peers, and other professionals; inadequate educational, mentorship, and

---

BOX 16.1   Characteristics of Quality Practice Environments

Quality practice environments identified in the "Canadian Nurses Association & Canadian Federation of Nurses Unions Joint Position Statement" demonstrate the following characteristics:

1. *Communication and collaboration*—Quality practice environments promote effective communication and collaboration throughout the system: Among nurses, between nurses and clients, between nurses and other health and non-health professionals, between nurses and unregulated workers, and between nurses and system managers and employers.
2. *Responsibility and accountability*—Nurses are professionals; they are responsible and accountable for their practice. Therefore, nurses must be supported in their practice environments to participate in decision making that affects their work, including developing policies, allocating resources, and providing client care.
3. *Realistic workload*—Quality practice environments support continuity of care and enable nurses to maintain competence, develop holistic therapeutic relationships, and create work-life balance. There must be sufficient nurses to provide safe, competent, and ethical care. Together with supportive employer policies and effective relationships with team members, sufficient time will allow nurses to practice at their full level of competence, to meet the "Code of Ethics for Registered Nurses," and to meet jurisdictional standards of practice.
4. *Leadership*—Effective leadership is important in all nursing roles and is an essential element for quality practice environments. Nurses who are employers have a direct impact on nurses' work environments, but nurses who act as collaborators, communicators, mentors, role models, visionaries, and advocates for quality care also play a leadership role.
5. *Support for information and knowledge management*—Quality practice environments include enabling technologies to support optimal information and knowledge management as well as critical thinking (e.g., electronic health records and decision support tools). Adequate time for nurses to access these technologies is important.
6. *Professional development*—Quality practice environments must be adequately funded to allow nurses to access professional development opportunities to develop and maintain competence. These opportunities include continuing education, formal education, online learning, and mentoring.
7. *Workplace culture*—A quality practice environment creates a workplace culture that values the well-being of clients and employees. The culture must be continually assessed and evaluated with an interest in improving client, nursing, and system outcomes. Contributions to a positive workplace culture include, but are not limited to, policies that address ethical issues, support safety, promote employee recognition, and ensure adequate resources.

From: Canadian Nurses Association (CNA) & Canadian Federation of Nurses Unions (CFNU). (2006). *Practice environments: Maximizing client, nurse and system outcomes* [Joint Position Statement]. Retrieved from http://www.cna-aicc.ca

---

substantive orientation programs for new nurses; decreased levels of support for professional development; and the failure of governments and the public to recognize and support the need for change in nurses' workplaces. Despite the well-documented lack of control over their work and work environments, nurses continue to be held accountable for and, in some cases, hold themselves accountable for providing quality practice environments and safe, competent, and ethical care. The following sections contain an expanded discussion of these issues.

Professional Accountability and the Issue of Workplace Bullying

The lack of documentation about the history of acts of bullying behavior might suggest that bullying, as we currently understand it, is on the increase within the profession. However, all we can accurately know is that bullying is a topic that is emerging in the nursing literature. As research becomes available on the experience of people being bullied, and of others observing and reporting bullying in the work place, with limited action being taken on behalf of the victims (Laschinger et al., 2010) the urgency of this issue is apparent.

In a 2011 issue of *Canadian Nurse* (Eggertson, 2011) an article told of accounts of numerous nurses facing bullying so intense that it disrupted their personal lives and health, and in some instances led to nurses leaving the profession. This same article reports that, "in 2010, Toronto

> ## BOX 16.2   Common Bullying Behaviors
>
> Recent studies report that the most common bullying behaviors among nurses are:
>
> * Being allocated an unmanageable workload
> * Being ignored or excluded
> * Having rumors spread about you
> * Being ordered to carry out work below your competence level
> * Having your professional opinion ignored
> * Having information relevant to your work withheld
> * Being given impossible targets or deadlines
> * Being humiliated or ridiculed about your work

Adapted from: Cleary, M., Hunt, G., & Horsfall, J. (2010). Identifying and addressing bullying in nursing. *Issues in Mental Health Nursing, 31,* 332.

researcher Claire Mallette led a study on horizontal violence with the University Health Network. Of the 160 nurses involved in the study, 95 per cent had observed horizontal violence and 71 per cent identified themselves as targets" (p. 18). In addition, the publication and national circulation of this article resulted in an unprecedented number of letters to the editor from a groundswell of Canadian nurses dealing with bullying in the workplace either currently or in their previous practice settings.

So what is workplace bullying and how would one recognize this behavior? Drawing on recent research, Cleary et al. (2010), provide a useful overview of common bullying behaviors, listed herein Box 16.2. Additional behaviors referred to throughout the literature include excessive criticism, over-checking, sabotaging, being ignored, given "the silent treatment," and being blamed for things that are beyond the person's control. Kathleen Bartholomew, a Seattle-based RN and the author of *Ending Nurse-to-Nurse Hostility* cited in the Eggertson's (2011) article wisely reminds us "The biggest thing I want nurses to know is that bullying is not OK...tolerating the abuse helps to entrench it in the workplace—and that makes the environment unsafe for everyone" (p. 21).

Problematic Experiences of New Graduates

A particular group of nurses for whom the professional practice environment, including susceptibility to bullying, is an issue, is that of new graduates. It is well known that a nurse's first year of work is stressful and that the number of nurses leaving the profession in the first year of practice is high. After more than a decade of research on this topic, what Viens claimed in 1996, that new graduates continue to suffer when "the work situation proves to be very different from what they have been taught" (p. 44), continues to be relevant today. Canadian researchers (Rhéaume et al., 2011, p. 498) claim that a little under half (45%) of the 348 new graduate nurses in their study, conducted in eastern Canada, were considering leaving their current employer. As with the 1996 study, the authors of the 2011 study report that new graduates are less likely to leave practice when they are "able to practise in an environment supportive of a nursing philosophy...Thus, a work environment allowing these nurses to give patient care according to how they were taught in their educational programs is a priority." Put another way, these researchers maintain that new graduates "able to practise in an environment which allows them to apply the skills, knowledge and values acquired in school is imperative" (Rhéaume et al., 2011, p. 498).

Significant findings echoed in numerous studies include the need for support of new graduates in the form of orientation programs, mentorship, and nurse manager leadership (Rhéaume et al., 2011; Scott et al., 2008). Numerous innovative programs across Canada support new graduates and their mentors through the provision of release time and reduced responsibilities for both participants. An outstanding of such a program is found at St. Michael's Hospital in Toronto where the "New Graduate Internship Program offers a three to six month orientation, mentoring, and onboarding program that assist new graduate nurses to make the transition from nursing students/graduates to confident and independent practitioners" (recruitment—nursing—graduates.pdf, www.stmichaelshospital.com/careers/index.php).

The Changing Demands of Nurses' Work

Although one can cite many examples of the increasing volume of nurses' work, it is important not to overlook the demands of increasing acuity and complexity of patient care. Baumann et al., (2001) conclude that the discrepancy between the work demanded of nurses and what nurses can reasonably give because of increased patient acuity and complexity of care creates an imbalance that threatens the health of nurses and "puts patients throughout Canada at risk" (p. 4).

The care provided by nurses is thought to be more complex than ever before. O'Brien-Pallas et al. (2001) reported that the acuity of patients has increased steadily since 1994. Nurses have the added responsibility of providing care not only to individual patients but also to families and communities; this suggests that nurses' work is increasingly physically, intellectually, and emotionally demanding (Baumann et al., 2001). Studies also show that, in addition to the increased demands brought on by patient acuity and complexity of care, the effects of hospital downsizing and restructuring of the last decade continue to intensify nurses' work (Choiniere, 2011). The ways in which healthcare restructuring participates in the changing demands of nurses' work is addressed later in this chapter under the discussion of lack of control over nurses' work.

Although the work of Gaudine is more than a decade old, the compelling message of nurses workload is as relevant and meaningful as when it was first published in 2000. In a descriptive study in which 31 nurses were interviewed, Gaudine offers narration of the experiences of workload—and work overload—from the nurses' accounts. Although nurses' descriptions of what constituted work overload varied significantly, the message was clear as can be seen in the following narrations.

Simultaneous demands were apparent in situations in which study subjects talked about being expected to do more than one thing at a time and to be in more than one place at a time:

> A doctor is asking me questions.... Meanwhile a patient's relative is standing beside me and wants something, and the phone is ringing. I have to get a patient ready to go to X-ray. Then the doctor wants a dressing changed and I know the vitals need taking on my patient receiving blood.
> *(Gaudine, 2000, p. 24)*

In a second example of work overload, Gaudine (2000) describes "qualitative work overload," in which the nurses' experiences of work overload are attributed by the nurses to the unfamiliar nature of the work. The following example richly illuminates one nurse's experience with this:

> It was the night shift, and I had never done [total parenteral nutrition (TPN)] before. I had eight charts to look over. The TPN lines hadn't been changed on days and had to be done for around 8 PM. I spent a half hour with the procedure manual, which for me is useless. I want to see it, not just read it. The dressing set didn't have what the procedure book said it would. It was 9:30 PM by the time I finished it, and I hadn't even looked at the other patients' charts (p. 25).

"Heavy load" is another dimension of the work that Gaudine (2000) describes. Heavy load involves situations in which there is just too much work to do and is exemplified by this nurse's response:

> I can't believe we have to be here for twelve hours and often have to miss our breaks. And I just get the expectations of nurses is really, like super nurse, to do an incredible amount, and I think it is just too much. To work twelve hours, and I can't even go out to lunch, like at any other job (p. 25).

The final example of work overload is illustrated by a situation in which nurses are, by virtue of their competence and experience, responsible directly for the care of the patients assigned to them and also responsible indirectly for the patients assigned to other nurses on their unit. One of the nurses in Gaudine's (2000) study talks about this dilemma in a way that resonates with other accounts throughout the literature: "Most [nurses] are more junior than me and may have trouble doing new things...Just to be cautious, I stayed on the unit at break today, because there was a very sick child and so many new nurses" (p. 25).

Many researchers and practicing nurses identify workload as the most significant issue for nurses directly and indirectly because of links between nurses' work, nurses' health, and the health of patients in their care (Baumann et al., 2001; Burke & Greenglass, 2000; Cockerill & O'Brien-Pallas, 1990; Laschinger & Leiter, 2006; O'Brien-Pallas et al., 1997; Shullanberger, 2000; White, 1997).

Lack of Control Over Nurses' Work

Commitment and Care: The Benefits of Healthy Workplaces for Nurses, Their Patients and the System, by Baumann et al. (2001), makes an important contribution to our understanding of issues arising from the nature of nurses' work in Canada. Although this seminal work is now more than a decade old, the findings remain relevant today. Drawing on the earlier work of Kristensen (1999), Baumann identified six principles that constitute an optimal work environment for nurses' social and psychological well-being. Baumann's work incorporates a review of literature, including relevant policy documents on the topic as well as the findings of focus group discussions with nurses in practice across Canada. The term *control* as it is used here can be understood as both control over the work that nurses do and control over the ways in which that work is organized in practice. Since Baumann's research in the area, nurse scholars have continued to develop understandings of the increasing lack of control nurses' have over their work, particularly in the face of the ongoing effects of reorganization of healthcare to align with a business model of healthcare delivery (Choiniere, 2011).

This business model of care raises tensions for nurses between professional accountability for patient care and institutional demands for financial accountability. Beginning in the 1990s and continuing today, institutional financial accountability dramatically overshadows accountability for patient care. The reform initiatives that have led to this restructured focus of fiscal accountability reflect the values implicit in the "competitive, market-based principles of the private sector" (Choiniere, 2011, p. 330). The pressure for nurses to practice under these market-based principles erases the possibility for nurses to practice according to nursing philosophy, or to provide care in the way in which they were educated to do and highlights the incompatibility of these two competing approaches to accountability.

In another discussion, "the incommensurability of nursing as a practice and the customer service model" (Austin, 2011) is framed as a threat to the discipline itself. Austin evocatively suggests that what is sometimes labeled "compassion fatigue" is in fact the effect of nurses being denied the opportunity to practice in a way that is congruent with the compassion they intend. Links are made between the barriers that separate nurses from compassionate care and the system wide move toward market-based principles in health care (Austin, 2011).

In the 2001 study, Baumann et al. (2001) reported that research participants strongly supported the need for nurses to have input into the "patient-care decisions related to their practice" (p. 9). Similarly in 2011, Choiniere finds that ongoing reorganization of practice threatens both the quality of care and the health of nurses. Nurses stressed the importance of having their say in "all aspects of care within their scope of practice, including serving as patient advocates" (Baumann et al., 2001, p. 9). Nurses in the 2001 study experienced difficulty in playing "significant roles in policy-making" or in communicating "effectively with decision makers" because of being "under-represented in institutional hierarchies" (p. 10). A decade later, nurses continue to identify the accountability gap of healthcare administrators who act without adequate consultation, or collaboration in advance of reforms, as well as take responsibility for the ongoing monitoring of the effects of these reforms. In this same study, nurse participants "identified a serious accountability gap in their descriptions of managers who are absent for both patients and nurses as their focus has been reorganized away from the point of care" (Choiniere, 2011, p. 342).

For nurses to experience control over their work, they must be central in the policy decisions that direct work-life issues, such as scheduling full-time to part-time staff ratios, casual nurses, and auxiliary workers. The failure to gain control over and have meaningful input into one's practice influences nurses' commitment to their practice and the decisions they make about remaining in practice. Nurses who are satisfied with their work and the organization of their work show a higher commitment to their practice. Research shows that the job satisfaction level of the nursing staff strongly determines the satisfaction level of the patients in their care (Baumann et al., 2001).

Analyzing Issues Arising from the Nature and Conditions of Nurses' Work

Issues arising from the nature of nurses' work and the conditions within and under which this work is performed are not new. Although the rationale for making nurses' work-related issues a priority has varied across time, overall, governments, employers, and even nurse leaders have failed to address these issues in a way that resulted in lasting effects.

Clearly, more than the temporary provision of resources or superficial changes in nurses' working conditions is at stake in this issue. Each of these elements—numbers, working conditions, and work satisfaction—incorporates underlying and unexamined assumptions about the nature of nurses' work, nursing knowledge, and the relationship of each to power structures in healthcare and society. What follows is a discussion of different frameworks for analysis and the possibilities they generate for understanding issues arising from the nature and conditions of nurses' work.

Historical Understandings of Nurses' Work

In reviewing historical literature, one gets a sense that the nature of nurses' work has always been idealized—and less than ideal (Gibbon & Mathewson, 1947). What we can learn from historical analysis is how the issues have been sustained over time and the implications this has for the current situation and for long-term planning of healthcare provision.

Despite the evidence of declining enrollments and an inadequate supply of nurses to fill current positions, many employers continue to assume that one can still "recruit women interested in self-denial, servitude and the expression of their natural qualities as women...the workplace still operates to some extent on that basis—expecting nurses to work harder than ever for less and less" (Stuart, 1993, p. 22). Although many nurses in the past expressed a deep dissatisfaction with nurses' work, what has changed is that, today, nurses are more likely to view themselves as professional and their work as a career rather than to understand nursing as a calling to servitude. With this view of professional work, nurses who stay in the profession do so knowing they have choices. Nurses now have many more opportunities to leave the profession and work elsewhere than they did in the past.

Social and Cultural Analysis

Priorities placed on nurses' work and the value attributed by society and by nurses to this work have often been linked to economic rather than social realities (Choiniere, 2011; Donner et al., 1994). The issues arising from the nature of nurses' work would benefit from a social and cultural analysis that considers the social realities of nurses' lives, nurses' health, and the quality of patient care.

A social and cultural analysis reminds us that considering the realities of nurses' lives must include consideration of the realities of the lives of women in our society. Nurses facing issues of increasing demands and lack of support for their work simultaneously experience the demands of the multiple roles in their nonworking lives as women. Prevailing attitudes in society suggest that work and personal lives are separate domains. This attitude privileges particular members of society and fails to take into account the realities of the lives of women as mothers, care providers, community supporters, and volunteers juggled alongside their paid work as nurses. Issues that arise from mandatory callback, overtime, and the increased workload demands of nursing compromise the quality of nurses' lives, their well-being, and their energy to participate fully in both their personal and professional lives.

Professional organizations and individual nurses have lobbied, and continue to lobby, government representatives for changes that would empower nurses to control their workplaces and that would provide the resources needed for safe, competent, and ethical nursing care. Yet as our history unfolds, it is the values and priorities of the dominant culture rather than those that are representative of nursing or the recipients of nursing care that continue to influence this issue.

Despite a growing awareness of how professions whose members are predominantly women are disadvantaged, decisions about nurses' work and their workplaces continue to be made by non-nurses. Decisions about nurses' work and nurses' work environments are increasingly based on criteria derived from business, management, and economic models rather than on the needs of the populations nurses serve (Choiniere, 2011; Taft & Steward, 2000; White, 1997).

Nurses and their managers continue to hear explanations of budget cuts that have forced them to reconceptualize services without the opportunity for nurses or their leaders to provide input about what patients need in terms of care. Moreover, nurses have insufficiently understood and critiqued the ways in which these values and priorities put the needs of the dominant culture over other members of society (Davies, 1995). As the culture of healthcare delivery shifts to that of a market-driven model, the work of managers becomes further and further removed from nursing at the point of care. When managers are co-opted by the agenda of a market-driven or business model of care, nurses are unsupported in delivering care that is congruent with their professional values (Austin, 2011).

Political Analysis

Typically, issues arising from the nature of nurses' work come to the foreground when recruitment and retention issues arise, but these issues tend to fade from public awareness and concern once the numbers (shortages) problem is averted. Significantly, once vacant positions are filled, concern about nurses' work tends to be put aside as a topic for serious debate. The failure of governments, employers, professional organizations, and nurses to address adequately the issues arising from the nature of nurses' work is linked to the failure to understand the implications of such conditions and their significance for the health of Canadians.

A political analysis asks who benefits from this issue being resolved and who benefits from things staying the same. Nurses and the patients they care for stand to benefit from the resolution of issues arising from the nature of nurses' work. Employers, however, may benefit from some of these issues remaining as they are. For example, the lack of clarity between nursing and non-nursing work allows employers to exploit nurses in assigning multiple roles to them. This exploitation serves managers as well as nurses to take on the work of other professionals and clerical staff when needed but it undermines the control that nurses have over what constitutes nurses' work. When nurses are engaged in non-nursing work in addition to their patient care, it is the patient care, the real work of nurses, that is compromised.

Ethical Analysis

Professional codes, such as the CNA "Code of Ethics" and the provincial and territorial scope of practice guidelines, direct nurses to advocate for patients in the provision of healthcare. Legislative acts, such as the Canada Health Act and the Health Professions Act, mandate nurses as professionals to provide competent, ethical care. Collective bargaining and labor laws are in place to protect nurses from the demands of overwork, to control the hours of work, and to ensure safe practice standards. Despite these multiple levels of regulation of nurses' work, governmental agencies and employers continue, uninterrupted, to demand work of nurses that erodes these guidelines.

Ethical questions are raised about the health of nurses and the subsequent healthcare provided to patients. These quandaries include the risks to patients when a nurse who has worked many shifts without leave or entire shifts without a break becomes vulnerable to fatigue and a consequent increased risk for making errors. Ethical questions may also evolve from the added responsibility felt by nurses when they are working with other nurses whose competence is compromised by unfamiliarity with the work demanded of them or with the fatigue of overwork.

Economic Analysis

An economic analysis highlights how the forces of supply and demand work in a particular issue. For issues related to nurses' workplaces, one may explore the influence nurse leaders have in challenging purely cost-containment strategies when the health of Canadians is thought to be at risk. A purely economic analysis of these issues could lead, and has led to nurses being asked to do with less. Sochalski (2001, p. 15) reminds us that "economics provides the framework for the allocation of resources," and the economics question facing nursing is not what the value of nursing care is but rather "how to allocate this valuable resource to best meet the health care needs of our patients and our population."

The difficulty with talking about healthcare and nursing care in purely economic terms is that it overlooks other costs. What needs to be made more transparent to the public is the high cost and incredible waste of resources resulting from the short-term slashing of funds, the closure of needed health facilities, and the withdrawal of life-sustaining services. A point to consider here is that the position statement obligating nurses to demand quality practice environments includes a phrase suggesting that this be done "within the costs and quality framework mandated by the organization where the care is provided" (CNA, 2001, p. 1). The concern is that such wording supports the claim that governments would provide differently if they could, a point that, in many cases, has been accepted without question.

BARRIERS TO RESOLVING WORK AND WORKPLACE ISSUES

Perhaps the most significant barrier to the resolution of workplace issues is the reality that many decisions that affect the quality of nurses' work environment are beyond the control of nurses themselves. The environmental influences that contribute to nurses' work as rewarding, satisfying, and engaging, for new graduates and others, is well known. The barriers to the changes that are needed to establish or return to satisfying work places are largely seen as systemic. Issues such as the organization of nurses' work and the distance of people in nursing leadership and management positions from the point of care can currently be seen as resting on decisions made by people other than nurses themselves. The failure to recognize the impact of the current situation on the health of patients and of nurses, by the decision makers in health care, is in itself a serious barrier. While on one hand these barriers might seem insurmountable, the costs of nurses leaving the profession, for the discipline, and for the Canadian healthcare system, mandate that nursing must mobilize to engage with these issues.

STRATEGIES FOR RESOLVING WORK AND WORKPLACE ISSUES

Research studies over the previous decade provide compelling evidence that the issues arising from the nature of nurses' work can and must change (Baumann et al., 2001; Choiniere, 2011). They challenge the notion that these issues are a problem for nurses to address; instead, the studies assign responsibility for the current situation of nurses' work and the threat of a system-wide shortage of nurses to governments, employers, and professional organizations.

Strategies to overcome the existing barriers to resolving issues that arise from the nature of nurses' work are those that "enable nurses to practice in a way that optimizes the use of their knowledge and expert judgment" in their practice (Laschinger et al., 2001, p. 240). "Work environments that provide opportunities to learn and grow" and "support creative strategies" in nurses' work are those that will be considered health promoting for nurses and those to whom they provide care (p. 240). Strategies increasing "decision-making latitude" (the extent to which a worker has control over the job and how it is done) will "moderate the effects of high levels of psychological demands" (p. 239) and enhance the quality of nurses' work lives.

In her research on work overload, Gaudine (2000) stressed the importance of administrators listening carefully to the accounts of nurses' experiences of workload as part of verifying what a particular workload might be. Although one can make use of the tools available to get some indication of workload, one should not interpret the findings of such tools without considering the particularities of the nurse or nurses involved. An additional insight gained from Gaudine's study was that even in situations in which it is not possible to alter the workload or change the conditions at that particular time, taking the time to understand a particular nurse's experience of workload or work overload can make a contribution to the quality of a nurse's work life through validation and support.

In their work on "moral climate," understood as "the implicit and explicit values that drive healthcare delivery and shape the workplaces in which healthcare is delivered" (Rodney et al., 2006, p. 24) offer valuable insights for addressing many of the workplace issues discussed earlier in this chapter. Drawing on their studies with nurses on the enactment of moral agency and ethical policy and practice, these researchers have made a significant contribution to the knowledge needed for change to occur. This group of authors note that nurses in practice already know what is needed to create a moral climate: What is required is "the opportunity for self-reflection and for true collaboration with their colleagues in management, administration, and other health-care disciplines to make it happen" (p. 27) (Box 16.3).

The issue of bullying in nursing practice has recently gained increased prominence in the nursing literature. Some authors suggest that bullying behavior can be linked to healthcare restructuring, a sense of powerless among staff, and the increasing distance of nurse managers from the point of care (Cleary et al., 2010). Strategies to address workplace bullying have been suggested (see Box 16.4), although what is most important and often overlooked is that everyone who is aware of bullying behavior becomes complicit in the abuse if it is not addressed.

In making reference to the many challenges and limited benefits that nursing offers, the report of Baumann et al., (2001) on the benefits of a healthy work experience for nurses predicts that if nursing is to "remain a viable profession, its status must be enhanced and the welfare of nurses promoted" (p. 13). In their policy synthesis on the benefits of a healthy work experience for nurses and the patients they care for, Baumann et al., (2001) stressed that governments, professional organizations, employers, educators, and researchers must act together to promote patient welfare by facilitating healthy work experiences for nurses. What

BOX 16.3 Creating a Safer Moral Climate in the Workplace

- An explicit ethical and moral (value-based) dimension must be included in research on nursing practice and nurses' workplaces.
- The moral climate of healthcare workplaces shapes the safety of patients and the safety of healthcare providers.
- Nurses in all facets of the profession need to be supported in using the language of ethics to name problems in nursing practice and in the quality of care they deliver, including matters of patient safety.
- To improve ethical practice, nurses must work proactively with other disciplines to identify problems in the moral climate in which they practice and to come up with solutions.
- Nurses in advanced practice and in other leadership positions are well situated to identify problems in the moral climate of nursing and interdisciplinary practice.
- In the current moral climate, nurses in direct-care delivery roles often feel powerless when confronting problems with the structural and interpersonal resources available to them. These nurses must be actively and systematically involved in planning, implementing, and evaluating changes in their practice environments.
- Nurses in all facets of the profession (practice, research, management, and education) need more opportunity to reflect on their practice, on the quality of their interactions with others, and on the resources they need to maintain their own well-being.
- While personal reflection and individual action are important, collective action is necessary if meaningful changes are to be made to work environments. This collective action must involve nurses in direct care and in leadership roles.

Adapted from: Rodney, P., Doane, G., Storch, J., et al. (2006). Toward a safer moral climate. *Canadian Nurse, 102*(8), 27.

follows are a selection of the key points identified by this research team (Baumann et al., 2001).

Key points for governments include the following:

- Revise funding formulas to better support the many dimensions of nursing practice.
- Set rules for using the funds, and monitor how they are spent.
- Support the welfare of nurses by providing funds to increase staff so managers can assign workloads that consider the acuity and complexity of patient care.
- Ensure the supply of nurses in the future by investing in continuing education, including baccalaureate and postgraduate education.

Key points for professional associations and councils include the following:

- Continue to advocate for nurses and advise governments and employers to allow nurses to practice to their full scope.
- Share recruitment and retention strategies, and promote nursing through advertising and marketing strategies.

BOX 16.4 Strategies for Managing Bullying Behaviors

Six steps necessary for the prevention of workplace bullying:

1. Develop a policy or unit specific code of conduct
2. Create awareness of acceptable and unacceptable workplace behavior
3. Recognize risk factors and support those at risk
4. Inform, instruct, and train all staff including managers
5. Control risks by developing a strong sense of community in the workplace
6. Promote speaking out and safe reporting to bodies with the power to act

Modified from: Cleary, M., Hunt, G., & Horsfall, J. (2010). Identifying and addressing bullying in nursing. *Issues in Mental Health Nursing, 31,* 331–335.

Key points for employers include the following:

- Address staffing issues by hiring sufficient nurses to ensure a reasonable workload.
- Address issues of staff mix and full-time and part-time statuses.
- Work with unions to develop flexible scheduling that suits both nurses and employers.
- Engage nurses on units in the recruitment and hiring processes.
- Adopt the most effective tools for measuring and allocating workload.
- Recognize effort and achievement with economic remuneration and other rewards.
- Support nursing leadership and professional development.
- Monitor nurses' health.
- Promote recruitment and retention of graduates into the workforce.

Key points for educators include the following:

- In partnership with employers, governments, and nursing associations, integrate new nurses into the workplace through such strategies as clinical internships and cooperative programs.
- Ensure a match between the curriculum and the skills required in the workplace.
- Teach leadership skills, healthcare policy, and work-life health issues for nurses.
- Work with nursing associations on scope-of-practice issues.

Key points for researchers include the following:

- Develop databases, workload-measurement instruments, and human resources forecasting tools.
- Conduct studies to evaluate the effectiveness of strategies to improve nurses' well-being.

The strategies suggested in this chapter are directed toward individuals and groups with the power to sustain or to revise the structures and ideologies that underlie the issues arising from the nature of nurses' work. Societal and cultural analysis, in particular, helps us to recognize that the burden for the resolution of these issues does not rest with individual nurses but with governments, professional groups, employers, and labor groups.

What, then, is the role of the individual nurse in coping with and contributing to the establishment of a healthier work experience for nurses and, subsequently, to improved patient care? Perhaps the most powerful action that individual nurses can take is to disrupt or to interrupt the dominant discourse in society regarding the assumption that healthcare organization could benefit from the market driven values of the private sector. Rather nurses must continue to articulate the alternative discourse of nursing as the provision of compassionate individualized care for patients. Critical reflection on the disjuncture between the values of nursing and those of a market-driven system can move nurses toward what Pauly et al. (2009) refer to as "deepening political consciousness" (p. 122). When given the opportunity, nurses can make their voices heard with governments, professional associations, and labor groups by broadcasting the issues of justice and health arising from the nature of nurses' work as it is currently experienced.

SUMMARY

Although historically the nature of nurses' work has been less than ideal, the changes in nurses' work and the issues that have arisen from this work in the past decade have seriously compromised nurses' ability to provide quality care in some circumstances and even adequate care in others. Nurses' work has undergone dramatic changes without corresponding support to moderate the effect of these changes. Increased workloads and work overload, higher patient acuity and care complexity, and increased job insecurity in the workplace have had an overwhelming effect on how nurses experience their work. The impact of the issues that arise from the nature of nurses' work can be seen in the way nurses care for their patients and ultimately contributes to both the quality of nurses' work and the quality of care they are able to provide.

There is significant research evidence presented in this chapter to support the links between nurses' work, nurses' health, quality of nursing care, and patient outcomes. Studies support the link between the practice of nursing and hospital mortality and nurses' work satisfaction with better patient care (Aiken et al., 1994; Laschinger et al., 2001).

Barriers to resolving the issues arising from the nature of nurses' work are significant, but the need to overcome these barriers and begin to address these issues has never been more urgent. Strategies for resolution involve the cooperation of governments, professional organizations, employers, educators, and researchers. The time to act is now.

Add to your knowledge of this issue: *Online*

Canadian Federation of Nurses Unions	**www.nursesunions.ca**
Canadian Nurses Association	**www.cna-nurses.ca**
International Council of Nurses	**www.icn.ch**

R E F L E C T I O N S *on the Chapter...*

1 From your own experiences in practice, describe situations that support or challenge what you have read about the nature of nurses' work.

2 How do you account for the current issues arising from the nature of nurses' work in your practice or practicum areas? Who might you ask or where might you look to gain an understanding of these current issues?

3 Researchers have located the responsibility for the issues arising from the nature of nurses' work with governments, employers, and professional organizations. Support or challenge this view.

4 The idea of strengthening the moral climate has emerged from recent studies with nurses in practice. Reflect on your practice experiences in which there might have been evidence of moral distress.

5 What other strategies might you suggest for resolving issues related to the nature of nurses' work?

Want to know more? Visit the Point, for additional helpful resources:

• Journal Articles
• Learning Objectives
• Nursing Professional Roles and Responsibilities
• Bonus chapters:
  ◦ Health and Nursing Policy: A Matter of Politics, Power and Professionalism
  ◦ The NP Movement: Recurring Issues
  ◦ When Difference Matters: The Politics of Privilege and Marginality

References

Aiken, L.H., Smith, H.L., & Lake, E.T. (1994). Lower Medicare mortality among a set of hospitals known for good nursing care. *Medical Care, 32*(8), 771–787.

Austin, W. (2011). The incommensurability of nursing as a practice and the customer service model: An evolutionary threat to the discipline. *Nursing Philosophy, 12*(3), 158–166.

Baumann, A., O'Brien-Pallas, L., Armstrong-Strassen, M., et al. (2001). *Commitment and care: The benefits of health workplaces for nurses, their patients and the system. A policy synthesis.* Canadian Health Research Foundation. Ottawa, ON: Government of Canada.

Burke, R.J., & Greenglass, E.R. (2000). Effects of hospital restructuring on full time and part time nursing staff in Ontario. *International Journal of Nursing Studies, 37*(2), 163–171.

Canadian Nurses Association. (2001). *Position statement: Quality professional practice environments for registered nurses.* Ottawa, ON: Author. Retrieved from http://www.cna-nurses.ca/CNA/documents/pdf/publications/PS53_Quality_ Prof_Practice_Env_RNS_NOV_2001_e.pdf.

———. (2006). *Joint position statement: Practice environments: Maximizing client, nurse and system outcomes.* Joint CNA and CFNU Position Statement. Ottawa, ON: Author. Retrieved from www.cna-aiic.ca

Ceci, C., & McIntyre, M. (2001). A "quiet" crisis in health care: Developing our capacity to hear. *Nursing Philosophy, 2*(2), 122–130.

Choiniere, J. (2011). Accounting for care: Exploring tensions and contradictions. *Advances in Nursing Science, 34*(4), 330–344.

Cleary, M., Hunt, G., & Horsfall, J. (2010). Identifying and addressing bullying in nursing. *Issues in Mental Health Nursing, 31*, 331–335.

Cockerill, L., & O'Brien-Pallas, L. (1990). Satisfaction with nursing workload systems: Report of a survey of Canadian hospitals. Part A. *Canadian Journal of Nursing Administration, 3*(2), 17–22.

Davies, C. (1995). *Gender and the professional predicament in nursing.* Philadelphia, PA: Open University Press.

Donner, G., Semogas, D., & Blythe, J. (1994). *Towards an understanding of nurses' lives: Gender, power and control.* Toronto, ON: Quality of Nursing Worklife Research Unit.

Eggertson, L. (2011). Targeted: The impact of bullying and what needs to be done to eliminate it. *Canadian Nurse, 107*(6), 18–22.

Gaudine, A.P. (2000). What do nurses mean by workload and work overload? *Canadian Journal of Nursing Leadership, 13*(2), 22–27.

Gibbon, M., & Mathewson, M. (1947). *Three centuries of Canadian nursing.* Toronto, ON: MacMillan.

Kristensen, T.S. (1999). Challenges for research and prevention in relation to work and cardiovascular diseases. *Scandinavian Journal of Work, Environment and Health, 25*(6), 550–557.

Laschinger, H., & Leiter, M. (2006). The impact of nursing work environments on patient safety outcomes: The mediating role of burnout and engagement. *Journal of Nursing Administration, 36*(5), 259–267.

Laschinger, H., Leiter, M., Day, A., & Gilin, D. (2009) Workplace empowerment, incivility, and burnout: Impact on staff nurse and retention outcomes. *Journal of Nursing Management, 17*, 302–311.

Laschinger, H., Grau, A., Finegan, J., Wilk, P. (2010) New graduate nurses' experiences of bullying and burnout in hospital settings. *Journal of Advanced Nursing, 66*(12), 2732–2742.

Laschinger, H., Finegan, J., Shamian, J., & Almost, J. (2001). Testing Karasek's demands-control model in restructured health care settings: Effects of job strain on staff nurses' quality of worklife. *Journal of Nursing Administration, 31*(5), 233–243.

O'Brien-Pallas, L., Irvine, D., Peereboom, E., & Murray, M. (1997). Measuring nursing workload: Understanding the variability. *Nursing Economics, 15*(4), 171–182.

O'Brien-Pallas, L., Thomson, D., Alksinis, C., et al. (2001). The economic impact of nurse staffing decisions: Time to turn down another road? *Hospital Quarterly, 4*(3), 42–50.

Pauly, B., MacKinnon, K., & Varcoe, C. (2009). Revisiting "who gets care": Health equity as an arena for nursing action. *Advances in Nursing Science, 32*(2), 118–127.

Rhéaume, A., Clément, L., & LeBel, N. (2011). Understanding intention to leave. *International Journal of Nursing Studies, 48*, 490–500.

Rodney, P., Doane, G., Storch, J., & Varcoe, C. (2006). Toward a safer moral climate. *Canadian Nurse, 102*(8), 24–27.

Saint Michaels Hospital. (2012). Nursing new graduate information. Recruitment—nursing—graduates. pdf Retrieved from www.stmichaelshospital.com/careers/index.php

Scott, E., Engelke, M., & Swanson, M. (2008). New graduate nurse transitioning: Necessary or nice? *Applied Nursing Research, 21,* 75–83.

Shullanberger, G. (2000). Nurse staffing decisions: An integrative review of the literature. *Nursing Economics, 18*(3), 124–132, 146–148.

Sochalski, J. (2001). Nursing's valued resources: Critical issues in economics and nursing care. *Canadian Journal of Nursing Research, 33*(1), 11–18.

Stuart, M. (1993). Nursing: The endangered profession. *Canadian Nurse, 89*(4), 19–22.

Taft, K., & Steward, G. (2000). *Clear answers: The economics and politics of for-profit medicine.* Edmonton: Duval House.

Viens, C. (1996). The future shock of nursing graduates. *Canadian Nurse, 92*(2), 40–44.

White, J.P. (1997). Health care, hospitals, and reengineering: The nightingales sing the blues. In A. Duffy, D. Glenday, & N. Pupo (Eds.), *Good jobs, bad jobs, no jobs: The transformation of work in the 21st century.* Toronto, ON: Harcourt & Brace.

Chapter

17 The Nursing Shortage: Assumptions and Realities

Marjorie McIntyre and Carol McDonald

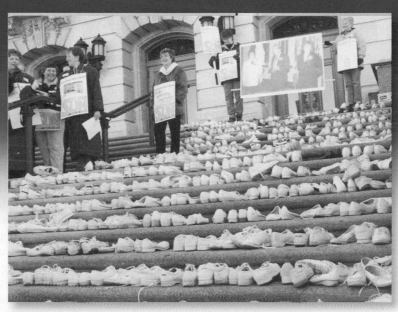

Nurses in Saskatchewan took public steps to communicate their response to nursing cutbacks and other work environment issues. They marched and left their shoes as a calling card to "run a mile in (a nurse's) shoes." (Used with permission of Saskatchewan Union of Nurses.)

Critical Questions

As a way of engaging with ideas in the chapter, consider the following:

1. What are your views about whether or not there is a shortage of nurses in Canada?

2. What, if anything, have you read in the media about the nursing shortage?

3. Is there evidence from your practice experience of a shortage of nurses currently?

Chapter Objectives

At the completion of this chapter, you will be able to:

1. Identify relevant issues in relation to the nursing shortage.

2. Articulate selected frameworks for analyzing issues arising from the nursing shortage.

3. Analyze selected strategies to address these issues.

4. Identify past and current barriers to resolution of the nursing shortage.

5. Discuss strategies for resolution of the nursing shortage.

309

This chapter challenges existing assumptions about the nursing shortage in order to generate new ways of understanding it and new possibilities for resolving it. At the outset, it is assumed that the recurrence of nursing shortages relates directly to an inability to see beyond the immediate problem of not enough nurses to the larger issues that have sustained and perpetuated shortages. The chapter then challenges the acceptance of the inevitability of recurrent shortages and the ethos of nurses as expendable, interchangeable, and easily replaced. Finally, questions are raised about the relationship between recurrent shortages and the conceptualization of nurses' work, women's work, and nursing knowledge. The arguments proposed in these pages resist the notion that the predicted scarcity of nurses is a problem that can be solved by simply increasing the numbers of graduating nurses. Instead, different perspectives on the issue are presented in an effort to generate new possibilities for its resolution.

NATURE OF THE NURSING SHORTAGE

The Canadian Nurses Association (CNA) has highlighted an impending shortage of nurses who have the skills and knowledge to meet the healthcare needs of the Canadian population, a shortage, according to the CNA, that has been unequaled in past decades (2002, 2009). Historically, nursing shortages have alternated with periods when too many nurses were available for the positions offered by employers. The question that arises, then, is what, if anything, is different now? Before answering the question, we must consider how the complexity of the issue precludes finding quick solutions, such as hiring more nurses, recruiting more students, or paying higher wages.

Hospital administrators, board members, leaders in professional nursing organizations, collective bargaining groups, and all people involved in staffing nursing positions have been and continue to be concerned with the numbers of nurses available for work. When the inability to fill vacant positions is conceptualized simply in terms of shortage, as a temporary and easily corrected mismatch of supply and demand, mainly instrumental or quick-fix solutions suggest themselves. The concern with these quick-fix solutions is that there is an element of distress that remains unaccounted for, suggesting perhaps that nurses' suffering and their concomitant exodus from the workforce "may arise not only from the conditions of their work but also more existentially, from having one's way of understanding the world unacknowledged" (Ceci & McIntyre, 2001, p. 123).

Oulton (2006), the Canadian chief executive officer of the International Council of Nurses, notes that there is "both a real shortage and a pseudo-shortage, in which there are enough nurses but not enough willing to work under available conditions" (p. 35S). This view suggests that if we increase the number of new graduate nurses without addressing the working conditions for nurses, the situation will remain the same. It is important here to view the working conditions not only as the physical environment in which the work is carried out but also as including the factors that sustain the professional and personal well-being of the nurses themselves.

The issue of nursing shortages will ultimately be discussed many times in this book in relation to many other topics. This chapter provides a critical analysis of the way in which the nursing shortage has been conceptualized and of the strategies aimed at its resolution.

FRAMING AND ANALYZING THE ISSUE

Like other complex issues, the nursing shortage can be best understood as multiple problems—all raising issues for nurses, healthcare providers, and Canadians seeking healthcare. Viewed simply as a problem of numbers, the nursing shortage could be resolved by producing more nurses. Viewed as a problem of working conditions, the issue could be resolved by mobilizing resources to improve working conditions. Viewed as a problem of work satisfaction, the issue could be resolved by addressing nurses' concerns about salaries and other contractual issues. Studies on work satisfaction for nurses have identified alleviating work pressures, security and workplace safety, support of managers and colleagues, opportunities for education, professional identity, control over practice, scheduling, and leadership as elements that are as important to nurses as remuneration (Baumann et al., 2001).

Clearly, more than the provision of resources or changes in nurses' working conditions is at stake in this issue. Each of these elements—numbers, working conditions, and work satisfaction—incorporates underlying and unexamined assumptions about the nature of nurses' work, nursing knowledge, and the relationship of each to power structures in healthcare and society. What follows is a discussion of different frameworks for analysis and the possibilities they generate for understanding the nursing shortage, its recurrence, and its resolution.

Historical Analysis of the Nursing Shortage

> The point is to write about and render historical what has hitherto been hidden from history.
> (Joan Scott, 1992)

The purpose of a historical analysis is to show how a particular issue has evolved and how it has been, and continues to be, analyzed in relation to different points of view. If we draw on the work of feminist historians, such as Joan Scott (1992), we quickly realize that histories are written from different perspectives. Historical analysis helps us to understand the views we currently hold or could hold about an issue. It may also provide insights into how we have come to hold those views.

What exactly constitutes a shortage? Who decides that a shortage is a shortage? These are questions to be addressed through historical analysis. To begin these discussions, consider the following comments that appeared in a 1943 issue of the *Canadian Nurse*:

> How would you answer the age-old imponderable —Is there a shortage of nurses? A study made not long ago showed that on November 20, 1942, there were 986 vacancies for nurses reported in Canada. A statement from all registries revealed the fact that 1133 nurses were on call that same day. We do not know what a statistician would make of these figures... but, so long as these conditions persist, we must say there is a shortage of nurses in certain vital services. (Kathleen Ellis, p. 269)

Sounds familiar? What makes these words, now written 70 years ago, so relevant today is that there is still no consensus about what constitutes a shortage and the relationship between persistent vacancies and the apparent availability of nurses to fill them. Despite the confusion about whether or not there is a shortage, Ellis feels bound to say there is a shortage as long as there are vacancies in particular areas.

What has continued since, and likely preceded, Ellis's clear conceptualization of the confusion about what constitutes a shortage is this: Until we know better what is going on when faced with vacancies in nursing positions, we will continue to talk about the situation as a shortage. To support what Ellis brings into question, it is not just that the shortage is expressed in numbers that must be challenged but that the number often reflects vacant positions as opposed to nurses available.

The literature contains ample evidence that shortages are recurrent in nursing history. What is less clear and never really made explicit is whose and what authority defines a shortage? Does what we mean by a shortage depend to some extent on the authority of the speaker? That is, does what actually counts as a shortage in nursing rely less on what is happening at a particular moment in history and depend more on *who* claims that a shortage exists? You may ask, for example, if one nurse is doing the work that to be done competently should be done by two, is there a shortage? Or, if nurses are mandated to work past their 12-hour shift, on days off or holidays, is there a shortage? Or, if nurses on a particular unit are overworked, but there are no vacant positions for nurses, is there a shortage? Whether these situations represent a problem of numbers or a problem of workplace is unclear.

In many instances, nurses are excluded from important decisions about the number of nurses needed, how nursing positions are best managed to provide care, and even what constitutes adequate care. In situations in which well-qualified nurse managers are present, the best-planned staffing can be undermined by the so-called cost-containment strategies. Thus, it is not always clear to others or even to nurses what it is that we are short of when we talk of shortages (Ceci & McIntyre, 2001).

In considering how shortages come about in the first place, we need to take into account how strategies for dealing with shortages, such as unfilled registered nurse (RN) positions, are commonly based on the assumption that not enough nurses are being produced or maintained in the system. In some ways, this assumption is true. In other ways, it is a limited understanding of how shortages are created.

Another way to illuminate the picture of how shortages come about is to consider the relationship between shortages and surpluses. For example, the nursing shortages of the 1980s can be linked to the development of new technologies leading to increasing demand for medical services. The expansion of services and increased use of medical technologies increased the demand for nurses, who were now needed to administer and monitor the new technologies. Given that nurses could also take on the care provided by other nursing personnel, the numbers of licensed practical nurses and orderlies decreased. These shortages, created by demand for more nurses to incorporate the advances in technology into patient care, became, in the context of health-care restructuring and government cost-containment strategies, the nursing surplus of the 1990s (Donner et al., 1994).

What is important to grasp here is that there was no significant change in the number of nurses available. More often, what changed was the demand for nurses, not a decline in the supply of nurses. Increased medical services increased the number of RN positions needed. Later, the reduced funding available for structures that provided nursing positions, such as hospitals and health units, created the impression that a surplus of nurses existed where once there was a shortage. In reality, the number of nurses available for work had scarcely changed.

Across Canada, the previous decades of restructuring and downsizing have had profound effects. Without a plan of how care would be provided and concern for the welfare of nurses whose positions were cut or those nurses who remained in a system decimated by the cuts, extensive layoffs of nursing positions took place. Nurses struggled and continue to struggle to provide care in environments characterized by heightened patient acuity, intensified workloads, and limited resources. Experienced RNs and new graduates were abandoned by the system they had prepared themselves to serve through advanced education and years of clinical service. Recurrent shortages and surpluses continue to be viewed in relation to numbers of nursing positions left vacant. What remains unacknowledged are the underlying conditions that created the surplus and the conditions—now about a decade later—that have led to a predicted nurse shortage of crisis proportions. What also remain unacknowledged are the effects of all this on nurses. The problem for nurses who make these claims and who continue to gather data to support these claims is that the predictions, however, compelling, were not and are not accompanied by authority to act. The concerns of nurses have not been heard (Ceci & McIntyre, 2001).

Ethical Analysis of the Nursing Shortage

In addition to the ethical issues raised for individual nurses when they are not able to practice in accordance with the CNA's Code of Ethics (2008) in the provision of safe, competent, and compassionate care, an ethical issue of great concern is the recruitment of nurses internationally to fill positions in Canada. Bourgeault (2012) notes that recruitment of nurses from other countries is viewed as an immediate strategy for issues of supply. "In 2010, member states of the World Health Organization, including Canada, formally adopted the WHO Global Code of Practice on the International Recruitment of Health Personnel, which strongly encourages countries to mitigate the negative effects of international recruitment" (Bourgeault, 2012, p. 44). It should be no surprise that the circumstances that contribute to a nursing shortage in Canada, that is increasing demands on nurses in a troubled work environment, are also present in countries around the world. An appealing standard of living contributes at least in part to Canada's ability to recruit nurses from international countries, who have not only invested in those nurses' education but themselves suffer from even more extreme shortages of nurses.

Social and Cultural Analysis of the Nursing Shortage

The purpose of social and cultural analysis is to provide the background to how particular issues develop in particular contexts that influence both the way the issue is understood by others and its possibilities for resolution. Important questions to guide social and cultural analysis include, but are not limited to, the following:

- What are the prevailing attitudes in society about this issue?
- What values and priorities of the dominant culture influence this issue?
- In what ways, if any, do these values and priorities privilege the dominant culture over other members of the society?

The topic of the nursing shortage is prevalent in the literature and media discussions both within and beyond the discipline of nursing. Since 2002, the global nursing shortage has, in fact, been termed a "global crisis"; "in developing countries the situation is dramatic—a chronic nursing shortage is worsened by the migration of nurses in search of better working conditions and quality of life" (Oulton, 2006, p. 35S). In her paper on the global nursing shortage, Oulton (2006) identifies factors contributing to the increasing demand and decreasing supply of nurses. Demands include shortened hospital stays and increased acuity of care, a shift to ambulatory and community care, and publicizing the aging of the population. The decreased supply of nurses is influenced by the aging and retiring workforce, fewer applicants and new graduates, and nurses leaving the profession citing unfavorable work environments.

The disparity between what the society believes it means to be a nurse—a belief that draws many students into nursing—and the reality of the nature and conditions of nurses' work continues to grow. Although the nature and conditions of nurses' work have not changed significantly over time, the attitudes toward the nature of work, the conditions of nurses' work, and the availability of other possibilities for work have changed. In fact, the reasons given for leaving the profession by nursing students in the 1940s, such as mandatory overtime, the valuing of non-nursing tasks over the delivery of nursing care, and reproach for sick time taken (Cohen, 1948, as cited in West et al., 2007), are not dissimilar from current day workplace realities.

The attitudes discussed above, particularly the aging nursing workforce, are those commonly held by societal members, including nurses, as the "reasons for the shortage." What is less understood are the assumptions and discourses that underlie these conditions, the values that are attached to nurses' work that perpetuate unsatisfactory or, in many cases, intolerable working conditions. Oulton (2006) reports that "nurses are changing jobs, leaving the country, and leaving nursing" (p. 37S), as she gives voice to nurses' parting comments: "I'm leaving because of understaffing, because we don't have the human resources, because the skill mix is not right, because I go home at night and I am frustrated and unhappy and dissatisfied with myself that I cannot give the kind of care that I want to give" (p. 36S). Other voices say, "I am frustrated and tired because of the lack of support, because I do not have professional parity, because there is not the team work I wanted to see, because my salary and benefits are not what I want. There is not the opportunity for autonomy and for control of workload" (p. 37S). This international work by Oulton raises many issues that are relevant for Canadian nurses; the remaining question is, why, for over 50 years, have unsatisfactory working conditions for nurses prevailed?

An additional topic is the culture *within* healthcare, where the presumed versatility of nurses to competently take on the work of others interferes with the accomplishment of nurses' work. That it is unimaginable that a pharmacist, physiotherapist, or physician would be asked to take on a role usually assigned to others, suggests that nurses are viewed differently from their contemporaries in practice. Other professionals clearly have the same ability with minimal supervision for a wide range of duties outside their practice fields, and yet no one would consider this possibility, making it clear that a nurse's work is viewed differently from the work of other professionals (Fawcett, 2007).

Ivy Bourgeault, who holds the CIHR/Health Canada Research Chair in Human Health Resource Policy, suggests that the issue of nursing shortage would be better viewed from a perspective of "human resources for health" (2011). This approach suggests that a dispassionate assessment of the work that needs to be done and an appraisal of who is best prepared to accomplish that work would provide a way out of the ongoing challenges of human health resources (Bourgeault, 2012). Importantly, and as Bourgeault points out, these are not political or economic decisions to reorganize care, but informed decisions made by qualified managers at the point of care.

Economic Analysis of the Nursing Shortage

An economic analysis can highlight how the forces of supply and demand work in a particular issue. What some call a nursing "shortage" may manifest itself principally as a "problem of numbers," which, in turn, can be most effectively addressed by managing or rebalancing supply and demand. Put another way, nurses are viewed as "an application of technology, as objects to be controlled, managed, and understood primarily in practical instrumental ways" (Ceci & McIntyre, 2001, p. 123).

Although understanding the economic elements of any issue is important, this point of view has limitations. Its effects have created problems for nursing—particularly in relation to nursing shortages. What makes an economic analysis so useful is not just what the numbers are telling us but what they do not tell us. For example, vacancy rates are frequently cited as evidence of a shortage of nurses. However, vacancies only indicate "the inability to recruit people or retain them in a particular position" (Ross, 1996, p. 201). There is no analysis of how the numbers of needed nursing positions are determined or of who determines this. New RN positions can be created for many reasons. Ideally, positions are created or added in response to an identified need for the knowledge and skills an RN provides. What is notable is that numbers tell us very little about the different knowledge, skills, and experience that the new positions require. In addition, what an analysis of numbers of nurses or numbers of positions may overlook is the hidden and non-nursing work incorporated in what many positions involve.

In an interesting forum, speaking of the United States nursing shortage, Fawcett (2007) suggests that efforts to rapidly increase seats for nursing students in the "shortest and least professionally focused programs" (p. 98) will flood the market and contribute to the undervaluing of professional nurses in the market place. In Canada this is played out with increasing education and workplace opportunities for Licensed Practical Nurses (LPNs). The educational requirements of LPNs now approach those of diploma prepared nurses who are still in practice. This reality points to the need for informed assessment of allocation of work, outside of those with economic or political agendas.

In other words, knowledge of the discipline and professional nursing practice is critical to analyzing the shortage. We must ask how are the decisions to create new nursing positions or to cut back on the number of nurses made? Who makes these decisions? It is not so much that a good economic analysis is not useful in making these decisions, but rather, how are other perspectives taken into account? How much influence do nurse leaders have in challenging purely cost-containment strategies when the health of Canadians is thought to be at risk? Influence is discussed further in the following section on political analysis.

Political Analysis of the Nursing Shortage

Politics is often talked about as the art of influencing another person. When individuals and groups with disparate values enter into decision-making processes, politics shapes the content of what is discussed and the decision-making process itself. Although some nurses claim they are not political, others insist there is no escaping politics. A political analysis can be useful in highlighting the relationship between knowledge and power. To be able to persuade others that nurses working to their full capacity will produce different outcomes, that practice could be restructured to maximize nurses' skills and knowledge, and that nurses are a scarce resource that cannot be spared to do non-nursing tasks is to have power. Put another way, knowledge is power and may be nurses' greatest source of power. Although many nurses have recognized the importance of developing political skills, using their knowledge to influence health and nursing policy has not been that easy. What structures keep nurses from using what they know to influence others?

Ideologies are the voices of power and of authority within a culture. Ideologies are how we come to know who we are, what we are to think, and how we are to behave. Ideologies are ways through which we come to understand ourselves. The power of ideologies lies in the authority they have to define many of our social arrangements as obvious or natural (Althusser, 1971). How do dominant ideologies keep a nurse from accepting one's own ideas or the ideas of one's leader over those imposed by other authorities? The concept of power is not generally associated with nursing. The concept usually refers to the power of major corporations, politicians, trade unions, medical associations, and male-dominated organizations. Despite nurses' numbers and roles in healthcare, it is not that common for the nursing profession and nurses to be considered powerful.

A political analysis points to the conditions that influence us to act or not on that which we know. What follows are examples of changing conditions that have enabled nurses to use knowledge to pursue or influence decision making and policy development. In many provinces, nurses have, through changing legislation, acquired legal powers that legitimize various nurse roles. In several provinces, roles such as the nurse practitioner and clinical nurse specialist have been created, accepted by the public, and integrated into the healthcare system. In addition to the clinical expertise nurses in these roles provide, these advanced practitioners also contribute to the larger system. Through serving on advisory boards and acting as preceptors, these nurses are able to monitor and influence course content in schools of nursing. Through their involvement in research, evidence-based practice, and quality assurance, these nurses have opportunities to monitor activities and facilitate change in service settings. Most importantly, through these changing conditions, nurses' power base is expanded. Nurses have begun to encourage and support nurse candidates for political office and are increasingly involved in professional organizations' lobbying efforts.

Critical Feminist Analysis of the Nursing Shortage

A feminist analysis looks beyond the experiences of a particular nurse—man or woman—to the structures and ideologies that influence these experiences. Although one could use many different approaches to guide feminist analysis, the questions selected for this chapter are the following:

- What are the structures and ideologies in our world that contribute to errors or myths about a nurse's abilities or realities?
- Is this issue influenced by the power inequities or the hierarchic or patriarchal structures of institutions over patients?
- In this situation, is expert power given authority over the right to be the subject of one's life?

Despite our significance in healthcare settings, nurses are thought by many to be "marginal players, and this marginality affects our sense of ourselves and our possibilities for practice" (Ceci & McIntyre, 2001, p. 128). Nowhere is this more apparent than in discussions of how to address the current so-called nursing shortage. Discussions of shortage are all too easily transformed into arguments concerning what constitutes an adequate nursing education. Shortages are and have always been accompanied by discussions of how to shorten the time needed for nursing education, assuming that "skilled and intelligent nursing care may be accomplished in the absence of a broad and substantive knowledge base. Not only does it seem that anyone can be a nurse but that any nurse is better than no nurse—again a claim hard to argue with but one that merely reinforces the intellectual subordination of nurses" (Ceci & McIntyre, 2001, p. 128).

Although the nursing literature and other human care literature highlight the importance of relationship accompanied by an ethic of care in the work of nursing, there is still an unquestioned assumption that implicitly or explicitly nursing is an expression of women's natural capacities, a view that effectively erases the knowledge required by nurses to comprehend and respond to the needs of another (Ceci & McIntyre, 2001). Still "other discourses obscure or slide over the emotional labor and stress involved in nurses' work and instead emphasize the instrumentality (of nurses' work), the tasks that need to be done and (the) pairs of hands" (p. 128) needed to perform them.

BARRIERS TO RESOLUTION OF THE NURSING SHORTAGE

That nurses are considered expendable as evidenced by cost cutting in the 1990s (1993 to 1996) was, in no sense, inevitable but rather the result of values, beliefs, and choices among possibilities. An outcome of these choices that seems not yet to be appreciated by the public or by policymakers, at least not in any deep sense, is the way in which these actions and policies have precipitated a certain suffering among nurses, a suffering which needs to be understood as now contributing to both a scarcity of nurses and a deficiency of nursing care (Ceci & McIntyre, 2001). One of the most important strategies for moving an issue toward resolution is identifying barriers that may impede the resolution process. Once the barriers are identified, the chances for resolution through mediation, collaboration, and negotiation increase. What makes identifying barriers so useful in issue resolution is that we may lack awareness of the taken-for-granted assumptions that sustain an issue and obstruct its resolution. Nowhere is this truer than in the nursing shortage issue.

The biggest barrier to resolving what has been called a nursing shortage is the way this issue has been conceptualized and understood. Typically, shortages have been viewed as short-term problems solved temporarily either by educating more nurses or by recruiting nurses internationally (Bourgeault, 2012). Although it can be argued that a focus on the recruitment and retention of student and graduate nurses would go a long way in addressing the current shortage, history has shown that it does not effectively address many of the underlying issues that sustain and perpetuate the ongoing cycle of surplus and shortage.

A second barrier that follows from the first is viewing nurses as temporary workers created to fill a gap in services. In this view, the gap is thought to be easily addressed by accelerating training, increasing head counts, and adding full-time equivalent positions, actions that undermine attempts at long-term recruitment and retention (Brush, 1992).

A third barrier to resolving the nursing shortage is the incongruity between the complex nature of nursing practice and the status of nurses' work and nurses' knowledge. In nursing history and today in practice, it is disturbing how "significant knowledge, insight, and experience that nurses require in their practices can be so effortlessly rendered invisible. How does this trivialization of the knowledge of nursing work itself contribute to what is called a nursing shortage?" (Ceci & McIntyre, 2001, p. 124).

We would like to suggest that it is the persistent undervaluing of nurses' knowledge and the status of nurses' work that accounts for the increased attrition of students and new graduates, and continuing difficulties with retention. This failure to acknowledge the disciplinary knowledge required for professional nursing practice keeps the focus on numbers of nurses needed to fill vacant positions, assuming that any nurse will fill any position and undermining the need to seriously address the quality of workplace environment issues.

A fourth barrier is government's failure to consider the long-term ramifications of cost cutting on healthcare and of the nurses who are central to its provision. One cannot overlook the possibility that the negative impacts on the health and well-being of nurses contribute to nurses leaving the profession, nurses not being available for work, and nurses not being able to contribute effectively at work. We should consider the possibility that nurses are refusing to tolerate work environments that "invalidate their concerns, which fragment their practices, and disallow their understandings" (Ceci & McIntyre, 2001, p. 126). Perhaps a large part of the current situation in nursing has to do with how these conditions of practice conflict with "nurses' beliefs about what is necessary in terms of care. Nurses, it seems, are refusing to accept such unreasonableness as part of what it means to be a nurse" (p. 126).

STRATEGIES FOR RESOLUTION

Nurses, when they have a choice, will go where they are respected, rewarded for their competencies and problem-solving skills, challenged appropriately, and given opportunities for personal and professional development. Creating those conditions need not be costly and will go a long way to resolving the nursing shortage. (Oulton, 2006)

Following the articulation, analysis, and discussion of barriers to resolution of a nursing issue, strategies for resolution must be generated. Although there are a wide variety of effective strategies to choose from, complex issues such as the nursing shortage call for particular strategies for resolution. As the analysis of the nursing shortage in this chapter clearly shows, long-term strategies are most important in moving this issue toward resolution. Also, given that the focus on numbers and instrumental solutions has been conceptualized as part of the problem, the strategies section deliberately highlights other possibilities for resolution. Finally, given the concern that nurses have been left out of many of the discussions involving the nursing shortage, emphasis is placed on the contributions that nurses have to make in its resolution. Strategies that nurses can carry out are central, beginning with what nurses must change to move the nursing shortage issue to resolution.

A first and, likely, a pivotal strategy is to acknowledge that nurses' concerns have been largely ignored in the past decades. There is no point in continuing strategies that history clearly shows have not worked. Concerns about the knowledge and skills needed for entry to practice, predicted shortages due to an aging workforce and declining enrollments, and the restructuring of the healthcare system in the 1990s have been articulated clearly by nurses and supported with research. Professional organizations have lobbied all levels of government on behalf of nurses, the health of Canadians, and the healthcare system. History tells us that nurses have not been heard.

The specific action that would follow would be to challenge ourselves and others to hear what nurses have to say as significant. Put another way, we need to insist that concerns, which are sometimes dismissed as groundless complaints, be seen as the "beginnings of a critique...of the dominant modes of thinking that organize the work of health care" (Ceci & McIntyre, 2001, p. 126). The term *critique,* as used here, is not to suggest that nurses are right and that dominant modes of thinking are somehow misinformed. Rather, the point is to suggest that there is room in the discussion of healthcare concerns for the different perspective that nurses can bring. To sum up this first strategy then, nurses are well positioned by their knowledge and experience of the healthcare system to critique dominant ways of thinking that inform healthcare decisions. The point is not that dominant ways of thinking are wrong, but that they are simply insufficient to handle important issues in the Canadian healthcare system, of which the nursing shortage is one example.

Emanating from this first strategy of listening to what nurses have to say and hearing their views as significant among others' views is the second strategy to dispassionately assess the work to be accomplished in healthcare and to ask who is best qualified to undertake this work.

Moving the debate of a nursing shortage to the broader perspective of human resources and quality work environments more accurately addresses the numerous complex realities that underlie human health resource issues (Bourgeault, 2012).

SUMMARY

Those who understand nurses as something more than a pair of hands or more than technical support for the real work of medicine will recognize the need to question the current situation that has been named the nursing shortage. As we have discussed in numerous ways throughout this chapter, nurses' views of the world are both overshadowed and undermined by more dominant views that define who nurses are; the work they do; and, in many cases, the knowledge and skill needed to do this work. Until we can move beyond thinking of recurrent nursing shortages as inevitable; of the ethos of nurses as expendable, interchangeable, and easily replaced; and of the immediate problem of not enough nurses to the larger issues that have sustained and perpetuated shortages, the current situation is unlikely to change. Questions raised about the relationship between recurrent shortages and the conceptualizations of nurses' work, quality work environments and human health resource issues must be addressed.

Add to your knowledge of this issue:	
Canadian Nurses Association	**www.cna-nurse.ca**
International Council of Nurses	**www.icn.ch**
National League for Nurses	**www.nln.org**
Canadian Association of Schools of Nursing	**www.casn.ca**
Canadian Institute of Health Information	**www.cihi.ca**

Online

REFLECTIONS *on the Chapter...*

1 The Canadian Institute for Health Information (CIHI) Office of Nursing Policy has published a document called Regulated Nurses: Canadian Trends 2006–2010 highlighting numbers on relevant topics for nursing. Visit this document online and identify ways in which the use of these numbers both supports and obscures your understanding of the nursing shortage.

2 How do you understand the ethics of internationally recruiting nurses, who are greatly needed in their own countries?

3 In this chapter there are several examples of working conditions that nurses have found intolerable. Which of these in your opinion is the most important for nurses and the profession?

4 Identify an additional barrier to the resolution of the nursing shortage that has not been discussed in the chapter.

5 Suggest a strategy for the barrier you have named above.

Want to know more? Visit thePoint for additional helpful resources:

- Journal Articles
- Learning Objectives
- Nursing Professional Roles and Responsibilities
- Bonus chapters:
  - Health and Nursing Policy: A Matter of Politics, Power and Professionalism
  - The NP Movement: Recurring Issues
  - When Difference Matters: The Politics of Privilege and Marginality

References

Althusser, L. (1971). Ideology and ideological state apparatuses. In L. Althusser (Ed.), *Lenin and philosophy and other essays* (B. Brewster, Trans., pp. 123–173). London: New Left Books.

Baumann, A., O'Brien-Pallas, L., Armstrong-Strassen, M., et al. (2001). *Commitment and care—the benefits of a healthy workplace for nurses, their patients and the system: A policy synthesis.* Ottawa, ON: Canadian Health Services Research Foundation.

Bourgeault, I. (2012). If the answer is "more nurses", what is the question? *Canadian Nurse, 108*(2), 44.

Brush, B. (1992). Shortage as shorthand for the crisis in caring. *Nursing & Health Care, 13*(9), 480–486.

Canadian Nurses Association. (2002). *Planning for the future: Nursing human resource projections.* Retrieved from www.cna-nurses.ca/cna/documents

———. (2009). *Human Health Resources: Tested Solutions for Eliminating Canada's Registered Nurse Shortage.* Retrieved from www.cna-aiic.ca/CNA/issues/hhr

Ceci, C., & McIntyre, M. (2001). A quiet crisis in health care: Developing our capacity to hear. *Nursing Journal of Nursing Philosophy, 2*(2), 122–130.

Donner, G., Semogas, D., & Blythe, J. (1994). *Towards an understanding of nurses lives: Gender, power and control.* Quality of Nursing Worklife Research Unit Monograph Series. Toronto, ON: University of Toronto.

Ellis, K. (1943). Some pertinent questions. *Canadian Nurse, 39*(4), 268–271.

Fawcett, J. (2007). Nursing qua nursing: The connection between nursing knowledge and nursing shortages. *Journal of Advanced Nursing, 59*(1), 97–99.

Oulton, J. (2006). The global nursing shortage: An overview of issues and actions. *Policy, Politics and Nursing Practice, 7*(3), 34S–39S.

Ross, E. (1996). From shortage to oversupply: The nursing workforce pendulum. In J. Kerr & J. McPhail (Eds.), *Canadian nursing: Issues and perspectives* (pp. 196–207). St. Louis, MO: Mosby.

Scott, J. (1992). Experience. In J. Butler & J. Scott (Eds.), *Feminists theorize the political.* London: Routledge, 22–40.

West, E., Griffith, W., & Iphofen, R. (2007). A historical perspective on the nursing shortage. *Medsurg Nursing, 16*(2), 124–130.

18 Rural Nursing in Canada

Karen MacKinnon

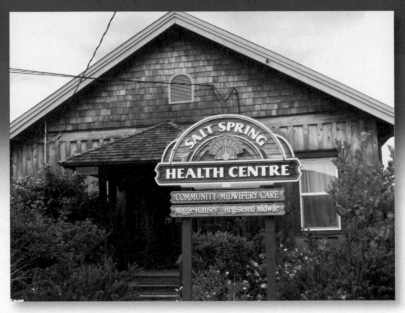

Nurses and other healthcare providers respond to needs in rural communities. (Used with permission. Photographer Carol McDonald.)

Critical Questions

As a way of engaging with the ideas in this chapter, consider the following:

1. What do you already know about rural nursing? Why is rural nursing important for the health of Canadians?

2. What do you think it would be like to work as a nurse in a rural, remote, northern, or Aboriginal community? What knowledge and skills are required?

3. How does the rural setting of practice influence nursing work? What are the similarities and differences between rural, remote, and northern nursing?

4. What social and institutional factors affect rural nursing work and the recruitment and retention of rural nurses?

Chapter Objectives

After completing this chapter, you will be able to:

1. Identify relevant issues in relation to rural nursing and the health of rural Canadians.

2. Explore one longstanding rural nursing issue using the issues articulation framework.

3. Appreciate how different understandings of this issue affect the recruitment and retention of skilled rural nurses.

4. Identify past and current barriers to resolving this issue.

5. Identify possibilities for working toward resolution to ensure the provision of safe, accessible, and appropriate rural health services.

*Y*ou know that you are rural if there is no Starbucks or Second Cup…You know you are remote if there is no Tim Horton's.

(J. Roger Pitblado, 2005)

Rural Canadians have been identified as a vulnerable group because they lack access to health services and have overall poorer health outcomes. Life expectancy is significantly lower for both women and men, the incidence of respiratory disease is significantly higher, and rural residents have high mortality rates due to injuries, suicide, and circulatory diseases (Canadian Institute for Health Information [CIHI], 2006). Rural residents also travel greater distances to receive all services and have high death rates due to motor vehicle accidents (Kulig, 2010).

Rural geography is varied across Canada but weather, mountain ranges, coastal hazards, and large distances pose significant barriers to health service access and delivery. Rural Canadians have lower income and educational levels but describe a greater sense of belonging to their community (Kulig, 2010). In addition, more than half of Canada's Aboriginal people (including First Nations, Métis, and Inuit people) live in rural, remote, and northern Canada. Aboriginal people face unique health challenges (Smith et al., 2005) that are explored in this volume (see Chapter 4.)

No universally agreed-on definitions of "rural" exist in the literature but population counts indicate that the percentage of Canadians living in rural communities ranges from 21% to 30% (Hanvey, 2005). The way "rural" is defined, for statistical purposes, is important because it affects health service decision making and the allocation of resources. Small, geographically isolated towns that may not meet the common definition of rural (less than 10,000 people) also experience acute stress in providing appropriate health services. MacLeod et al. (1998) propose a more encompassing practical definition of rural that focuses on the "skills and expertise needed by practitioners who work in areas where distance, weather, limited resources and little backup shape the character of their lives and professional practice" (p. 72).

In this chapter, the author explores the nature of rural nursing, the knowledge and skills required, the experiences of rural nurses, and the influence of the rural setting for nursing practice. In addition, one longstanding nursing issue, the recruitment and retention of skilled rural nurses, is discussed using the issues articulation framework. Finally, barriers that influence rural nursing work will be identified along with strategies for working toward a more sustainable future for health service delivery to rural Canadians.

UNDERSTANDING THE ISSUES

In this section four questions are addressed:

1. Where do rural nurses work in Canada?
2. What is it like to provide nursing care in a rural, remote, northern, or Aboriginal community?
3. How does the local context for care influence rural nursing work?
4. What are the differences and similarities in rural, remote, and northern nursing?

Work Settings: Where Do Rural Nurses Work in Canada?

Rural nurses work in a variety of settings across Canada and their nursing work reflects this diversity. Examples of rural nursing practice include working as a public health nurse, a home care nurse, or a hospital nurse in rural communities and geographically isolated small towns. Nurses also work in more remote and/or northern communities, sometimes alone as the only healthcare provider in an outpost setting. Outpost nurses provide essential health services to isolated and northern communities who have little or no access to medical care.

> Anne, a band-employed nurse in southern Ontario, has worked with community members to develop residential workshops on learning to live with diabetes. June, a home care nurse and the only healthcare practitioner in a small southern prairie community, helped a drop-in client to her weekly foot care clinic to gain a timely referral to an urban specialty clinic. The clinic confirmed June's assessment of advanced congestive heart failure. Barbara, a nurse in a small hospital in a coastal community, tells about travelling by snowmobile to the site of a violent crime and having to attend to both victim and perpetrator—neighbors of hers—in a snowstorm. Claire, a nurse in northern Canada, tells about how she and her colleague, the only nurses in a small community, handled a cardiac arrest by drawing on the only resources available, including the patient's adult children, to perform CPR and the "attending" physician, 600 km away on the speakerphone. (MacLeod et al., 2004, p. 27)

Stories like these help us to understand the nature of nursing practice in rural and remote Canada.

In Canada, hospital-based nurses are the largest group of rural nurses (Stewart et al., 2005). Rural nurses provide emergency care for people injured in car accidents or requiring care following a mental health crisis. They also provide care for older adults experiencing complications of their chronic illnesses; including some who require intensive monitoring. In addition, these nurses may be required to provide nursing care for healthy women during labor and/or for women experiencing pregnancy complications, such as preterm labor or birth, until transport to a regional center can be safely accomplished (MacKinnon, 2008). Rural nursing in small acute care hospitals has been described as a form of "multi-specialist practice" (MacLeod et al., 2008). Rural nurses also tell us that much of their work in small acute care hospitals focuses on "safeguarding" or keeping their patients safe (MacKinnon, 2011).

The Nature of Rural Nursing Work

What is it like to be a rural nurse? In the last few years, the experiences of rural nurses have been studied by nurse researchers (Lee & McDonagh, 2010; Long & Weinert, 2010; Rosenthal, 2010). "Nursing practice in rural and remote Canada is characterized by its variability, complexity, and the need for a wide range of knowledge and skills in situations of minimal support and few resources" (MacLeod et al., 2004, p. 2). Rural nurses are also expected to do the work of both nonprofessionals, such as housekeepers and dietary aids, and other professionals, such as physiotherapists and pharmacists, particularly on night shifts and weekends when these workers are not available. Based on her research, Scharff (2010) has eloquently described the meaning of being a rural nurse:

> Being rural means being a long way from anywhere and pretty close to nowhere. Being rural means being independent or perhaps just being alone. Being a rural nurse means that when a nurse saves a life, everyone in town recognizes that she or he was there, and that when a nurse loses a life, everyone in town recognizes that she or he was there. Being rural means turning inward for answers, because there may be nobody to turn to outward. Being rural means that when a nurse walks into the emergency room, it may be her or his spouse or child who needs a nurse, and at that moment, being a nurse takes priority over being anyone else. Being rural means being able to deal with what she or he has got, where she or he is, and being able to live with the consequences. (p. 181).

Rural nurses work as "expert generalists" in many rural communities settings (Troyer & Lee, 2010). One of the Public Health Nurses (PHNs) who participated in a pilot study described being a generalist nurse.

On most days, I guess, I love the generalist model. I always have. I love the variety of the day. And that's really challenging and it keeps me fresh and I don't get bored very easily. The down side of that (is) some days I just want to be a specialist. I just want to be responsible for one area and really sink my teeth into that one area and really feel completely confident and competent in that area. Because when you're responsible for everything, that's challenging too. (Focus group, PHNs; MacKinnon et al., 2007)

Although rural and remote nursing can be very different, there are also important commonalities across rural settings of practice. Studies of the experiences of rural nurses reveal that rural nursing is rewarding work. Rural nurses are proud of the work they do and demonstrate passion, commitment, and creativity in their everyday work (MacKinnon, 2008). Historically, nurses living and working in rural communities have taken on additional responsibilities to ensure that the health needs of rural Canadians have been addressed (MacLeod et al., 2004).

Rural nurses' sense of responsibility and commitment to their local communities is evident in how they practice nursing in their communities. For example, in one relatively isolated small town the two remaining operating room nurses in the community worked out between themselves an informal on-call system so that one or the other would always be available should a local woman require an emergency cesarean delivery. Sometimes this commitment was visible in the willingness of rural nurses to learn new things to better meet the needs of people living in their community (MacKinnon, 2008).

Although privacy concerns are acknowledged, rural nurses consistently describe knowing the people in the community as a way to enhance local health services. This commitment can lead to an increased sense of responsibility for ensuring that people living in their communities have access to the health resources they need. One PHN, who resides in a rural community, talked about how her work intersects with her life.

When you're in the small community, especially something like Public Health, where we're talking about healthy lifestyles and we're talking about good decisions and all this sort of stuff, you sort of have to be more of a "walk the walk" sort of person. (Focus group, PHNs; MacKinnon et al., 2007)

Nurses working in small rural communities need to be skilled in maintaining professional boundaries between their home and their work responsibilities. At the same time, rural nurses demonstrate considerable creativity mobilizing community resources and developing/delivering local programs and health services (Bushy, 2002; MacKinnon, 2008). Rural nurses have mobilized community strengths by knowing about and living alongside the people in their communities. Feminist researchers (DeVault, 1991) have described "relationship work" as a form of important, yet invisible, work done by women in our society. This kind of nursing work is grounded in knowing their rural community. The centrality of relationships in rural nursing work and the importance of knowing their community also makes visible the difficulties of practice models where nurses "from away" are flown into isolated rural and remote communities for relatively brief periods of time (Minore et al., 2005). Vukic and Keddy (2002) have also described invisible aspects of rural nursing work such as "integrating into an indigenous setting" (p. 542).

Consistently, researchers hear of the complexity of rural nurses' work (MacLeod et al., 2004). In a recent study of rural nurses' experiences of providing maternity care, rural hospital nurses were able to clearly identify situations in which their work required advanced assessment and decision-making skills such as delivering the baby and resuscitating a preterm neonate until the neonatal transport team arrived (MacKinnon, 2008). Performing complex tasks, even if only rarely, requires accessible skill rehearsal continuing education programs, preferably in an interprofessional format (Horner, 2008).

Areas identified as particularly challenging for rural nurses working in hospital settings included providing emergency and maternity care and dealing with complex mental health challenges (MacKinnon, 2008). Working alone can also mean being the designated maternity nurse in a small rural hospital. Being alone can be a scary experience, particularly for new and less experienced registered nurses. Understanding the knowledge and skills required by rural nurses makes the experiences of new nurses understandable and provides support for the need for nursing internships models and for continuing professional education (MacKinnon, 2010).

While the resources in rural and remote communities vary considerably, many rural nurses do share a sense of marginalization or identify a lack of understanding about rural nursing issues from nurses and educators working in urban and suburban settings (Medves & Davies, 2005; Drury et al., 2005).

The Context for Rural Nursing Work

The characteristics of the local community, including available resources, amenities, people, and community needs, directly influence nursing work in these settings. Rural nurses describe needing to know who lives in their community, what their skills are, and whether they are available to address local health needs and respond in emergency situations (MacKinnon, 2008). Rural settings can be very different across the country; the context for nursing work becomes increasingly significant as the size of the community decreases. For example, the nature of nursing work in settings where the nurse is the sole healthcare provider differs considerably from nursing work in small towns where peer support and mentoring are available (Andrews et al., 2005).

Differences in rural nursing work are heavily influenced by the context for care and the human, material, social, and educational resources available for the nurse to draw upon when caring for people living in a particular community (Howie, 2008a; Misner et al., 2008). For example, mobilizing available resources might include knowing who has taken a First Aid course and could "help out" when a serious motor vehicle accident involving several people occurs.

SITUATING THE TOPIC: FRAMING THE ISSUE

The shortage of available healthcare providers who are able and willing to work in rural, northern, and remote communities across Canada continues to worsen (Stewart et al., 2005). The intensifying nursing shortage and increasing regionalization of healthcare services requires new and creative approaches to provide nursing and health services for rural Canadians (McBride & Gregory, 2005).

Explicating Assumptions

As a nurse educator and researcher who has practiced nursing in both geographically isolated small towns and large urban settings, it is important to articulate the assumptions about rural nursing that underpin the issues analysis that follows. Based on a review of the literature and research conducted in partnership with rural nurses, it is assumed that rural nursing is influenced by:

- The context for care and the availability of social, material, educational, and human resources.
- Perceptions about the nature and importance of rural nursing work which influences decisions about the allocation of resources.
- How nursing work is organized by textually mediated work processes and institutional work practices.

Examining rural nurses' work of caring for childbearing women and their families allows us to explore many of the factors that influence rural nurses' satisfaction with their work and their willingness to work in rural and remote communities. Finally, better support for rural nurses' work could address the longstanding issues surrounding recruitment and retention of rural nurses.

Articulating the Issue

The issue that we will explore is how to ensure that there are enough skilled nurses available to provide appropriate nursing care for people living in rural and remote communities across Canada. What are the factors that influence the recruitment and retention of rural nurses?

Analyzing the Issue: Ways of Understanding

The issue of recruitment and retention of skilled nurses is one of the most longstanding and multi-faceted issues affecting rural nurses in Canada. It involves complex community factors such as community services and job opportunities for nurses and their family members. Many rural communities in Canada are experiencing job losses due to mill closures, decreases in fish and lumber resources, and the consolidation of many services in larger urban centers (Hanlon & Halseth, 2005). The tourism industry also presents unique challenges for rural nurses because of fluctuations in health service requirements and increased safety needs when rural nurses work alone with strangers (Fitzwater, 2008). The availability of maternity care in rural communities has also been shown to influence young families' willingness to relocate to rural and remote communities (Klein et al., 2002). The issues articulation framework is used to explore historical, political, economic, ethical/legal, social/cultural, postcolonial, and feminist understandings.

Understanding the Issue Historically

The Victoria Order of Nursing (VON) was founded in 1897 by the National Council of Women of Canada. These women were convinced that the lack of medical and nursing services for pioneer women contributed to high maternal and infant mortality rates. VON began by providing prenatal and postnatal care in small cottage hospitals across Ontario and visiting nurse services in country districts. Although the rural program was not continued because of the lack of secure funding, this early work convinced health and medical officials that nurses were able to provide care in the home and therefore improve the health of rural families. VON also established "training homes" in Ottawa, Montreal, Toronto, and Halifax, which provided nurses with the opportunity to take a formal course in public health and visiting nursing in Canada. Because employment in this nursing specialty required skills beyond those obtained in hospital training programs, PHNs were later counted among the profession's elite (McKay, 2005).

The first PHNs in rural and northern Canada often worked alone, were assigned to large geographic districts where travel was difficult, and were more likely to be expected to provide emergency medical care. Nurses' stories about early rural public health nursing speak to the difficulties nurses experienced traveling in rural and remote communities. "Nurses travelled on foot, by car, on horseback, by dogsleds, on airplanes and trains, and on snow-shoes. They braved dangerous road and weather conditions to travel to families in need of care" (McKay, 2005, p. 109).

Unlike their counterparts in urban settings, the first rural PHNs were often generalists. They delivered programs in health education, dental health, communicable disease control, prenatal and postnatal care, prevention of chronic illness, and medical/surgical nursing. In addition, they delivered babies and provided emergency medical, dental, and even veterinary assistance on frequent occasions when these professionals were not available. Although the work was arduous and seemingly never ending, the sense of satisfaction in both a career and a way of life was sufficient reward for many nurses (McKay, 2005, p. 119).

After World War I (WWI), interest grew in the role nurses could play improving the health of Canadians. Concerns were once again raised about Canadians living in rural and remote areas of the country where public health programs were not available. Although there was also a need for primary care services in rural communities, local governments did not have the resources to fund child welfare nurses. Nurses who had struggled to establish themselves in rural communities knew that when they left the rural community nobody was going to take their places. Their exit meant the end of both public health programs and essential primary healthcare services (McKay, 2005). Prior to the introduction of the Hospitals Act and medical care funding, which positioned doctors as the "gatekeepers" to the Canadian healthcare system, most "graduate" nursing work was community-based practice (McPherson, 2003).

Outpost nursing began as early as the 1890s and was well established in Canada by the 1920s (Dodd et al., 2005). Outpost nurses provided essential health services to isolated and northern communities who had little or no access to medical care. Following WWI, the Canadian Red Cross Society set up a chain of outpost nursing stations and hospitals in remote areas with 43 outposts eventually being established in Ontario alone. Similar services, modeled after the pioneering work of VON, were established in Newfoundland, Labrador, Alberta, and Quebec. These pioneering programs also demonstrated that public funding was needed to ensure access to essential health services in remote and, typically, poor communities that could not afford or were unable to attract a physician. Because of need, outpost nurses frequently undertook tasks that were beyond the sanctioned scope of nursing practice and gained gratitude and respect from their local communities.

The work of outpost nurses included managing deliveries, suturing victims of farm accidents, battling epidemics of influenza and diphtheria, and holding makeshift "clinics" at local dances to provide opportunities for rural people to consult the nurse about their health concerns. These nurses were on call 24 hours a day to provide advice and treatment, sometimes consulting with distant physicians. Outpost nurses also organized traveling dental, eye, and tonsil clinics, bringing needed health services to their remote communities (Dodd et al., 2005). Because the needs of the community commonly shaped the roles and responsibilities of the community-based nurse, the boundaries between district, outpost, and public health nursing have always been blurred. PHNs, however, focused their efforts primarily on the prevention of illness and the promotion of health rather than on the provision of direct nursing care (McKay, 2005).

Beginning in 1904, the Canadian government, because of its responsibilities for Aboriginal healthcare, placed a few outpost nurses in arctic and sub-arctic regions of Canada. This placement was deemed necessary "for humanitarian reasons … and to prevent the spread of disease to the white population" (Dodd et al., 2005, p. 144). Maternity care was one of the primary motivators for establishing outposts but posed problems because midwifery was illegal in most provinces. The federal government preferred to hire nurses with midwifery experience (usually from Britain) to provide care in northern communities partly because they were less expensive than PHNs. Few outpost nurses received obstetrical training and many simply learned on the job or from "lay" midwives in the community. In Alberta, the Public Health Nurses Act of 1919 granted nurses the authority to practice midwifery in remote areas where no doctors were available.

Understanding the Political Nature of the Issue

Although rural nursing is practiced locally, it is affected by political decisions usually made in larger urban centers. When resources are allocated proportionate to population, rural communities are disadvantaged. Since it costs more to live and to provide health services in small rural and remote communities, allocating resources in this way can result in health inequities and affect the willingness of nurses and other healthcare providers to work in rural and remote communities (Howie, 2008b).

Decisions made about resource allocation are political decisions that are influenced by perceptions about the nature and importance of rural communities and rural nursing work. The relative invisibility of rural nurses' work also contributes to misunderstandings by the public and by other nurses. For example, many people do not know that rural nurses frequently deliver babies when the primary maternity care provider (physician or midwife) is not available at the local hospital and the woman arrives in active labor (MacKinnon, 2008).

Health professionals' scopes of practice are also negotiated politically. The practice of many rural and remote nurses overlaps with medicine and rural nurses are frequently "certified" to provide medical diagnostics (such as Pap smears and testing for sexually transmitted infections) and minor procedures such as suturing (College of Registered Nurses of British Columbia [CRNBC], 2011). Nurse practitioners are increasingly being prepared to provide primary healthcare in rural and remote settings (McDonald & McIntyre, 2010). However, power differentials between nursing and medicine remain and warrant our thoughtful consideration.

The reintroduction of midwives into the Canadian healthcare system also required the renegotiation of scope of practice boundaries between providers of maternity care. While many rural nurses welcomed midwives to their communities, lack of understanding about the knowledge and skill of midwives and nurses makes collaborative relationships more difficult. Shared interprofessional education has been proposed as one strategy for fostering collaboration (Zimmer, 2006).

Many of the policies and practice guidelines that influence rural nursing work are developed for urban and suburban practice settings. For example, the number of required continuing education programs and certifications for nurses in generalist practice can be overwhelming. Educational programs that utilize "train-the-trainer" models may also be difficult to implement in settings where the nursing resources are stretched to capacity. As the list of required certifications and mandatory education programs grows for RNs, we need to be aware of the implications for generalist rural nurses working in resource-limited facilities and communities (MacKinnon, 2010). This continual increase in the demands and scope of practice influence the recruitment and retention of nurses willing and able to practice in rural and remote settings.

Economic Understandings

In the late 1990s reductions in federal spending on healthcare resulted in regionalized healthcare services and, consequently, health services were centralized for fiscal reasons (Pauly, 2004). Although it may make economic sense to centralize some acute and/or highly specialized services, unrecognized costs are borne by Canadians living in rural and remote communities. These costs include travel to and from regional referral centers—and the dangers associated with travel, particularly in winter months—as well as the emotional, social, and family costs of leaving their home communities to access healthcare (Kornelsen & Grzybowski, 2005; Moffitt & Vollman, 2006). These costs can also affect the willingness of nurses to work in rural and remote communities.

For example, since 2000, maternity services were closed in 17 communities across British Columbia, echoing a trend that has also occurred in Ontario, Nova Scotia, and abroad (Kornelsen & Grzybowski, 2006). Although maternity care can be thought of as a "specialized" health service, the need to provide care for healthy women and families and the unpredictability of childbirth also make maternity care an essential component of primary healthcare services (Multidisciplinary Collaborative Primary Maternity Care Project [MCPMCP], 2006). Decision makers need a complex understanding of the effects of their decisions on rural communities and awareness of the contribution of maternity care to the sustainability of small communities (Miewald et al., 2011). Closing small rural hospitals or decreasing the availability of primary healthcare services also has a cost that may be borne disproportionately by Canadians, including Aboriginal people, living in rural and remote communities (Kornelsen & Grzybowski, 2005).

Another hidden cost that needs to be taken into account is the cost of continually needing to recruit and provide orientation for nurses (American Federation of State, County, and Municipal Employees [AFSCME], 2011). One nurse manager noted the considerable time involved, as rural nurses need a combination of education and experience, often in more than one nursing specialty. Although she recommended building teams of nurses with different areas of expertise, she also lamented the retirement of many skilled rural nurses and identified the costs associated with supporting new nurses to develop the knowledge and skills needed for rural nursing work (MacKinnon, forthcoming).

Ethical and Legal Understandings

The fact that both successes and failures in nursing practice are more visible in small rural and remote communities has been documented (Scharff, 2010). Stories of moral distress experienced by nurses who lost a community member in an emergency or a baby in the delivery room have surfaced in studies of nurses' experiences with working and living in rural and remote communities. Although most rural nurses report good relationships with physicians and other healthcare providers, tensions can arise when others do not respond to the nurses' calls for assistance or do not respect the nurses' knowledge and skills (MacKinnon, 2011).

Previous research has also documented that healthcare providers and rural and remote community members may have different understandings of risk—including legal risks. Within medicine and nursing, taking risks during childbearing or with the lives of neonates and children is understood as an unacceptable practice (MacKinnon & McIntyre, 2006). In many remote and northern communities across Canada, childbearing women are routinely evacuated in the last month of pregnancy so that they can give birth in larger, regional hospitals (Moffitt & Vollman, 2006). Because nurses with midwifery background are less available to provide care in small outpost settings today, some nurses also feel less confident about supporting normal childbirth. Tensions arise when First Nations' women, who understand birth as a "community, social and spiritual act" (Daviss, 1997, p. 441), want to reclaim birth in their communities. Nurses can experience ethical distress when they are caught between wanting to advocate for community needs and their own beliefs about "acceptable" risks.

Currently, the predominant discourses of legal risk are very loud (MacKinnon & McCoy, 2006), discouraging nurses from taking professional risks by stepping outside the sanctioned scope of nursing practice. Rural nurses are also held to the same standard of care as nurses working in urban and suburban settings. When the context for nursing care is not taken into account, concerns about losing one's "registration" can also influence the willingness of nurses to work in rural and remote communities. For example, outpost nurses also face overwhelming workloads and isolation when working as the sole health service providers in Inuit and First Nations communities. Lack of adequate staff, backup, and resources increase rural nurses' concerns about their legal and ethical risks (Andrews et al., 2005).

Rural nurses tell us that much of their work in the hospital setting involves protecting patients from harm (MacKinnon, 2011). They are concerned about having sufficient human and material resources available for them to do their "safeguarding" work and are particularly concerned about ensuring that a skilled nurse (a nurse who had the requisite knowledge and skills for the situation "at hand") is always available. Rural nurses' work of staffing their local hospital could also be seen as a form of safeguarding and of advocating for the people living in their rural community (MacKinnon, forthcoming).

Social and Cultural Understandings

Rural residents value independence, hardiness, and self-reliance, which can affect their willingness to seek and accept healthcare (Bales et al., 2010). Some rural residents believe that community cohesiveness is enhanced by living in an isolated or remote community (Findholt, 2010). The differentiation between "newcomers" and "old timers" has been well documented and rural nurses need to establish both relationships and their credibility before they will be trusted professionally (Scharff, 2010). Privacy is also more difficult in small rural communities with some nurses reporting that they feel like they are constantly "on duty" and under the gaze of community residents. Rural nursing practice "emerges as a lifestyle, not merely an occupation" (Howie, 2008a, p. 35).

Rural nurses' job satisfaction has been linked to retention in both acute care and community agencies (Roberge, 2009). Penz et al. (2008) identified the following predictors of job satisfaction for rural nurses working in the hospital setting: Having available and up-to-date equipment and supplies, satisfaction with scheduling and shifts, lower psychological demands or stress in the workplace, and higher satisfaction with the home community. Zibrik et al. (2010) learned that rural acute care nurses equated adequate equipment, education, and staffing with professionalism. Understanding rural nurses' experiences with professionalism helps us to identify sources of job satisfaction and create practice environments that support professional nursing practice. Rural nurses' job satisfaction is also intertwined with their satisfaction with living in a particular rural community.

Nursing also has a culture. Much of the leadership for the profession originates in educational institutions and professional organizations, which tend to be organized around urban and suburban centers. Areas of practice have been contested within nursing but the trend has been for increasing education and specialization. For example, the Canadian Nurses Association (2011) currently recognizes and provides certification for 19 nursing specialties. Preparing generalist nurses within an increasingly specialized healthcare environment is a growing challenge. Nowhere is this more apparent than in maternity care, which is both a nursing specialty and an essential component of primary healthcare services.

RNs make an important contribution to Aboriginal health services in many rural and remote First Nations and Inuit communities. "Since 1994 the First Nations and Inuit Health Branch (FNIHB) of Health Canada has been committed to handing over responsibility for direct service delivery to First Nations and Inuit people" (Kulig et al., 2007, p. 14). Although there are some required components, such as public health, this decentralization has resulted in more local flexibility to deliver health services that are tailored to Aboriginal health needs. For rural nurses, this means that more RNs will be employed by First Nations' communities and fewer by FNIHB. Rural nurses need to be prepared for working in a "politically charged organizational environment" (Kulig et al., 2007).

Many Aboriginal people value relationships and want to receive care from people they know, people who understand their unique cultures and who provide culturally safe and responsive care. The concept of cultural safety moves beyond notions of cultural sensitivity to identify how historical power imbalances and institutionalized racism affects health service provision today (Browne, 2005; Browne et al., 2009). Some nurses may not be aware of how their own cultural background influences the assumptions they make about people living in their rural communities. Self-awareness and willingness to learn from and with Aboriginal people about their strengths and ways of knowing are very important skills for rural nurses working with Aboriginal people (Tarlier et al., 2007).

Postcolonial and Critical Feminist Understandings

In Canada about 4% of the population is Aboriginal, while Aboriginal nurses comprise less than 1% of the nursing workforce (Smith et al., 2011). A postcolonial lens is helpful for understanding why Aboriginal people are underrepresented in the nursing workforce and in nursing education programs. Increasing the proportion of Aboriginal nurses working with First Nations' communities has been suggested as an important strategy for providing culturally relevant health services in these communities (Kulig et al., 2006). A "decolonizing multiple intervention and evaluation approach, and commitment from Aboriginal–university partnerships, governments and health professions" has been recommended (Smith et al., 2011).

The gendered nature of family caregiving has been well described in the feminist literature (DeVault, 1991). Many healthcare services are constructed around assumptions made about families (Smith, 1999) in which women are expected to provide care for family members throughout their lives. Rural women have verbalized their concerns about how the shift from institutional care to the community and the home has increased their work, yet provided little recognition for the stresses placed on women caregivers (Petrucka & Smith, 2005). Recognizing women's family caregiving contributions as work (MacKinnon, 2006) makes the need for access to respite care and home support services more visible to health service planners.

Does the lack of women's and family health services affect the recruitment and/or retention of rural nurses? Although there are few studies of the health needs of rural nurses, the health needs of rural women have been studied. Health concerns identified by women living in rural communities include: Dealing with stress and emotional problems, smoking cessation, limited access to programs and facilities that promote physical and mental health, and the lack of services for older women (Paluck et al., 2006). Bales (2010) interviewed women living in communities with 850 people or less who described navigating distance as both a way of life and as a disadvantage in an emergency. These women put the health of their children first but expressed a desire for preventive, holistic health services and "reasonable access" to medical care.

RESOLUTION: CONSTRAINTS AND POSSIBILITIES

This final section focuses on identifying barriers that influence rural nursing work and creative possibilities or solutions that may address some of these concerns. A global crisis in health and human resources has once again brought attention to the lack of nurses and other healthcare providers who are willing and able to work in rural and remote settings across Canada. Specific challenges include physical isolation, heavy workloads, fewer social amenities or opportunities for spousal employment, smaller professional networks, fewer treatment services, and increased costs of living in rural and remote communities (Kosteniuk et al., 2006).

Internal migration patterns of Canadian-educated rural RNs have been studied using information from the Registered Nurses Database and a national survey (Pitblado et al., 2005). Researchers learned that most RNs who leave their rural community for work or for school do not return home. They concluded that mobility may result in greater losses of nurses than retirement. Communities lose more than healthcare providers when nurses leave rural and remote communities. They also lose "community members who directly contribute to the social and economic well-being and therefore the sustainability of those communities" (Pitblado et al., 2005, p. 119). Proposed recruitment and retention strategies then involve investing in local communities and investing in local healthcare providers (Table 18.1).

Table 18.1 Articulating the Challenges and Recognizing the Possibilities for Supporting Rural Nursing Work

CHALLENGES	POSSIBILITIES
Lack of recognition for the variability and complexity of the work	Listening to the voices of rural nurses who know their work and their communities
Lack of resources including nursing staff & opportunities for continuing education	Creative recruitment incentives and flexible distance/blended learning opportunities
Urban-centric policies, guidelines, and educational programs	Developing policies and programs that reflect the realities of rural nursing practice
Being visible in the community and feeling responsible for needed health services	Developing creative programs based on knowing their community, knowing how to mobilize resources, and knowing how to promote intersectoral collaboration
Difficulty working together when conflict is experienced in interprofessional relationships	Relationship building opportunities, nursing leaders who support "new" nurses, and opportunities for interprofessional education
Generalist/specialist tensions, particularly in hospitals	Building areas of "expertise" within generalist practice over time

Nurses educated in rural communities or small towns are more likely to stay in their communities (Bushy & Leipert, 2005; Lea et al., 2008). Another proposed strategy for recruiting more rural nurses is providing opportunities to live, learn, and work in a rural community as part of preregistration professional education programs (Neill & Taylor, 2002; Van Hofwegan et al., 2005). Communities have rallied around these projects, sometimes providing accommodation and support for students. Because local resources are limited, providing support for rural RNs as preceptors of nursing students has also been identified as essential to ensuring success for rural placements (Yonge, 2007). Creating a consortium that allows nursing students and new graduates to rotate between different rural and remote health services to gain experience has also been recommended (Hegney et al., 2002a).

Rural nurses place high value on building and maintaining competency in clinical skills, particularly in being able to perform rarely used emergency skills (Hegney et al., 2002b; Horner, 2008). Continuing education opportunities, then, become an important retention strategy for rural and remote nurses. Barriers to continuing education that have been identified include staffing shortages and the resultant inability to replace rural nurses so that they can attend education sessions (Jukkala et al., 2008; MacKinnon, 2010). Other barriers include the lack of employer or administrative support, workplace budget constraints, family responsibilities and limited access to childcare, and time and financial constraints for tuition and travel (Penz et al., 2007).

Kosteniuk et al. (2006) proposed that employers can facilitate access to information and knowledge exchange by providing education, travel support, opportunities for knowledge sharing, and promoting physical access to peripheral information sources (such as the Internet and journals) during work time. Scholarships and bursaries for both nursing students and rural and remote nurses have been recommended (MacLeod et al., 2004).

Supporting nurses through providing opportunities for continuing professional education in their local communities has been identified as an important retention strategy for rural nurses. Lindsey (2007) conducted interviews and focus groups with rural nurses from across British Columbia to develop an education program that was tailored to the needs and concerns of rural nurses. The rural nursing certificate program was then developed collaboratively with participation from nurse leaders, nurse educators, and front-line nurses working in rural and remote communities. This module-based, distance education program uses blended learning technologies to deliver educational opportunities as close to home as possible. (See the University of Northern British Columbia's Website for further details.)

Kulig (2005) noted that a number of nursing education programs with a rural focus are being developed across Canada. Recruitment and retention of rural nurses have become an important priority for employers, and a variety of recruitment incentives are being proposed and used. These incentives include student loan repayment incentives, housing and northern cost of living allowances, and systems that facilitate relocation of spouses and partners. Marketing a rural lifestyle and the advantages of community support might also be an effective recruitment strategy (Hegney et al., 2002b).

However, nurses working as the *only* healthcare provider warrant special consideration. A recent study of 412 RNs working alone in rural and remote Canada described these nurses and the communities they work in and identified predictors of work satisfaction (Andrews et al., 2005). Barriers to continuing education and emotional stressors associated with high workloads were identified as negatively related to job satisfaction. Face-to-face contact with other healthcare providers (not necessarily RNs) and "decision latitude," or the discretion needed to make decisions, organize their work, and use their skills, were positively related to work satisfaction. Given the importance of continuity of care and relationships in remote communities, this study has important implications for employers who recruit and attempt to retain nurses who work alone.

MacLeod et al. also identified the need to pay special attention to supporting nurses working with Aboriginal communities and to "the ways in which continuity of care and culturally appropriate care can be provided" (2004, p. 3). Creative models with respite from isolated remote communities may also be required (Minore et al., 2004). Henderson-Betkus and MacLeod (2003) have also identified strategies for retaining PHNs in rural British Columbia.

Nursing regulations and scope of practice documents also influence nursing practice in rural and remote communities. Negotiations around scope of practice and "who can do what" are also political acts that tend to ignore the impact of these decisions on rural and remote communities. For example, PHNs working in northern British Columbia identified a number of barriers (including economic, scope of practice limitations, and power relations) to their ability to offer health promotion and early risk identification for women living in their communities (Leipert, 1999). These rural PHNs believed that their ability to listen, to respect, and to provide care in a nonjudgmental way meant that they could provide more comprehensive and holistic women's health services, including sexual health services and Pap screening. Flexible boundaries and overlapping scopes of practice may be more appropriate for healthcare providers working in rural and remote communities.

Interprofessional willingness to embrace new and creative models for collaborative practice may come from carefully listening to the experiences and concerns of all rural healthcare providers. Union and management structures and practices can also be a barrier in rural settings. The disappearance of front-line nursing leaders (e.g., head nurses) within hospital administrative structures has made visible the need for front-line leadership for nurses working in rural communities. For example, negotiating a delay in a "routine" induction when skilled nursing staff are not available may be difficult for inexperienced rural nurses who do not have the support of a more experienced nurse available to them (MacKinnon, 2010). However, closer relationships between managers, nurses, and other healthcare providers in local rural and remote communities also increase the possibilities for collaborative resistance against centrally imposed cutbacks in personnel or health services (MacKinnon, forthcoming).

Within nursing education there are also competing priorities between community health and acute care nursing, and between specialty practice as needed for urban and suburban settings and primary healthcare which may be more appropriate for nursing in rural and remote communities. Nursing education programs that focus on rural and remote health services are being developed in several locations across the country, which may allow more sustained attention to the knowledge needed for rural and remote nursing practice.

Along with embracing the full scope of nursing practice, creative programs that provide educational opportunities for advanced practice nurses with additional skills in primary healthcare, such as NPs, are also being developed to address health needs in rural and remote communities (Higuchi et al., 2006; Tilleczek et al., 2005).

The World Health Organization [WHO] (2010) has recently released evidence-based recommendations for the retention of health workers in rural and remote areas globally. These recommendations address education, regulation, financial incentives, and both personal and professional support (Rourke, 2010).

SUMMARY

Rural communities are extremely different from one another so it is likely that "one-size-fits-all" solutions will not work for all rural and remote communities across Canada. Learning to listen well to rural nurses, other healthcare providers, and community members, and sustaining attention through rural health research should help to ensure that policies and practices that influence health and health services in rural communities are identified. Working collaboratively with rural nurses, decision makers can identify and address barriers that influence the recruitment and retention of skilled nurses who work in rural and remote communities. Community partnerships that mobilize local resources can help to ensure that Canadians living in rural and remote communities across Canada are also recipients of our global attention to "Health for All" (WHO, 2007).

Add to your knowledge of this issue:		*Online*
Aboriginal Nursing Association of Canada	http://www.anac.on.ca	
Canadian Association for Rural and Remote Nursing (CARRN)	http://www.carrn.com	
Rural Nursing Program at the University of Northern British Columbia	http://www.unbc.ca	

REFLECTIONS *on the Chapter...*

1 Is rural nursing a specialty? If so, what kinds of education and experience do rural nurses need?

2 What does it mean to practice the "full scope" of nursing in rural and remote communities?

3 How can we make continuing education programs for rural nurses affordable and accessible?

4 What role do/could advanced practice nurses, such as NPs, play to address health needs in rural and remote communities?

5 How can nurses provide culturally safe and responsive care when working with First Nations' communities?

6 How could interprofessional teams of healthcare providers work together to ensure that rural health services are available as close to home as possible for Canadians living in rural and remote communities?

7 What assumptions are currently being made about women's family caregiving work in rural and remote communities? How could women, families, and nurses work together to lobby for resources?

8 What assumptions are currently being made about rural nursing work and what can we learn from nurses working in rural and remote communities?

Want to know more?   Visit the Point for additional helpful resources:

- Journal Articles
- Learning Objectives
- Nursing Professional Roles and Responsibilities
- Bonus chapters:
  - Health and Nursing Policy: A Matter of Politics, Power and Professionalism
  - The NP Movement: Recurring Issues
  - When Difference Matters: The Politics of Privilege and Marginality

References

American Federation of State, County, and Municipal Employees (2011). *Solving the nursing shortage* Retrieved from http://www.afscme.org/publications/1193.cfm

Andrews, M., Stewart, N., Pitblado, R., Morgan, D.G., Forbes, D., & D'Arcy, C. (2005). Registered nurses working alone in rural and remote Canada. *Canadian Journal of Nursing Research, 37*(1), 14–33.

Bales, R. (2010). Health perceptions, needs, and behaviors of remote rural women of childbearing and childrearing age. In H. Lee & C. Winters (Eds.), *Rural nursing* (3rd ed., pp. 91–104). New York: Springer Publishing.

Bales, R., Winters, C., & Lee, H. (2010). Health needs and perceptions of rural persons. In H. Lee & C. Winters (Eds.), *Rural nursing* (3rd ed., pp. 57–71). New York: Springer Publishing.

Browne, A. (2005). Discourses influencing nurses' perceptions of First Nations patients. *Canadian Journal of Nursing Research, 37*(4), 62–87.

Browne, A., Varcoe, C., Smye, V., Reimer-Kirkham, S., Lynam, M.J., & Wong, S. (2009). Cultural safety and the challenges of translating critically oriented knowledge in practice. *Nursing Philosophy, 10*(3), 167–179.

Bushy, A., & Leipert, B. (2005). Factors that influence students in choosing rural nursing practice: A pilot study. *Rural and Remote Health (online), 5*(2), 387. Retrieved from http://www.rrh.org.au

Bushy, A. (2002). International perspectives on rural nursing: Australia, Canada, USA. *Australian Journal of Rural Health, 10*, 104–111.

Canadian Institute for Health Information. (2006). *How healthy are rural Canadians? An assessment of their health status and health determinants.* Ottawa, ON: Author. Retrieved from www.phac-aspc.gc.ca/publicat/rural06/pdf/rural_canadians_2006_report_e.pdf

Canadian Nurses Association. (2011). *Certification for nursing specialties.* Retrieved from http://www.cna-aiic.ca/CNA/nursing/certification/specialties/default_e.aspx

College of Registered Nurses of British Columbia. (2011). *Remote Nursing Certified Practice.* Retrieved from https://www.crnbc.ca/Standards/CertifiedPractice/Documents/RemotePractice/493Introductionto RemoteCP.pdf

Daviss, B. (1997). Heeding warnings from the canary, the whale and the Inuit. In R. Davis-Floyd & C. Sargent (Eds.), *Childbirth and authoritative knowledge* (pp. 441–473). Berkeley, CA: University of California Press.

DeVault, M. (1991). *Feeding the family: The social organization of caring as gendered work.* Chicago, IL: University of Chicago Press.

Dodd, D., Elliott, J., & Rousseau, N. (2005). Outpost nursing in Canada. In C. Bates, D. Dodd, & N. Rousseau (Eds.), *On all frontiers: Four centuries of Canadian nursing* (pp. 139–152). Ottawa, ON: University of Ottawa Press.

Drury, V., Francis, K., & Dulhunty, G. (2005). The lived experience of rural mental health nurses. *Online Journal of Rural Nursing and Healthcare, 5*(1), 19–27.

Findholt, N. (2010). The culture of rural communities: An examination of rural nursing concepts at the community level. In H. Lee & C. Winters (Eds.), *Rural nursing* (3rd ed., pp. 373–384). New York: Springer Publishing.

Fitzwater, A. (2008). The impact of tourism on a rural nursing practice. In J. Ross (Ed.), *Rural nursing: Aspects of practice* (pp. 137–146). Dunedin, NZ: Rural Health Opportunities. Retrieved from http://www.moh.govt.nz/moh.nsf/pagesmh/8310/$File/rural-nursing-aspects-of-practice-mar08.pdf

Hanlon, N., & Halseth, G. (2005). The greying of resource communities in northern British Columbia: Implications for health care delivery in already-underserviced communities. *The Canadian Geographer/ Le géographe canadien, 49*(1), 1–24.

Hanvey, L. (2005, September). *Rural nursing practice in Canada: A discussion paper.* Ottawa, ON: The Canadian Nurses Association.

Hegney, D., McCarthy, A., Rogers-Clark, C., & Gorman, D. (2002a). Why nurses are attracted to rural and remote practice. *Australian Journal of Rural Health, 10*(3), 178–186.

———. (2002b). Retaining rural and remote area nurses. *Journal of Nursing Administration, 32*(3), 128–135.

Henderson-Betkus, M., & MacLeod, M. (2003). Retaining public health nurses in rural British Columbia: The influence of job and community satisfaction. *Canadian Journal of Public Health, 95*(1), 54–58.

Higuchi, K.A., Hagen, B., Brown, S., & Zieber, M.P. (2006). A new role for advanced practice nurses in Canada: Bridging the gap in health services for rural older adults. *Journal of Gerontological Nursing, 32*(7), 49–55.

Horner, C. (2008). Emergency health provision and maintaining competency. In J. Ross (Ed.), *Rural nursing: Aspects of practice* (pp. 125–136). Dunedin, NZ: Rural Health Opportunities. Retrieved from http://www.moh.govt.nz/moh.nsf/pagesmh/8310/$File/rural-nursing-aspects-of-practice-mar08.pdf

Howie, L. (2008a). Contextualized nursing practice. In J. Ross (Ed.), *Rural nursing: Aspects of practice* (pp. 33–52). Dunedin, NZ: Rural Health Opportunities. Retrieved from http://www.moh.govt.nz/moh.nsf/pagesmh/8310/$File/rural-nursing-aspects-of-practice-mar08.pdf

———. (2008b). Rural society and culture. In J. Ross (Ed.), *Rural nursing: Aspects of practice* (pp. 3–18). Dunedin, NZ: Rural Health Opportunities. Retrieved from http://www.moh.govt.nz/moh.nsf/pagesmh/8310/$File/rural-nursing-aspects-of-practice-mar08.pdf

Jukkala, A., Henly, S., & Lindeke, L. (2008). Rural perceptions of continuing professional education. *The Journal of Continuing Education in Nursing, 39*(12), 555–563.

Klein, M.C., Johnston, S., & Christilaw, J., & Carty, E. (2002). Mothers, babies, and communities. Centralizing maternity care exposes mothers and babies to complications and endangers community sustainability. *Canadian Family Physician, 48*, 1177–1179.

Kornelsen, J., & Grzybowski, S. (2005). The costs of separation: The birth experiences of women in isolated and remote communities in British Columbia. *Canadian Woman Studies, 24*(1), 75–80.

———. (2006). The reality of resistance: The experiences of rural parturient women. *Journal of Midwifery & Women's Health, 51*(4), 260–265.

Kosteniuk, J., D'Arcy, C., Stewart, N., & Smith, B. (2006). Central and peripheral information use among rural and remote Registered Nurses. *Journal of Advanced Nursing, 55*(1), 100–114.

Kulig, J. (2005). What educational preparation do nurses need for rural and remote Canada? *The nature of rural & remote nursing, 2*. Retrieved from http://www.ruralnursing.unbc.ca/factsheets/factsheet2.pdf

———. (2010). Rural health research in Canada: Assessing our progress. *Canadian Journal of Nursing Research, 42*(1), 7–11.

Kulig, J., MacLeod, M., & Lavoie, J. (2007). Nurses and First Nations and Inuit community-managed primary health services. *The nature of rural & remote nursing, 5*. Retrieved from http://www.ruralnursing.unbc.ca/factsheets/factsheet5.pdf

Kulig, J., Stewart, N., Morgan, D., Andrews, M.E., MacLeod, M.L., & Pitblado, J.R. (2006). Aboriginal nurses: Insights from a national study. *The Canadian Nurse, 102*(4), 16–20.

Lea, J., Cruickshank, M., Paliadelis, P., Parmenter, G., Sanderson, H., & Thornberry, P. (2008). The lure of the bush: Do rural placements influence student nurses to seek employment in rural settings? *Collegian, 15*(2), 77–82.

Lee H., & McDonagh, M. (2010). Updating the rural nursing theory base. In H. Lee & C. Winters (Eds.), *Rural nursing* (3rd ed., pp. 19–40). New York: Springer Publishing.

Leipert, B. (1999). Women's health and the practice of Public Health Nurses in northern British Columbia. *Public Health Nursing, 16*(4), 280–289.

Lindsey, E. (2007). *Rural focused nursing education: Post-basic nursing education in northern and rural British Columbia* (Phase 2 Report). Prepared for the B.C. Nursing Directorate.

Long, K., & Weinert, C. (2010). Rural nursing: Developing the theory base. In H. Lee & C. Winters (Eds.), *Rural nursing* (3rd ed., pp. 3–18). New York: Springer Publishing.

MacKinnon, K., & McCoy, L. (2006). The very loud discourses of risk in pregnancy! In P. Godin (Ed.), *Risk and nursing practice* (pp. 98–120). Basingstoke, UK: Palgrave Publishers.

MacKinnon, K., & McIntyre, M. (2006). From Braxton Hicks to preterm labour: The constitution of risk in pregnancy. *Canadian Journal of Nursing Research, 38*(2), 52–72.

MacKinnon, K. (2006). Living with the threat of preterm labor: Women's work of keeping the baby in. *Journal of Obstetrical Gynecologic & Neonatal Nursing, 35*(6), 700–708.

———. (2008). Labouring to nurse: the work of rural nurses who provide maternity care. *Rural and Remote Health, 8*(4), 1047.

———. (2010). Learning maternity: Rural nurses experiences. *Canadian Journal of Nursing Research, 42*(1), 38–55.

———. (2011). Rural nurses' safeguarding work: Re-embodying patient safety. *Advances in Nursing Science, 34*(2), 1–12.

———. (2012). We cannot staff for "what ifs": The social organization of rural nurses' safeguarding work. *Nursing Inquiry, 19*(3), 259–269.

MacKinnon, K., Yearley, J., Ondrik, C., Kornelsen, J., & Thommasen, H. (2007). *Pilot study for rural nurses' experiences with the provision of maternity care.* Report prepared for the B.C. Medical Services Foundation, the Canadian Nurses' Foundation and the Nursing Care Partnership Program.

MacLeod, M., Browne, A., & Leipert, B. (1998). Issues for nurses in rural and remote Canada. *Australian Journal of Rural Health, 6*(2), 72–78.

MacLeod, M., Kulig, J., Stewart, N., et al. (2004). *The nature of nursing practice in rural and remote Canada.* Retrieved from http://www.chsrf.ca/Migrated/PDF/ResearchReports/OGC/macleod_final.pdf

MacLeod, M., Lindsey, E., Ulrich, C., et al. (2008). The development of a practice-driven, reality-based program for rural acute care Registered Nurses. *The Journal of Continuing Education in Nursing, 39*(7), 298–304.

McBride, W., & Gregory, D. (2005). Aboriginal health human resource initiatives: Towards the development of a strategic framework. *Canadian Journal of Nursing Research, 37*(4), 89–94.

McDonald, C., & McIntyre, M. (2010). The NP movement: Recurring issues. In M. McIntyre & C. McDonald (Eds.), *Realities of Canadian Nursing: Professional, practice, and power issues* (3rd ed., pp. 166–179). Philadelphia, PA: Wolters Kluwer/Lippincott Williams & Wilkins.

McKay, M. (2005). Public health nursing. In C. Bates, D. Dodd, & N. Rousseau (Eds.), *On all frontiers: Four centuries of Canadian nursing* (pp. 107–123). Ottawa, ON: University of Ottawa Press.

McPherson, K. (2003). *Bedside matters: The transformation of Canadian nursing. 1990–1990.* Toronto, ON: University of Toronto Press.

Medves, J., & Davies, B. (2005). Sustaining rural maternity care: Don't forget the RNs. *Canadian Journal of Rural Medicine, 10*(1), 29–35.

Miewald, C., Klein, M., Ulrich, C., et al. (2011). "You don't know what you've got till it's gone": The role of maternity care in community sustainability. *Canadian Journal of Rural Medicine, 16*(1), 7–12.

Minore, B., Boone, M., & Hill, M. (2004). Finding temporary relief: Strategy for nursing recruitment in northern Aboriginal communities. *Canadian Journal of Nursing Research, 36*(2), 148–163.

Minore, B., Boone, M., Katt, M., et al. (2005). The effects of nursing turnover on continuity of care in isolated First Nations communities. *Canadian Journal of Nursing Research, 37*(1), 86–99.

Misner R., MacLeod M., Banks K., et al. (2008). There's rural, and then there's rural: Advice from nurses providing primary healthcare in northern remote communities. *Journal of Nursing Leadership, 21*(3), 54–63.

Moffitt, P., & Vollman, A. R. (2006). At what cost to health? Tlicho women's medical travel for childbirth. *Contemporary Nurse, 22*(2), 228–239.

Neill, J., & Taylor, K. (2002). Undergraduate nursing students' clinical experiences in rural and remote areas: Recruitment implications. *Australian Journal of Rural Health, 10*(5), 239–243.

Paluck, E., Allerdings, M., Kealy, K., & Dorgan, H. (2006). Health promotion needs of women living in rural areas: An exploratory study. *Canadian Journal of Rural Medicine, 11*(2), 111–116.

Pauly, B. (2004). Shifting the balance in the funding and delivery of healthcare in Canada. In J. Storch, P. Rodney, & R. Starzomski (Eds.), *Toward a moral horizon: Nursing ethics for leadership and practice* (pp. 191–208). Toronto, ON: Pearson/Prentice Hall.

Penz, K., D'Arcy, C., Stewart, N., Kosteniuk, J., Morgan, D., & Smith, B. (2007). Barriers to participation in continuing education activities among rural and remote nurses. *The Journal of Continuing Education in Nursing, 38*(2), 58–66.

Penz, K., Stewart, N., D'Arcy, C., et al. (2008). Predictors of job satisfaction for rural acute care Registered Nurses in Canada. *Western Journal of Nursing Research, 30*(7), 785–800. DOI: 10.1177/0193945908319248.

Peterson, W., Medves, J., Davies, B., & Graham, I. (2007). Multidisciplinary collaborative maternity care in Canada: Easier said than done. *Journal of Obstetrics and Gynaecology Canada, 29*(11), 880–886.

Petrucka, P., & Smith, D. (2005). Select Saskatchewan rural women's perceptions of health reform: A preliminary consideration. *Online Journal of Rural Nursing and Healthcare, 5*(1), 59–73.

Pitblado, J. R. (2005). So, what do we mean by "rural," "remote," and "northern"? *Canadian Journal of Nursing Research, 37*(1), 163–168.

Pitblado, J., Medves, J., & Stewart, N. (2005). For work and for school: Internal migration of Canada's rural nurses. *Canadian Journal of Nursing Research, 37*(1), 102–121.

Roberge, C.M. (2009). Who stays in rural nursing practice? An international review of the literature on factors influencing rural nurse retention. *Online Journal of Rural Nursing and Health Care, 9*(1), 82–94.

Rosenthal, K. (2010). The rural nursing generalist in the acute care setting: Flowing like a river. In H. Lee & C. Winters (Eds.), *Rural nursing* (3rd ed., pp. 269–283). New York: Springer Publishing.

Rourke, J. (2010). WHO recommendations to improve retention of rural and remote health workers— important for all countries. *Rural and Remote Health (Online)*, *10*(4), 1654.

Scharff, J. (2010). The distinctive nature and scope of rural nursing practice: Philosophical basis. In H. Lee & C. Winters (Eds.), *Rural nursing* (3rd ed., pp. 249–268). New York: Springer Publishing.

Smith, D., McAlister, S., Gold, S., & Sullivan-Bentz, M. (2011). Aboriginal recruitment and retention in nursing education: A review of the literature. *International Journal of Nursing Education Scholarship*, *8*(1), DOI: 10.2202/1548-923X.2085.

Smith, D., Varcoe, C., & Edwards, N. (2005). Turning around the intergenerational impact of residential schools on Aboriginal people: Implications for health policy and practice. *Canadian Journal of Nursing Research, 37*(4), 38–60.

Smith, D.E. (1999). The standard North American family: SNAF as an ideological code. In D. Smith (Ed.), *Writing the social: Critique, theory, and investigations.* Toronto, ON: University of Toronto Press.

Stewart, N., D'Arcy, C., Pitblado, R., et al. (2005). A profile of registered nurses in rural and remote Canada. *Canadian Journal of Nursing Research, 37*(1), 163–168.

Tarlier, D., Browne, A., & Johnson, J. (2007). The influence of geographical and social distance on nursing practice and continuity of care in a remote First Nations community. *Canadian Journal of Nursing Research, 39*(3), 126–148.

Tilleczek, K., Pong, R., & Caty, S. (2005). Innovations and issues in the delivery of continuing education to Nurse Practitioners in rural and northern communities. *Canadian Journal of Nursing Research, 37*(1), 146–162.

Troyer, L., & Lee, H. (2010). The rural nursing generalist in community health. In H. Lee & C. Winters (Eds.), *Rural nursing* (3rd ed., pp. 285–298). New York: Springer Publishing.

Van Hofwegan, L., Kirkham, S., & Harwood, C. (2005). The strength of rural nursing: Implications for undergraduate nursing education. *International Journal of Nursing Education Scholarship, 2*(1), 1–13.

Vukic, A., & Keddy, B. (2002). Northern nursing practice in a primary healthcare setting. *Journal of Advanced Nursing, 40*(5), 542–548.

World Health Organization. (2007). *The World Health Report: Conclusions and recommendations.* Retrieved from http://www.who.int/whr/2007/conclusion/en/index.html

———. (2010). *Increasing access to health workers in remote and rural areas through improved retention: Global policy recommendations.* Geneva: World Health Organization. Retrieved from http://www.who.int/hrh/retention/guidelines/en/

Yonge, O. (2007). Preceptorship rural boundaries: Student perspectives. *Online Journal of Rural Nursing and Healthcare, 7*(1), 5–12.

Zibrik, K., MacLeod, M., & Zimmer, L. (2010). Professionalism in rural acute-care nursing. *Canadian Journal of Nursing Research, 42*(1), 20–36.

Zimmer, L. (2006). *Seeking common ground: Experiences of nurses and midwives.* Doctoral dissertation, University of Alberta, Edmonton, AB.

19 The Challenges of Holistic Nursing Practice

Noreen Frisch

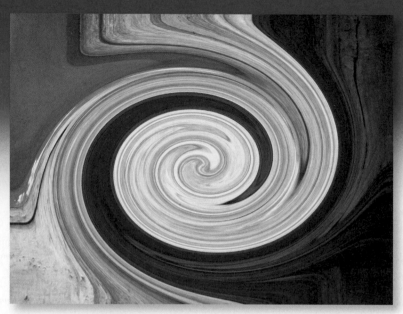

Spiral imaging reminds us of the nonlinear interconnections of holistic nursing. (Used with permission. Photographer Larry Frisch.)

Critical Questions

As a way of engaging with the ideas in this chapter, consider the following:

1. What comes to mind when you think of holistic nursing practice?

2. Do you assume that all nursing practice has the potential to be holistic in nature?

3. Have you thought about how you might look after yourself as an "instrument of healing" throughout your nursing career?

4. What are your assumptions about electronic health records (EHRs) and the ways in which

holistic care might be documented on such records?

5. How do you think the calls for "evidenced-based and evidenced-informed practice" influence your ability to practice holistically?

6. How does commitment to holism interface with nursing contributions to interprofessional practice?

Chapter Objectives

After completing this chapter, you will be able to:

1. Describe the development of holistic thought in the discipline of nursing.

2. Explore the influences of holistic philosophy and nursing theory on holistic practice.

(continued on page 339)

Chapter Objectives (continued)

3. Compare and contrast differing approaches to and definitions of holistic nursing.

4. Examine the challenges to implementation of broadly defined holistic care.

5. Define holistic nursing within your own nursing practice.

Holistic nursing has been defined as an approach to care, a theory of practice, a philosophy of life, a nursing specialty, and an integral part of all nursing practice. Also, holistic nursing is viewed by many healthcare consumers and nurses alike as that practice which incorporates complementary and alternative modalities. Nursing literature includes descriptions of differences between holistic care and comprehensive care. Also, in some cases, holistic approaches are cited as the distinguishing difference between technical care and professional care. There is little doubt that the term *holistic nursing* will lead to confusion and misunderstanding among many. The purpose of this chapter is to review the development of holism in nursing and to provide the reader with enough background from which to make informed judgments about the personal and professional meaning of holistic nursing.

WHAT IS HOLISTIC NURSING?

While there are competing definitions of holistic nursing, there seems to be general agreement that the practice of holistic nursing has to do with an understanding of the person as a whole. Nurses have long been taught that one does not care for the disease or illness, but rather must give care to the *person* with the condition. Most nurses remember the instructions to "address the patient by name," "individualize care," "put yourself in the bed," "understand your patient as a person," and the like. Any approach that calls for nurses to individualize care and to see each client as a unique person calls for some understanding of the person as a whole being. At its very basic level, holistic nursing care means that the nurse addresses more than the client's disease state or physical needs and requires the nurse to give care to the client as a unique individual.

Introductory nursing texts offer differing perspectives on holistic care. Authors of a popular fundamentals of nursing book state that, "when applied to nursing, the concept of holism emphasizes that nurses must keep the whole person in mind and strive to understand how one area of concern relates to the whole person" (Berman, Snyder, Kozier, & Erb, 2008, p. 271). These authors go on to state that nursing interventions aim to restore harmony and serve a client's sense of meaning and purpose in life. To define holistic nursing, these authors simply state, "holistic nursing is nursing practice that has as its goal the healing of the whole person" (p. 1546), taking their definition from that of the American Holistic Nurses Association (AHNA). In contrast, another introductory nursing text states that holism in nursing means "that individuals function as complete units that cannot be reduced to the sum of their parts" (Daniels, 2004, p. 1546). The words *whole*, *complete,* and *harmony* provide descriptors that assist in understanding a broad approach to care that can be called holistic.

At a more advanced level, holistic nursing is the embodiment of the role of "nurse healer." In 1992, Quinn, in her effort to bring clarity to the concept of holism in nursing, noted that our word *heal* stems from the Greek word *hael* "to make sound or whole." Thus, Quinn encouraged nurses to conceptualize a relationship between nursing the whole and healing. She stated, "wholeness as it relates to human beings is much too big, too comprehensive, and too encompassing to be constrained by/in the physical…healing and health are about body-mind-spirit" (p. 553). She went on to present a perspective that wholeness requires people to be in relationship with others. Further, she states that healing is about becoming whole and the locus of healing is within each person. Quinn believed that the holistic nurse becomes one who assists innate healing to occur, perhaps reflecting on nursing heritage and the Nightingale directive to "put the patient in a place where nature can act upon him" (Nightingale, 1946, p. 79).

Understanding the concept of holistic nursing requires knowledge of the development of holistic nursing thought in the discipline. Though, since the time of Nightingale, nursing has addressed aspects of holism, there were events in the 20th century that called attention to holism and affirmed nursing's role in holistic care. These developments will be summarized in the following section.

HOLISM IN NURSING: 20TH CENTURY DEVELOPMENTS

Nurse-theorist Myra Levine is credited with being the first person to use the words "holistic nursing" in her writings. In 1971 she wrote: "The logic of all human experience tells us that we are *whole,* and yet the concept of *holism* is labeled esoteric, elusive and even impractical" (Levine, 253). She was presenting work on her developing nursing theory and recognized that modern scientific thought brought a reductionistic view of all phenomena. Research, scientific findings, and technological advances not only provided many startling benefits to people, but also suggested a view that people could be "reduced" to a series of physiochemical equations. Science brought explanations about disease, molecules, and treatment but could not bring explanations about cure, recovery, and endurance that accounted for individual differences. Levine focused on concepts of integration, interdependence with the environment, change, and adaptation and believed that nursing care should assist in establishing or re-establishing individual integrity (Levine, 1969, 1971).

Levine, however, was not the only nurse scholar of her time who expressed concern over the real or potential dehumanization of care that modern technology could bring. Nor was she alone in calling attention to a holistic paradigm that refused to define nursing as a science of sickness and disease. In 1970, Martha Rogers stated that "human beings are more than and different from the sum of their parts" (p. 46). Others, most notably Jean Watson, developed and expanded the idea that nursing involved caring and was grounded in an important person-to-person relationship between client and nurse. These nursing theorists took a clearly holistic view different from the prevailing scientific view held by many nurses, physicians, and scientists of the time. Reflecting on nursing's past, Erickson (2007) describes the developments this way: One group of nurses was advocating for the advancement of the profession through the specialization of nurses in the care of specific organs or disease conditions (i.e., medical–surgical nurses, neurology nurses, and nephrology nurses). This group believed that people were "*wholistic*"—that people had parts such as a psychosocial part, a biological part, or a cognitive part—but also believed that nursing care could be delivered to one part of the person in isolation from the others. Thus, "*wholistic*" came to mean the view that the whole is the sum of the parts and that the parts are independent. Erickson reports that those skilled in this view became experts in technology, objectivity, and scientific treatments. The other group of nurses, represented by the theorists mentioned above as well as others, argued for a "*holistic*" paradigm that understood the whole as greater than the sum of the parts. This view guided nurses to become concerned with the client's perceptions. These nurses focused on the caring and comforting aspects of nursing (those aspects that the profession inherited from Florence Nightingale) and developed into the true *art* of nursing practice. Erickson (2007) describes the work of these early holistic nurses:

> [They]…recognized the importance of stimulating the five senses as a way of facilitating balance and harmony in themselves and their clients. They used touch, music, massage, soft voice

tones, quiet, and other nursing techniques and strategies that helped people regain balance in body, mind, and spirit. They talked about the person, their perceived needs, and what nurses could do to help the person feel connected and comfortable (p. 144).

The 1970s and 1980s marked a dramatic turning point in the development of nursing as a discipline, as there were four simultaneous movements that later would have huge impacts on holistic nursing. These developments were: (1) Presentation of holistically oriented nursing theories, (2) development of nursing language and classification systems, (3) writings by practitioners who used holistic nursing approaches in actual practice settings, and (4) the establishment of a number of nursing organizations committed to advancing the profession. These developments were followed in the 1990s by the popular discovery of holism—holistic, alternative, and complementary care. Each of these issues is addressed in the following sections.

Holistically Oriented Nursing Theories

Throughout the 1970s and 1980s, academic nurses published theoretical perspectives on the discipline, and students in graduate nursing programs studied and developed various aspects of these theories. Most prominent in the 1970s were Rogers' *Nursing: The Science of Unitary Man* and Watson's *Nursing: The Philosophy and Science of Caring.* Other theorists followed with books, such as Newman's *Health as Expanding Consciousness;* Parse's *Human Becoming;* and Erickson and colleagues' *Modeling and Role-Modeling.* While these theories are distinct from one another, each incorporates aspects of the *holistic* view defined above. Each presented a distinct definition of nursing and a distinct view of the person: Watson emphasized "human care," the caring–healing relationships between nurse and client; Rogers defined the person, not as merely more than and greater than the sum of the parts but as an irreducible whole—a human energy field; Parse also emphasized the notion of the person as irreducible (i.e., that which cannot be reduced to parts and is inseparable from and in mutual process with the environment and nursing as both a science and an art); Newman emphasized health as expanding consciousness that includes an individual's total energy field pattern and nursing as a caring support for people experiencing disruptive processes that can resolve in new patterns; and Erickson and colleagues emphasized *modeling the client's world,* meaning understanding the world from the client's perspective and modeling health behaviors from within the client's worldview. As nursing theory continues to develop today, it provides clear direction for *holistic* care and considerations about care that are grounded in holistic philosophy, nursing science and research, and thoughtful reflections. Table 19.1 presents a summary of these theoretical perspectives on the person and on nursing as presented in the early work of these theorists.

Nursing Language and Classification Systems

In 1972 a different group of nurses came together to define nursing's phenomenon of concern. These nurse leaders were attempting to define that which is nursing and that which a nurse is licensed to do independently, recognizing that much of nursing had been undocumented and undefined. They sought to describe aspects of care that could assist in understanding the discipline as a whole. While some of the nurse theorists were initially involved in this work, the nurse theorists did not continue with this effort and individuals such as Marjorie Gordon and Linda Carpenito became prominent in this field. They sought to establish a nursing language and classification system that would give voice to nursing's work and they certainly believed that nurses' work encompassed care of the whole person. Those involved ultimately established the North American Nursing Diagnosis Association (NANDA), which has become NANDA-International (NANDA-I) today. The NANDA taxonomy became a list of nursing's concerns and, from the beginning, included a call for nurses to document practice areas of physical, cognitive, emotional, spiritual, and family and community care. Criticisms emerged that these systems and

Table 19.1   Theoretical Perspectives on Holism in the 1970s and 1980s

THEORIST (YEAR)	THEORY	HOLISTIC VIEW: PERSON	HOLISTIC VIEW: NURSING
Rogers (1970)	Science of unitary man	Irreducible whole; human energy field	The scientific study of human and environmental energy fields
Watson (1979)	Theory of human care	A holistic being that is greater than and different from the sum of its parts; each person is valued to be cared for and cared about	Mediated by human care transactions that are professional, personal, scientific, aesthetic, and ethical
Parse (1981)	Man–living–health (later renamed as the Theory of human becoming)	Human energy field that is open, indivisible, unpredictable, and ever-changing; in mutual process with the universe and co-constituting rhythmical patterns of relating	A basic science, the practice of which is an art
Erickson et al.(1983)	Modeling and role-modeling	Greater than the sum of the parts; having biophysical, cognitive, psychological, and social components with a genetic base and a spiritual drive	A process that involves interpersonal and interactive relationships and includes facilitation, nurturance, and acceptance
Newman (1986)	Health as expanding consciousness	Dynamic energy field; humans are identified by their field patterns	A profession moving toward an integrated role; nursing is caring

related developments (such as the Nursing Interventions Classification [NIC] and the Nursing Outcomes Classification [NOC], which came later) were following a *wholistic* model that merely listed comprehensive aspects of care without addressing the true *holistic* nature of nursing's work (Mitchell, 1991). Others argued that the classification systems were atheoretical and could be used with any nursing theory to provide *holistic* care. They believed that the nursing language provided a means to describe and document the holistic components of care in a "shorthand" language system as necessary for charting and payment for nursing services (Frisch & Kelley, 2002; Kelley et al., 1995; Potter & Guzzetta, 2005; Potter & Frisch, 2007). These writers also noted that a majority of nursing diagnostic categories described and defined in the taxonomy were of a psychosocial and spiritual nature, requiring the nurse to address the client as a whole person. These debates about the use of standardized language systems in the delivery of holistic care are unresolved today and remain a critical challenge in the 21st century, particularly for holistic nurses entering the world of EHR.

Writings of Nurses Who Applied Holistic Care and Modalities in Practice Settings

Practicing nurses who were discovering holism began to write about their experiences with nursing practice that truly touched themselves and their patients alike. In 1981, Kenner et al. (1981) wrote the first nursing text describing applications of holistic principles and interventions in critical and intensive care nursing settings. They described use of touch, sound, music, and relaxation techniques as part of nursing care and gave nurses guidelines for use of these modalities. At the time, the ideas expressed in this work were revolutionary in critical care settings. Within 2 years, Dossey et al. (1983) published the first edition of their now popular text, *Holistic Nursing: Handbook for Practice.* This book emphasized not only the holistic nursing interventions (touch, massage, imagery, and movement), but also addressed the role of "nurse self-care" in one's personal development and professional readiness for holistic practices. In these writings, for the first time nurses were able to see how others used interventions and strategies to provide comfort and support to treat the whole person in the context of nursing's work. This work was followed by the establishment of newsletters (*Beginnings*) and professional journals (*Journal of Holistic Nursing, Australian Journal of Holistic Nursing,* and *Holistic Nursing Practice*) that continued to provide information, research findings, advice, and opportunities for dialogue for nurses embracing holistic care.

Nursing Organizations

The period of the 1970s and 1980s may well be described as the pinnacle of nursing organizations. Before that time, a few national organizations had prominence in the profession. In the 1970s and 1980s, nurses established and joined a number of specialty organizations. It was a time of excitement and hope as nurses participated in these organizations to move the profession to new heights. This period marks the establishment of several nursing organizations devoted to development of theory (e.g., the Society of Rogerian Scholars), organizations devoted to the use of modalities (e.g., Nurse Healers Professional Associates), and nursing organizations to support the nurse desiring to enter holistic practice (e.g., the AHNA). These organizations each had a unique perspective on holism, and *holistic nursing* took on different connotations as the work of these organizations continued and newer organizations emerged in the decades that followed.

Popular Culture and Interest in Holism

To further complicate the meaning of holistic nursing, the popularization of complementary modalities in the 1990s drew public attention to alternative and holistic practices. In a United States study, Eisenberg's initial survey reported an astounding two thirds of the people surveyed used complementary and unconventional remedies and did not report the use of these remedies to their care providers (Eisenberg et al., 1993). Eisenberg's work pointed out that a significant number of well-educated people were searching for something not included in conventional medical practices, and at least some of their search outside conventional practices was related to their desire for humanistic care that involved relational practices. Holistic nurses were in a position to provide some of the care demanded by the public, but so were other care providers, such as chiropractors, herbalists, acupuncturists, and massage therapists. For many consumers, the search for holism became the search for modality-based providers. Nurses who were developing holistic practices were also gaining knowledge and skills in alternative and complementary modalities and many carried modality-based certification. Thus, nurses who were certified in modalities such as aromatherapy, guided imagery, hypnosis, reflexology, or healing touch were developing what they called *holistic nursing practices,* whether or not these practices were based on holistically oriented nursing theory and whether or not these practices documented care in a nursing model. By 1998, in a survey of over 700 holistic nurses, researchers found that interventions such as acupressure, aromatherapy, biofeedback, guided imagery, presence, healing touch modalities and therapeutic touch, massage, music, and sound therapy, and relaxation were commonly used in practice (Dossey, Frisch, Forker, & Lavin). Some of these nurses stepped into a market with "skills" and developed themselves as holistic nurse entrepreneurs in nurse-owned businesses providing consultation, healthcare assessments and treatment recommendations, life coaching, nurse professional development activities, and direct provision of specialized modalities to clients.

Thus, in the 21st century, nursing is left with a rich tradition of thought that developed nursing's art and continues to expand the theory of nursing in an abstract and conceptual manner. This tradition is steeped in academic nursing, theory development, and critique, and is being carried forward by organizations devoted to the use of nursing theory. Nursing is also enriched by languages and classification systems that have evolved worldwide through NANDA-I and through the work of others that came later to develop the International Classification for Nursing Practice (ICNP). These systems give language to nursing's phenomenon of concern and provide a means to document and reflect on all areas of nursing practice. Many of the terms used in these systems (e.g., *therapeutic presence, spiritual support, grief counseling*) describe aspects of care that are relational, humanistic, and meet the psychosocial and spiritual aspects of care typically associated with holistic interventions. Lastly, many nurses have become experts in alternative modalities that support care of the whole person and have sought modality-based certification. So it is not readily apparent what holistic nursing really is today and what it means to nurses.

MODERN HOLISTIC NURSING: WHAT WE CAN LEARN FROM PROFESSIONAL ORGANIZATIONS

The official voice for nurses is often spoken through national professional associations, so it makes sense to review documents and publications of such organizations for an understanding of how holistic nursing is taken up. Therefore, we will begin by examining the work of the Canadian Holistic Nurses Association (CHNA) and compare its philosophy and approach to organizations in the United States and Australia as these two other approaches are quite different.

The Canadian Holistic Nurses Association

Nurses in Canada who were committed to holism joined to form an organization to further the development of holistic nursing practice. In 1986 they formed the CHNA to ensure that professional health maintenance and promotion services are made available to the people of Canada. The philosophical statement of the association begins with a quotation from Leddy (2003) and states, "we believe that each person is a whole, unitary human being, and a unitary human essence field in continuous mutual process with the environmental essence field" (CHNA, 2006). The association quotes the work of nurse theorist Martha Rogers in describing nursing as an art that is the creative use of science for human betterment and well-being and that has values that include compassion and unconditional love. The goals of nursing listed by the association include to "strengthen the coherence and integrity of the human-environment essence field...stimulate mind-body-spirit healing...[and] facilitate empowerment through the health patterning process" (CHNA, 2006). According to CHNA, holistic nursing practice is grounded in health patterning as described by Barrett's pattern manifestation knowing and mutual patterning process (1990, 1998) and Cowling's pattern manifestation knowing process (1990). The CHNA has taken an exclusively Rogerian view and the representative of the association's specialization committee (Dobbie) writes, "we believe that a nursing conceptual framework based on unitary human science, human environmental essence field theory and energy based nursing practice is the foundation of holistic nursing practice" (retrieved April 30, 2011 from http//:www.chna.ca/specialization.htm).

CHNA provides specialty determination for holistic nursing and provides a framework to guide practice based on unitary human universal essence field theory and unitary energy-based nursing practice. Without question, this approach to holistic nursing has taken the work of Rogers's theory and its expansion and development over the years and built a credible specialty practice and specialization program grounded in this theoretical point of view. The educational program for the specialty begins with coursework on Rogers's theory, field theory, and energy-based and other modalities. Progression requires completion of Level 1 Healing Touch (an introduction to the practice of energy work) or Reiki and further develops theories derived from and consistent with Rogers's work. Lastly, the final phase of the educational program expands to the study of nurse-theorists presenting unitary human wholeness and human–universe mutual process perspectives. A nurse completing the educational program and meeting requirements of the association carries specialization from the CHNA.

Reflecting on the literature of holistic nursing and holism and then examining the approach embraced by our Canadian organization, it is clear that the CHNA takes up one view of holistic nursing—that it be exclusively defined as theory-based practice and be firmly grounded in Rogers's Science of Unitary Human Beings (UHB). Probably no one would dispute that a practice such as that described and supported by CHNA represents holistic nursing. However, a comparison of the CHNA approach to that of other holistic nursing organizations raises important questions about the meaning of the term and its application to practice in settings that function outside the theory of UHB.

There have been two other major movements in holistic nursing—in the United States and in Australia. Each of these countries developed their own holistic nursing organizations and implemented practices, supports, and definitions of holistic nursing that are quite different from each other and stand as a contrast to the approach taken in Canada. Each will be described briefly.

The AHNA was founded in 1980 with a mission "to unite nurses in healing with a focus on holistic principles of health, preventive education, and the integrations of allopathic and complementary caring-healing modalities to facilitate care for the whole client..." (Dossey, 2000, p. xv). AHNA's description of holistic nursing includes the basic statement that "holistic nursing embraces all nursing that has enhancement of healing the whole person from birth to death as its goal" (Dossey, 2000, p. xxvi). Further, the AHNA statement includes the ideas that holistic nursing can be practiced using more than one theoretical perspective; that the holistic nurse is an instrument of healing; and that practicing holistic nursing requires self-care and personal self-responsibility, reflection, and spirituality. Thus, the organization has taken on two simultaneous foci: The development of holistic nursing practices through research and education and assistance to its members in their own personal and professional development through networking groups, conferences, supports, and opportunities to "nurture the nurse." This organization has established the Standards of Holistic Nursing Practice (Frisch et al., 2000; Mariano, 2007) grounded in core values of holistic nursing. The association members had many discussions on whether or not holistic nursing was truly a specialty area of practice or represented what all professional nurses do. The issue was simply that all registered nurses (RNs) have the obligation to carry out professional nursing care in keeping with their scope of practice and, in doing so, any professional nurse can (and should) have as a goal to address the needs of the whole person. However, it was also clear that there is a body of knowledge that is necessary to expand one's professional, legal practice in areas that demonstrate consistency with a specialty practice going beyond the practices legally required for RNs and tested for safe practice on the initial licensing exam. Therefore, the specialty certification is a means to document that individual nurses have knowledge, competencies, and skills beyond what is required for entry into practice as an RN. In 2006, much like the efforts of the CHNA and the Canadian Nurses' Association, the AHNA and the American Nurses Association joined in a mutual effort to recognize holistic nursing as a specialty in the United States. In distinct contrast to the approach taken by the CHNA, the definition of holistic nursing presented by AHNA is broad and designed to encompass much of nursing practice and varying nursing theories. The emphasis on nurse self-care underpins the view that holistic nursing is a way of life.

Nurses in Australia have had a longstanding interest in and commitment to holistic nursing. They established two organizations: The Australian College of Holistic Nurses, Inc. (ACHN) and the Holistic Nurses Association (HNA) of New South Wales. These organizations are no longer active but did attract, support, and launch holistic nurses in their work and their quest for knowledge about holism and complementary modalities. The ACHN was devoted to education and support of nurses performing holistic practices. A former president of the organization,

Rosalie Van Aken (personal communication, June 12, 2008) reports that the 1990s were the most active period for membership. The college sponsored annual conferences that included speakers on theory, complementary modalities, and self-care practices. In collaboration with Southern Cross University, the organization supported the *Australian Journal of Holistic Nursing,* a biennial, peer-reviewed publication that was printed from 1994 to 2005. The mission of the journal reflected the mission of the organization: To document the trends and issues that emerged from contemporary nursing practice. The second Australian organization, the HNA of New South Wales, was founded in the 1990s as well (Redmond, 2000). This organization was inspired by a national conference in natural therapies, and grew out of a "disenchantment with the mechanistic and reductionistic methods of modern healthcare" (Redmond, p. 95). It was founded with an intent to support nurses wishing to undertake holistic practices. The organization had a focus on assisting nurses to develop competence in complementary and alternative modalities. The HNA met its goals of supporting nurses by teaching complementary modalities and working with the regulatory bodies to gain legal support for use of these modalities in nursing practice. Thus, the HNA represented the point of view that holistic nursing is the use of alternative interventions in the practice of nursing for the purpose of meeting client needs.

The fact that these two organizations are no longer active does not necessarily mean that their interests are no longer relevant or valued in Australia. According to Dr. Van Aken, there are probably multiple factors that contributed to the closure of these organizations. Among these were two significant developments: The fact that many holistic nurses became active members of organizations related to complementary modalities (such as Healing Touch or Aromatherapy) and no longer maintained membership in the nursing organizations and the fact that the nurses in Australia (including the Royal College of Nursing) adopted the broader view that all nursing is holistic. In Australia, nurses have not sought to make holistic nursing a specialization as their counterparts in Canada and the United States have done. Many holistic nurses in Australia carry certification in various complementary modalities and continue to build nursing practice on holistic theory.

International Comparison

The holistic nursing movements in these three countries represent very different perspectives and quite diverse views of holistic nursing. Understanding the divergent views may bring nurses to a better understanding of the complexities of determining "what is holistic" and may, in turn, stimulate nurses to consider their personal and professional need to confront the differences.

Canadian nurses may ask themselves to what degree is holistic nursing:

- A specialty rather than an expectation of all nurses,
- Defined narrowly through adopting one theoretical perspective or more broadly based accepting several theoretical perspectives,
- Defined by the theory guiding the practice or by the goal of the care provided, and
- Related more to a philosophy of care or the performance of complementary modalities.

All of the perspectives are legitimate and supported in the literature and each brings value in nursing practice. Given that the CHNA defines holistic nursing according to one theory, Canadian nurses certainly may question if that perspective represents the totality of holistic nursing or if one could practice holistic nursing without being an adherent of Rogerian science.

PRACTICING HOLISTIC NURSING TODAY: ISSUES AND CHALLENGES

Modern nursing work is complex and challenging. The shortage of nurses in Canada (Maddalena & Crupi, 2008) and worldwide has attracted attention to what nurses actually do and plays into the discussions of what nurses will do in the future. Nursing theories have advanced in their development and contribute to nursing reflection and practice. However, nurses in practice see the results of mechanistic and reductionistic care. Nurses' work has been described as a series of tasks to complete, with little time to devote to client education, surveillance, and compassion (Tucker & Spear, 2006; Tucker, 2003). Writers have addressed the silencing of nurses (Gordon, 2005) and the emotional exhaustion felt by many nurses (Aiken et al., 2001). If nurses are to continue to serve as the "front-line" patient contact, holistic nurses must be in a position to provide care true to the "art" of nursing practice—those aspects of care described by Erickson (citedabove) as the work of early holistic nurses who refused to accept nursing as a science of disease and illness. There are four important developments in current practice that should be addressed as one considers the role of holistic nursing today. These are the use of holistic principles in the evidence-based practice (EBP) environment, the use of holistic principles with EHRs, the call for interdisciplinary and interprofessional practice, and the need for nurse self-care to sustain professionalism throughout a 21st century nursing career.

Challenge 1: Evidence-Based Practice

Modern healthcare is steeped in a continuous search for quality through clinical practice guidelines and standardization based on sound research and an evaluation of the evidence. These are very good developments and have certainly helped to raise care standards so that people in one city or locality have the same access to quality care as people on other areas. There is, as is described, the "national standard" of care that requires all providers to accept the prevailing view of "best practice" and provide such care to all. In healthcare, the 21st century arrived with a call for "evidence-based practice" (EBP) and a mandate to perform based solely on that evidence.

The challenge with this development for holistic nurses is that the EBP movement neither defines what evidence is nor does it readily examine the limits of the evidence one has. In modern medicine, evidence is usually determined by the randomized controlled clinical trial (RCT) (Frisch, 2007). The RCT certainly provides clear data on the average response to clinical or experimental interventions and can set parameters for the use of those interventions. Few, however, question if the RCT is the best research method to provide data, not for experimental purposes but for application to actual clinical situations in which clients do not meet the standard of homogeneity required of experimental subjects in clinical trials. Holmes and colleagues pointed out that the operationalization of EBP gives an unquestioned privilege to research designs that prioritize frequency-based methods over qualitative ones (Holmes et al., 2006).

Challenge 2: Electronic Health Records

The second challenge for holistic nurses is the inevitable move from paper to computerized patient care records. This move is in process now as health systems across the country seek to document all aspects of client care through various electronic systems. There is no question that these electronic systems provide an efficient means to record client data and client progress. In addition, they provide a means to track outcomes across client populations. EHR is viewed by most as an interdisciplinary record so that each health professional can enter data into the system and that data can be retrieved by other professionals.

A challenge for nurses, particularly holistic nurses, is the decision of how nursing will be documented electronically. Current nursing language and classification systems provide a very shorthand means of describing nursing's phenomenon of concern. These phenomena may include (among many others): Spiritual distress or spiritual well-being, anxiety, fear, states of grieving, states of coping, and issues related to sleep quality, nutritional status, family relationships, and health promotion. A review of the ICNP (International Council of Nurses [ICN], 2009) and the current NANDA-I taxonomy (Herdman, 2009) indicates that over half of the terms used in these systems are psychosocial and/or spiritual in nature. These terms provide the basis for a very full documentation of nurse and client concerns. Electronic record systems have been developed to make full use of these nursing terms in documenting nursing assessments and care planning, but most of these systems exist outside of Canada. Canadian nurses have developed the Canadian Health Outcomes for Better Information and Care (C-HOBIC) which at the time of this writing is a system to document and initial assessment for an adult client in acute care and track readiness toward discharge. This system is excellent for establishing guidelines for a focused area of practice but leaves the holistic nurse without a formal means to identify the full range of information, actions, and outcomes involved in providing holistic care. Nursing narrative records can be placed into electronic record systems, but these leave nurses' contributions to care irretrievable later.

As stated previously, there has been dissension regarding the use of standardized nursing languages, and many holistic nurses have rejected the process of documentation through standardized nursing terms. At the same time, many have strived to make the standardized languages inclusive so that every area of nursing could be recorded. Today, holistic nurses who may have preferred narrative documentation are faced with the challenge of either using the standardized languages to give voice to nursing's work or to become silent in a system that will include only electronic entries based on coded terms. The challenge for holistic nurses may become to learn to use the standardized languages to their fullest extent and to engage as leaders in activities that promote recording of holistic practices in systems that could easily omit nursing and result in electronic medical records rather than EHRs.

Challenge 3: Holistic Nursing Practice in an Interprofessional Environment

Currently, there is strong interest in having teams of health professionals work together for the betterment of patient care. The impetus for attention to interprofessional practice is the current (perhaps long overdue) effort to provide care that is truly patient centered. Patient-centered care means that not only is the patient a member of the interprofessional team, but also that the patient is very central as the team's source of patient knowledge and as the decision maker about choice of treatments.

The move to provide patient-centered care is highly consistent with the values and approaches taken in holistic practice, as is knowing one's own discipline and its unique contribution to the interprofessional team. Some suggest that the most important contribution that professional nursing makes to the interprofessional team may be nursing's intimate knowledge of each patient and nursing's expertise and ability to reflect on the individual's unique experiences when planning and administering care. One group of writers suggest (after a review of holistic nursing theories) that the unifying focus of professional nursing includes attention to ensuring a humanizing environment, assisting the patient in finding meaning and quality of life, providing for patient choice, and expressing a goal for healing in living and dying (Willis et al., 2008). Thus, one could conclude that the nurse's contribution to the interprofessional team resides not only in holistic values and attitudes but also in the ability to implement care processes that incorporate them. Nurses are the healthcare providers that work most closely with the patients as nurses are with hospitalized patients around the clock and are the most common health professional to visit patients in their homes. Quinn writes, "One of the most powerful tools for healing is the presence of the nurse in the patient's environment" (2009, p. 97). Quinn is describing the nurse acting with intentionality and consciously shifting from "doing to" to "being with" the patient in order to facilitate healing. It is from such a presence that nurses gain the ability to understand and interpret their patients' experiences to other members of the team and influence the care decisions. Other writers suggest that nurses bring their disciplinary perspective of ethical and moral reasoning that, as distinct from that of other health professionals, provides a framework for understanding patient experiences and needs. (Wright & Brajtman, 2011). As nurses attend to individual needs, feelings, and subjective experiences they are often in the best position to interpret for the team members what is important to the patient and, as follows, what is the right action to take.

As nurses reflect on their holistic practices, it is not sufficient to claim that nurses are the only holistic members of interprofessional teams. However, nurses can articulate their contribution to the team if they describe that they bring a therapeutic presence and support to the patient that forms the basis of a nurse–client relationship. This relationship, in turn, permits the nurse to see the patient as unique and encourages understanding of the patient's experiences of living with the illness or condition. Thus, a nurse's contribution to the healthcare team rests on the nurses' ability to engage in relational practice, understand the patient, and bring a unique contribution to the team's thinking. In short, the nurse's contribution to the interprofessional team is the nurse's ability to practice holism.

Challenge 4: Sustaining Self Over the Course of a Nursing Career

One of the definitions of holistic nursing discussed previously is that holistic nursing is a way of life. This perspective means that holistic nursing entails adopting a philosophy of holism, that is, a "philosophy based on a perspective that acknowledges and values the connectedness of the body-mind-spirit, the inherent goodness of human beings, and the ability of each person to find meaning and purpose in his or her own life, and the nurse's role of support to each client so that the client may find comfort, peace, and harmony" (Frisch, 2000, p. 1). Having adopted such a philosophy of nursing, the nurse recognizes in herself or himself that person who is whole and who has the capacity for growth, development, and healing. The holistic nurse becomes an instrument of healing when using unconditional presence and intention to support the healing process of another (Quinn, 2000). To do so, however, the nurse must attend to his or her own personal awareness and self-care. Self-care practices that assist the nurse to sustain health begin with an honest assessment of one's life demands and personal needs, one's risks for health problems, and the formation of a life pattern aimed at supporting one's own health. Secondly, holistic nurses must cultivate awareness and understanding of the deeper meaning and purpose of life and the connectedness with self and others, perhaps aided through ongoing reflections on their own nursing practice.

The importance of self-care for nurses was supported recently by a study conducted by a group of nursing students and their faculty member (Christiaens et al., 2010). The students approached experienced nurses who self-identified as holistic nurses and asked the experienced nurses for advice about how to best enter into the profession. The most frequent response given by the experienced nurses was related to self-care. The students were told that a nurse must care for self first in order to be ready and able to care for others.

Self-care practices are highly individualized, such that practices that support one nurse may not be those that support another. However, all self-care practices give the nurse a strength and a balance or harmony that help one to deal with the stressors, uncertainties, and demands of nursing's work-life. Considering the fact that nurses are at significant risk for vocational "burnout" and emotional exhaustion (Aiken et al., 2001; Beebe & Frisch, 2009), self-care practices may be the distinguishing difference between those who thrive in nursing and those who are unable to sustain the work-life demands. Box 19.1 lists examples of nurse self-care activities.

BOX 19.1   Examples of Nurse Self-care Activities

- Engaging in health-promoting behaviors and health-protecting behaviors
- Empowering self to modify attitudes and develop healthy life patterns
- Creating satisfying interpersonal relationships
- Using wellness programs
- Creating social networks
- Engaging in activities to awaken the inner spirit
- Developing a healthy self-outlook
- Ongoing reflection on one's own professional practice

SUMMARY

This chapter has presented multiple views and definitions of holism and the meaning of holistic nursing. The 20th century was a time of considerable change and advancement in nursing and health science. That period was associated with advances in medical science and a concurrent need to articulate that which is nursing as distinct from the reductionistic view of a medical science of illness and disease. Holistic nursing theorists wrote prolifically and presented views about nursing's philosophy and outlook, successfully challenging the accepted worldview of other healthcare professionals. Similarly, nurses sought to establish nursing standardized languages to give voice to that which had been silent. Nurses experimented with the application of holistic principles and modalities in acute and chronic care settings and began to share their practice experiences with one another. By the end of the century, nurses had established professional organizations to provide support, networking, scholarly exchange, and a collective voice of the discipline.

There have been a number of holistic nursing organizations; one is in Canada. Each is committed to the general ideals of holism and each carries or carried out its work in a manner unique to the organization and its location. Nurses should consider each of the perspectives presented to gain a full understanding of the complexities of holism and its meaning for nursing.

Nursing as a discipline has many challenges on entering the 21st century. How holistic nurses negotiate those challenges will dictate, in many ways, the future of the entire profession. The challenges discussed include: (1) The need to articulate holistic principles in a system devoted to EBP, (2) the requirement of documenting nursing in an electronic patient care record, (3) the contributions of professional nursing to the interprofessional team, and (4) the nurse's need for self-care practices to sustain one's work over the course of a career.

The overriding issue for readers of this chapter may be deciding how holism fits with one's individual worldview and perspective on nursing. In many ways, all nursing care that is professional and compassionate is holistic care. Yet, there are certifications and specialty designations in holistic nursing. Each individual must consider the philosophy of holism and the work of nursing theorists who serve as guides to holistic practices. The questions at the end of the chapter are suggested for further exploration of the issues.

Add to your knowledge of this issue:		Online
Canadian Holistic Nurses Association	**www.chna.ca**	
American Holistic Nurses Association	**www.ahna.org**	

REFLECTIONS on the Chapter...

1 Write you own definition or description of *holistic nursing*. What is the essence of holistic nursing? What perspective do you take regarding your own practice?

2 In what ways is your nursing practice holistic? In what ways is it not?

3 Do you subscribe to a theory of practice? If so, which one? Why is the theory thought to be holistic?

4 Do you have experience with any modality or nursing intervention that may be considered alternative or complementary? Which one(s)?

5 Have you looked at the ICNP or NANDA-I taxonomy of nursing and the NIC and NOC? Try to document the humanistic aspects of your care in this language. Does it work for you?

6 Do you practice self-care techniques and modalities? What do you believe is the single most important factor in sustaining yourself in a nursing career?

7 In what ways are you currently connected to other nurses in supportive ways? How will you continue those connections over time?

Want to know more? Visit thePoint for additional helpful resources:

- Journal Articles
- Learning Objectives
- Nursing Professional Roles and Responsibilities
- Bonus chapters:
  - Health and Nursing Policy: A Matter of Politics, Power and Professionalism
  - The NP Movement: Recurring Issues
  - When Difference Matters: The Politics of Privilege and Marginality

References

Aiken, L.H., Clarke, S.P., Sloane, et al. (2001). Nurses' reports on hospital care in five countries. *Health Affairs, 20*(3), 43–53.

Barrett, E. (1990). *Visions of Rogers' science based nursing.* New York: National League for Nursing.

———. (1998). Theoretical concerns: A Rogerian practice methodology for health patterning. *Nursing Science Quarterly, 11*(4), 136–138.

Beebe, R., & Frisch, N. (2009). Development of the Differentiation of Self and Role Inventory for Nurses (DSRI_RN): A tool to measure internal dimensions of workplace stress. *Nursing Outlook, 57*(5), 240–245.

Berman, A., Snyder, S.J., Kozier, B., & Erb, G. (2008). *Fundamentals of nursing: Concepts, process and practices* (8th ed.). Upper Saddle River, NJ: Prentice Hall.

Canadian Holistic Nurses Association. (2006). *Canadian holistic nursing practice standards.* Author.

Christiaens, G., Abegglen, J.A., & Gardner, A. (2010). Expert holistic nurses' advice to nursing students. *Journal of Holistic Nursing, 28*(3), 201–208.

Cowling, W.R. (1990). A template for unitary pattern-based nursing practice. In E.A.M. Barrett (Ed.), *Visions of Rogers' science-based nursing* (pp. 45–65). New York: National League for Nursing.

Daniels, R. (2004). *Nursing fundamentals: Caring and clinical decision making.* Clifton Park, NY: Delmar Thomson Learning.

Dossey, B. (2000). Introduction. In N. Frisch, B. Dossey & C. Guzzetta, et al. (Eds.), *AHNA Standards of Holistic Nursing Practice* (pp. xv–xxiii). Gaithersburg, MD: Aspen.

Dossey, B., Frisch, N., Forker, J., & Lavin, J. (1998). Evolving a blueprint for certification: Inventory of professional activities and knowledge of a holistic nurse. *Journal of Holistic Nursing, 16*(1), 33–56.

Dossey, B., Keegan, L., & Guzzetta, D. (1983). *Holistic nursing: Handbook for practice.* Sudbury, MA: Jones and Bartlett.

Eisenberg, D.M., Kessler, R., Foster, C., Norlock, F.E., Calkins, D.R., & Delbanco, T.L. (1993). Unconventional medicine in the United States: Prevalence, costs and patterns of use. *New England Journal of Medicine, 328*(4), 246–252.

Erickson, H. (2007). Philosophy and theory of holism. *Nursing Clinics of North America, 42*(2), 139–163.

Erickson, H., Tomlin, E., & Swain, M.A. (1983). *Modeling and role-modeling: A theory and paradigm for nursing.* Englewood Cliffs, NJ: Prentice Hall.

Frisch, N. (2000). Holistic philosophy and education. In N. Frisch, B. Dossey & C. Guzzetta, et al. (Eds.), *AHNA standards of holistic nursing practice* (pp. 1–22). Gaithersburg, MD: Aspen.

————. (2007). Preface, EBP. *Nursing Clinics of North America, 42*(2), xi–xiv.

Frisch, N., Dossey, B., Guzzetta, C., et al. (2000). *AHNA standards of holistic nursing practice.* Gaithersburg, MD: Aspen.

Frisch, N., & Kelley, J. (2002). Nursing diagnosis and nursing theory: An exploration of factors inhibiting and supporting simultaneous use. *Nursing Diagnosis, 13*(2), 53–56.

Gordon, S. (2005). *Nursing against the odds.* Ithaca, NY: Cornell University Press.

Herdman, T.H. (2009). *NANDA – International, Nursing diagnoses: definitions and classification 2009–2011.* Chichester, West Sussex, UK: Wiley-Blackwell.

Holmes, D., Perron, A., & O'Bryne, P. (2006). Evidence, virulence, and the disappearance of nursing knowledge: A critique of the evidence-based dogma. *Worldviews, Evidence Based Nursing, 3*(3), 95–101.

International Council of Nurses (ICN). (2009). *ICNP® Version 2.* Geneva: Author.

Kelley, J., Frisch, N., & Avant, K. (1995). A trifocal model of nursing diagnosis: Wellness reinforced. *Nursing Diagnosis, 6*(3), 123–128.

Kenner, C., Dossey, B., & Guzzetta, C. (1981). *Critical care nursing: Body-mind-spirit.* Boston, MA: Little Brown.

Levine, M. (1969). The pursuit of wholeness. *American Journal of Nursing, 69*(1), 93–99.

————. (1971). Holistic nursing. *Nursing Clinics of North America, 6*(2), 253–264.

Maddalena, V., & Crupi, A. (2008) *A renewed call for action: A synthesis report on the nursing shortage in Canada.* Ottawa, ON: Canadian Federation of Nurses Unions.

Mariano, C. (2007). Holistic nursing as a specialty: Holistic nursing—scope and standards of practice. *Nursing Clinics of North America, 42*(2), 165–188.

Mitchell, G.J. (1991). Diagnosis: Clarifying or obscuring the nature of nursing. *Nursing Science Quarterly, 4*(2), 52.

Newman, M. (1986). *Health as expanding consciousness.* St. Louis, MO: Mosby.

Parse, R. (1981). *Man-Living-Health: A Theory for Nursing.* New York: John Wiley & Sons.

Potter, P., & Frisch, N. (2007). Holistic assessment and care: Presence in the process. *Nursing Clinics of North America, 42*(2), 213–228.

Potter, P., & Guzzetta, C. (2005). The holistic caring process. In B. Dossey, L. Keegan & C. Guzzetta (Eds.), *Holistic nursing: Handbook for practice* (4th ed., pp. 341–372). Sudbury, MA: Jones and Bartlett.

Quinn, J.A. (2000). Holistic nurse self-care. In N. Frisch, B. Dossey & C. Guzzetta (Eds.), *AHNA Standards of holistic nursing practice* (pp. 55–74). Gaithersburg, MD: Aspen.

Quinn, J.F. (1992). On healing, wholeness and the haelan effect. *Nursing Outlook, 10*(10), 552–556.

————. (2009). Transpersonal Human Caring and Healing. In B.M. Dossey & L. Keegan (Eds.), *Holistic nursing: A handbook for practice* (5th ed., pp. 91–100). Boston, MA: Jones and Bartlett.

Redmond, C. (2000). The Holistic Nurses Association of New South Wales: Our history, our present and our future. *Contemporary Therapies in Nursing and Midwifery, 6*(2), 95–97.

Rogers, M. (1970). *An introduction to the theoretical basis of nursing.* Philadelphia, PA: F.A. Davis.

Tucker, A. (2003). *Organization learning from operational failures.* Doctoral dissertation, Graduate School of Business, Harvard University.

Tucker, A., & Spear, S. (2006). Operational failures and interruptions in hospital nursing. *Health Services Research, 41*(3), 643–662.

Watson, J. (1979). *Nursing: The Philosophy and Science of Caring.* Boston: Little Brown.

————. (1988). *Human science and human care.* New York: National League for Nursing.

Willis, D.G., Grace, P.J., & Roy, C. (2008). A central unifying focus for the discipline: Facilitating humanization, meaning, choice, quality of life and healing in living and dying. *ANS, 31*(1), E28–E40.

Wright, D., & Brajtman, S. (2011). Relational and embodied knowing: Nursing ethics within the interprofessional team. *Nursing Ethics, 18*(1), 20–30.

20 Opening Conversations: Dilemmas and Possibilities of Spirituality and Spiritual Care

Anne Bruce

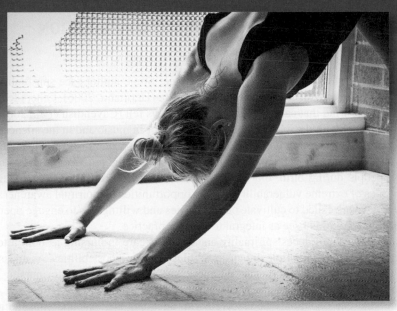

Ancient spiritual practices offer nursing new possibilities for understanding spirituality.
(Used with permission from Heather Macleod of Moksha Yoga Victoria.)

Critical Questions

As a way of engaging with the ideas in this chapter, consider the following:

1. What are the different ways we speak of our spiritual natures and our philosophies of life? What makes your life worth living?

2. If faced with a life-limiting illness, what do you think you might identify as most important in your life?

3. In the ordinariness of your days, what do you yearn for? Do you see yearning as linked to health?

Chapter Objectives

After completing this chapter, you should be able to:

1. Understand the relevance of spirituality for nursing practice.

2. Reflect on your own assumptions about the meaning of spirituality and the effects of these assumptions in your practice of spiritual care.

3. Articulate barriers to providing spiritual care.

4. Generate possibilities for meeting the mandate of providing spiritual care to patients and families.

Spirituality is that part of human beings that is responsive to beauty, searches after truth, appreciates kindness and compassion, accepts the obligations to care for fellow beings, motivates our efforts, energizes our lives, and opens the gates to laughter and tears. Spirit has little to do with religion, or as much, as he or she who has it, wishes.

(Bevis & Watson, 1989)

INTRODUCTION TO THE TOPIC: OPENING THE CONVERSATION ABOUT SPIRITUALITY

Spirituality is difficult to contain within language. Some authors see spirituality as a personal journey of discovering meaning and purpose in life (Hermann, 2006). Others feel spirituality as a force like the wind that cannot be seen but is always felt (Cavendish et al., 2004). And yet others hear spirituality in the whispers of forest groves or in music and in the silences before words. I acknowledge a view that no single understanding of spirituality can adequately embrace all human experience (Box 20.1) and yet also recognize that the practice of nurses includes accompanying people during birth, old age, sickness, and death. As nurses, we engage with people during times of extreme vulnerability—when opportunities for spiritual awareness present themselves, and we are called to cultivate our capacities and willingness to engage openly with people at a spiritual level; this I see as integral to nursing practice.

This chapter introduces spirituality and spiritual care in nursing as both a topic of interest and a conundrum with multiple dimensions, dilemmas, and possibilities. As an issue, spirituality is of widespread concern to the general public and poses challenges for nursing practice as we grapple with nurses' roles and capacities in providing spiritual care. However, unlike nursing problems that can commonly be resolved with adequate analysis and consultation, spirituality as a nursing issue is not seen as something to be solved but rather as a multifaceted topic that requires personal awareness, critical analyses, and the powers of curiosity and "unknowing" to open possibilities for understanding and engaging spiritual connectedness.

My intention in writing this chapter is to open a conversation about what I identify as some of the relevant questions that emerge with the topic of spirituality and spiritual care in nursing practice. The purpose is not to convince you, the reader, of anything at all about spirituality but rather to open spaces for you to wonder about and to explore the meaning that the topic of spirituality holds in your nursing practice. My belief is that we bring ourselves to each encounter with patients and families. Although this may seem an obvious and taken-for-granted idea, it holds important assumptions that are central to the writing and reading of this chapter.

BOX 20.1   How Other People May Refer to Spirituality

Philosophy of life	Connection
	Love
Search for meaning	Peace
	Contentment
Inner resources	Personal strength
Personal beliefs	Religious beliefs/practices
Faith	Opening to the universe
Relationship with a higher power/god/goddess/nature	

BOX 20.2 **Personal Assumptions**

The lens through which I view the world is multihued. In part, my world view is shaped by my connection with the natural world and, in part, by my interest and practice in Buddhist interpretations of life and suffering.

SITUATING THE TOPIC: PERSONAL AND PROFESSIONAL ASSUMPTIONS

Each of us comes to the conversation about spirituality with a history and a particular "situatedness" in the world. Our history is constructed of past experiences, beliefs, and values that have brought us to our current understandings of spirituality. From this position, I hold assumptions about the place and purpose of spirituality in my own life and in the lives of others (Box 20.2). These assumptions are present in my nursing practice. Although some people may believe that we can extricate ourselves as nurses from ourselves as people, it is not always clear that we can or would even want to do this. And so, our assumptions about spirituality and spiritual care are with us in our conversations and in the practice of spirituality and nursing. At this juncture, it may be useful to think about the assumptions that are present for you as you engage with this chapter, assumptions derived from your personal and professional histories, and your current "situatedness" in the world.

SITUATING THE TOPIC: UNDERSTANDING SPIRITUAL PRACTICES HISTORICALLY

As well as the individual assumptions that accompany us to this conversation, our understandings of spirituality and, in particular, our understandings of the dilemmas that arise when considering spirituality in nursing practice are influenced by the ways in which spirituality and nursing have intermingled historically. You might wonder what this history has to do with your current nursing practice. I would suggest that our history is, in a sense, inescapable and that, although historical practice may not be clearly visible, it remains present and influences the ways in which nursing is understood by nurses and others.

The history of nursing in the Western world has a close alliance with spirituality and spiritual practices. Long before the era of Florence Nightingale, credited with the founding of modern Western nursing, individuals who were organized around religious or spiritual ideals practiced care of the sick. According to nurse scholars and historians, nursing's inception can be traced backward through the 19th-century Sisters of Mercy and Sisters of Charity and the 17th-century origins of the Daughters of Charity to the early Christian doctrine of St. Benedict, who elevated the care of the sick as service imbued with spiritual value (Nelson & Rafferty, 2010; O'Brien, 2008). Nightingale is said to have studied with the Daughters of Charity in Paris, France, and to have "learned from them, how to become, and how to form a nurse" (Nelson, 1995, p. 37). Nightingale's so-called secular schools of nursing ascribed to ideals originating with Christian ideology. The influence of particular spiritual ideals is readily recognizable in our Canadian nursing history, in which the earliest organized nursing practice arrived in the form of Augustine nuns from France in August 1639, centuries before a Nightingale-model nursing school was established in Canada in June 1874. "For the Augustine nuns, caring and healing work was central to their Christian beliefs" (Carr, 2003, p. 472). The "training regimen" of Nightingale's schools and of nursing schools well into the 20th century sought to build capacity in nursing students for service and duty, building on a thinly veiled Christian morality.

Nelson (1995) asserts that Christian doctrine remains embedded in particular nursing discourse, now reinscribed as ideologies of humanism. "Humanism in nursing has resurrected the religious discourse and the spiritual dimension of nursing...Salvation has been redrafted to self-actualization" (Nelson, 1995, p. 37). Entire nursing curricula embrace humanism's ideals as foundational to nursing practice: Valuing individual uniqueness, empowerment, freedom, and the caring relationship. Perhaps the most visible reinterpretation of spirituality in nursing from the 20th century onward is the widely held and seldom critiqued ideal of nursing practice as a "holistic" endeavor.

This brief look at the history of the alliance of nursing and spirituality is important for a number of reasons, not the least of which is the recognition of the position from which this history has been written. Much of what we take to be an unbiased account of our past can also be understood as an interpretation of historical proceedings, recorded through the lens of people who are situated within particular social, cultural, political, and spiritual realities. Our nursing history has been written and interpreted from a position of Eurocentrism, in this case meaning that history has been interpreted through a Western world perspective that privileges Judeo-Christian ideology. Embedded in this position is the notion that kindness, compassion, charity, faith, hope, and service which historically underpin the nursing profession, are primarily Christian attributes. My intent here is not to argue against kindness or other attributes, but to suggest that hope, for example, may not hold the same meaning and importance in spiritual, philosophical, or social knowledge systems unrelated to Judeo-Christian ideology. Yet nurses increasingly encounter people from diverse spiritual traditions and religious backgrounds. How might nursing's history be understood differently through the lens of other positions in the world, positions that have been less privileged in the recorded history of the Western world?

SIGNIFICANCE OF THE TOPIC FOR NURSING: EMBRACING THE TENSIONS

Several considerations underlie the relevance of spiritual practice for nurses, including our position of access to patients' lives during times of spiritual crisis or suffering, the subscription of nursing discourse to "holistic care," and a growing mandate to categorize and account for spiritual care.

As was highlighted in the introduction to this chapter, nurses often have opportunities to be with people during birth, old age, sickness, and death, and, as nurses, we have privileged access to people during times of extreme vulnerability—when opportunities for spiritual awareness present themselves. These opportunities do not necessarily announce themselves as spiritual crises or awakenings, prompting us to plan for or execute "spiritual care," but they unfold in the ordinariness of days and evenings and nights, when we as nurses are already present and engaged with patients as they live out their lives. It is with the knowledge that these occurrences are surely and repeatedly lived by patients and families and nurses that we are invited to cultivate our capacities and willingness to engage openly with people at a spiritual level.

A "holistic" approach to nursing practice is a central tenet in many nursing school curricula and is embedded in the philosophies of practice of countless individual nurses. One interpretation of the beliefs underlying holistic practice is "the mind, body and spirit are interdependent; the human spirit is the core of the person; a person's attitude and beliefs toward life are major etiological factors in health and disease" (Freeman, 2004, p. 165). In spite of the predominant understanding of holistic practice as inclusive of spiritual practices, many nurses do not feel adequately prepared to provide spiritual care to patients—and spiritual aspects of care are poorly represented in Canadian nursing school curricula (Olson et al., 2003; Pesut & Reimer Kirkham, 2010).

Last, the relevance of spiritual practice in nursing is underscored when we recognize the provision of spiritual care as mandated both ethically and through overt and pragmatic means. The Canadian Nurses Association (CNA) "Code of Ethics" asserts that nurses work with persons, families, groups, and populations and "take into account their unique values, customs and spiritual beliefs" (CNA, 2008, p. 13). The impetus to attend to spiritual care grows as practicing nurses face increasing pressure to categorize and document all nursing practice, including practice that is spiritual in nature. For example, the Joint Commission on Accreditation of Healthcare Organizations (JCAHO) in the United States now requires that every patient receive spiritual assessment on admission along with appropriate care for those who request it (JCAHO, 2004).

ARTICULATING THE TOPIC AS AN ISSUE: PRACTICE DILEMMAS

This chapter also invites you into a conversation on the topic of spirituality and nursing practice. I have selected one particular dilemma around which to focus the analysis and conversation. The issue, reflected in the nursing literature on spirituality, is the *gap between positive attitudes toward spiritual care among nurses and the lack of spiritual care that is actually being provided by nurses*. It seems that, although assessing and attending to the spiritual needs of patients and families is valued by nurses, many of us do not feel comfortable doing so.

Analyzing the Issue: Multiple Understandings

There are multiple ways of understanding the tension that arises between the ideal and the reality of spiritual care in nursing practice. Pesut and Thorne (2007) explore one way by analyzing the issue based on understanding spirituality as a personal and private concept that is being brought into the public domain of nursing care. They view spirituality as primarily a personal concept that must now be engaged publicly, and this tension evokes unique dilemmas and ethical risks for nurses. Olson et al. (2003) present another way of analyzing the issue, which will frame the analysis in this chapter. The issue will be analyzed by exploring different ways of understanding what contributes to the existing discrepancy between the valuing of spirituality in nursing discourse and the inadequacy of nurses' preparation and ability to address spiritual care in practice. I will engage with three understandings, or positions, that inform this issue. Embedded in each of these positions are barriers to, as well as strategies that will promote resolution. In the following sections I will analyze the following understandings:

1. The nonscientific nature of spirituality does not easily fit within a science-based approach to nursing care (Price et al., 1995).
2. There is ambiguity about what is included in spiritual care in nursing (White et al., 2011).
3. Nurses do not believe they have the knowledge necessary to adequately approach spiritual care (Chadwick & Piles, cited in Olson et al., 2003).

Engaging in a critical conversation about spirituality and spiritual care requires questioning the assumptions embedded within each of these ways of understanding the issue. I situate this discussion in a constructivist view; that is, knowledge is not perceived as unbiased or detached but as always generated, formed, and constructed within particular social, cultural, political, and material realities. This means that knowledge is never neutral but is always developed and situated within a particular view of the world. One approach to making the "situatedness" of knowledge visible is to identify the taken-for-granted assumptions on which the knowledge is shaped or constructed. My intention, then, is not to resolve the challenges of how to provide spiritual care but to analyze and critique the issue with the view of opening spaces for you to develop your own interpretations.

Ways of Understanding: Scientific and Nonscientific

The non-scientific nature of spirituality does not easily fit within a science-based approach to nursing.

(Price et al., 1995)

Historical Influences of Science: Privileging a De-Spirited Body

Although a spiritual heritage has been claimed in nursing, Wojnar and Malinski (2003) suggest that this spiritual legacy has been challenged by the separation of body from spirit in science. Interestingly, this was not always the case, as, when around the 8th century, the body and spirit were established as connected yet separate in the Christian tradition (Burkhardt & Nagai-Jacobson, 2002). Later, in the 17th century, the philosopher René Descartes proposed that the body and spirit are mutually exclusive. This belief became accepted in Western thought and paved the way for biologic and medical knowledge to become the dominant scientific view that persists today in many parts of the world. The body became the exclusive domain of science, whereas the spirit and soul were relegated to philosophers, theologians, and priests. The modern era is marked by an unprecedented growth of scientific knowledge and power of the natural sciences.

This view of the world also reinforced oppositional thinking, a view where binaries or opposites are set up, known as *dualism*. In dualism, emphasis is given to separateness rather than to interconnectedness of phenomena. For example, dualistic thinking sees opposite positions of this versus that: Science versus nonscience, body versus spirit, and good versus bad, for example. Although oppositional thinking is useful in distinguishing differences and categories, it is often inadequate when addressing complex human experiences. The complexity of human suffering or spirituality, for example, cannot be contained in simple categories. Instead, the messy, ambiguous nature of living and dying, of feeling health within illness, also needs to be acknowledged and valued. However, ambiguity, uncertainty, and unknowing have not often been valued in nursing.

In the name of science, oppositional thinking has become almost uncritically accepted. Scientism, as distinguished from science, is a matter of putting too high a value on science as a branch of learning in comparison with other ways of knowing (Haack, 2003). With scientism, the belief is that science is the most beneficial form of learning and, as such, it is good for all domains, including spirituality and philosophy, to be placed on a scientific footing. Consequently, we see that scholars claim to have made history, politics, ethics, or aesthetics into a science and assume that these claims of scientific status are desirable. In nursing, Kikuchi and Simmons (1994) provide examples in which nurse researchers attempt to answer philosophical questions such as, "what is the nature of health?" and "what is the purpose of caring?" using exclusively scientific means, thereby demonstrating nursing's vulnerability to scientism. In recent years, however, many of the long-held tenets of science and ways of obtaining knowledge have been questioned. Previously held assumptions about reality and the nature of truth have been challenged both within traditional scientific communities and by feminists, critical theorists, and postmodern thinkers. Even so, science and, perhaps, scientism remain the dominant view within healthcare professions. The dominance of scientific knowledge has led to almost unquestioned acceptance of technology and secularism in social, political, and educational institutions.

Until recently, spirituality as a human phenomenon that is separate from the body and material world has been neglected by scientific inquiry. Increasingly, however, spirituality is receiving scientific attention as the body–mind–spirit split is challenged and shown to be too limited in understanding human health and well-being. Consequently, spirituality is being conceptualized in ways that promote distinctions and measurements that are congruent with the assumptions of scientific world views. Without minimizing the importance of scientific knowledge, the risk of scientism must also be attended to as we see the call in nursing for standardized language and interventions for spiritual care. Clearly, we must avoid the pitfalls of according science a privileged view at the expense of other ways of knowing spirituality, while at the same time valuing the contributions of scientific knowledge.

In analyzing science, it is not my intention to throw out science or situate spirituality in opposition to science. Nevertheless, different ways of generating knowledge will shape our nursing practice differently. Through critical analysis, we can distinguish what kinds of knowledge and practices are left out, which are ignored or perhaps not legitimized, and where particular beliefs and knowledge become dominant.

Natural Science and Human Science: Differing Approaches to Knowledge

In the academic milieu of the early 1980s, nursing attempted to legitimize its position as a discipline of science by privileging the natural sciences of medicine over what became known as human sciences (Johnson & Webber, 2005). The natural sciences support a view where people are made up of different components continuously interacting with one another and the environment. This concept of person as an assemblage of traits and variables is inconsistent with a human science view. Rather than seeing a person with components, the view from a human science perspective sees the person as a complex, evolving being, interconnected with the universe. The personal meanings of people's realities are considered of central importance in the investigations and practices of human science disciplines.

This is not to suggest that there is a single perspective of nursing theory and practice that draws on the human science view. Numerous nursing theories within human science value spirituality in nursing practice, among them the diverse approaches of Jean Watson, Margaret Newman, Martha Rogers, and Rosemarie Parse. Consider the effect that differences in underlying assumptions have on how spirituality is understood and practiced. For example, to view spirituality as a component of a person would lead to different ways of practicing than would seeing each person as spirit and spirituality as integral to our nature.

Ways of Understanding: Clarity and Ambiguity

There is ambiguity about what is included in spiritual care in nursing.
(Price et al., 1995)

Embedded in this position is an assumption that clarity is required to overcome current ambiguity about what spirituality means in nursing practice. As with the underlying assumption of the first position, a binary of "clarity versus ambiguity" is inferred in the language of this position. That is, it is assumed that clarity concerning spirituality is preferred over the existent situation of multiple and diverse understandings. Is it possible, or even desirable, to construct a single, clear, concise definition of spiritual practice that will adequately encompass all perspectives from ecologic, Aboriginal, religious, and humanistic views as well as from those views that cannot be easily identified? This assumption and its oppositional thinking are challenged as we explore other ways of approaching this dualism. In particular, I will consider differences between and the interdependence of spirituality and religion followed by a discussion of differences between spirituality understood as a concept and as lived experience.

Religion and Spirituality: Vehicle and Destination

According to Paley (2008), viewing spirituality as a separate concept outside of particular religions is a relatively recent shift in thinking. Nevertheless, it could be said that religion and spirituality are interconnected for some people some of the time, whereas for others they are always interconnected, and for still other people religion and spirituality are two separate entities. Given this variability, it seems important to understand them as separate, yet sometimes related, concepts. A great deal of the research before the year 2000 has examined *religion* and *spirituality* as if they were synonymous (George et al., 2000). Increasingly, however, nurses and others understand the importance of teasing apart the differences between religious traditions and our many interpretations of spirituality. Although religion and spirituality are seen as related concepts,

BOX 20.3   **How People May Identify Spiritual Practice**

Yoga		Conversation
Meditation		Reminiscing
Prayer		Being in nature
Practicing kindness		Chanting
Listening		Singing
Ceremonies	Rituals	Traditional dance
Silence	Solitude	Sacred space
Making offerings		Sharing meals
Reading sacred text		Sacred art
Celebrations		Listening to/making music
Being close to important others		Mantra repetition

religion is often linked to formal religious institutions whereas spirituality is seen as a broader idea that does not depend on institutional contexts. Arguably, spiritual practices are more varied than, although certainly overlapping with, religious ones (see Box 20.3). Religion is like a train journeying through and toward spirituality in which we are cautioned not to mistake the vehicle for the destination (Borysenko, 1999). While for some, spiritual experience is not separate from religious beliefs and practices, this is not the case for many who consider themselves spiritual yet not at all religious.

Spirituality as a Concept and as a Lived Experience

Just as religion and spirituality are closely linked, yet also very different, the interdependence of experience and concept can also be suggested. The nature of spirituality is complex as an experience and as a concept. This distinction between experience and the conceptual representation of experience—how we understand spirituality through language—is rarely distinguished in current discussions of spirituality (Bruce et al., 2011). Nevertheless, this distinction is important and may assist us in sifting through the many ways of understanding (conceptualizing) spiritual phenomena.

As with experiences of pain, many authors suggest that the experience of spirituality is unique to each person and can only be known by that person. From this perspective, the understanding of a particular person's spirituality is whatever the person says it is. Although our experiences are unique, at the same time there are also common themes and patterns of spiritual understanding that extend across groups of people. Through systematically examining how people describe their experiences, researchers generate categories and theories to better understand this human experience. The caution, however, is to avoid confusing individual experience (of each distinct patient and family) with a generalized understanding generated in concepts about spirituality. In nursing, we require embodied knowledge from the unique experiences of patients and families along with diverse sources of generalized conceptual knowledge, including nursing knowledge and empirical research.

If we accept the assumption that no single expression of spirituality can embrace all human experience, then it cannot reasonably be anticipated that nurses will know how to recognize or interpret the multiple possible expressions of spirituality or spiritual need. However, what nurses can do (and often do very well) is enter into and engage with the unique experiences of patients. From this standpoint, the central questions may not be, "what is spirituality?" but rather "how is spirituality lived between this patient and family and the illness, and how can we engage there with families?" Nurses do not necessarily need to possess broad understandings of religious practices, theology, or cultural studies to provide spiritual care. Instead, nurses can be willing and able to engage patients with spiritual awareness about values, beliefs, and their experiences of illness.

Paterson and Zderad (1976) also emphasize the relationality of nursing in their focus on where nursing happens rather than what it is. "Nursing is an experience lived between human beings" (p. 3) "and is concerned with, 'the between' of nurses and their others" (p. 44). Here, "the between" refers to a merging of nurse–patient boundaries into a space of authentic presence while maintaining one's capacity to question.

> When I reflect on an act of mine (no matter how simple or complex) that I can unhesitatingly label "nursing," I become aware of it as goal-directed (nurturing) being with and doing for another. The intersubjective or interhuman element, "the between," runs through nursing interactions like an underground stream conveying the nutrients of healing and growth. In everyday practice, we are usually so involved with the immediate demands of our "being with and doing with" the patient that we do not focus on the overshadowed plane of "the between." However, occasionally, in beautiful moments, the interhuman currents are so strong that they flood our conscious awareness. Such rare and rewarding moments of mutual presence remind us of the elusive ever-present "between" (Paterson & Zderad, 1976, pp. 21–22).

This perspective resonates closely with definitions of spirituality and notions of spiritual care. According to Paterson and Zderad, it is important to explore and describe the nature of in-between experiences. This exploration is significant, according to Paterson and Zderad, if we are to better understand how our interactions with others can have both humanizing and dehumanizing effects.

How we conceptualize spirituality within nursing discourse also shapes our clinical practice. The way we talk and write about spirituality shapes knowledge about the phenomenon—through writing and reading, we are making real, so to speak, and establishing what spirituality is (Boxes 20.4 and 20.5). However, healthcare institutions are also mandating nurses to provide spiritual

---

BOX 20.4   Reflection Poem

Momentarily awake, pale gray-blue eyes washed out by morphine.
Pin-point pupils, beady eyes peering into space.
You didn't want this, but are at the mercy of night guardians.
Well meaning, yet inattentive . . . or unable to see?
"Good morning Martin".
.. .. You startle,
eyes flitting, seeking recognition,
hands grasping invisible objects in space.
"Hi, how are you" you whisper through dentureless jaws.
About to respond, but you're gone
drifting rudderless
eyes rolling upward
and away.
Are you able to be present
for the journey?
You moaned and groaned too loudly,
so they took away
their pain
and hushed you into slumber
where we cannot go or witness,
you journey there alone. .. .. ..

Bruce, A. (2002). *Abiding in liminal spaces: Inscribing mindful living/dying with(in) end-of-life care.* (Unpublished doctoral dissertation). University of British Columbia. Used with permission.

> ### BOX 20.5 Reflection on Nursing
>
> I am aware of the dance between definitive and nondefinitive language. Although the question remains, how is this relevant for nursing practice, I hope to elude the pitfall of prescriptive discourse as my intention has always been otherwise. Death is not a problem to be remedied. Accompanying those in this journeying is also seeing the interplay of y/our dying and the limits of prescribed 'doing'.. .. . and yet. .. .

Bruce, A. (2002). *Abiding in liminal spaces: Inscribing mindful living/dying with(in) end-of-life care.* (Unpublished doctoral dissertation). University of British Columbia. Used with permission.

care. What conceptualization of spirituality do we want to support and foster? How might we proceed in a healthcare system and society that privileges "interventions" that can be measured and documented? An all-encompassing definition would be congruent with a science-based approach to nursing while the ambiguity of diverse and multiple definitions would more closely reflect differences encountered in people's experiences.

Is it possible to hold a space open in our thinking, where spirit and spirituality in nursing practice are understood in multiple ways, as experience and concept, rather than narrowing our thinking to reach a clear and concise definition? I would suggest that in our wish to find simple definitions to these complex experiences, we risk generalizing and relying too heavily on the power of already privileged religious ideologies in our society. Rather than creating space for a range of spiritual practice, the search for "clarity" can lead us to marginalize, ignore, or trivialize spiritual practices that fall outside of the dominant norm. Perhaps then, developing comfort with the inevitable ambiguity of complex human experiences is also important.

Ways of Understanding: Knowing and Unknowing

> *Nurses do not believe they have the knowledge necessary to adequately approach spiritual care.*
> *(Chadwick & Piles, cited in Olson et al., 2003)*

Without minimizing the question of what nurses need to know to provide spiritual care, I would like to question the underlying assumptions embedded in this third position that infer an emphasis on knowing versus not knowing. Attending to knowledge, as this question implies, renders a valuing of "doing" and knowing in opposition to "being" and not knowing. The following discussion of these tensions may provide alternative ways of looking at spirituality.

The quest to know and define phenomena can be seen as part of a larger ideology or belief system. As mentioned, the model for generating nursing knowledge and practice has been embedded within a discourse of science. Although this model is changing, the push toward standardization of spiritual care and measurements of spirituality illustrates both the usefulness and continued dominance of this view. Once again, the issue is not that different ways of knowing are beneficial but rather that we need to be aware of and question the privileging of particular views at the expense of others. One such privileging arises in valuing knowing over unknowing and is explored here for other possible interpretations.

Unknowing as a Way of Knowing

Recognizing different modes of reality (such as spirit as supernatural) is difficult within the limited scope of language and ways of knowing in science and health care (Diddle & Denham, 2010). For example, conventional scientific knowledge focuses on what is said, thereby excluding what is unsaid, or unsayable. By concentrating on what is certain and knowable, we often exclude the ambiguous, unknowable, and paradoxical. Conventional models of scientific knowledge depend on exclusion and function to privilege one voice or perspective over another. Through valuing what we can know of spiritual experience within a fixed idea of what is acceptable, we may ignore that which is "unknowable" or indescribable within spiritual experience. When exploring spirituality in nursing practice, careful attention to language and discourses can guide us to help people to live within the reality of their own spiritual experiences.

The question of what nurses need to know to provide spiritual care has practical implications when we consider that many nurses do not feel comfortable attending to the spiritual needs of their patients (McSherry & Ross, 2002), and nursing students seek guidance for developing spiritual awareness and engaging in spiritual discussions with patients and families (Pesut, 2002). Addressing spirituality from a scientific or a modernist view emphasizes knowing through establishing clear definitions that may lead to assessment tools and concept clarification. This could help to differentiate spirituality from other phenomena, such as a sense of coherence, caring, or connectedness. Although these ways of knowing contribute to nursing knowledge and practice, they also raise many other questions, including, "How are definitions determined?" "Who decides what definitions we will rely on?" "What world view or belief system is embedded within this knowledge?" "What happens when patients and families do not fit into particular views of spirituality?" Even though themes related to spiritual experience may be identified across groups and aggregates, if spirituality, as some authors suggest, is whatever people say it is for them (Malinski, 2002), what pitfalls and potential harms do we face in privileging the views that are dominant or most commonly held?

Alternative ways of knowing may complement and yet put into question modernist approaches to spirituality. Whereas the modernist approach is based in a historical era when there was increased growth in the valuing of freedom, individuality, and scientism, views from a postmodern perspective challenge the nature of modern assumptions. Modernism, although largely located in the 19th and early 20th centuries, continues to inform some schools of thought, particularly those of the natural sciences; whereas postmodernism critiques of modern thought are increasingly prevalent in nursing scholarship.

Holtslander (2008) and Munhall (1993) challenge modernist assumptions about knowledge in exploring unknowing as a way of knowing. Munhall introduces "unknowing" as a state of mind and a way of knowing that brings another dimension to understanding complex human experience. Unknowing is viewed not simply as a gap in knowledge that must be filled but as an ability and way of knowing that is interconnected with conventional knowing. After all, knowing that we do not know opens us to learning and new possibilities. Munhall calls for unknowing to be included as another pattern of knowing (Box 20.6).

Cultivating Abilities to Engage with Spiritual Openness: A Way of Being

I support the view of nurse scholars who suggest that spiritual care is multifaceted and wide-ranging, much of which does not demand or require specialized knowledge (Pesut & Reimer-Kirkham, 2010). If we are practicing nursing in an interdisciplinary setting, what aspects of care are within the purview of nursing and what areas can best be referred to other healthcare and spiritual care practitioners, such as Aboriginal healers, pastors, shamans, and priests? And what aspects of spiritual care can be attended to within direct nursing care?

Research reports that patients and families appreciate and see spiritual care from nurses more as a way of being rather than as specific interventions (Sellers, 2001). The most frequently identified descriptors of spiritual care included being treated with kindness and respect ("it's the little things"), talking and listening, praying, connecting (e.g., being genuine and showing interest), providing quality temporal care (e.g., keeping the room tidy and not letting the patient suffer), and mobilizing religious and spiritual resources (e.g., providing referrals to clergy and providing spiritual music or readings [Taylor, 2003, pp. 587–588]).

BOX 20.6   Unknowing May Be a Way of Knowing

Let us not talk *about* death,
Let us talk. .. with/in
.. .. open-endedness
forming and dissolution.
trans/forming, per/forming,
constantly dissolving
becoming anew
abiding in spaces between thoughts.
Let us talk
Nursing
as witnessing
mindful of empty spaces and places
of self/no self
of birth, old age, sickness, and death.
Mindful of basic impermanence
of living and dying,
abiding in spaces
of ceaseless transitioning. .. ..

Bruce, A. (2002). *Abiding in liminal spaces: Inscribing mindful living/dying with(in) end-of-life care.* (Unpublished doctoral dissertation). University of British Columbia. Used with permission.

Some patients have reported that they do not want nurses to be spiritual care providers based on the perception that nurses are not qualified and an assumption that differing beliefs between patients and nurses would be a barrier to spiritual care (Taylor, 2003). Other participants in the same study saw nurses as appropriate spiritual care providers because nurses were perceived as those who are there during vulnerable experiences and recognize experiences that would prompt a desire for spiritual care. Patients without family or particular spiritual or religious support were seen to particularly benefit from nurses with spiritual awareness. Taylor identifies several prerequisites to the provision of spiritual care from the perspective of patients in her research (Box 20.7). Most significantly, patients stated that "nurses need to establish some respect and relationship with patients prior to providing spiritual care" (Taylor, 2003, p. 589). This finding supports an understanding that spiritual practice may be most effectively delivered through a "way of being" with patients rather than through the influences of scientific or modernist knowledge.

IDENTIFYING BARRIERS: FURTHERING OUR UNDERSTANDING

The following are some barriers to nurses providing spiritual care:

1. Our lack of knowledge of our nursing history and the influence of this history on our current understandings of spiritual care in nursing practice.

BOX 20.7   Prerequisites to Spiritual Care

Personal: Having a spiritual awareness; establishing trusting relationships
Relational: Possessing a caring attitude; developing rapport first; conveying warmth and interest; assessing patient receptivity
Professional: Meeting patients' expectations for what nurses might do; having appropriate training if needed

2. An unexamined Eurocentric perspective of spirituality that privileges Judeo-Christian ideologies.
3. The dilemma of defining *spirituality* and *spiritual care* (Definitions and clarity, regarding both concepts and interventions, lend themselves to accounting for evidence-based practice and meeting mandated requirements for care. However, this kind of clarity is located within a particular world view and understanding of knowledge that may not move us any closer to the actual provision of meaningful spiritual care for patients and families).
4. The idea that there is, or should be, a single understanding of spirituality and of approaches to spiritual care in the face of the lived realities of multiple understandings and meanings of spirituality.

GENERATING STRATEGIES: FUTURE POSSIBILITIES

The following are some possibilities for nurses to remain open and provide spiritual care:

1. Make clear our personal and professional assumptions about spirituality and recognize the influence that these hold on our practice.
2. Always search for the taken-for-granted assumptions on which knowledge is shaped or constructed.
3. Pay careful attention to language and discourse because it is important in helping others live within their own spiritual realities.
4. Develop curricula and opportunities for nurses in practice to expand their comfort with the inevitable ambiguity of complex human experiences.
5. Potential questions to consider if appropriate when opening conversations with patients and families about spirituality*:
   How would you describe your philosophy of life?
   What type of spiritual/religious support (if any) would you like?
   Do you have a clergy, minister, chaplain, pastor, rabbi, imam that you would like us to be aware of?
   What does suffering mean to you?
   Do you have spiritual goals that you'd like us to be aware of?
   Is there a role of church/synagogue/mosque that is important in your life?
   How does your faith help you in coping with your illness?
   What helps you to keep going day after day?
   How has illness affected you and your family?

SUMMARY

Through this chapter's conversations, poems, and reflections on the literature, I have intended to open the possibilities for multiple understandings of spiritual practice for nurses. One might assume from the language used in the literature regarding spiritual care (*kindness, gentleness, caring*) that good nursing care is spiritual in nature. However, as you consider this evocative idea, we are left with the notion that it is something more—that spiritual practice involves accompanying patients and families on their journeys of suffering and hope and joy in ways that allow them to be present to the journeys themselves.

---

*These questions are modified from JCAHO's elements for Spiritual Assessments. Retrieved June 29, 2011 http://www.jointcommission.org/standards_information/jcfaqdetails.aspx?StandardsFaqId=290&ProgramId=1

> **Add to your knowledge of this issue:**
>
> | | |
> |---|---|
> | American Holistic Nurses Association | **www.ahna.org** |
> | Canadian Holistic Nurses Association | **www.chna.ca** |
>
> *Online*

R E F L E C T I O N S *on the Chapter...*

1 Does everyone have spiritual experience? What words do you use to refer to your spiritual life and practices?

2 In your practice, what have you observed about the spiritual nature of people and how does that fit with nurses' practice?

3 Identify the assumptions and beliefs you hold about spirituality and the provision of spiritual care to patients and their families.

4 How do your assumptions align or differ from those held by the author of this chapter and the literature she included?

5 Is there a mandate for nurses to provide spiritual care in your province? If so, how does this compare with the CNA "Code of Ethics" mandate?

Want to know more? Visit the**Point** for additional helpful resources:

- Journal Articles
- Learning Objectives
- Nursing Professional Roles and Responsibilities
- Bonus chapters:
  - Health and Nursing Policy: A Matter of Politics, Power and Professionalism
  - The NP Movement: Recurring Issues
  - When Difference Matters: The Politics of Privilege and Marginality

References

Bevis, E.O., & Watson, J. (1989). *Toward a caring curriculum: A new pedagogy for nursing.* New York, NY: National League for Nursing.

Borysenko, J. (1999). *A woman's journey to god: Finding the feminine path.* New York: Riverhead Books.

Bruce, A. (2002). *Abiding in liminal spaces: Inscribing mindful living/dying with(in) end-of-life care.* (Unpublished doctoral dissertation). University of British Columbia, Vancouver, British Columbia, Canada.

Bruce, A., Sheilds, L., & Molzahn, A. (2011). Language and the (im)possibilities of articulating spirituality. *Journal of Holistic Nursing, 29*(1), 44–52. doi: 10.1177/0898010110381116

Burkhardt, M., & Nagai-Jacobson, M.G. (2002). *Spirituality: Living our connectedness.* Albany, NY: Delmar Thomson Learning.

Canadian Nurses Association. (2008). Code of ethics for Registered Nurses. Retrieved from http://www.cna-nurses.ca/CNA/documents/pdf/publications/Code_of_Ethics_2008_e.pdf

Carr, T. (2003). The spirit of nursing: Ghost of our past or force for our future? In M. McIntyre & E. Thomlinson (Eds.), *Realities of Canadian nursing: Professional, practice, and power issues.* Philadelphia, PA: Lippincott Williams & Wilkins.

Cavendish, R., Luise, B.K., Russo, D., et al. (2004). Spiritual perspectives on nurses in the United States relevant for education and practice. *Western Journal of Nursing Research, 26*(2), 196–212.

Diddle, G., & Denham, S.A. (2010). Spirituality and its relationships with the health and illness of Appalachian people. *Journal of Transcultural Nursing, 21*(2), 175–182.

Freeman, J. (2004). Holistic healing modalities. In B. Kozier, G. Erb & A. Berman, et al. (Eds.), *Fundamentals of nursing: The nature of nursing practice in Canada.* Toronto, ON: Prentice Hall.

George, L., Larson, D., Koenig, H., & McCullough, M.E. (2000). Spirituality and health: What we know, what we need to know. *Journal of Social and Clinical Psychology, 19*(1), 102–116.

Haack, S. (2003). *Defending science within reason: Between scientism and cynicism.* Amherst, NY: Prometheus Books.

Hermann, C.P. (2006). Development and testing of the spiritual needs inventory for patients near the end of life. *Oncology Nursing Forum, 33*(4), 737–744.

Holtslander, L. (2008). Ways of knowing hope: Carper's fundamental patterns as a guide for hope research with bereaved palliative caregivers. *Nursing Outlook, 56*(1), 25–30.

Johnson, B.M., & Webber, P.B. (2005). *An introduction to theory and reasoning in nursing.* Philadelphia, PA: Lippincott Williams & Wilkins.

Joint Commission of the Accreditation of Healthcare Organizations. (2004). Available from http://www.jointcommission.org/standards_information/jcfaqdetails.aspx?StandardsFaqId=290&ProgramId=1

Kikuchi, J., & Simmons, H. (1994). *Developing a philosophy of nursing.* Newbury Park, CA: Sage.

Malinski, V. (2002). Developing a nursing perspective on spirituality and healing. *Nursing Science Quarterly, 15*(4), 281–287.

McSherry, W., & Ross, L. (2002). Dilemmas of spiritual assessment: Considerations for nursing practice. *Journal of Advanced Nursing, 38*(5), 479–488.

Munhall, P. (1993). "Unknowing": Toward another pattern of knowing in nursing. *Nursing Outlook, 41*(3), 125–128.

Nelson, S. (1995). Humanism in nursing: The emergence of the light. *Nursing Inquiry, 2*(1), 36–43.

Nelson, S., & Rafferty, A.M. (2010). *Notes on Nightingale: The influence and legacy of a nursing icon.* Ithaca, NY: Cornell University Press.

O'Brien, M.E. (2008). *Spirituality in nursing: Standing on holy ground.* (3rd ed.). Sudbury, MA: Jones and Bartlett Publishers.

Olson, J., Paul, P., Douglass, L., Clark, M.B., Simington, J., & Goddard, N. (2003). Addressing the spiritual dimension in Canadian undergraduate nursing education. *Canadian Journal of Nursing Research, 35*(3), 94–107.

Paley, J. (2008). Spirituality and nursing: A reductionist approach. *Nursing Philosophy, 9*(1), 3–18.

Paterson, J., & Zderad, L. (1976). *Humanistic nursing.* New York: National League for Nursing.

Pesut, B. (2002). The development of nursing students' spirituality and spiritual care-giving. *Nurse Education Today, 22*(2), 128–135.

Pesut, B., & Reimer-Kirkham, S. (2010). Situated clinical encounters in the negotiation of religious and spiritual plurality: A critical ethnography. *International Journal of Nursing Studies, 47*(7), 815–825.

Pesut, B., & Thorne, S. (2007). From private to public: Negotiating professional and personal identities in spiritual care. *Journal of Advanced Nursing, 58*(4), 396–403.

Price, J.L., Stevens, H.O., & LaBarre, M.C. (1995). Spiritual caregiving in nursing practice. *Journal of Psychosocial Nursing, 33*(12), 5–9.

Sellers, S.C. (2001). The spiritual care meanings of adults residing in the midwest. *Nursing Science Quarterly, 14*(3), 239–248.

Taylor, J.E. (2003). Nurses caring for the spirit: Patients with cancer and family caregiver expectations. *Oncology Nursing Forum, 30*(4), 585–590.

White, M., Peters, R., & Schim, S.M. (2011). Spirituality and spiritual care: Expanding self-care deficit nursing theory. *Nursing Science Quarterly, 24*(1), 48–56.

Wojnar, D., & Malinski, V. (2003). Developing a nursing perspective on spirituality and healing: Questions and answers following a letter to the editor. *Nursing Science Quarterly, 16*(4), 297–300.

21 Ethical and Legal Issues in Nursing

Nancy A. Walton

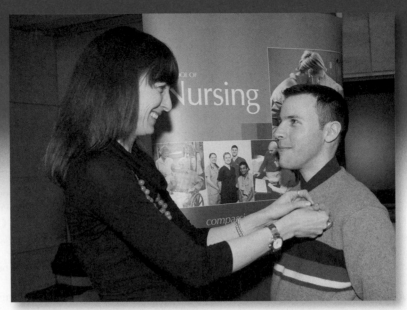

Chapter author, Nancy Walton (left) at student pinning ceremony. (Used with permission. Photographer Dave Upham.)

Critical Questions

As a way of engaging with the ideas in this chapter, consider the following:

1. What kinds of ethical dilemmas have you encountered in your own practice?

2. What has best prepared you to deal with complex ethical dilemmas in practice? What would help you feel better prepared to deal with these kinds of issues?

3. Think about the current trends and issues in healthcare today. What do you see as the most important ethical challenges in the near future for healthcare?

4. Reflect upon the values and beliefs you hold about contentious issues such as end-of-life care, maternal–fetal conflicts, the use of embryos and stem cells in research, the allocation of scarce healthcare resources, and the rights and treatment of marginalized or institutionalized patients. How are your personal values and beliefs about these issues reconciled with your professional role?

Chapter Objectives

After completing this chapter, you will be able to:

1. Identify an ethical issue or dilemma.

2. Articulate the overlap between ethical and legal perspectives, and identify the differences between these two perspectives.

3. Demonstrate a beginning understanding of common legal issues in practice.

4. Acknowledge the implications for nurses, the nursing profession, and the public if complex ethical and legal issues are not addressed and resolved.

(continued on page 369)

5. Identify some potential barriers to, and strategies for, approaching ethical issues in practice.

6. Use a decision-making framework to help work through complex ethical dilemmas.

Nurses do not practice in a vacuum. They practice in a wide variety of areas and contexts, with diverse clients. Much of what they do is affected by political, economic, and social structures that exist in the healthcare environment and society. What is most important to remember is that nursing always takes place within the context of relationships: Relationships with clients, colleagues, other healthcare professionals, families, groups, and communities. Within these relationships between the individuals and groups involved, ethical issues are often encountered. Healthcare and the delivery of care occurs in a complex, sociopolitical landscape that, despite our best intentions, marginalizes and oppresses some while helping many. As nurses, we are often witness to situations, incidents, and relationships that we find ethically problematic, and we must address them in a knowledgeable, ethically competent, and informed way. Doing so also requires that we have knowledge of the legal obligations that accompany our professional role and how these obligations "fit" alongside our ethical duties.

In our professional roles, we are moral agents, which means that we have an obligation to ensure integrity and ethical soundness in the care we provide and in our interactions with others (Canadian Nurses Association [CNA], 2008). As we conduct ourselves with integrity and are aware of ourselves as moral agents, we help to create ethical workplaces and moral communities in which we are more able to provide ethically sound and reflective care. In this chapter, you will be introduced to legal and ethical issues in nursing as well as to some fundamental ethical principles and theories from which you can adapt strategies and reflect upon ethical and legal issues in your own practice and the healthcare environment in which nurses provide care.

Consider the following case:

Case Study

Amanda is a nurse practitioner on a busy cardiac postsurgical ward. She has a long-time patient, Rudy, who had a serious postoperative infection of a sternal incision, which has required surgical debridement and deep dressings to pack the wound. The dressing changes are very painful and frequent, necessitating pain medication. Rudy has become withdrawn and depressed, dreading the dressing changes every 6 hours. Before the surgery, Rudy lived in a men's shelter with no family or close friends. Today, the unit manager tells Amanda to prepare Rudy for discharge tomorrow with home care nursing to continue dressing the wounds. Amanda is surprised and tells the manager that Rudy cannot possibly cope in the shelter with his complex needs. The manager insists, adding that an unexpected heart transplant was carried out last night and the Intensive Care Unit is now full. In order to keep the flow of patients moving from the operating room to the ICU and then to the ward, beds must be freed up on the ward. Rudy has been on the ward the longest and is the most stable, even with his complex postoperative infection. Amanda knows that home care may be difficult to obtain for frequent complex dressing changes and she is also concerned about Rudy's mental health. When she tells the manager this, the manager responds with a sigh, "Look, Amanda, they wanted to discharge him today.

(continued on page 370)

Case Study (continued)

I've given you an extra day but he has to go. The OR is on my case. He's stable medically. Work with him and get some home care nursing in place. Look at it this way, at least he's had his bypass surgery—he's better than when he came in." Amanda isn't sure she agrees with that, and is distressed at having to discharge Rudy into what she knows is not an ideal situation. She doesn't feel, however, as if she has a choice. She could stand her ground and refuse to discharge Rudy, but she also understands the demands of the system and the expectation to free up beds as soon as possible. She has always promised herself that she would not abandon a patient, and to her, this feels as if she will be abandoning Rudy.

Like many nurses, Amanda has been confronted with an ethical dilemma in her practice. This situation is not a unique or rare one, but one faced by nurses time and time again in a variety of settings. In situations like this, nurses like Amanda are driven to reflect not only on their own values and beliefs, but also on the political, institutional, and social structures within which they deliver care. Amanda clearly knows how she would like to resolve this situation but the constraints of the environment in which she works will not support that resolution. In other words, a very significant gap exists between what Amanda wants for her patient and what is required by the hospital. Instead, Amanda must decide what options she has and which action is most ethically sound. She feels a sense of fidelity and obligation to her patient, Rudy. However, she also understands the challenge that her manager faces in ensuring beds are available to facilitate the movement of patients, all of whom are owed a standard of care, just as Rudy is owed. She also understands that, somewhere, there is a patient she does not know whose surgery may well be canceled if she does not discharge Rudy. Amanda is faced with a dilemma with multiple dimensions and more than one stakeholder; however, Amanda feels strongly that her role must be to advocate for her patient in this case. Nurses have a unique role in that they are often faced with their duty to consider, as a primary responsibility, the best interests of their individual patient but must also always be mindful of the balance between individual best interests and the resources and cost constraints of the system in which they work (Yeo et al., 2010). It is an arduous task to balance competing demands while wanting to make the *right* decision for an individual patient with whom we have a relationship based on trust. But for many nurses like Amanda, confronting this balancing act is a part of their everyday practice. It takes time, energy, and a willingness to constantly reflect upon our values, beliefs, and professional obligations to try to sort out each ethical problem we, as nurses, are faced with.

SITUATING THE TOPIC: WHAT IS ETHICS?

Ethics can be defined as the process of carefully thinking through what is *right* or *wrong* in behavior, decision making, and values. The study of ethics is not only about thinking and reflecting upon what we consider to be good but also examining critically the social norms, practices, moral issues, and ethical foundations of our societies. Many people use the term *morality* interchangeably with ethics. Morality can be defined as beliefs about what we consider to be right or wrong in our actions and behaviors toward those around us and is, in essence, very similar to *ethics*. While the terms are almost identical in meaning for some, there is a tendency to associate the term *ethics* more with the academic and philosophical study of right and wrong and the term *morality* more with individual and more general social norms, values, and beliefs (Fisher, 2009). What is clear, however, is that each of them can be applied to the kinds of problems or issues in which we find ourselves thinking about what *ought to happen, what should be done,* or *what is fair and just.* Nurses are faced with these kinds of problems frequently and studying ethics enables nurses to have a strong foundational knowledge from which to begin to approach such problems, in a professional, informed, and reasonable way.

Within the study of ethics, the field of *bioethics* focuses on the study of ethical issues surrounding human lives, health, and illness. It encompasses matters such as euthanasia and assisted suicide, the use and allocation of new technologies, stem cell research, and maternal–fetal conflicts, among many others. This is one of many fields of applied ethics, in which theories, principles, and value judgments are used to approach and work through ethical dilemmas in particular contexts. Other examples of applied ethics include medical ethics (the study of the ethical dimensions of medical care), environmental ethics (concerned with our obligations toward the land, water, and animals), and business ethics (addresses questions of how corporations and other businesses should deal with problems such as conflicts of interest, product safety, and the rights of consumers).

Many discussions in bioethics relate more often to situations that are extraordinary, singular, or tragic situations. But much of what nurses experience in terms of ethical issues in human lives, health, and illness are related to the everyday kinds of challenges, and practice issues that arise when engaging in therapeutic relationships with other persons. Nursing is, indeed, a "moral endeavour" (Smith & Godfrey, 2002, p. 302) and as one author notes, "every nursing act is a moral statement" (Levine, 1989). Levine goes on to explain that, while there are times in which nurses face ethical dilemmas and situations that are significant or major, much of the moral work of nursing is found in the *everyday* activities of nursing care and that nurses, as a result of being engaged in a moral practice, are constantly making ethical decisions that appear, to others, to be straightforward practice decisions. Often these decisions are fraught with uncertainty and distress for the nurses who are challenged with deciding what they feel is best for patients in complex and dynamic situations (Johns, 1999). These decisions are often less significant than the grander or more devastating decisions such as whether or not to withdraw life-sustaining technology from a comatose patient or to discontinue futile treatment of a terminally ill child. Rather, these kinds of decisions arise in the ethically important kinds of day-to-day situations that nurses like Amanda, in our case study, face in their practice on an ongoing basis. Levine (1989) goes on to note:

> Although nurses may occasionally confront a genuine dilemma—a situation where clearly no answer is entirely acceptable—most of the day-by-day activities of nurses pose moral questions that can be answered in ways that are entirely satisfactory. If this were not the case, no nursing intervention would ever be successful. (p. 125)

Much of the field of healthcare ethics has been shaped by the topics in bioethics that, arguably, garner the most attention: End-of-life care, futility, extraordinary measures, the use of new technologies, stem cell and genetic research, etc. Yet, less attention has been paid in the literature to the kinds of ethical issues that are encountered far more often by far more practitioners. These are the kinds of everyday problems issue nurses face that are sometimes dismissed, labeled as practice issues or practical problems, or ignored by virtue of being, simply put, too ordinary (Varcoe et al., 2004). They are the problems and challenges grounded in nursing practice and the special nature of the nurse–patient relationship. Nursing ethics calls our attention to this and can be considered to be somewhat distinct from bioethics or medical ethics in that it is rooted in the unique sphere of practice of the nurse. Much of the study of nursing ethics focuses on the noteworthy relationships that are a part of nursing practice: The nurse–patient relationship is only one of them. The nurse–nurse relationship and the nurse–physician relationship also create unique moral responsibilities and, sometimes, result in conflicts or competing duties. Nurses often occupy an "in between" position (Storch et al., 2004, p. 2) in which the nurse strives to maintain balance and to meet the needs of more than one stakeholder. This unique position implies a need for a unique field of inquiry that acknowledges both the multidimensional role of the nurse and the complex relationships that surround this role. Additionally, implicit within the study of nursing ethics is the understanding that nurses face ethical issues across a wide spectrum of contexts and situations. Many people assume that ethical dilemmas only occur within the context of highly technological acute care or with life-and-death situations. However, nurses in public health, long-term care, community settings, and rural and remote settings as well as in clinics and health promotion settings, all face ethical dilemmas in their practice. Nurses in a variety of roles, from a school nurse to a palliative care nurse, each face ethical challenges. While technology-driven and life-and-death ethical dilemmas often capture the headlines, nurses in all kinds of settings must deal with complex ethical issues.

The kinds of ethical issues that nurses face are manifold and vary according to context. No one situation is the same as another, although the key issue and principles may be similar. This is why it is often so difficult to recognize an ethical dilemma when faced with one. Sometimes, it is obvious that a problem has an ethical dimension, while at other times it may not be clear that the problem is, in fact, an ethical one. We may well recognize that we are facing an ethical dilemma when we have a problem without an obvious solution and in which each possibility might be supported by clear ethical rationale or in which each possible solution may well compromise an ethical principle (Beauchamp & Walters, 1999; Collier & Haliburton, 2011). In other words, the *right* solution, in an ethical dilemma, is never obvious and is often obscured by other possibilities.

ARTICULATING THE ISSUE

How we first approach an ethical problem is just as important as how we work through it and talk about it with others involved. The first step is recognizing that we are facing an ethical dilemma and critically reflect upon what we think are possible options, as well as what we think we ought to do, and why. But another key step is recognizing our own values and beliefs and how they might have an impact upon the kinds of decisions we make when faced with ethical dilemmas. As professional nurses, we cannot simply leave our values and beliefs behind when we are working, but instead must learn to be aware of and reflect upon the values and beliefs we hold, our own moral responses, and the subsequent effect upon our ethical decision-making abilities.

There are three levels of moral responses to ethical problems: An expressive level, a pre-reflective level, and a reflective level (Thomas & Waluchow, 1990). At an expressive level, we may simply state the way we feel about something without providing justification or rationale for beliefs. A statement such as "I'm against euthanasia because killing is wrong" is an example of an *expressive* response. At a *prereflective* level, we may well justify our response by citing legal, religious, or professional norms without critical reflection upon those norms. The statement "I oppose euthanasia because my professional duty requires me to do no harm" is an example of a prereflective statement. Finally, a *reflective* response is one in which the justification for our position is based upon principles or values that we have reflected upon, critically, and made a decision to use as a basis for our stance. Consider the following example of a reflective response: "I oppose euthanasia as the sanctity of all life and the principle of not doing harm takes precedence over the autonomy of a person to choose." While reasoning at a reflective level does not guarantee easier resolutions or agreement, it provides more opportunity than reasoning at a merely expressive level, for discussing views between those who might disagree.

ANALYZING ISSUES: WAYS OF UNDERSTANDING

Ethical Theories

A key skill in the articulation and analysis of ethical issues is the ability to provide a rationale, based on principles, to help back up our positions. Learning about ethical theories can help us in communicating our viewpoints to others. While the effectiveness of ethical theories for assisting nurses in finding solutions to real life ethical dilemmas is limited, a basic knowledge of ethical theories is necessary to help us in approaching and framing complex issues with multiple perspectives. Two specific types of theories are widely discussed in applied ethics: Deontological and consequentialist theories. Both of these have rich philosophical histories; we will only sketch them in outline here. *Deontological* ethics is mainly concerned with the duties we have toward others. From the point of view of deontology, adherence to these duties and consistency are what makes an action morally right. For example, from a deontological point of view we might regard telling the truth to patients as an absolute duty, rooted in the principle of respect for persons, which we must adhere to regardless of consequences. There are three difficulties with deontological theories. First, it is often difficult to determine what our duties are. Some duties and obligations are clearer, dictated by law or policy, while others are less obvious. In our first case study at the outset of the chapter, we see that Amanda is faced with more than one obligation or duty. While her primary obligation is to advocate for her patient, she also realizes that she has other kinds of obligations. These might include ensuring the system allows for the movement of patients to facilitate high-quality and efficient care, and working as a member of a nursing team and cooperating with policies and procedures that are in place to meet the needs of patients. A second difficulty with deontological theories is that we often find ourselves facing multiple and competing duties. Deontological theories offer little practical advice for how to deal with competing duties and demands. Finally, to pay attention only to duties and to fail to consider possible outcomes or consequences of adhering to our duties is, in a real-life context, problematic and often irresponsible. We are using deontological reasoning when we act according to a duty that we hold absolutely, such as not lying to a patient or not causing intentional harm to a patient.

In contrast to deontological or duty-based theories, *consequentialist* theories state that the rightness or wrongness of an action is determined by the outcomes, or consequences, of a particular action. Utilitarianism is the most commonly identified consequentialist theory and we will be discussing it here. In utilitarianism, an action is deemed to be ethically sound if it minimizes the negative outcomes (e.g., sadness, grief, distrust) and maximizes positive outcomes (e.g., pleasure, happiness, trust). From a utilitarian perspective, deciding upon the most ethically sound option is straightforward: Consider the possible options, "calculate" the relative balance of good and bad outcomes from each option, and choose the one that produces, for example, the most happiness and the least sadness for the most people concerned. While apparently simple—since it requires adherence to just a single principle—this utilitarian calculation poses three inherent difficulties. First, our ability to predict outcomes is imperfect as we are always making predictions about a future that is unsure. Second, measuring abstract and subjective notions such as goodness, happiness, or sadness is very difficult. Finally, what one person may consider to be a good outcome another person may evaluate quite differently. Universal agreement on what is "good" and "bad" can never be reached, so who gets to decide? In real life, utilitarian reasoning is widely used in public health. Quarantine and vaccination are two examples of utilitarian measures used to produce the most good for the most people. Amanda is, to some extent, pulled between doing "good" for Rudy, her patient, and considering the needs of other patients who are in need of a bed on the unit. From a utilitarian perspective, Amanda needs to consider how to produce the most "good" for each of the persons involved in the situation. She needs to consider more than simply what would produce the most good for Rudy in order to decide what is the most ethically sound course of action.

Criticisms that apply to the two most common ethical theories include the criticism that they are difficult to apply in real-life healthcare challenges and that they lack any kind of guidance for what principles should be used to make decisions, across a variety of contexts, times, and places. Thomas Beauchamp and James Childress, in response to some of this criticism, drew on the basic wisdom contained in those two theories to conceptualize a fundamental set of four principles (autonomy, beneficence, nonmaleficence, and justice) called *principlism* to guide ethical decision making for healthcare providers dealing with ethical problems (Beauchamp & Childress, 2008). Of the four, autonomy is very likely the most strongly emphasized in modern Westernized thinking about healthcare ethics, as the authors originally intended. Autonomy refers to the ability of a competent person to make decisions regarding his or her own life and health. Beneficence refers to the obligation of the healthcare provider to act for the good of the patient, protect the patient from harm, and promote the best interests or welfare of the patient. Nonmaleficence refers to the duty to not do anything that might harm a patient. Of course, this obligation to prevent harming others needs to be balanced with the obligation to do good. Consider, for example, the pain caused by a vaccine injection. While many might construe the pain as harm, the benefit gained from the vaccination outweighs the pain of the injection. Finally, justice is always an important principle to always consider in the provision of healthcare. Questions about what is *just* may arise in discussions of what is fair or what is owed to a patient, how scarce resources might be allocated, or the rights of patients. The most challenging aspect of considering the principle of justice in an ethical dilemma is reaching consensus or agreement on what is *fair* or just. Even among reasonable or fair-minded persons, there may be disagreement on what is considered to be fair (Daniels, 2000). Principlism is often viewed as more contextual and relevant to today's healthcare environment; a criticism of this theory is that it can be very limiting to think about ethical problems by considering only these four principles. For many who are learning about ethics and principles, principlism is an attractive theory. It is fairly easy to apply to scenarios and cases encountered in the provision of healthcare; however, it is often applied by new learners in a very pragmatic and inflexible way. Principlism often is most effective at helping to highlight key issues within an ethical case study by providing an overarching structure, or starting point, for considering all the facets of a problem or dilemma. It also, however, has limitations in effectively applying the theory in situations involving diverse cultures or communities outside of a more Westernized context.

As we have noted, ethical theories don't necessarily provide an "answer" to an ethical problem. However, what they can do is allow us to better understand the values and attitudes of others by highlighting the different ways that diverse people approach the same problem. Taking time to reflect on whether you are supporting a particular option for the best outcome, to adhere to a duty, or to ensure a principle like autonomy is protected is an important step in working with others to resolve ethical problems.

Codes of Ethics

A profession is, in part, defined by having a code of ethics that provides public documentation of the expectations of ethical practice. It is an essential aspect of professional practice to adhere to the responsibilities and duties, as outlined in a code of ethics. In Canada, the Canadian Nurses Association has developed a *Code of Ethics for Registered Nurses,* a living document that is continually revised (CNA, 2008). The code outlines seven "nursing values and ethical responsibilities."

A code of ethics outlines, in a very general way, expectations of ethical practice. Unlike a law, a code of ethics cannot be legally enforced by courts. However, every profession has the legal right to sanction members for failure to adhere to their ethical responsibilities and duties. Provincial regulatory bodies have disciplinary committees that include members of the lay public. Typically, the activities and minutes of such committees are publicly available. Internal regulation and sanctioning of members who do not act in accordance with the code of ethics is the responsibility of a professional regulatory body. What a code of ethics does not do, however, is prescribe particular actions to take in specific situations where ethical problems have arisen. It is expected that a professional nurse can apply the principles, values, and responsibilities outlined in the code in particular situations. For many novice nurses, this can be challenging as constructs or notions such as "dignity" and "respect" are highly interpretable. What the newest revision of the *Code of Ethics for Registered Nurses* has done is outline some real responsibilities that are in keeping with the seven values. This is a step toward making the *Code of Ethics* a more easily applicable, less abstract, and more clinically relevant document. This most recent revision of the code also includes a helpful appendix that addresses how to apply the values and responsibilities of the code in special circumstances, such as in interactions with nursing students, when job action (i.e., a strike) is involved, in the context of a pandemic or natural disaster, when a nurse is being asked to do something that is in opposition to her values, or in a situation in which a nurse is aware of unethical or unsafe care. These situations are commonly encountered by nurses and involve contextual considerations, along with considerations of the political, social, and environmental structures in which they occur. Practical applications of the code are helpful in illustrating to nurses (and to the public) what tangible responsibilities are implied by the more abstract and idealistic values.

Ethics and the Law

The relationship between ethics and the law is a dynamic relationship in which there are some overlaps as well as some clear points of divergence. What we know to be legal may not be ethical. It is not against the law to spread malicious gossip or to talk badly about co-workers behind their backs, although most of us would consider those actions to be unethical. Alternatively, it may be illegal to speed or go through a stop sign in a car; however, if you are rushing a critically ill child to a hospital, that may be considered an ethical exception to a legal rule. As a profession, nurses are affected by laws to which they must attend and adhere. Consider the ethical principle of maintaining confidentiality of patients, an obligation emphasized in our *Code of Ethics*. While we are ethically and legally bound to maintain confidentiality of patient information, there are situations in which breaching confidentiality is allowed and even required. Situations such as child abuse or neglect or a patient intending to do imminent harm to self or others are reasons to breach confidentiality. A further example: In Ontario, the Mandatory Gunshot Wounds Reporting Act (2005) requires that any patient with a gunshot wound be reported to police. While many healthcare professionals, including nurses, support this from a patient and community safety perspective, many others have found themselves uncomfortable, and even resistant to the legal requirement to report, feeling that it may present an increased risk to the patient and create an environment of mistrust, thus discouraging others from seeking help (MacKay, 2004; Ovens & Borgunvaag, 2008). Mandatory gunshot wound reporting is a good example of balancing the needs of communities and the safety of societies against the best interests of an individual patient. For many nurses, this is, understandably, a difficult challenge.

Nurses have three kinds of legal obligations: To have knowledge of the legal boundaries of their jobs, to protect patients' rights, and to protect themselves from liability. Nurses must provide a reasonable and competent standard of care to their patients. Sometimes this is referred to as a *fiduciary* duty, a trust-based duty that implies a higher duty of care to others. Those in fiduciary roles are required to place the needs of another person ahead of their own needs. Implied trust in both the nurses' knowledge and integrity are part of a fiduciary relationship. Legal concepts important to think about within the sphere of professional competence include: *Professional misconduct, negligence,* and *duty of care.* These kinds of legal concepts are usually found under the category of unintentional torts. A tort refers to an act of wrongdoing that results in harm or injury. In the aftermath, the injured party makes a claim for damages and in order to deter further similar wrongs. Torts may be intentional or unintentional. Intentional torts include examples such as assault, battery, false imprisonment, or invasion of privacy. Unintentional torts are divided into two kinds: *Liability* and *negligence.* In nursing and healthcare, most of the cases that arise are cases of unintentional negligence. Unintentional negligence occurs when any treatment or aspect of care clearly falls below an acceptable level and causes injury to a patient.

Nurses are legally regarded as having a *duty of care,* that is, they have an obligation to not act in a particular way that causes harm, either intentionally or unintentionally (through being careless or having a lack of knowledge or skill). When the care provided is not consistent with the duty of care, or falls below the duty of care (i.e., the nurse fails in his or her duty of care), and injury of any kind results, this is referred to as negligence and also falls under the umbrella of professional misconduct. While the actions of the nurse may be unintentional, in cases of negligence, they are unreasonably unsafe and result in injury. In order to determine that a situation is, in fact, one of negligence, four elements must be present. First, a duty of care must exist. Second, it must be evident that the duty of care was breached through the actions or conduct of the nurse. Third, there must be a resultant injury or harm. Finally, it must be clearly evident that the injury or harm resulted directly from the conduct or actions of the person entrusted with a duty of care. In cases of unintentional negligence, the legal focus is usually on some kind of compensation for the injury rather than on punishment of the nurse. However, a nurse who is found to be negligent will most likely also be subject to disciplinary action from their provincial professional nursing regulatory body.

Consider the following case: Lars is a new graduate RN who has been working on a medical unit for 3 months since his graduation. Today, the unit is poorly staffed due to illness and vacation. The nurse in charge gives Lars an assignment, which not only includes four additional complex patients beyond his typical assignment of five patients, but also the administration of chemotherapy to one patient and caring for another patient with a central venous line. Lars has not yet been certified in administration of chemotherapy or maintenance of central venous lines and is worried about his ability to care for nine complex patients when so far in his nursing career he has only looked after five patients in a shift. When he approaches the nurse in charge with his concerns, she responds by saying, "You'll be fine. Don't worry about it. I have no choice—there's no staff today! Just keep everyone status quo for 12 hours. And the certification for chemo and the central line—that's just a formality. You probably already know how to do it. The manual is there if you need to read up on anything, but just give the chemo—and be careful!—and flush the central line every few hours and after any meds. No problem!" Lars isn't confident about his ability to provide competent care, to prevent his patients from harm, and to ensure that they are kept safe and healthy, but he isn't sure what to do and, furthermore, he isn't sure he has a choice.

In this case, Lars does have a choice, albeit a difficult one. Professional competence requires that Lars not give chemotherapy or maintain a central venous line without proper training and certification. Furthermore, if he knows that he is not capable of competently caring for nine patients, he needs to be clear with the nurse in charge and work with her and other staff to find compromises and alternatives that keep patients safe and ensure competent care. Failure to do so, in this case, may well result in injury to the patient through incompetent or inexperienced care. It is also important to note in this case that, as a professional, Lars (as well as the nurse in charge) is expected, by virtue of their specialized knowledge, to have a degree of *foresight* that is greater than a layperson. Lars knows that if chemotherapy is provided incorrectly or a central line is flushed improperly, either of these actions may result in injury or harm to the patient. He also knows that his current level of skill and organization is not at a point yet where he can, with confidence and ease, care for nine complex patients safely. This case has both legal and ethical implications, yet involves a kind of situation that many new graduate nurses find themselves in, time and time again. Understanding both the legal and ethical obligations we have to patients as well as knowing one's own level of skill, knowledge, and limitations is an important part of providing safe, competent, and high-quality care.

BARRIERS TO RESOLVING ETHICAL DILEMMAS

While it is helpful to learn about ethical and legal obligations in a classroom, it is certainly different to be faced with ethical and legal challenges in the workplace. It can be difficult and even impossible to consistently maintain the highest ethical standards and never compromise. Often, factors beyond the control of individual nurses make it difficult to maintain moral integrity, even with the best intentions. Factors such as scarcity of resources, low staffing, lack of knowledge, or a real or perceived lack of power may all have an effect on an individual nurse's ability to be a moral agent. Moral distress was first defined by Jameton (1984) as resulting from knowing the right thing to do but being unable to do it, typically due to institutional constraints that make the desired actions difficult or impossible to carry out. Others have gone on to add to Jameton's definition, noting that inability to act in an ethically appropriate way may arise not only out of institutional constraints or factors related to the organization. Such inability might also be attributed to characteristics of the moral agent (e.g., lack of adequate knowledge, a perceived or real lack of power, moral fatigue, or fear) (Webster & Baylis, 2000). Moral distress has been shown to contribute to a desire to leave the profession and to feelings of powerlessness, fatigue, disrespect, and frustration (Ulrich et al., 2007).

Moral distress is a multifaceted problem that has been extensively investigated and discussed in the nursing literature (Corley 1995; Corley, 2002; Jameton, 1984; Jameton, 1993; Storch et al., 2004; Ulrich et al., 2007). While it is often discussed as a problem in nursing, it is evident in other healthcare professions as well (Walton et al., 2007). Moral distress that is not addressed or distressing situations that are not resolved can leave, over time, a *moral residue* (Webster & Baylis, 2000). Described as the remains of unhealed "moral wounds" (Epstein & Delgado, 2010, p. 2) that accumulate over time as a result of making moral compromises, experiencing lack of control, and dealing with constraints on moral autonomy, moral residue can seriously harm one's integrity and career. There are no easy solutions to the problem of moral distress but strategies such as creating ethically conducive environments, changing attitudes and structures to allow for challenging the status quo, increasing accountability, providing for safe and open discussion, and fostering active collaboration with identification of ethical nurse leaders are some ways to begin addressing moral distress (Corley et al., 2005).

STRATEGIES FOR RESOLVING ETHICAL DILEMMAS

In this section, we will address three strategies for resolving ethical problems that nurses are faced with in practice. In the first part of this section, we will discuss how *moral integrity* can contribute to being a more effective moral agent. Second, we will outline an *ethical decision-making model* that may help in approaching and addressing difficult ethical problems. Finally, we will address the idea of what it means to exemplify *ethical leadership,* demonstrate *moral courage,* and help to create more ethically sound workplaces.

Moral Integrity

The term "integrity" is widely used to describe a person of good moral standing. To say we know "a person of integrity," however, may mean something quite different to different people. On one hand, integrity may mean being of good moral character. On the other hand, it may refer to a sense of wholeness, completeness, and being morally intact. When an ethical problem becomes overwhelming, the ability of the nurse to maintain a sense of integrity may well be "pushed to a limit" (Yeo et al., 2010, p. 349) and her or his ability to be a moral agent may be compromised. Yeo et al. deal with this topic particularly well and outline four necessary elements of moral integrity: Moral autonomy, fidelity to promise, steadfastness, and wholeness. *Moral autonomy* refers to our developing a sense of who we are, in terms of the authentic and consistent values we hold. As children, our parents have moral authority over us and our values are prescribed by our families, culture, socioeconomic status, and friends. As we get older, and become braver and more willing to explore our own values and beliefs, we typically find ourselves examining long-held beliefs instilled by our parents and families, trying them on for size, and either rejecting them and adopting new ones or embracing them as our own. This means taking responsibility and ownership, and being accountable for our values and beliefs. With increased moral autonomy comes increased integrity.

Fidelity to promise involves two important aspects: Making a promise and then keeping it. Those who are less willing to make promises or keep promises that they have made are often viewed by others as having less integrity. Keeping a promise does not only demonstrate that we are willing to abide by social norms; it also shows trustworthiness and reliability, two fundamental elements of moral integrity.

Steadfastness might be described as "sticking to our moral guns," even in the face of adversity. Being steadfast is, for many of us, a "work in progress" as we learn over time to stand up for our values and beliefs and what we believe is *right,* even when it may be difficult or may pose a risk to ourselves. Some examples of steadfastness include:

- The nurse who questions the order for a painful, futile treatment that the patient does not want.
- The student nurse who reminds more senior nurses that discussing a patient's family in an elevator is not acceptable.
- The nursing professor who stands up for a student's rights when the university is not listening.
- The nurse who advocates for a marginalized or stigmatized client and finds herself "fighting the system."

The last element of moral integrity is wholeness. All nurses have multiple roles in their lives: They are not only professionals but they may also be sons, daughters, spouses, employees, students, parents, volunteers, church members, etc. It is often difficult for us to integrate all these roles into a morally consistent person who acts the same in every context. Consider the student nurse who is caring and compassionate toward his elderly patients but abrupt, unsupportive, and unfriendly with his grandparents. Or think of the rural nurse who spends much of her day counseling her patients on maintaining a healthy lifestyle, but spends many evenings drinking too much in the local bar. Furthermore, consider the nurse manager who is a sought-after volunteer mentor in the literacy and job-seeking work she does with homeless youth, but is exceptionally and unfairly hard on new student nurses on her unit. Why is it so difficult to maintain wholeness in all that we do? Integrity requires that we try to incorporate our values and beliefs across the many dimensions, roles, and relationships in our lives. While not an easy task, the constant work we do to maintain this is part of moral integrity (Yeo et al., 2010).

Ethical Decision-making Models

The two most difficult parts of approaching ethical problems are (1) figuring out that, in fact, you do have an ethical problem and (2) deciding how to go about working through it. Using an ethical decision-making model can help structure the activity of working through such a problem and provide a framework for dealing with complex and multidimensional problems. No ethical decision-making model can provide a guarantee that all decisions will be good ones, nor does such a model replace thoughtful reflection and consideration of what is at stake in a situation. Remember that an ethical dilemma is one in which there are opposing views or principles that each support reasonable but contradictory actions. In an ethical dilemma, reasonable people can typically see "both sides" of the problem but only one outcome is possible and often the challenge is moving from the point where someone recognizes that a problem has a moral dimension to figuring out a resolution. So, how then do we approach ethical problems? MacDonald (2010) provides a straightforward and easy-to-use *Guide to Moral Decision Making* which consists of nine steps (MacDonald, 2010). Taking time to think through each of these steps in an attempt to resolve an ethical dilemma will at least ensure that you have taken time to consider a range of relevant factors in reaching your decision. There are a number of ethical decision-making models that have been developed for use. Many of them share similar properties and foundational principles. Some other examples include *A Framework for Ethical Decision-Making* (McDonald et al., 2001) and *Storch's Circle Method for Ethical Decision-Making* (CNA, 2002). The key is finding one that reflects the reality of your own practice, and then referring to it when faced with an ethical problem or situation in which you may benefit from some structure to facilitate working through the problem.

Creating Ethical Workplaces

One fact that is evident from the nursing literature is that nurses feel strongly about having workplaces and supervisors that support ethically sound and principled care, that allow nurses to advocate for what they feel is right, and that make space and time for ethical reflection. It is clear that the *ethical culture* or *ethical climate* of an organization is important to nurses. Ethical climate can be defined as the sustained or consistent conditions, cultural norms, and practices, within an organization, that have an effect upon how the way commonly encountered difficult ethical problems are identified, addressed, and resolved (Hart, 2005; Olson, 2002). Having a climate that allows those working there to be able to enact positive change, to challenge the status quo, and to stand up for principles and values, all in a safe and ethically sensitive environment—these are all very important attributes of an organization that nurses value and that are likely to be important ingredients to achieving ethically good outcomes. Poor ethical climates are tied to more frequent reports of moral distress for nurses and are clearly linked to both low retention and high turnover rates (Corley et al., 2005; Hart, 2005; Olson, 2002; Pauly et al., 2009).

Clearly, the *culture* of an organization is important in establishing an ethical climate. Sims (1991) refers to organizational culture as the "social glue that helps hold an organization together" (p. 502). While Sims is referring most especially to large organizations or corporations, his insight can clearly be applied to nursing units. Without a culture that supports strong ethical standards and values, those within the organization can be left feeling isolated, worried, or unable to make positive changes or to advocate for change. When the values and standards of an organization are explicitly known and shared by all who work there, a positive working environment can be created (Graf & Halfer, 2002).

In nursing scholarship on ethical climate, it has been demonstrated that nurses, when talking about the ethical climate of their workplace, are typically talking about how difficult or challenging patient care issues are discussed, handled, and addressed by peers, managers, and other healthcare professionals (Olson, 1998). In other words, the relationships that nurses have with others and how these relationships withstand difficult ethical problems may be an important factor in deciding whether or not the ethical climate of nursing organizations is a positive one (i.e., a climate more conducive to ethically sound practice). Nurses note that an environment in which there are overly rigid policies, unresolved conflict, and inappropriate use of resources can lead to moral distress (Storch et al., 2002). Certainly, more work needs to be done to help us understand the complicated relationships between ethical climate, organizational culture, moral distress, ethical practice, and rates of nursing turnover and retention. It is clear, however, that with such high turnover rates for nurses, especially those who are in the first 2 years after graduation (Lavoie-Tremblay et al., 2008), a better understanding of these relationships and a focus on how ethical climates can be created and sustained is an important priority for the profession.

Ethical Leadership

Throughout this chapter, we have identified the kinds of ethical issues and challenges that nurses face and have also highlighted some barriers and some strategies for approaching these kinds of problems effectively and with integrity. Despite the identified challenges and barriers to ethical action, the presence of environments and workplaces that do not support advocacy and positive change, and the prevalence of moral distress and moral residue, there are still many opportunities for nurses to demonstrate ethical leadership. Nurse leaders are also moral leaders, and can act as a "moral compass for nurses, using their power as a positive force to promote, provide, and sustain quality practice environments for safe, competent, and ethical practice." (Storch et al., 2002, p. 7). Storch and colleagues go on to note that moral leadership implies both commitment and *moral courage*—to address inequities, to engage in resolving conflicts, and to facilitate a strong and sustainable connection between moral intent and moral action. But moral courage is never easy. Defined as a willingness to stand up for what is right in the face of adversity, moral courage, in practice, involves the ability to advocate for others despite forces or pressures to act differently (Lachman, 2010). Courage is considered to be a virtue and like other virtues, can be learned, taught, and further developed in practice. Aristotle posited that courage involves wisdom, emotional control, and an ability to manage risk and that it exists somewhere along a spectrum between rashness and cowardice (Aristotle, 350 BCE/1998). In nursing, the virtue of moral courage means overcoming fears, resisting pressures to act differently, and standing up for what nurses, after careful consideration, believe to be right. Moral courage can be supported in ethical workplaces, through education and the active promotion of clear reasoning, wisdom, and knowledgeable advocacy by nurses. Through the development of virtues such as moral courage, nurses, as moral agents, can become mentors and moral leaders.

If we return to Amanda's situation presented at the outset of the chapter, it is clear that Amanda has a choice to demonstrate moral courage by speaking up and advocating for Rudy's unique needs and best interests to prevent him from being discharged from hospital at this time, despite the pressures she and others around her feel to "move patients through the system efficiently." Moral courage would imply that Amanda advocates for Rudy, using her knowledge and experience to endorse the promotion of the best, safest, and most ethical care for her patient. In an environment that supports ethical practice and allows for individual nurses to safely demonstrate ethical leadership and moral courage, Amanda would not feel either silenced or oppressed. In advocating for her patient, Amanda would effectively be developing the virtue of moral courage. Nurses who do not feel silenced, but who instead seize opportunities to speak out for what they believe in, to engage in advocacy for others, to have an active voice in promoting positive change can, over time, help to create environments in which all nurses can develop and exercise moral courage.

SUMMARY

Nurses, as professionals, have legal and ethical duties that flow from their obligation to serve both individual patients and the common good. In this chapter, we have addressed the importance of having an awareness of the ethical and legal obligations that being part of a profession, like nursing, involves. What is also clear is that it is equally important to have a way to discuss and approach difficult ethical problems that are encountered in practice. While there are barriers to resolving ethical problems that exist across the spectrum of nursing workplaces, strategies to address these barriers do exist. Knowing your legal obligations, having a working knowledge of ethical theories, fostering an ethically sound workplace, and becoming a responsible and accountable moral agent are all strategies to address ethical problems and ensure safe, high-quality, ethically sensitive care.

REFLECTIONS *on the Chapter...*

1 From your own practice, identify examples of ethical issues. What helped you know that an issue was, in fact, an ethical one? Did others view the issue as involving ethics? Was there an opportunity to discuss it and work through it as a group, or did you approach the problem on your own?

2 What are examples of legal issues in your practice? Do you feel as informed as you should about legal obligations in your practice?

3 How does your workplace deal with ethical issues that arise in everyday practice? Are there resources available to you? Do you feel that your place of work is one that supports discussion and resolution of difficult ethical issues? How would you change or improve the workplace to better address the needs of nurses dealing with ethical issues in practice?

4 Reflect upon the two main ethical theories introduced in this chapter: Deontology and consequentialism. Do you consider yourself as acting in a particular way that is more frequently aligned with one of these theories? Think about some examples from your own practice.

5 Consider a common ethical issue in healthcare such as: Truth-telling in practice, how to best support patients through a difficult or serious diagnosis or health setback, or dealing with patients who might not wish to follow the instructions of the healthcare team. Now think about your education and training. Do you feel prepared to deal with these kinds of common ethical issues in practice? If not, what would have helped you feel better prepared?

6 Think about your personal values and beliefs you hold and how these fit with your practice. Have you ever had to compromise your personal values and beliefs as you have provided care to patients? Think about how this made you feel. Did this change how you now approach these kinds of issues in practice?

Want to know more? Visit thePoint for additional helpful resources:

- Journal Articles
- Learning Objectives
- Nursing Professional Roles and Responsibilities
- Bonus chapters:
  - Health and Nursing Policy: A Matter of Politics, Power and Professionalism
  - The NP Movement: Recurring Issues
  - When Difference Matters: The Politics of Privilege and Marginality

References

Aristotle. (350 BCE/1998). *The Nicomachean ethics* (W.D. Ross, Trans.). Oxford, UK: Oxford University Press (original work published c. 350 BCE). Retrieved from http://classics.mit.edu/Aristotle/nicomachaen.html

Beauchamp, T., & Childress, J. (2008). *Principles of biomedical ethics*. London: Oxford University Press.

Beauchamp, T., & Walters, L. (1999). *Contemporary issues in bioethics*. Belmont, CA: Wadsworth.

Canadian Nurses Association. (2002). *Everyday ethics: Putting the code into practice*. Ottawa: Canadian Nurses Association.

———. (2008). *Code of ethics for registered nurses*. Ottawa: Canadian Nurses Association.

Collier, C., & Haliburton, R. (2011). *Bioethics in Canada: A philosophical introduction*. Toronto: Canadian Scholar's Press.

Corley, M. (1995). Moral distress of critical care nurses. *American Journal of Critical Care, 4*, 280–285.

———. (2002). Moral distress: a proposed theory and research agenda. *Nursing Ethics, 9*(6), 636–650.

Corley, M.C., Minick, P., Elswick, R.K., & Jacobs, M. (2005). Nurse moral distress and ethical work environment. *Nursing Ethics, 12,* 381–390.

Daniels, N. (2000). Accountability for reasonableness: Establishing a fair process for priority setting is easier than agreeing on principles. *British Medical Journal, 321,* 1300.

Epstein, E., & Delgado, S. (2010). Understanding and addressing moral distress. *OJIN: The Online Journal of Issues in Nursing, 15*(3), 1–12.

Fisher, J. (2009). *Biomedical ethics. A Canadian focus.* Toronto: Oxford University Press.

Graf, E., & Halfer, D. (2002). Creating great places for nurses to work. *Chart, 99*(6), 4–5.

Hart, S.E. (2005). Hospital ethical climates and registered nurses' turnover intentions. *Journal of Nursing Scholarship, 37,* 173–177.

Jameton, A. (1984). *Nursing practice: The ethical issues.* Englewood Cliffs, NJ: Prentice Hall.

———. (1993). Dilemmas of moral distress: Moral responsibility and nursing practice. *AWHONN, 4*(4), 542–551.

Johns, C. (1999). Unraveling the dilemmas in everyday nursing practice. *Nursing Ethics, 6*(4), 287–298.

Lachman, V. (2010). Strategies necessary for moral courage. *OJIN: The Online Journal of Issues in Nursing, 15*(3).

Lavoie-Tremblay, M., O'Brien-Pallas, L., Gelinas, C., Desforges, N., & Marchionni, C. (2008). Addressing the turnover issue among new nurses from a generational point of view. *Journal of Nursing Management, 16,* 724–733.

Levine, M.E. (1989). Beyond dilemma. *Seminars in Oncology Nursing, 5*(2), 124–128.

Mackay, B. (2004). Gunshot wounds: The new public health issue. *Canadian Medical Association Journal, 170*(5), 780–781.

MacDonald, C. (2010). Retrieved October 12, 2012, from www.ethicsweb.ca/guide/<http://www.ethicsweb.ca/guide/>

McDonald, M., Rodney, P., & Starzomski, R. (2001). A framework for ethical decision-making: Version 6.0 Ethics Shareware. http://www.ethics.ubc.ca/upload/A%20Framework%20for%20Ethical%20Decision-Making.pdf

Olson, L. (1998). Hospital nurses' perceptions of the ethical climate of their work setting. *Image—The Journal of Nursing Scholarship, 30*(4), 345–349.

———. (2002). Ethical climates as the context for nurse retention. *Chart, 99*(6), 3,7.

Ovens, H.J., & Borgunvaag, B. (2008). Bill 110: An evaluation of the impact of Canada's first mandatory gunshot wound reporting law. *Annals of Emergency Medicine, 51*(4), 537.

Pauly, B., Varcoe, C., Storch, J., & Newton, L. (2009). Registered Nurses perceptions of moral distress and ethical climate. *Nursing Ethics, 16*(5), 561–573.

Sims, R. (1991). The institutionalization of organizational ethics. *Journal of Business Ethics, 10,* 493–506.

Smith, K.V., & Godfrey, N.S. (2002). Being a good nurse and doing the right thing: A qualitative study. *Nursing Ethics, 9*(3), 302–312.

Storch, J., Rodney, P., & Starzomski, R. (2004). *Toward a moral horizon: Nursing ethics for leadership and practice.* Toronto: Pearson.

Storch, J., Rodney, P., Pauly, B., Brown, H., & Starzomski, R. (2002). Listening to nurses' moral voices: Building a quality health care environment. *Canadian Journal of Nursing Leadership, 15*(4), 7–16.

Thomas, J.E., & Waluchow, W. (1990). *Well and good: Case studies in biomedical ethics.* 2nd ed. Peterborough: Broadview Press.

Ulrich, C., O'Donnell, P., Taylor, C., Farrar, A., Danis, M., & Grady, C. (2007). Ethical climate, ethics stress, and the job satisfaction of nurses and social workers in the United States. *Social Science and Medicine, 65,* 1708–1719.

Varcoe, C., Doane, C.G., Pauly B., et al. (2004). Ethical practice in nursing: Working the in-betweens. *Journal of Advanced Nursing, 45*(3), 316–325.

Walton, N., Martin, D., Peter, E., Pringle, D.M., & Singer, P.A. (2007). Priority setting in cardiac surgery: A qualitative study. *Health Policy, 80,* 444–458.

Webster, G.C., & Baylis, F.E. (2000). Moral residue. In S.B. Rubin & L. Zoloth (Eds.), *Margin of error: The ethics of mistakes in the practice of medicine.* (pp. 217–230). Hagerstown, MD: University Publishing Group.

Yeo, M., Moorhouse, A., Khan, P., et al. (2010). *Concepts and cases in nursing ethics* (3rd ed.). Peterborough: Broadview Press.

22 Issues in Healthcare for an Aging Population

Angela Gillis

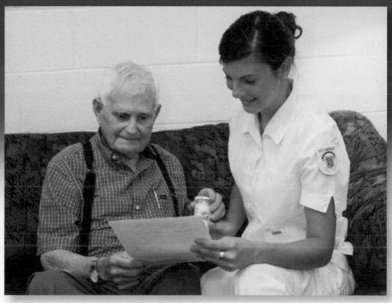

Gerontology plays an increasingly vital role in nursing education. (Used with permission of School of Nursing, St. Francis Xavier University.)

Critical Questions

As a way of engaging with the ideas in this chapter, consider the following:

1. Reflecting upon your experience as a nursing student, how are older adults portrayed in the healthcare system, in the media, and in society at large?

2. What is healthy aging and how do you understand it in the context of chronic illness?

3. What factors facilitate and hinder healthy aging in Canada's healthcare system?

4. Can the goal of healthy aging be achieved for older adults?

Chapter Objectives

After completing this chapter, you will be able to:

1. Discuss diversity in older adults as reflected in Canada's aging population.

2. Identify issues of relevance to older adults seeking to age well in Canada.

3. Explore healthy aging as an issue for older adults.

4. Appreciate how different understandings of aging and what is important in healthcare for

older adults can impact achievement of healthy aging.

5. Identify barriers to healthy aging for older adults.

6. Describe strategies for addressing barriers to healthy aging and moving forward toward the provision of care that is responsive to the needs of older adults.

*L*isten to the aged for they will tell you about living and dying. Listen to the
aged for they will teach you how to be courageous, loving and generous. They
are distinguished faculty without formal classrooms, tenure, sabbaticals. They
teach not from books but from long experience in living.

—*Irene Burnside*

INTRODUCTION

This chapter discusses the phenomenon of population aging and the challenges in healthcare
that an aging population presents. In particular, it explores the issue of healthy aging and how to
promote it within the context of the Canadian healthcare system. Every report on the future of
healthcare that has been penned in the last decade has discussed implications of an aging population and proposed strategies to deal with the increasing complexity that such a seismic shift
presents. In keeping with the title and focus of the text, this chapter is an attempt to accurately
reflect the realities of issues in healthcare for our aging population. It explores the taken-for-
granted view of healthcare for the elderly and examines a range of factors impacting it. The
complexity of the issue of healthy aging is examined and barriers to and strategies for achieving
healthy aging are explored.

SITUATING THE TOPIC

Older Canadians are a growing phenomenon in healthcare. This is due in large measure to a drop
in fertility rates, improvements in health status, an increase in life expectancy, and the impact of
the baby boomer generation (individuals born between 1946 and 1965; they are the parents of
most nursing students reading this chapter today). It is assumed that this group by virtue of their
numbers will exert increased demands for nursing and healthcare, as well as needs for a whole
spectrum of services ranging from transportation and assistance with personal care to management of complex chronic illnesses. The conundrum becomes how to promote healthy aging in
a place of choice, and provide the widest range of service options to this population amidst a
system of care that, still in 2011, focuses on cure rather than disease prevention or health promotion. This chapter presents students with an opportunity to explore this conundrum. In so doing,
negative stereotypes of aging are dispelled, as the complexity of health issues of older adults and
the challenge of responding to them are examined.

FRAMING THE ISSUE

Framing the issues of older adults in healthcare requires one to make explicit assumptions
that are held about the topic, and to uncover what is written or known about the issue. Hence,
for purposes of this chapter responses to the following questions are basic to a discussion of
issues in healthcare for older adults: What is aging? What is healthy aging? Who and what
defines the older adult? Before responding to these queries, the author wishes to acknowledge
that any discussion of issues of older adults as a group requires that some generalizations
and simplifications be imposed on the discussion because of the heterogeneity of the group.
Indeed some authors caution that the one universal characteristic that unites today's aging
population is diversity (Segall & Fries, 2011). To understand what it is like to be a senior

seeking care and services to achieve healthy aging let us consider the story of Alice and Andrew Greer.

An Aging Exemplar: Meet Alice and Andrew Greer

Alice and Andrew are 85 and 87 years old, respectively, leading normal lives and living in their own home. Alice has arthritis, hypertension, and recent cataract surgery but copes very well, and Andrew has hypertension and diabetes controlled with diet and medication. They live close to their oldest daughter and family who provide help and companionship but the Greers prefer to be independent. While Alice and Andrew worry that someday they may have to go into a nursing home, their aim is to stay in their own home as long as possible, and continue to contribute to their family and community through their volunteer activities.

The Greers are typical of many older Canadians who view their health on the whole as very good. Research indicates that more than 90% of seniors 65 years and older live in the community and 80% of all care for older seniors is provided by close friends and relatives. Less than 10% are in nursing homes despite seniors' fears of long-term institutional care (Chappell, 2010). While Alice and Andrew enjoy a sense of good health and are able, at present, to maintain a comfortable lifestyle in their rural community, they fear the common losses associated with aging such as reduced vision, hearing, and mental functioning. Their healthcare needs require long-term help and support services rather than the expensive, short-term medical interventions that Canada's healthcare system is mainly designed to provide. While it is a popular misconception that health declines as part of normal aging, seniors like Alice and Andrew are examples of how many older people have learned to adapt to the changes that chronic disease has brought. Furthermore, chronic disease, disability, and loss of independence are not inevitable consequences of aging. A vision of healthy aging can help seniors like Alice and Andrew manage their chronic illnesses, prevent the onset of further illnesses, and embrace a positive approach to living so that they enjoy more years in good health. This ultimately will reduce their long-term care needs and save healthcare costs. In light of this, it is important to us as nurses to understand the factors that both impede and promote healthy aging for older Canadians so they can influence the health agenda to achieve this goal.

Stories about couples like Alice and Andrew help us to appreciate the nature of issues confronting the older adult in healthcare today, and the need to advocate, along with seniors, for a new vision for healthy aging. There is no clear consensus in the literature as to what the healthcare needs of the baby boomer generation will be. Some suggest that this generation who will follow Alice and Andrew will exert increased demands for services and redefine the senior years, as they are expected to have longer life expectancies (Alzheimer Society of Canada [ASC], 2010). Others argue that seniors of the future will be healthier than their predecessors; they will be better informed health consumers; and they will use fewer healthcare services (B.C. Ministry of Health [BCMH], 2005). Hence, the impact of the baby boomer generation on future healthcare remains a paradox. Given this paradox, it is prudent to address the issue of healthy aging now, so that current and future seniors can be supported to maintain optimal health and quality of life, and in so doing pressures on the health system can be better managed (Special Senate Committee on Aging, 2009).

APPRECIATING DIVERSITY IN AGING AND HEALTH

The one characteristic that can be used to describe Canada's aging population is that it is heterogeneous. While older adults share common characteristics and concerns, they differ significantly on many issues of importance to achievement of healthy aging. There has been a history in program planning and policy development in Canada to treat older adults as a homogenous group. Consequently, important distinctions among older adults that impact health needs and requirements for service are obscured. This section provides a description of Canada's aging population and highlights some of the common characteristics, as well as some of the important and unique differences among older adults. It begins with a discussion of age, a characteristic that all too frequently is used to systematically categorize older adults inappropriately into categories that enable differences to go unrecognized.

The diversity of Canada's aging population requires a shift in thinking from a narrow understanding of aging as a biological process that begins with birth and ends with death, to a more holistic view of it. Aging is too complex a process to be defined only by birth date. In reality, most people define aging in terms of personal meaning and experience. Aging is a relative term, commonly associated with how one acts and feels physically, emotionally, socially, and culturally than with one's chronological age. If we go back to our example of Mr. and Mrs. Greer, it is apparent that the traditional use of chronological age to define who is old, in the case of the Greers, may lead to negative stereotypes of this couple that do not bear out in reality.

For healthcare professionals whose practice focuses on care of the older adult, as well as for most older adults, the important indicators of age are physiologic health, psychological well-being, and the ability to function and perform activities of interest to the individual (Christenson et al., 2009). On the basis of this perspective of aging, the use of functional age has emerged as a worldwide concept to explain aging. Functional age represents a focus on positive attitudes toward aging and is associated with higher levels of well-being. Miller (2012) notes that functional age is a more rational basis for determining care and service requirements than number of years since birth, and she adds that the question, "How functional?" is more relevant than "How old?" when one is trying to promote healthy aging in older adults. From a holistic perspective, this conceptualization of aging is more in keeping with nursing's bio-psycho-social-spiritual view of person than is a narrow focus on biological aging and physical functioning.

Historically, the chronological age of 65 years has heralded receipt of the Old Age Pension and it has become the designated marker for classification as a senior or older adult in Canada (Special Senate Committee on Aging, 2009). Having said that, the author of this chapter questions whether 65 years of age serves a useful purpose today, given the changing nature and diversity of the baby boom generation. Research evidence would support the claim that chronological age by itself is not a good proxy for predicting either aging progress or decline, or understanding this age group (Martin et al., 2010). Baby boomers themselves argue that turning 65 years of age does not alter their lives. In fact, those 65 years and older may vary as much as 30 to 40 years in age from one another, creating subcategories of seniors similar to those of the World Health Organization (WHO). These categories include the young-old (65 to 74 years) who for the most part are healthy and fit, the middle-old (75 to 84 years) who may have less financial and other resources and are beginning to experience a slow down, and the old-old (85 years and older) who may be labeled "frail" and characterized as having special social and physical needs (Murray, Zctncr, Pengman, & Pengman, 2006). This division of the older adult into chronological subdivisions, while an important improvement over the categorization of all adults over 65 years as one homogenous group, has the persistent disadvantage of creating negative stereotypes and age biases that we see played out in the healthcare system. Again we go back to our example of the Greers who would not fit into the label of "frail," so frequently assigned to the old-old group by health professionals.

In recent years, nurses, particularly those in the field of gerontological nursing, have been concerned about the tendency of health professionals, policy advisors, and others to essentialize older adults around chronological age rather than work to understand the important differences and distinctions among members of birth cohorts. Differences exist in terms of health status, lifestyles, income, independence, mobility, place of residence, relationships, etc. All of these factors impact perceived health, quality of life, and the need for health services.

Ethnicity

Canada's older population differs from previous generations in terms of its ethnicity and cultural makeup. Recent changes in immigration patterns across Canada have created a richer repertoire of peoples from Asia, Africa, and the Middle East, in addition to traditional migrants from continental Europe and the United Kingdom. Aboriginal elders are also growing in numbers and are expected to triple in population by 2016 from their numbers in 1996. It is well known that culture has important implications as a determinant of health. The result is diversity in terms of language, cultural beliefs, values, and religious identities, all of which are important reference points for individuals seeking healthcare and support services. These differences impact the health needs and demands of the ethno-culturally diverse minority groups for service and present unique challenges for achieving healthy aging. In particular, the premature aging and death of Aboriginal peoples represent a challenge to healthy aging.

A demographic profile of the senior population sheds additional light on the diversity of older adults and the context within which decisions about healthy aging are made. Canada's population is aging quickly as the first of the baby boomer generation turned 65 in 2011. This trend will continue over the next three decades. By the year 2015, Canadians aged 65 and over will be more numerous than children under 15 years of age. In 2009 there were 4.7 million Canadians over the age of 65, but by 2031, there will be approximately 9 million over 65 years, and they will account for 25% of the total population. This will be almost double the current proportion of 13.9% (Statistics Canada, 2005, 2010).

Gender

Gender differences are also present in Canada's aging population with the percentage of female seniors outnumbering male seniors. As a group, women in Canada tend to live an average of 4 years longer than men, and they now represent 60% of the senior population. This proportionate increase in women with advancing age is referred to as the "feminization of later life" (DiBartolo, 2008). Most seniors are married and with the tendency for women to live longer and marry men older than themselves. Approximately one third of older Canadians are widowed, with more likely to be women (40%) than men (14%). Living arrangements reflect this difference with 47% of women living with a spouse, versus 78% of men (Public Health Agency of Canada [PHAC], 2009). In summation, seniors differ tremendously in terms of marital status, geographical residence, age, income, social support, lifestyles, personal circumstances, etc. Because seniors differ so much in terms of these factors, they differ in their needs. The challenge is how to promote healthy aging and provide appropriate services to meet the diverse needs of this population through the widest range of options.

Health Issues

Health status is the final area examined in discussing diversity in aging. Contrary to popular opinion, the majority of older Canadians, like Alice and Andrew Greer, are living their later years in good health. Most Canadians over 65 years of age rate their health as good to excellent on self-reported measures of health status despite the increasing prevalence of chronic disease (Park, 2011). Although the incidence of chronic illness has increased in recent decades, the prevalence of disability resulting from it has declined. This is due in part to improved socioeconomic conditions, advances in treatments, technology, environmental designs, and support systems that help maintain independence. This latter trend has given rise to several new phenomena such as co-morbidity, compression of morbidity, and compression of disability. Co-morbidity refers to the high rate of co-occurrence of multiple chronic conditions in older adults. Compression of disability is the tendency for disability to be compressed into a shorter time span at the end of life (McPherson & Wister, 2008), and similarly compression of morbidity refers to the tendency for the onset of disease to occur toward the end of life (Segall & Fries, 2011). While different terms may appear in the literature to describe health status of older adults, the goal is consistent, namely to improve their quality of life and lessen the burden of chronic illness, so that older adults can enjoy more years without serious disability or restrictions of their activities of daily living. The majority of older adults have one chronic condition, and 33% (like Alice Greer) have three or more conditions such as arthritis, cardiac disease, hypertension, cataracts, etc. (Gilmore & Parks, 2006; PHAC, 2009; Schellenberg & Turcott, 2007).

One of the greatest health challenges facing an aging population is that of dementia. Currently there is no cure for dementia. It affects 8% of seniors over 65 years, and a range of 25% to 50% of those over 80 years of age. Without any intervention, it is anticipated that the current incidence of 500,000 older adults with this condition will increase to 1.1 million and affect 2.8% of all Canadians by 2038. There will be a 10-time increase in long-term care requirements and the direct and indirect cost to society over the next 30 years will be $872 billion (ASC, 2010). Dementia is an increasingly important health issue of the older adult for two reasons. First, age is a primary risk factor for dementia, so one can assume that the incidence of dementia will increase as the population ages, if no action is taken to prevent it. Second, the preference of older people to "age in place of choice" has translated into most people with dementia continuing to live in their own homes, and in community settings with the support of informal, often unpaid caregivers (Chappell et al., 2008; Ploeg et al., 2009). These caregivers often struggle with their own chronic health conditions, depression, and sense of isolation that comes with caring for cognitively impaired adults. Many caregivers themselves are elderly and experience significant burdens in their lives. Hence, dementia exerts as a double-barrel effect in older adults. The national voice for people living with dementia is the Alzheimer Society of Canada. It has called for a pan-Canadian response to address the impending dementia epidemic that will improve care at every level of the disease. Healthy aging is an important component of the strategy to prevent and manage dementia. See the website for the Alzheimer Society as a resource for more information.

In summary, there is a need to focus now on preventing and controlling co-morbidities and the consequences of chronic illness in older adults. One way to improve their quality of life is to prevent the onset of chronic conditions and minimize exacerbations through healthy aging strategies (Pangman & Pangman, 2010). This brief profile of diversity in older adults suggests that investment in healthy aging is a prudent strategy. Healthy aging strategies can delay and minimize chronic illness and disability in later life, consequently reducing long-term care needs and healthcare costs (WHO, 2005; PHAC, 2009). Experts believe the healthcare costs of an aging population can be managed through prevention or delay of chronic illness until later life. An anticipated outcome of this approach is that people will live longer in good health, and use fewer resources. It is anticipated that future cohorts will do so as well. This brings us to a discussion of the question, what is healthy aging?

HEALTHY AGING

The nursing profession embraces a holistic view of health as a positive resource for everyday living that includes attention to the physical, mental, social, and spiritual well-being of the individual (WHO, 2005). In relation to the older adult, it implies the importance of maximizing physical health, having a purpose in life, meaningful communication with others, and opportunities to maintain dignity and contribute meaningfully to society. As such, nurses believe that a system of care that promotes the health of Canadians as they age requires a holistic understanding of health with programs that focus as much on the promotion of mental health and social well-being as on physical health status (PHAC, 2009). Given this holistic understanding of health, healthy aging is defined as "a lifelong process of optimizing opportunities for improving and preserving health and physical, social and mental wellness, independence, quality of life and enhancing successful life-course transitions" (Health Canada, 2002). This definition is not new. It is over 10 years since Health Canada published this perspective, and indeed variants of it have been reported in the literature dating back over half a century (Dunn, 1958); yet, its enactment in today's healthcare system remains illusive.

To achieve healthy aging requires a reorientation of the system with direct attention paid to the promotion of healthy aging in addition to other health-related activities, so that older adults like Alice and Andrew Greer can live healthier lives. The PHAC (2009) proposed a new vision for healthy aging that values the contributions of seniors, celebrates diversity, and reduces inequities. It calls for age-friendly environments and resources that enable seniors to make healthy choices to enhance their independence and quality of life. This vision acknowledges the contributions of the broad determinants of health to healthy aging (health and social services, income and social status, social support networks, education, employment and working conditions, physical environment, social environment, biology and genetics, personal health practices, coping skills, and healthy development). In particular, it embraces action in five key areas, namely, the need to be socially connected as one grows older, the need to stay physically active, the value of healthy eating, the prevention of falls and injuries, and the avoidance of risky behaviors such as smoking. These five foci have been selected for action based on their demonstrated impact on seniors' health. They are not meant to diminish the contributions of the other determinants of health to healthy aging.

Three mechanisms are proposed to achieve this vision of healthy aging. They include:

1. Supportive environments referring to policies, services, and programs that enable healthy aging in places where older adults live, work, worship, etc.;
2. Mutual aid, which refers to actions people take to support each other emotionally and physically and their sharing of ideas, resources, and experiences;
3. Self-care, which includes choices and actions individuals take in the interest of their own health.

This vision of healthy aging builds on key national and international documents on healthy aging and health promotion (PHAC, 2009; BCMH, 2005). The implementation of this vision will not happen without informed political action on the part of nurses and others. It will require commitment from key stakeholders including all levels of government who can develop policy to support the healthy aging framework. Nongovernmental agencies can work in partnership with others including older adults and their families to advocate and support healthy aging programs and facilities. While the power to implement this vision does not rest primarily with nurses, nurses can contribute to its enactment through delivering quality care under current regulatory and organizational conditions and by working with their professional organizations, other professional groups, and key stakeholders to lobby for resources necessary to enact the vision.

Despite reports in the literature about the value of healthy aging, the Canadian healthcare system continues, in 2011, to focus on cure rather than on promotion of healthy aging and disease prevention. A focus on the latter is needed to help all Canadians and, in particular, older adults such as Alice and Andrew Greer to achieve healthy aging. It may well become a major means of managing current and future health system pressures. An analysis of this conundrum requires that we ponder questions such as: Who dictates what is important in healthcare for older adults? Who decides who is important in healthcare? What is the dominant discourse around healthcare decisions for the elderly? We can begin to explore these questions by examining some of the historical, political, economic, and gender influences on the provision of healthcare to our aging population. This will move us past the notion that older adults such as Alice and Andrew Greer will bankrupt the healthcare system. Unfortunately the rhetoric supporting this belief is much stronger than the evidence (Canadian Health Services Research Foundation [CHSRF], 2011).

Historical Understanding

A historical analysis ponders questions such as: Under what conditions did the current situation originate? What has contributed to the evolution of the issue over time? What factors have influenced the position that people have taken on the issue? The meaning of healthy aging, the situation of being older, and the extent to which older people are valued and supported in later years have varied as a function of the time in which people have lived (McPherson & Wister, 2008). In the past, both religious and secular movements influenced society's views on aging. For example, ancient Hebrews viewed long life as a blessing and Puritans thought the process of aging was a sacred pilgrimage to God (Ebersole et al., 2008; Segall & Fries, 2011). Before the industrial revolution, older adults were considered a valuable source of knowledge and elders held influential positions in social, political, and religious circles. With the arrival of the industrial revolution, the elderly lost power and status. Social changes emerging from this period of modernization included a break up of the extended family, a separation of work and home, a dependency on nonfamily employers for economic security, and a rapid growth in new knowledge that replaced the tacit knowledge held by older adults. This situation led to a decline in status of older people as they no longer played essential roles.

During the early to mid-1900s a biomedical approach dominated society's thinking of the elderly. This approach has been criticized for "over-medicalizing" people and viewing aging as a disease process. It perpetuates the idea that health status is caused by physiological and biological systems (Lange, 2012; McPherson & Weister, 2008). The medicalization of the study of aging continues to influence the public view of the older adult and the perpetuation of the negative images of aging—that later life is a time of disability, decline, and dependence.

The arrival of the baby boom generation and their ascendance to senior status beginning in 2011 marked a changing shift in attitudes toward aging. The pendulum is slowly moving again toward more positive views with an expectation by baby boomers to engage in healthy aging as they move through their senior years. In the second millennium, advances in the gerontology field have weakened the influence of the biomedical view of aging, which inevitably had been understood through the distorted lens of disease. It is now perceived as a complex but normal process with biological, psychological, social, and spiritual aspects that impact how individuals age. Yet, much remains to be understood about normal aging. Care of older adults continues to be influenced by longstanding negative attitudes held by some health professionals, and society continues to associate being old with disease, disability, and decline. A historical analysis reveals how these persistent patterns of erroneously attributing undesirable characteristics and disease patterns to normal aging have influenced healthcare decisions for this age group. Interrupting this discourse is important to the delivery of holistic care for older adults and the achievement of the vision of healthy aging now and into the foreseeable future.

Political Understanding

A political analysis ponders the relationship between power and knowledge, and the location of influence within the particular issue. When differing beliefs enter into decision making, politics will help determine what is discussed and decided. Powerful beliefs or ideologies shape the way we understand the world and the way we come to see our actions based on these beliefs as normal (McIntyre & McDonald, 2010). In relation to healthy aging, decisions are influenced by multiple stakeholders with competing values and interests such as health administrators, government, physicians, nurses, and older adults themselves. Assumptions have been made by the privileged in healthcare that aging inevitably accompanies a decline in health. This has led to the adoption of a disease management approach to care rather than a health promotion approach that embraces healthy aging. The result is that health issues of the older adult have been falsely managed as acute medical problems, rather than persistent life challenges that call for continuous attention to health promotion (Canadian Association on Gerontology [CAG], 2011). These powerful ideologies that value cure and acute care over older people and health promotion and prevention need to be interrupted. Nurses can use their knowledge of gerontology to challenge ideologies resulting from ageism and the medicalization of aging. Enlightened nurses can lead the way in facilitating a critical attitude shift that will be required to reframe the concept of healthy aging. It is unlikely that other groups such as healthcare administrators or physicians, who are threatened by radical reform of the acute care and hospital system and who stand to benefit from the status quo, will lead the way. The pendulum is slowly moving toward positive support for healthy aging as accurate information about the difference between aging and disease emerges.

Economic Understanding

Questions of economics, cost effectiveness, and efficiencies play a role in understanding the issue of healthy aging for seniors. Common beliefs to be challenged are those such as the aging population is to blame for uncontrollable healthcare costs and the needs of the baby boomers will bankrupt the health system. The curiously persistent myth that the aging population, by itself, is a major contributor to the increase in demand for healthcare, and thus total health spending, needs to be dispelled. The CHSRF, in 2002 and again in 2011, provided evidence contrary to these views. They showed convincingly that although healthcare costs will rise as baby boomers age and access more services, the impact of this increase will be modest in comparison to that of other cost drivers such as technological innovation and drug costs (CHSRF, 2011). Other researchers have reported similar results and conclude that growth in healthcare costs due to population aging will be about 1% per year between 2010 and 2036 (McKenzie & Rachlis, 2010). This evidence begs the question, whose interests are driving healthcare costs and who is profiting?

When economic discourse frames an issue, nurses are often caught in the tension between limited resources to respond to the needs of the older adult for appropriate care. This point is made powerfully in Chapter 17 by drawing on the work of Ceci (2006) who cautions that economic discourse has the capacity to limit other ways of understanding practice. The majority of healthcare dollars in Canada continue to be spent in acute care and in the hospital sector. We know we need to change this scenario in order to invest where it counts for the elderly.

To invest in healthy aging, changes will be required in policy, care delivery, and health promotion and disease prevention. The need to invest more in services that make sense for the older adult and disinvest in others is critical. A move away from acute episodic care for the elderly to integrated continuing care delivery can produce cost savings and improve the quality of care, but it will require significant investment to support a stronger continuing care sector and an investment in the education and recruitment of caregivers to meet the needs of older adults. The good news is that there is no need to be gloomy about the coming of an aging society. The problems expected to arise from population aging can be managed with strategic changes to care delivery for the older adult. It is the other cost drivers such as technological innovations and drug costs that require attention.

In summation, the language of markets that is efficiency, effectiveness, and individual autonomy is often used in discussing healthcare for older adults. This language reflects a neoliberal paradigm that places responsibility for healthy aging with the individual, shifting responsibility away from government. Canada's universal public healthcare system was designed to ensure that the healthcare needs of all Canadians, including the older adult, would not be sacrificed for the benefit of the powerful and wealthy. While individuals do bear significant responsibility for decisions and actions that impact healthy aging, government must be prepared to invest in healthy aging, including health promotion, disease prevention, and home, community, and long-term care so that universality and the values of the Canadian healthcare system are protected for all Canadians. The need for a pan-Canadian investment in healthy aging is paramount.

Feminist Understanding

A feminist understanding of aging issues in healthcare (and in particular of healthy aging) questions how the notion of gender has influenced older adults as clients, and their relationship with others in the healthcare system. It considers how traditional structures based on gender divisions of power have shaped health issues. This perspective would argue that aging has been conceptualized by the medical model that reinforces patriarchy and privileges the expertise of physicians over others. In this way aging has been viewed through the lens of disease, and later life has been characterized as a time of diminished capacity to perform important roles in the society. Negative images of aging endure and ageism continues to spread.

From a feminist perspective, healthy aging is a women's issue because so many more women survive into old age than do men and they face significant challenges as they age. Women live longer, often alone, and face more poverty than their male counterparts. Structural inequalities create different life chances for them. These structural inequalities include pay disparity, caregiving responsibilities, longer life expectancy, and women's work patterns, all of which reduce pension earnings and personal savings (Moody, 2010).

The shift from institutional to community and home care settings for seniors is based on assumptions about families in which women are expected to be caregivers, most of them unpaid and volunteer. From a feminist perspective, caregiving for the older adult became politicized in the 1990s when a new vision of health reform and a redefined model of home care emerged. This model focused on short-term, post-acute care rather than long-term care for older adults, and recognition of informal caregivers (mainly women) was imbedded in the new model. The distinction between informal and family care, on the one hand, and community care on the other, was not made and this has proven problematic. The lack of distinction continues to be troublesome with the new discourse around "aging in place." The distinction is critical because if it is assumed that community care is equivalent to family care, an increased burden is placed on informal caregivers, most of whom are women. Women willingly assume this burden at great personal cost.

Community care calls for resources to build infrastructure such as homemaking services, transportation services for appointments, and community support groups. It includes opportunities for older adults to engage in socially meaningful ways and it calls for attention to health promotion, disease prevention, and building the formal community system of care. Presently, the resources are not present to do this although the current discourse assumes informal caregivers, the majority of whom are women, will fill this void.

BARRIERS TO HEALTHY AGING

An important strategy for moving the vision of healthy aging forward is to identify barriers that impede its progress. Ageism is a major barrier to implementation of the healthy aging agenda. It is a socially constructed way of thinking about and acting toward older adults. It includes any attitude, action, or institutional structure that infers older people are inferior to those who are younger, and results in negative stereotypes and prejudicial beliefs about older adults (Lange, 2012; Morgan & Kunkel, 2011; Murray et al., 2006). It is subtle, but pervasive in society, and is reflected in many stakeholders' underlying beliefs about the older adult. It is defined as discrimination against individuals solely on the basis of chronological age.

Ageism is common in all societies but especially in North America where dominant cultural beliefs perceive the individual as an autonomous agent, youth are venerated, and people are valued on the basis of their economic worth. This is in contrast to cultures where for example, interdependence is valued over independence, and the Confucian precept that children should respect and support their parents is in vogue (Miller, 2012). Ageism may be self-adopted or covert, manifesting itself at the level of the individual and at the level of the institution. The former influences our thinking and behavior, and the latter our legislation and public policies with both leading to inequalities across society for the elderly.

As a barrier, ageism is a prevalent form of exclusion that can impact achievement of healthy aging and increase the older adult's sense of vulnerability. Exclusion disenfranchises the older adult and perpetuates isolation, which negatively impacts quality of life, participation in lifestyle behaviors that affect health, and one's overall sense of health status (PHAC, 2009). Numerous age-related stereotypes are pervasive in society such as older adults are socially incompetent, lonely, in poor health, frail, dependent, and economic and familial burdens. These views influence older adults' sense of self and can discourage older adults from participating in activities that are integral to healthy aging.

Negative images and stereotypes of the elderly influence how others perceive them, and can shape public policy about the older adult. For example, ageist beliefs can influence which public health programs get funded and which do not and they can negatively impact the potential of adults as they move through their senior years. The media, in particular, can contribute to the phenomenon of a self-fulfilling prophecy whereby older adults begin to think and act the way they are portrayed in media and in socially constructed stereotypes. As a result, this can lead to a loss of self-esteem and to older adults withdrawing from participation in healthy practices such as exercise and social gatherings, delaying treatment for health problems, and labeling themselves as old.

In brief, ageism and negative attitudes toward the older adult lead to suboptimal care for the older adult. At best, older adults will not experience the benefits of engaging in healthy aging strategies, and at worst, they will experience unnecessary decline (Morgan & Kunkel, 2011; Segall & Fries, 2011). The vision of healthy aging is an ideal based on a holistic view of the older adult as a complex biological, psychological, social, and spiritual being. This view is congruent with the view of the person described in nursing theories, but it is in opposition to the views of other professionals that are focused more narrowly on physical health and functioning. Strategies for resolution will need to consider these conflicting perspectives.

A second barrier to achieving the vision of healthy aging is the competition between the interests of the acute care and the long-term care sector for resources and their different visions of how best to deliver services to older adults. The 1980s witnessed a movement across Canada to provide care for the elderly in integrated care delivery systems that included home care, home support, community services, residential care and acute care (Special Senate Committee on Aging, 2009). Different visions of how best to deliver care services to the elderly emerged. Home care was envisioned as part of a broader integrated system of care, often referred to as continuing care that would form the third largest component of Canada's healthcare system after hospital care and medical services. However, the cost-cutting efforts of the 1990s redefined this model, and in particular, the home care component became focused on short-term, post-acute replacement home care provided by professionals. The current federal policy as noted in the Romanow Commission and the Kirby Report has again redefined home care with an emphasis on short-term post-acute replacement home care. This misguided shift in focus signals a lack of understanding of the needs of the older adult to achieve healthy aging. It isolates home care from continuing care services, and increases the likelihood that long-term care for seniors, who suffer more from chronic illness than acute diseases, will be provided by for-profit interests (Hollander et al., 2007; Morgan & Kunkel, 2011). This current policy focus may ultimately serve to disenfranchise the elderly from care they need over the longer term, and reduce the home support that allows them to remain independent longer and achieve healthy aging.

A third barrier to the achievement of healthy aging is limited access to human resources with the appropriate knowledge and expertise to promote healthy aging. In particular, inadequate staffing levels, and inappropriate mix and preparation of professional and nonprofessional care providers to meet the needs of an aging population, interfere with the achievement of healthy aging and the provision of appropriate services to this population. The need for a holistic assessment of the complex needs of the elderly requires a high level of understanding of this age group, and knowledge and insight into the needs of this special population; yet, too often care providers with minimal levels of preparation and education are primarily assigned to this group. This paradox is pervasive in all sectors of health and social care.

Pressures are particularly acute for professional caregivers such as registered nurses, gerontologists, and social workers (Special Senate Committee on Aging, 2009). Recruitment into these areas is weak and supply is much less than the demand due in part to ageist beliefs and the negative image of this clinical practice area. A lack of qualified faculty with the necessary level of gerontological expertise contributes to the problem, as does an insufficient number of gerontological education programs or core courses in this content area in education programs. In addition, the traditional manner of educating health professionals by disciplinary models is no longer appropriate. Healthy aging consists of biological, psychological, social, and spiritual dimensions calling for a change in the way that we educate care providers so that they have the necessary knowledge and skills to provide holistic care to this population.

In addition, healthy aging is not just about preventing illness but also about meeting the needs of people in their homes and in their communities through a continuum of nonprofessional paid and nonpaid home care workers and support service providers. In many situations informal care providers provide the majority of care to seniors, yet their needs are rarely considered. There are no standardized qualifications or training requirements for these caregivers. This lack of a national human resource strategy and training standards for this sector is a barrier to the provision of quality care for seniors.

STRATEGIES FOR RESOLUTION

The final section of this chapter focuses on possibilities for addressing barriers to healthy aging and the provision of appropriate services for older adults. A variety of short-and long-term strategies are necessary to achieve healthy aging. It is obvious that participation by multiple stakeholders including government at various levels, health authorities, health professional groups, family and community members, and older adults themselves will be necessary to achieve healthy aging. A full discussion, however, is beyond the scope of this chapter. This section is limited to those strategies in which nursing can play an important role. Some strategies involve individual actions by nurses, whereas others require collective action by nurses working with their professional organizations, unions, government and nongovernment organizations, and other interest groups. Given the complexity of issues surrounding healthy aging, and the multiple ways of understanding them, nurses have an important opportunity to contribute to change both in societal attitudes toward the older adult and in care provided.

As caregivers and educators, nurses can provide accurate information about aging to clients, family members, government officials, and the public that will overcome the myths, misperceptions, and taken-for-granted views of aging. Through education attitudes can be changed. This begins with recognition of the effects of ageism and an examination by nurses of their own attitudes toward the older adult. Knowledge is a powerful instrument for addressing ageism and the negative attitudes that interfere with holistic care of the older adult. Nurses can challenge assumptions about the older adult and provide evidence that contradicts these unexamined ageist views.

Older adults themselves need accurate information about normal aging and knowledge of programs and supports to promote healthy aging so that they do not fall prey to a self-fulfilling prophecy based on negative stereotypes. Nurses are in ideal positions to provide this information and empower older adults to implement strategies directed toward improved health, functioning, and quality of life. Through their daily encounters with older adults, nurses have opportunities to teach them about healthy aging, as well as opportunities to learn from adults to whom they are providing care. Examples include family practice nurses working with chronic disease management and prevention, community health nurses offering fall prevention programs or smoking cessation initiatives, school nurses working with children and youth to promote intergenerational partnerships and communication with elders in classroom settings, or gerontological nurses overseeing care in long-term care settings (Canadian Nurses Association [CNA], 2008).

A major focus of a healthy aging approach is addressing the body–mind–spirit connectedness of each older adult as a unique, valued, and respected individual (Miller, 2012; Roach, 1997). While this approach is challenging especially for adults with multiple chronic illnesses, it is an achievable ideal to which nursing strives. Even in the midst of serious challenges, nurses can implement interventions with older adults to promote healthy aging. Nurses can challenge ageist attitudes including their own; assess each older person from a holistic perspective; recognize their potential for improved health and functioning, as well as psychological and spiritual growth (Miller, 2012).

As educators, nurses can campaign for inclusion of gerontological content in undergraduate and graduate programs. In particular, they can call for integration of core content on healthy aging into the curriculum early in nursing programs so that students embrace the concept of healthy aging and develop positive attitudes toward the older adult. As healthy aging consists of biological, psychological, social, and spiritual dimensions, it calls for a change in the way that we educate nurses and other care providers so that they have the necessary knowledge and skills to provide holistic care to this population. Nurses can advocate with other disciplines and professional associations for interprofessional education on healthy aging aimed at improving the quality of life for this population. Nurses can accomplish this by working with their national organizations such as the Canadian Association of University Schools of Nursing (CASN) and other accrediting agencies to include in their accreditation standards and criteria the requirement for interdisciplinary components about aging as core aspects of professional programs to improve the ability of nurses and other professionals to deliver age-appropriate services to this population.

As a collective, nurses can spearhead lobbying efforts to address disparities in service provision and problems with access to appropriate care for healthy aging. They can work through their professional organizations with government representatives to call for a renewed emphasis on long-term care and home support services with a rebalancing of long- and short-term home care and home support services. These should be universally accessible through our publicly funded healthcare system. This approach would restore and enhance services to the older adult, thereby reducing or delaying their need for institutional care and enabling older adults to age in their place of choice with appropriate support services.

Finally, nurses can promote wellness for caregivers and those who provide care to older adults. They can teach caregivers about strategies to promote health and functioning of the older adult, as well as strategies to improve their own quality of life. Collectively, nurses can work with different sectors and levels of government to have family caregivers formally recognized as part of the care team in long-term home care. Their needs should be assessed jointly with those of the older adult and integrated into the policy and delivery of healthcare services. This strategy would allow family members to continue to provide care to their loved ones, and allow older adults to remain in their homes, which is the "place of choice" for most, as long as possible. According to Hollander et al. (2007), this strategy has the potential to stop the current trend of increasing demands on informal caregivers, provide appropriate services that will assist informal caregivers in their role, and begin the possibility of a comprehensive cost-effective approach to meeting the needs of Canada's aging population.

SUMMARY

This chapter explored issues in healthcare for an aging population with a particular focus on the vision of healthy aging. Factors impacting the issue of healthy aging were examined from a historical, economic, political, and feminist perspective, making visible the complexity of the issue. A number of barriers to and strategies for resolution of the issue were explored. While the power to implement the vision of healthy aging does not rest exclusively with nurses, the chapter disrupts the notion that promotion of healthy aging will happen without informed political action on the part of nurses. This chapter challenges nurses to use their expert knowledge and regulatory power collectively and individually, to advocate for this new vision of healthy aging. Nurses are challenged to work with their professional and regulatory bodies, as well as other groups and key stakeholders including all levels of government, to implement strategies identified in the chapter. In doing so, nurses will contribute to shaping healthcare in a manner that is responsive to the needs of older adults. Our ability to successfully resolve this issue will ultimately affect the lives of all Canadians as we strive to build a better, more inclusive society.

Add to your knowledge of this issue:	
Alzheimer Society	www.alzheimer.ca
Canadian Association On Gerontology	www.cagacg.ca
Building on Values: The Future of Health Care in Canada. Final Report	http://www.cbc.ca
Canadian Coalition for Seniors Mental Health	http://www.ccsmh.ca
Canadian Women's Health Network	http://www.cwhn.ca
Canadian Gerontological Nurses Association	http://www.cgna.net
Public Health Agency of Canada	http://www.phac-aspc.gc.ca
Special Senate Committee on Aging	http://www.parl.gc.ca
Statistics Canada	http://www.statcan.gc.ca
The Health of Canadians-The Federal Role	http://www.parl.gc.ca

Online

REFLECTIONS *on the Chapter...*

1 Do you believe age is an appropriate criterion for framing public policy around health issues of older adults?

2 What impact will the baby boomers have on the Canadian healthcare system now and in years to come?

3 Are older adults more similar or more different when it comes to health issues?

4 How should decisions around allocation of health resources be made for older adults? Who should decide?

5 What assumptions are made about women as caregivers of older adults?
6 What role can nursing play in advancing a vision of healthy aging for older adults in Canada?

Want to know more? Visit the Point for additional helpful resources:

- Journal Articles
- Learning Objectives
- Nursing Professional Roles and Responsibilities
- Bonus chapters:
  - Health and Nursing Policy: A Matter of Politics, Power and Professionalism
  - The NP Movement: Recurring Issues
  - When Difference Matters: The Politics of Privilege and Marginality

References

Alzheimer Society of Canada. (2010). *Rising tide: The impact of dementia on Canadian society.* Toronto: Author. Retrieved from www.alzheimer.ca

B.C. Ministry of Health. (2005). *Healthy aging through healthy living: Towards a comprehensive policy and planning framework for seniors in B.C.: A discussion paper.* British Columbia Ministry of Health Population Health and Wellness Division. Retrieved from www.healthservices.gov.bc.ca

Canadian Association on Gerontology. (2011). *Policy statement: Health promotion for individual seniors.* Retrieved from http://www.cagacg.ca

Canadian Health Services Research Foundation (CHSRF). (2011). *Mythbusters: Using evidence to debunk common misconceptions in Canadian health care.* Retrieved from http://www.chsrf.ca

Canadian Nurses Association. (2008). CAN leads dialogue on healthy aging. *Canadian Nurse, 104*(6), 22.

Ceci, C. (2006). Impoverishment of practice: Analysis of effects of economic discourses in home care case management practice. *Canadian Journal of Nursing Leadership, 19*(1), 56–67.

Chappell, N., McDonald, L., & Stones, M. (2008). *Aging in contemporary Canada* (2nd ed.). Toronto, ON: Pearson-Prentice Hall.

Chappell, N.L. *About Canada: Aging and the Canadian population.* (2010). Retrieved from http://www.mta.ca/canada/aging/index.htm

Christenson, K., Doblhammer, G., Rau, R., & Vaupel, J.W. (2009). Aging populations: The challenges ahead. *Lancet, 374*(9696), 1196–1208.

DiBartolo, M. (2008). The demographic tidal wave: Are we ready? *Journal of Gerontological Nursing, 34*(4), 3–4.

Dunn, H. (1958). Significance of levels of wellness in aging. *Geriatrics, 13*(1), 51–57.

Ebersole, P., Hess, P., Touhy, T., Jett, K., & Schmidt Luggen, A. (2008). *Toward healthy aging. Human needs and nursing response* (7th ed.). St. Louis, MI: Mosby.

Gilmore, H., & Park, J. (2006). Dependency, chronic conditions and pain in seniors. *Health Reports Supplement.* Statistics Canada, Catalogue 82-003, 8, 33–45.

Health Canada. (2002). Division of Aging and Seniors. Dare to Age Well: Workshop on Healthy Aging. Ottawa: Government of Canada.

Hollander, M., Chappell, M., Prince, M., & Shapiro, E. (2007). Providing care and support for an aging population: Briefing notes on key policy issues. *Healthcare Quarterly, 10*(3), 34–45.

Lange, J.W. (2012). *The nurse's role in promoting optimal health of older adults: Thriving in the wisdom years.* Philadelphia, PA: F.A. Davis.

MacKenzie, H., & Rachlis, M. (2010). *The Sustainability of Medicare. Canadian Federation of Nurses Unions.* Retrieved from http://www.nursesunions.ca

Martin, L., Schoeni, R., & Andreski, P. (2010). Trends in health of older adults in the United States: Past, present, future. *Demography, 47*(suppl), S17–S40.

McIntyre, M., & McDonald, C. (2010). *Realities of Canadian nursing: Professional, practice and power issues* (3rd ed.). Philadelphia, PA: Lippincott, Williams & Wilkins.

McPherson, B., & Wister, A. (2008). *Aging as a social process: Canadian perspectives.* Toronto, ON: Oxford University Press.

Miller, C. (2012). *Nursing for wellness in older adults* (6th ed.). Philadelphia, PA: Lippincott, Williams & Wilkins.

Moody, H. (2010). *Aging: Concepts and controversies* (6th ed.). Thousand Oaks, CA: Pine Forge Press.

Morgan, L.A., & Kunkel, S.R. (2011). *Aging society and the life course* (4th ed.). New York: Springer.

Murray, R., Zenter, J., Pangman, V., & Pangman, C. (2006). *Health promotion strategies through the life span (Canadian edition).* Toronto, ON: Pearson Education Canada.

Pangman, V., & Pangman, C. (2010). *Nursing leadership from a Canadian perspective.* Philadelphia, PA: Lippincott, Williams & Wilkins.

Park, J. (2011). Retirement, health and employment among those 55 plus. Perspectives on Labour and Income. *Spring.* Statistics Canada, Catalogue. 75-001-XIE, *23*(1).

Ploeg, J., Denton, M., Tindale, J., et al. (2009). Older adults' awareness of community health and support services for dementia care. *Canadian Journal on Aging, 28*(4), 359–370.

Public Health Agency of Canada. (2009). *A guide to support the development of a comprehensive system of support to promote active aging.* Retrieved from http://www.phac-aspc.gc.ca/seniors-aines/publications/public/healthy

Roach, S. (1997). *Caring from the heart.* Mahwah, NJ: Paulist Press.

Schellenberg, G., & Turcott, M. (2007). *A portrait of seniors in Canada 2006.* Ottawa, ON: Statistics Canada. Catalogue no. 89-519-XIE.

Segall, A., & Fries, C. (2011). *Pursuing health and wellness: Healthy societies, healthy people.* Toronto, ON: Oxford University Press.

Special Senate Committee on Aging. (2009). *Canada's aging population: Seizing the opportunity (Final Report).* Ottawa, ON: Author. Retrieved from www.senate-senat.ca/age.asp

Statistics Canada. (2005). *Population Projections for Canada, Provinces, and Territories, 2005 to 2031.* Catalogue no. 91-520-XIE. Ottawa, ON: Author.

———. (2010). Seniors. Retrieved from http://www.statcan.gc.ca/pub/11-402-x/2010000/chap/seniors-aines/se

WHO. (2005). *Preventing Chronic Disease: A Vital Investment.* Geneva: Author.

23 Orientating to Difference: Beyond Heteronormative Sexualities

Carol McDonald

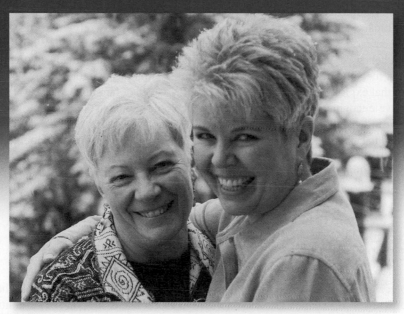

Societal changes call attention to long-standing heteronormative stereotypes in health care. This couple celebrates the legalization of their marriage in 2005, having lived together for years previously. (Used with permission of Photographer Bonny Johannson.)

Critical Questions

As a way of engaging with the ideas In this chapter, consider the following:

1. How would you describe your current knowledge of nonheterosexual people?

2. What do you imagine might be the issues for nonheterosexual people in the healthcare system?

3. How do you understand the difference between sexual orientation and gender identity?

Chapter Objectives

After completing this chapter, you will be able to:

1. Identify relevant issues for nonheterosexual people.

2. Understand the idea of the social construction of the categories of sexual orientation.

3. Describe the impact of medical discourses and classification for nonheterosexual people.

4. Understand the complexity of disclosure for gay, lesbian, bisexual, two-spirited, and transgendered (GLBTT) people.

5. Identify barriers to reducing assumptions and practices based on **heteronormativity**.

6. Articulate strategies to lessen stigmatization and discrimination.

This chapter presents the opportunity for you to consider the ways we have historically thought about ideas of sexuality in society, how ideas are changing, and the ways in which both historical and newer understandings influence nursing practice. Knowledge of different interpretations of sexualities and genders opens possibilities for us to provide health care informed by the realities of people's lived experience. As we delve into the knowledge of sexuality and gender, we are required, I would suggest, to question the assumptions that we hold about these topics. To have this conversation about sexuality, beyond what is commonly seen as the norm of heterosexuality and the binary genders of woman and man, we will necessarily rely on the use of categories. To draw on categories in our conversation is at once useful and problematic. While the use of categories or labels gives us language to talk about differences, we simultaneously run the risk of essentializing, meaning that we would view all people within the category as the same. In a previous chapter that explores difference as a feature of the world of nursing, Ceci (2009) reminds us, "As nurses we encounter people in their most vulnerable moments and so have the opportunity to cause harm by unthinking adherence to the false and damaging beliefs and assumptions often contained in categories and labels" (p. 358). And so while categories and labels are used as a way of understanding differences, it is always more important to see the gender and sexual identity of people as individually constituted; in other words, each person's life is formed through a particular set of experiences, and the meanings of those experiences are decided by the individual.

BEYOND HETERONORMATIVE SEXUALITIES: ARTICULATING THE TOPIC FOR NURSING

One place to enter this conversation is to establish a shared understanding of what is meant, for the purposes of this chapter, as heteronormative and nonheteronormative sexualities. In this process I would also hope to disrupt or to challenge the dual notion of sexual orientation as heterosexual and homosexual and the limited binary understandings of genders as woman and man and, instead, consider plural possibilities for the ways in which sexuality and gender are experienced and expressed (Box 23.1).

Sexuality Beyond the Binary

Sexuality is described by Health Canada as a "central aspect of being human throughout life and encompasses biological sex, gender identities and roles, **sexual orientation**, eroticism, pleasure, intimacy and reproduction" (Public Health Agency of Canada [PHAC], 2007). This description helps us to think of sexuality in a holistic way when we consider individuals of any sexual orientation. Consequently, while your sexual orientation may indicate the gender of the person you are sexually attracted to (object of desire), it is also intertwined with many other important aspects of your self and of the ways you relate to others in the world. Experiences of sexuality cannot be thought of as the same for all people who name themselves heterosexual, lesbian, bisexual, or gay. Some people who currently name themselves gay or lesbian may have, or have had, previous relationships with someone of the opposite sex. People who name themselves heterosexual may also engage in sexual behavior with someone of the same sex. There are people who name themselves heterosexual, gay, lesbian, or bisexual who are celibate (McDonald, 2009a, 2009b; McDonald, 2010). However, in the face of these multiple expressions and experiences of sexuality, the overwhelmingly dominant interpretation of sexuality in Canada is of heterosexuality, signifying the sexual and intimate relationships between women and men. The assumption of heterosexual relationships as representative of all sexuality underlies the idea of heteronormativity, the belief that all people are or wish to be in sexual and intimate relationships with a person of the opposite sex or gender. Oppressive action that privileges heterosexual people and positions

BOX 23.1   Glossary of Terms

This list describes the way some terms are used in the context of this chapter. They should not be taken as absolute definitions of the words.

- **Gender identity**—One's sense of oneself as feminine or masculine, commonly associated with categories of woman, man, or transgender.
- **Heteronormativity**—The assumption of heterosexual relationships as representative of all sexuality underlies the idea of heteronormativity; the belief that all people are or wish to be in sexual and intimate relationships with a person of the opposite sex or gender.
- **Heterosexism**—Oppressive action that privileges heterosexual people and positions nonheterosexual people in a position of "other."
- **Homophobia**—The irrational fear or hatred of, or aversion to, or discrimination against anyone who is not heterosexual.
- **Internalized homophobia**—When a nonheterosexual person accepts society's stereotypes and negative labels and internalizes them. The person is not always consciously aware of internalized homophobia.
- **Intersexed people**—People who have physical bodies outside the relatively narrow chromosomal, endocrinal, genital, and other physiological ranges associated with male or female. People may be born intersexed or become intersexed as a result of a medical intervention.
- **Queer**—An umbrella term used by people identifying with sexual minorities and/or non-traditional genders. "Queer" has been re-claimed by the LGBT community having previously been a derogatory term used against LGBT people.
- **Sexual Orientation**—The capacity to develop intimate emotional and sexual relationships with people of the same gender (lesbian or gay), the opposite gender (heterosexual), or either gender (bisexual). As these categories are limited, it is sometimes more useful to talk about nonheterosexual as the sexual orientation. In addition, some nonheterosexual people have reclaimed the word queer to identify their orientation as an inclusive term for all nonheterosexual people. Sexual orientation is distinct from gender and gender identity.
- **Transgender**—People whose sense of their gender (woman or man) is not congruent with the sexual characteristics of their physical body (female or male). People sometimes choose to transition to another gender while others opt to remain in the "gender-flux."

nonheterosexual people in a position of "other" is understood as **heterosexism** (Gray et al., 1996; Irwin, 2007). An important consideration for this chapter is that experiences of discrimination against GLBTT people continue to exist in contemporary society, both within and beyond the healthcare setting (Chinn, 2008; Irwin, 2007; McDonald, 2006; McDonald, 2008; Morgan & Stevens, 2008; Stevens, 1995; Stevens & Hall, 1988).

Gender Beyond the Binary

As I have discussed in Chapter 15 of this text, gender can be understood as the individual experience of femininity and masculinity in addition to the *expression* of that inner experience. While there is undoubtedly a relationship between biological sex and gender, we can consider gender as distinct from the biological sex of a person and as constructed through experiences of an individual in the social, physical, and discursive context of a life. The discursive contexts are the discourses we hear, full of assumptions about the "appropriateness" or "correctness" of particular ideas and expressions of gender. These discourses are, of course, reflective of the dominant values and beliefs at a particular time in a culture, and are by no means universal "truths." Beginning very early in our lives we each heard stories that conveyed to us what it meant to be a girl or a boy in our family and cultural setting. Throughout our lifetime we continue to receive messages from the media, popular culture, and many diverse sources depicting gender identities and gender expression. For the most part, the gender identities that are foregrounded in society are expressions of the binary categories of woman and man.

In reflecting on this dualistic or binary construction of gender, Butler (1990) suggests, "there is nothing about a binary gendered system that is given" (p. 282). Rather, we have come to rely on this association of gender with biological sex that supports the dominance of heterosexual reproduction. If, however, we move beyond this biologically driven system, "there is space to recognize the realities of people's lives that do not fit in the polarized and constructed categories. One example of people living beyond the binary understanding of gender is those who would name themselves transgendered" (McDonald, 2010). As we begin to move beyond the historical binary system of gender, the use of categories and labels becomes even less reliable. The label of **transgender** for instance, can mean different things to different people who take on the label. One common understanding of transgender suggests that it represents people whose sense of their gender (woman or man) is not congruent with the sexual characteristics of their physical body (female or male). Drawing on research conversations with transgender people, Morgan and Stevens (2008) caution us about the complexity of transgender people's experiences suggesting that we should not simply assume people are "in the wrong body" (p. 585). While some transgender people are interested in aligning their physical bodies or presentation more closely with their sense of their gender through surgical, endocrine, or cosmetic actions, other people live in the gender flux, avoiding the reinstatement (or compliance to) the historical gender dualism.

A couple of hypothetical examples might help to clarify: Jake was born as a biological female but self-identifies his gender as a man. He is in the process of transitioning to a male through the use of hormone therapy and plans to have a double mastectomy and chest reconstruction surgery. Kim was also born as a biological female but does not associate with the **gender identity** of "woman." Kim identifies with "trans" as gender, avoids aligning with either woman or man as a category, avoids the use of a gendered pronoun, such as "he" or "she," and presents with an androgynous appearance. It is, of course, beyond the scope of this chapter to explore the many possibilities of gender expression. A final thought for this section is a reminder that gender identity and sexual orientation are separate from one another. This reminder encourages us to avoid heterosexist assumptions with people of all genders and appearances; there is every possibility, for example, that a person who transitions from a feminine to a masculine gender is intimately and sexually attracted to men.

An additional idea worthy of discussion is the use of the term queer, as a signifier of gender and/or sexuality that does not fit into traditional categories. The term **queer** was reclaimed by the GLBTT community late in the 20th centrury, having previously been used as a derogatory term against GLBTT people. While for some "queer" is used as an umbrella term for sexual minorities (Cairns & Yoon, 2011), it has the additional advantage of being free from association with either of the traditional binary gender categories. In this way a queer identity frees one from identifying as either man or woman, while implying a non-traditional sexual orientation.

ARTICULATING THE TOPIC AS AN ISSUE

The preceding conversation is a useful way of establishing a shared understanding of the topics of sexual orientation and gender. The topic itself, however, is not an issue. The issue to be unpacked (systematically explored) in this chapter is that of heterosexism, in the healthcare setting and beyond, and the deleterious effects of such social conditions to health (Box 23.2).

BOX 23.2   Sexuality in the Healthcare System

"The health of a nation, physically and emotionally, can only be as good as the health of its most vulnerable and stigmatized citizens. While culture, class and religion are known to affect how illness may appear and be understood, sexual orientation has been less well researched or understood as a mediator of health and illness."

Source: Forstein, M. (2003). Introduction in A. Peterkin & C. Risdon (Eds.), *Caring for lesbian and gay people: A clinical guide.* Toronto, ON: University of Toronto Press.

The dominance of heteronormativity, in addition to the presence of actions fueled by systemic and individual heterosexism, is becoming increasingly well documented in the nursing literature (Chinn, 2008; Irwin, 2007; McDonald, 2008, 2009b; McDonald et al., 2011; Morgan & Stevens, 2008; Stevens, 1995; Stevens & Hall, 1988). While we might hope that individual acts of discrimination against nonheterosexual people are decreasing, literature suggests that full acceptance of nonheterosexual people varies considerably according to context and location. I would suggest that the assumptions of heteronormativity are so deeply entrenched in society, including in healthcare settings, that even when we intellectually accept the realities of GLBTT people, we continue to practice based on an assumption of heteronormativity. Systemic heteronormativity is reflected in the language and depictions used to convey sexuality, gender, and family life on forms, posters, and pamphlets in healthcare settings, in the textbooks of nursing education, and in the way we structure our conversations with clients, families, and one another.

The second important consideration in framing this topic as an issue is the idea that the social conditions of a person's life influence the experience of health and illness. In particular, Wilkinson and Marmot (2003) remind us that the World Health Organization states, "continuing anxiety, insecurity, low self-esteem, social isolation and lack of control over work and home life have powerful effects on health" (p. 12). We should specifically note that social exclusion resulting from "discrimination and stigmatization" has an injurious effect on health (p. 16). The Gay and Lesbian Medical Association (GLMA) put forth the following view: "Many avoid or delay care or receive inappropriate or inferior care, because of perceived or real homophobia, biphobia, transphobia and discrimination by healthcare providers and institutions" (retrieved July 20, 2008 from www.glma.org).

Given this knowledge, how might we influence the practice of nurses and other healthcare providers, which is underpinned by unconscious and unquestioned assumptions of heteronormativity and actions depicting heterosexism?

ANALYZING THE ISSUE: WAYS OF UNDERSTANDING

An analysis of the issue surrounding heteronormativity and heterosexism in health care begins with a historical analysis, raising questions for consideration in relation to the origin and evolution of the issue. Significantly for this chapter, a historical approach to analysis opens to questioning our taken-for-granted understanding of the issue, rather than simply recounting events as they have been recorded.

An ethical and legal analysis of the issue looks at the influence of Canadian law and the sections within the "Code of Ethics for Registered Nurses" (Canadian Nurses Association [CNA], 2008) that directly address gender and sexual orientation. The social and cultural analysis of the issue looks at the influence of language and culture on understandings of nonheterosexual orientations. Political analysis explores the relationship between knowledge and power. In the political analysis of nonheterosexual orientations, questions of disclosure, whom to tell and when, are raised and explored. Lastly, the issue will be viewed from a critical feminist perspective through which we question the value attached to particular sexual orientations and question the role of institutional power in our lives.

Understanding the Issue Historically

Have you ever wondered if there were lesbians around when your grandmother was a child? Do you imagine that the early immigrant settlers to Canada were all paired up in heterosexual relationships? How might people in same-sex relationships have been thought of in the early 1900s, or were they thought about at all?

It is fascinating for me to think of how much has changed for nonheterosexual people in my lifetime; as a young woman in the process of naming myself as gay in the 1970s I would never have imagined that I would one day legally marry a woman. Nor could I have imagined that my grandchildren would grow up in a society in which same-sex marriage would be a reality since before their birth. This reminder of recent history shows the way in which history is not just an account of events, but a view into the way categories and realities are shaped and remembered. Looking back on the accounts of intimate relationships, while holding in our awareness the recent changes for nonheterosexual people, the actual construction of what we currently accept as the categories of sexual orientations and genders come into focus. This look at historical evolution is not intended as a history lesson in dates but rather as an opportunity to think about the discourses and commonly held beliefs of society that influence and shape the way things come to be known or accepted.

Foucault (1990) in his book, *The History of Sexuality,* suggests that the very idea of sexualities came into language in the 19th century, shaped as they were by the efforts of institutionalized religion and the early practice of medicine, with the intention to persuade people to disclose or to confess the details of their intimate activities. As Foucault tells us, "sex was driven out of hiding…to lead a discursive existence" (p. 33). The medicalization of sexuality continued through the 19th and 20th centuries. In a medical practice that created a category of people, names long forgotten to us, such as "auto-monosexualists," were attached to nonheterosexual people. Through the influence of medical classification a category of people was constructed.

This categorical naming of a group of people is different, of course, from another historical reality that intimate practices and relationships have taken place between people of the same gender, likely for centuries. The names and the meanings of categories of sexual orientation have changed over time. The process, however, of the medical categorization and classification of people continued until late in the 20th century.

Nonheterosexual people have suffered from the medicalization of their health, including the pathologization of their relationships, and the oppressive experience of "curative" conversion therapies (Blackwell, 2008; Stevens & Hall, 1991). The medical construction of nonheterosexual people as psychopathological propagated and legitimated stereotypes of GLBTT people that fueled much of the discrimination against them. Under increasing pressure from the gay liberation movement and its supporters with new research findings, in 1973 the American Psychiatric Society removed homosexuality per se from the list of disorders in the *Diagnostic and Statistical Manual of Mental Disorders* (American Medical Association [AMA], 2002). What is less known, however, is that a number of related "disorders," including ego-dystonic homosexuality, remained in this influential medical text until as late as 1987.

As you begin your professional nursing practice in 2013 or beyond, the contents of a medical text published in 1987 might seem irrelevant or even obscure to you. Nonetheless, I would ask you to consider that many nurses you will encounter in practice, and an even larger number of citizens, were indoctrinated in the 20th century with the belief that homosexuality was pathological. Given the dominance of medical discourses in western society, it is in some ways remarkable that the ethical, legal, and social fabric of our society has changed as much as it has over the past three decades.

Ethical and Legal Understandings

Perhaps the Canadian law concerning the issues for nonheterosexual people that you are most familiar with is the national legalization of same-sex marriage in July 2005. This legislation followed several years of controversial activism and resistance, between and among individuals, political and religious organizations, and the provinces and territories, making Canada the fourth country in the world in which people of the same sex or gender can marry. And while this momentous legislation is changing the legal and social landscape of the country, at least one earlier piece of legislation can be seen as similarly notable. Any guesses what this socially relevant legislation might be? Perhaps you have heard the much quoted 1969 words of Pierre Elliot

> ### BOX 23.3   Promoting Justice
>
> Nurses uphold principles of justice by safeguarding human rights, equity, and fairness and by promoting the public good.
>
> #### Ethical Responsibilities:
>
> 1. When providing care, nurses do not discriminate on the basis of a person's race, ethnicity, culture, political and spiritual beliefs, social or marital status, **gender, sexual orientation**, age, health status, place of origin, lifestyle, mental or physical ability or socio-economic status or any other attribute. (Emphasis added).
> 2. Nurses refrain from judging, labeling, demeaning, stigmatizing, and humiliating behaviors toward persons receiving care, other healthcare professionals, and each other.
> 3. Nurses do not engage in any form of lying, punishment, or torture or any form of unusual treatment or action that is inhumane or degrading. They refuse to be complicit in such behaviors. They intervene, and they report such behaviors.
> 4. Nurses make fair decisions about the allocation of resources under their control based on the needs of persons, groups, or communities to whom they are providing care. They advocate for fair treatment and for fair distribution of resources for those in their care.
> 5. Nurses support a climate of trust that sponsors openness, encourages questioning the status quo, and supports those who speak out to address concerns in good faith (e.g., whistle-blowing).

Source: Canadian Nurses Association. (2008). *Code of ethics for registered nurses (2008 centennial edition)*. Retrieved from www.cna-nurses.ca

Trudeau, Justice Minister at the time in the liberal federal government: "There's no place for the state in the bedrooms of the nation." The government had just instituted sweeping changes in Canada's criminal law, which included decriminalizing homosexuality. Prior to that time, homosexuality was a criminal offence in Canada, which could result in long prison terms. Trudeau, speaking for the government stated: "It's bringing the laws of the land up to contemporary society I think. Take this thing on homosexuality. I think the view we take here is that there's no place for the state in the bedrooms of the nation. I think that what's done in private between adults doesn't concern the Criminal Code" (Makarenko, 2007).

While these legal advances have had both immediate and long-term influences on the people of Canada, I want to be clear to not conflate legal discourses with social acceptance. This distinction in part lies with the differences between legalization and socialization. Some people recognize same-sex marriage as an acknowledgment of equal rights for nonheterosexual people (Lannutti, 2005). On the other hand, real acceptance cannot be legally mandated—discrimination and prejudice are still lived realities for many GLBTT people. And further, there are many people who identify as nonheterosexual for whom marriage is not part of their reality, so we have to be careful not to view the legalization of marriage as evidence that the issues complicating the lives of nonheterosexual people have been resolved.

This complexity raises the question of where do we as nurses look for direction to mediate the tensions of the social and legal realities in this changing landscape? In the recent release of the "2008 Code of Ethics for Registered Nurses," section F: Promoting Justice clearly outlines the ethical responsibilities for practicing nurses (Box 23.3). As you might well know, codes of ethics are written to speak broadly to a profession; it is, however, up to each nurse to live this ethic as they work to understand difference.

Social and Cultural Understandings

As members of society, nurses and other healthcare professionals internalize the dominant discourses of the larger society. That said, nurses are, of course, not a homogenous group, but a very diverse group of people who are themselves influenced by their ethnic and cultural beliefs. It is these assumptions and beliefs that shape our intentional and unintended interactions with nonheterosexual people.

BOX 23.4   Reducing Heteronormative Bias

Language that reduces heteronormative bias includes questions such as:

Are you in a relationship or partnership?
Who is that you are with, and how do you define your relationship?
Who do you consider your immediate family?
Over your lifetime have your sexual partners been women, men, or both?
How would you like your partner or family to be involved in your care?

Source: McDonald, C. (2010). Sexuality and sexual practices. In B. Kozier, G. Erb, A. Berman, et al. (Eds.), *Fundamentals of Canadian nursing: Concepts, process, and practice* (2nd ed.). Toronto, ON: Pearson Education Canada.

I would suggest that we are not only talking about *other* people belonging to nonheterosexual orientation, we are talking about ourselves—nurses, physicians, and other healthcare professionals who may identify as nonheterosexual. In an article speaking to the stigmatization of gay and lesbian nurses, Chinn (2008) suggests "we will not realize our full potential as nurses, nor the full potential of our discipline as long as we allow the stigma of lesbian or gay identity to prevail within our own profession" (p. 552).

The language of the healthcare system, as we have touched on earlier, is based on the social norms of heterosexuality. The language is both based on and reinscribes, or reinforces, assumptions about the way things are in the world. These assumptions include the taken-for-granted assumptions of what constitutes a family, who might be a partner, and the gender of parents. Nonheterosexual people talk about the importance of seeing the realities of their own lives and relationships reflected in their environment (McDonald, 2006). It is difficult to know how to respond on a form in which your own reality is not reflected; further, it is difficult to have confidence in a system in which one is excluded by language. This exclusion extends to charts, admission forms, bathroom door signage, and even the so-called "innocent" inquiries or conversations (Box 23.4).

Understanding the Political Nature of the Issue

A political analysis explores the relationship between knowledge and power in a situation. We might think of a person's gender or sexual orientation to be personal knowledge, although increasingly this is knowledge that comes into the public domain. The holder of knowledge that is perceived of as personal and controversial is seen to hold, along with that knowledge, a component of power.

The idea of telling yourself or others of a nonheterosexual orientation has come to be known as "coming out." And, while coming out can be thought of as a one-time event in life, the action of disclosure of sexual orientation or of a transgender reality is an ongoing, repetitive experience. Every time GLBTT people meet someone new or encounter someone from their distant past, a decision is made of whether or not to disclose their current orientation. In everyday conversations with strangers, interviews with potential employers, and encounters with colleagues and healthcare providers, GLBTT people must decide how much to disclose about their lives (McDonald, 2006). These decisions are not only about what we might call "sex lives"; they are about sharing what they did on the weekend and with whom, the people who are important in their lives, and who they consider family.

And so how do people make decisions to disclose and how might we support people in these decisions? It's important to know that GLBTT people disclose for many different reasons. Although a considerable focus in the mental health literature associates disclosure with improved self-esteem, emotional health, and improved relationships (Jordan & Deluty, 1998; Morrow, 1996; Radonsky & Borders, 1995; Taylor, 1999), more recent studies suggest that each decision of disclosure must be made in the context of the lived life of the person disclosing (McDonald, 2006, 2008). That is to say that given the continued reality of discrimination and the heterosexual assumptions that influence safety, employment, and housing, the risks of disclosure must always be considered. Some people advocate disclosure as a political action that would disrupt taken-for-granted heteronormativity and, in a sense, reclaim our personal power (Chinn, 2008). "There is a belief that heteronormativity would topple and discrimination against homosexuals would plummet if people discovered that their mother/teacher/sister/friend/neighbour/professor/aunt/roommate/minister was a lesbian" (McDonald, 2006). Nonetheless, I would encourage you to keep in mind that disclosure is never unequivocally the right thing to do, and that the decision for disclosure always rests with the individual. As healthcare providers, we often have privileged access to personal knowledge of individual lives; with this privilege and power comes an obligation to understand the potential consequences of unintended disclosure.

Critical Feminist Understandings

To engage in a feminist critique of the issue, several important ideas come to mind. The first is the conflation that is often made between feminism and sexual orientation (lesbianism), often by people who value neither. To suggest that feminist thought, based on a body of knowledge, and what it means to be lesbian are interchangeable, is to undermine the possibilities for understanding both. Not only are there many feminists who are heterosexual, there are likely proportionally more lesbians who do not subscribe to feminist ideas. Indeed, confusing these two groups raises the question: Whose purpose is being served by this conflation?

A second point of feminist analysis brings to awareness the invisible power that institutional structures and hierarchies hold over nonheterosexual people. For example, accomplished nurse theorist Peggy Chinn relates an incident in which she was "advised by my chairperson that it would be prudent of me not to discuss openly the fact that I am a lesbian" (Chinn, 2008, p. 551). "Even in an academic community where the prevailing ethic is freedom of expression" nonheterosexual people can be silenced and manipulated to conform to heterosexual assumptions (p. 552). A feminist analysis asks, "Is expert power given authority over personal power and the right to be the subject of one's life?" Reflecting on the influence of the historical construction of categories and the power that medical discourses and institutional structures have exerted over nonheterosexual people, I would suggest that the answer is a resounding "yes!" In other words, heterosexism and heteronormativity in the healthcare system and beyond rob people of the right and the opportunity to be the subject of their own lives.

BARRIERS TO RESOLUTION

Given what you have read so far, can you imagine what some of the barriers are to the resolution of discrimination based on heterosexism and heteronormativity? Identifying these potential barriers is an important step in the process toward resolution of the issues.

1. There is a lack of visibility of the everyday life of nonheterosexual people in health care and in society generally.
2. Stigmatization reduces the safety for people in vulnerable positions to disclose nonheterosexual orientation.
3. A failure exists to understand all sexual orientations from a holistic view.
4. There is an absence of the knowledge needed about the lives of nonheterosexual people to provide professional care in the curricula of healthcare providers.
5. This lack of knowledge leads to decisions about the provision of care being based on assumptions that derive from heteronormativity and fuel heterosexism.

6. The dominant language of heteronormativity in the healthcare system does not reflect the realities of nonheterosexual people.
7. Outdated assumptions of the pathologization and medicalization of homosexuality remain present in health care.
8. The legalization of homosexuality is conflated with social acceptance of nonheterosexual relationships and lives.
9. There is continued reliance on the binary of genders (woman and man) and sexuality (heterosexual and homosexual).

STRATEGIES FOR RESOLUTION

"We cannot 'fix' the larger societal stigma associated with being GLBTT but we can make a commitment to address the internalized oppression of **homophobia** that affects us all. If for no other reason, our societal mandate to care for those who are sick, regardless of who they are, demands that we know, understand, and overcome the barriers of social stigma that affect health and well being" (Chinn, 2008, p. 552).

1. Position statements by professional organizations on gender and sexual diversity have the potential to positively inform and influence their membership. See Box 23.5 for an example.

BOX 23.5   Policy Statement on Sexual Diversity and Gender Identity—2002

1. **Sexual Diversity in Society**
   1.1 Homosexuality is defined as the sexual and emotional attraction to members of the same sex, and has existed in most societies for as long as sexual beliefs and practices have been recorded. The proportion of the population that is not exclusively heterosexual has been estimated at between 8% and 11%.
   1.2 Societal attitudes toward homosexuality have had a decisive impact on the extent to which individuals have been able to express their sexual orientation. In 1973 the American Psychiatric Association removed homosexuality from the *Diagnostic and Statistical Manual of Mental Disorders*. Subsequently, homosexuality was recognized as a form of sexual orientation or expression rather than a mental illness.
   1.3 Strong family connections are important to the health and well-being of individuals, and recently there has been greater recognition of the diversity of family structures that exist in our society. These family structures could include nuclear families, single parents, blended families from remarriages, as well as gay and lesbian parents.
2. **Discrimination**
   2.1 The term "heterosexism" has been used to describe the discrimination against gay, lesbian, bisexual, transgender, and intersex (GLBTI) populations. Heterosexism encompasses the belief that all people are and should be heterosexual and that alternative sexualities pose a threat to society. In this way heterosexism includes homophobia, a fear of alternative sexualities, and transphobia, a fear of alternative gender identities. It may also include a fear of intersex people who do not fit neatly into the binary categories of male and female.
   2.2 Discrimination may be overt as in verbal abuse and physical violence or as covert as the silence that surrounds talking about GLBTI issues. This affects all members of society as individuals comply with gender role stereotypes in order to avoid homophobic discrimination. It is a constraint on human behavior that serves to diminish individual potential for development as well as diversity in our community.
   2.3 The common experience of discrimination means that the health of GLBTI populations differs from that of the general population. For GLBTI individuals the impact of this discrimination can lead to a poorer general health status, diminished utilization of healthcare facilities, and a decreased quality of health services.

Source: Australian Medical Association. (2002). *Policy statement on sexual diversity and gender identity*. Retrieved from www.ama.com.au

2. Include knowledge regarding the everyday lives of nonheterosexual people in curriculum, faculty, and staff development in institutions, such as hospitals and universities, where outdated assumptions influence what is informing curriculum development and healthcare practice.
3. People in authority have the obligation to initiate policy reform including changes in the language used in forms and signage.
4. All nurses have the obligation and the opportunity to create social and relational space for the realities of nonheterosexual people.
5. Because of the impact of heterosexism on the health of nonheterosexual people, nurses have the obligation, wherever possible, to influence public policy related to the provision of safe and dignified care, access to employment, and housing.

SUMMARY

In this chapter we have explored and analyzed some of the issues facing people of nonheterosexual orientation. In particular, the assumption of heteronormativity and discrimination fueled by heterosexism has been discussed. The key notions in this chapter include the social and historical construction of categories of sexuality and the reality that many healthcare professionals are unwittingly complicit in heterosexism through practices based on inaccurate and outdated assumptions.

Unlike some issues, which require involvement from governments and authorities to make significant change, nurses in everyday practice can influence the issues faced by nonheterosexual people. By questioning our assumptions and being willing to examine our language and practices, nurses can reduce the dominance of heterosexism in the healthcare systems. Nursing students and new graduate nurses are perhaps in the best position to educate and mentor others, to question the historical assumptions that continue to be prevalent in educational and healthcare institutions.

Add to your knowledge of this issue:		
Gay and Lesbian Medical Association (GLMA)	**www.glma.org**	*Online*
Rainbow health Ontario about LGBT health	**www.rainbowhealthontario.ca**	
Parents and friends and lesbians and gays (PFLAG)	**www.pflag.org**	

REFLECTIONS on the Chapter...

1 How has the information you have read in this chapter affirmed or challenged the assumptions that you held prior to reading it?

2 Given what has been discussed in this chapter, what knowledge do you believe healthcare providers need to provide safe and dignified care to nonheterosexual people?

3 Explore the index in the back of at least three of your nursing textbooks, looking for information on transgender, gay, lesbian, or bisexual people. Does the nonheterosexual content in the text disrupt or reinscribe the idea of heteronormativity?

4 What other readings or resources have assisted you in understanding this issue?
5 After reading the chapter "Creating a Welcoming Clinical Environment" in *Guidelines for Care of Lesbian, Gay, Bisexual and Transgender Patients* at www.glma.org, assess your practice environment for its welcome of GLBTT people.
6 Referring to the same guidelines, how would you assess your school as a welcoming environment for GLBTT people?

Want to know more? Visit thePoint for additional helpful resources:

• Journal Articles
• Learning Objectives
• Nursing Professional Roles and Responsibilities
• Bonus chapters:
  ◦ Health and Nursing Policy: A Matter of Politics, Power and Professionalism
  ◦ The NP Movement: Recurring Issues
  ◦ When Difference Matters: The Politics of Privilege and Marginality

References

Australian Medical Association. (2002). *Policy statement on sexual diversity and gender identity.* Retrieved from www.ama.com.au

Blackwell, C. (2008). Nursing implications in the application of conversion therapies on gay, lesbian, bisexual, transgender clients. *Issues in Mental Health Nursing, 29*(6), 651–665.

Butler, J. (1990). Performative acts and gender constitution: An essay in phenomenology and feminist theory. In S. Case (Ed.), *Performing feminisms: Feminist critical theory and theatre* (pp. 270–282). Baltimore, MD: John Hopkins University Press.

Cairns, J., & Yoon, J. (2011). How to support LGBTTIAQQ students in the classroom. *Multiplicity: A biannual newsletter from the adviser to the provost on equity and diversity.* Victoria, VA: University of Victoria.

Canadian Nurses Association. (2008). *Code of ethics for registered nurses* (2008 centennial edition.) Retrieved from www.cna-nurses.ca

Ceci, C. (2009). When difference matters: The politics of privilege and marginality. In M. McIntyre & C. McDonald (Eds.), *Realities of Canadian nursing: Professional, practice, and power issues* (3rd ed.). Philadelphia, PA: Lippincott Williams & Wilkins.

Chinn, P. (2008). Lesbian nurses: What's the big deal? *Issues in Mental Health Nursing, 29*(6), 551–554.

Forstein, M. (2003). Introduction in A. Peterkin & C. Risdon (Eds.), *Caring for lesbian and gay people: A clinical guide.* Toronto, ON: University of Toronto Press.

Foucault, M. (1990). *The history of sexuality: An introduction.* New York: Vintage.

Gay and Lesbian Medical Association (GLMA) www.glma.org

Gray, P., Kramer, M., Minick, P., McGehee, L., Thomas, D., & Greiner, D. (1996). Heterosexism in nursing. *Journal of Nursing Education, 35*(5), 204–210.

Irwin, L. (2007). Homophobia and heterosexism: Implications for nursing and nursing practice. *Australian Journal of Advanced Nursing, 25*(1), 70–76.

Jordan, K., & Deluty, R. (1998). Coming out for lesbian women: Its relation to anxiety, positive affectivity, selfesteem, and social support. *Journal of Homosexuality, 35*(2), 41–63.

Lannutti, B. (2005). For better or for worse: Exploring the meanings of same-sex marriage within the lesbian, gay, bisexual and transgendered community. *Journal of Social and Personal Relationships, 22*(5), 5–18.

Makarenko, J. (2007). *Same-sex marriage in Canada.* Retrieved from www.mapleleafweb.com/features/same sex marriage

McDonald, C. (2008). Unpacking disclosure: Interrupting unquestioned practices. *Issues in Mental Health Nursing, 29*(6), 639–649.

———. (2009a). Issues of gender and power: The significance attributed to nurses work. In M. McIntyre & C. McDonald (Eds.), *Realities of Canadian nursing: Professional, practice, and power issues.* Philadelphia, PA: Lippincott Williams & Wilkins.

———. (2009b). Lesbian disclosure: Disrupting the taken for granted. *Canadian Journal of Nursing Research, 41*(1), 261–275.

———. (2010). Sexuality and sexual practices. In B. Kozier, G. Erb, A. Berman, et al. (Eds.), *Fundamentals of Canadian nursing: Concepts, process, and practice* (2nd ed.). Toronto, ON: Pearson Education Canada.

McDonald, C., McIntyre, M., & Merryfeather, L. (2011). Bringing ourselves into view: Disclosure as epistemological and ontological production of lesbian subject. *Nursing Inquiry, 18*(1), 50–54.

Morgan, S., & Stevens, P. (2008). Transgender identity development as represented by a group of female to male transgendered adults. *Issues in Mental Health Nursing, 29*(6), 585–599.

Morrow, D. (1996). Coming out for adult lesbians: A group intervention. *Social Work, 41*(6), 647–656.

Public Health Agency of Canada. (2007). Retrieved from www.phac-aspc.gc/publicat/cgshe-ldnemss/cashe

Radonsky, V., & Borders, L. (1995). Factors influencing lesbians direct disclosure of their sexual orientation. *Journal of Gay and Lesbian Psychotherapy, 2*(1), 49–63.

Stevens, P. (1995). Structural and interpersonal impact of homosexual assumptions on lesbian health care clients. *Nursing Research, 44*(1), 25–30.

Stevens, P., & Hall, J. (1988). Stigma, health beliefs and experiences with health care in lesbian women. *Image: Journal of Nursing Scholarship, 20*(2), 69–73.

——— (1991). A critical historical analysis of the medical construction of lesbianism. *International Journal of Health Services, 21*(2), 291–307.

Taylor, B. (1999). Coming out as a life transition: Homosexual identity formation and its implications for health care practice. *Journal of Advanced Nursing, 30*(2), 520–525.

Wilkinson, R., & Marmot, M. (Eds.). (2003). *Social determinants of health: The solid facts* (2nd ed.). Copenhagen: World Health Organization. Retrieved from http://www.euro.who.int/__data/assets/pdf_file/0005/98438/e81384.pdf

24 Environmental Health and Nursing

Andrea Monteiro, Carol McDonald, and Marjorie McIntyre

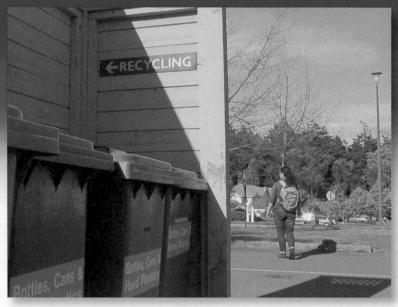

Recycling depot established at university family housing supports environmental health.
(Used with permission. Photographer Vitoria Monteiro.)

Critical Questions

As a way of engaging with the ideas in this chapter, consider the following:

1. What assumptions do you hold about the role of professional nurses in environmental health?

2. What knowledge would you need as a nurse to make a significant contribution to environmental health?

3. How might you account for the scarcity of knowledge in nursing curricula to support this area of nursing practice?

4. Given what you have read in earlier chapters, what contribution would you anticipate that professional organizations would play in creating healthy environments?

Chapter Objectives

After completing this chapter, you will be able to:

1. Identify some common environmental health hazards in your geographic region.

2. Examine the nursing profession's impact in addressing environmental issues.

3. Generate ideas about how individual nurses can affect issues of environmental health.

4. Evaluate how nursing curricula integrate health and the environment.

This we know…the earth does not belong to man, man belongs to the earth. All things are connected, like blood which connects one family. Whatever befalls the earth befalls the children of the earth. Man did not weave the web of life; he is merely a strand in it. Whatever he does to the web, he does to himself.
—*Chief Seattle, 1854 Suqwamish and Duwamish*

In a world that is increasingly affected by globalization and global warming, humans are as closely linked to the health of their environments as they were at the dawn of human history. Environmental hazards, the health of the earth, and the health of the earth's inhabitants are inseparable. The interdependence of all species on the earth and the physical environment cannot be overemphasized.

Although this chapter does not focus on the conservation of natural resources, it does underscore how environmental hazards contribute to adverse health outcomes for humans. We hope that readers will examine the regions and communities where they live and work to gain awareness of the connection between their own environments and the health of the people who live there. The need to be aware of how environmental hazards impact human health is important for nurses regardless of their practice settings—community, long-term, acute institutional care, or occupational health. Tragedies, such as the deaths from *Escherichia coli (E. coli),* bacteria resulting from contaminated water sources in Walkerton, Ontario (Ahluwalia, 2000), raise concerns for other communities about the possibility of similar events in their own neighborhoods.

There is no doubt that human health is affected when the environment or ecosystem is damaged (Canadian Nurses Association [CNA], 2008b, 2005). The term *environmental health,* as used in this chapter, refers to freedom from illness related to exposure to environmental contamination, hazards, and toxins that are detrimental to health. In the discussions that follow, the term *environment* includes the physical, social, political, legal, psychological, and cognitive environments of individuals, families, and communities. As scientific knowledge increases and social and political values change, the definition of, and factors related to, environmental health will also change. And further, "as our knowledge progresses about the etiology of disease, evidence of environmental contributions to disease also grows, particularly the environmental link to a number of chronic diseases" (CNA, 2005, p. 1). The disciplinary concepts of person, environment, health, and nursing, which form the metaparadigm of nursing, underscore the interdependence of the environment and health but a perusal of nursing curricula and textbooks uncovered a lack of focus on issues related to environmental health.

In 2005, the CNA developed a background paper titled, "The Ecosystem, the Natural Environment, and Health and Nursing: A Summary of the Issues," in which they made central the following issue: "The natural environment has a significant impact on our quality of life, our health and the sustainability of our planet. Increasing population, urbanization and industrialization…affect the quality of air we breathe, the water we drink and the food we eat" (p. 1). The World Health Organization [WHO] (2007) reminds us "to a large extent, public health depends on safe drinking water, sufficient food, secure shelter, and good social conditions. A changing climate is likely to affect all of these conditions." As part of the Centennial Celebrations (2008e), the CNA launched a project to support work in environmental health for nursing education, practice, research, and policy development. A group of nurses from across the country, the Environmental Health Reference Group, have guided and developed this impressive project. This group since has expanded to become the CNA emerging group: Canadian Nurses for Health and the Environment. In times of such pressing need for leadership in environmental health, in all sectors of society, this group of nurses has brought much needed attention to environmental issues. Their work includes a background paper, educational module, and video presentation on each critical area of environmental health, namely: Environmental health principles, greening the health system, and climate change. This information can be readily accessed through the CNA website. (See online resources at the end of this chapter.)

HISTORICAL LINKS BETWEEN ENVIRONMENT AND HEALTH

The effect that a healthy or, conversely, an unhealthy, environment has on human health is not a recent discovery. Early civilizations were aware of the impact of the environment on health. The Minoans (3000 to 1430 BCE), Mycenaeans (1430 to 1150 BCE), and Romans (509 BCE to 476 CE) all built extensive drainage and water systems, as well as baths and toilets (McGuire & Eigsti-Gerber, 1999) in response to related environmental health hazards of pestilence and disease. Early Hebrew writings included a code on hygiene, and the ancient Egyptians (3100 BCE to 600 CE) developed safe water and sewer systems. As civilizations rose and fell, this knowledge and the systems that had been developed were often forgotten or destroyed.

Plagues resulting from contamination of water sources and the spread of disease through animal vectors have been documented throughout history. Through the introduction of public health measures, such as providing a clean source of drinking water and disposing safely of sewage and other wastes, great improvements were made in the health of populations; these key elements remain as important as ever (Clark, 1999; McDevitt & Wilbur, 2002).

However, a major turning point in history, was the Industrial Revolution that began in Great Britain in the early 1700s and spread to Europe and North America. Industrialization resulted in a shift from what had been a rural, agricultural economy to one that was urban and factory-based with concomitant problems of pollution from large steel foundries and the burning of fossil fuels. The impact of the Industrial Revolution extended far beyond the production of goods and material to changes in governments, the use of resources in the world, material benefits for some of the world's population, and wars and exploitation of many populations. Modern transportation and communication, the globalization of markets, and the even more rapid destruction of habitats are evident today (Malcom et al., 2002). Nurses have been integral participants in examining and changing some of the harmful environmental conditions to improve public health.

In *Notes on Nursing,* Florence Nightingale (1860, p. 5) observed that environmental factors had a key impact on health and disease:

> In watching diseases, both in private homes and in public hospitals, the thing which strikes the experienced observer most forcibly is this, that the symptoms or the sufferings generally considered to be inevitable and incident to the disease are very often not symptoms of the disease at all, but of something quite different—of the want of fresh air, or of cleanliness, or of punctuality and care in the administration of diet, of each or of all of these.

Further, Nightingale (1860) noted that there were "five essential points in securing the health of houses" and, by extrapolation, the health of the population: "pure air, pure water, efficient drainage, cleanliness and light" (p. 14).

Other nurses who actively advocated for safe water, sewage, and sanitation systems, which they incorporated into their health promotion and education practices, included Lillian Wald in 1915 and Mary Breckenridge in 1952 (as cited in Eigsti-Gerber & McGuire, 1999). Wald was the founder of modern public health nursing, working in New York to improve the health of children in particular. Breckenridge incorporated principles of environmental health in her community health practice in rural Kentucky, which lowered infant mortality rates. Before the establishment of large hospitals and the focus on care in hospitals, most early nursing practice was carried out in the community. Nurses were cognizant of the environmental conditions in which their patients lived and worked. The shift to the majority of nursing practice being concentrated within institutions separated nurses from the environmental effects that had been more readily apparent.

CURRENT ENVIRONMENTAL ISSUES: CLIMATE CHANGE AND GLOBAL WARMING

Current environmental debates explore controversial issues such as global warming as a result of the continued rise of the use of fossil fuels and resultant greenhouse gas emissions (Foley, 2001; Jefferson, 2006; Last et al., 1998), and technological affluence at the cost of the destruction of natural habitat [Peace Out, 2011 (see educational resources)]. Multiple charters, agreements, summits, and conventions have been held to examine the health of the world's citizens, globalization and global issues related to the environment, access to safe water and food, climate change and global warming, the socio-political causes and impact of poverty, and the economic disparity that exists among nations within the context of a "sustainable global ecosystem" (Hilfinger Messias, 2001, p. 10). A proliferation of treaties and accords since the 1970s has resulted in more than 240 international agreements (Brown et al., 2001).

Brown et al. (2001) noted that the 1987 Montreal Protocol on Substances that Deplete the Ozone Layer led to the gradual phasing out of the use of chlorofluorocarbons that damage the stratosphere. The 1997 Kyoto Protocol to the 1992 United Nations (UN) Framework Convention on Climate Change was much more contentious, when the United States refused to ratify the treaty that required industrialized nations to cut carbon dioxide emissions by 6% to 8% between 2008 and 2012. It is important to note that carbon dioxide is the most significant anthropogenic greenhouse gas (Intergovernmental Panel on Climate Change [IPCC], 2007). At the 2008 G8 nations Summit on Climate Change, environmentalists were hopeful that the scientific evidence would influence world leaders to address the increasingly urgent issues around climate change. Although Russia and the United States did agree to some reduction in emissions by 2050, the conditions surrounding this agreement (e.g., the buy-in of China and India) and the timeframe for implementation have drawn significant criticism from environmentalists. Initially the Canadian Conservative federal government supported the Kyoto Protocol but later shifted its position to favor less onerous regulation of carbon dioxide emissions, favoring the continued expansion of the Alberta oil sands (Johnson, 2011). In December 2011, Canada withdrew from the Kyoto agreement, within the nation and worldwide. The Conservative government argues that Kyoto is ineffective since the United States and China, the biggest greenhouse gas emission countries, did not sign the agreement. They also argue that because Canada is not able to maintain the reduction rates that were agreed upon, the debt would be too large for Canada, affecting the Canadian economy (Zuydam, 2011). On the other hand, the official government opposition contends that the Canadian government is shaming Canadians by pulling out of a major international agreement (Fitzpatrick, 2011).

While recognizing positive global affects linked to health, sanitation, and urban reclamation, Berlinguer (1999) raises concerns regarding pollution, depletion of natural resources, global warming, and the declining quality of life—particularly in urban centers and in developing nations. He notes that people in the lowest socioeconomic classes suffer the greatest damage because they lack the resources and facilities to preserve their health. Put another way, it is the wealthiest countries and the wealthiest citizens of those countries who have benefited the most from industrialization.

In all nations, the poorest residents tend to live in substandard housing in densely populated communities in close proximity to industrial areas where the potential for contamination and hazardous waste leakage is the highest (Chaudhuri, 1998). Within Canadian society, Aboriginal people are four times more likely than non-Aboriginal Canadians to be living in crowded housing (Mikkonen & Raphael, 2010), a great concern with the spread of communicable diseases. In addition, members of First Nations communities are especially at risk for health problems related to unsafe drinking water, lack of adequate sanitation, and substandard housing (Health Canada [HC], 1999). Environmental contaminants such as polychlorinated biphenyls (PCBs) used in electrical and hydraulic equipment, dioxins from bleaching wood pulp with chlorine, and mercury from old industrial practices and long-range transport have been found in fish and marine mammals throughout the country. The result is a contaminated food supply, particularly for Aboriginal people in the north and those who follow a traditional diet.

In addition to the above-mentioned challenges, Nickels et al. (2005) argue that it is in the Arctic and sub-Arctic regions where the indication of global warming is initially expected to become most apparent. Increasing temperatures have already produced a variety of changes in the environment, and these changes are likely to become intensified. Some of these modifications include changes in the ecosystems that have sustained traditional Inuit life and ways of life for centuries. Major changes have occurred already including the order of migrating animals and the diminished time intervals for safe traveling on the land and ocean, limiting access to resources are current major challenges faced by Inuit. It is also important to note that Inuit hold specialized knowledge about the environment and the land (Nickels et al., 2005) and politicians, policy makers, and academics can greatly learn from their expertise.

ENVIRONMENTAL HEALTH HAZARDS

Around the world, life expectancy has increased and morbidity and mortality have decreased as a result of significant improvement in, and the availability of, safe water and sewage systems and better nutrition and housing. Individuals, communities, and governments need to be conscious that these gains do not overshadow current and developing environmental problems. WHO notes that about 2 million children younger than 5 years of age die annually because of unsafe drinking water and lack of sanitation. Air pollution is responsible for up to 20% of childhood mortality (World Health Organization [WHO], 2002). A WHO task force has been established to promote the identification, assessment, mitigation, and prevention of environmental hazards, specifically "to prevent disease and disability in children associated with chemical and physical threats" (Pronczuk, 2002, p. 495).

Various UN agencies participated in a global environmental assessment by providing data and information on environmental issues within their particular mandates (United Nations Environment Programme [UNEP], 1999). This assessment was undertaken in response to the need to build a consensus on priorities regarding the environment. According to this report, increased industrialization around the world has contributed to environmental deterioration resulting from air and water pollution, waste dumping, and increasing ill health, especially among the poor. Environmental contaminants include biologic agents, inorganic and organic chemicals, radiation, and particulate matter (Box 24.1).

Contaminants follow pathways from the time they are released into the environment until people, animals, or plants come in contact with them. These exposure pathways consist of five components that need to be examined when tracing sources of contamination (HC, 1998). The components are:

- Source of contamination (e.g., emissions, waste water and disposal sites, volcanoes, fires, and household products)
- Medium through which the contaminant travels (e.g., water, soil, air, and food products)
- Point at which people come into contact with the contaminant
- Person, animal, or plant that is the receptor of the contaminant
- Route of exposure (e.g., inhalation [gases, vapors, or particulate matter], dermal contact [working in contaminated soil or swimming in contaminated water], or ingestion [contaminated food or water]).

Many symptoms exhibited by people exposed to environmental contaminants can be attributed to other causes, making it difficult to establish an exact cause and effect. Therefore, it is

BOX 24.1   Selected Environmental Contaminants

Biologic Agents

Bacteria, such as *Escherichia coli,* protozoa, viruses, fungi, algae, molds, house dust mites, and pollen grains

Chemical Contaminants

Organic substances, such as fluorine, chlorine, bromine, iodine, nitrogen, sulfur, phosphorus, carbon, polychlorinated biphenyls, DDT, dioxins, benzene, malathion, toluene, and dioxane inorganic substances, such as ozone, nitrogen oxides, sulfur dioxide, lead, mercury, cadmium, arsenic, uranium, beryllium, and chromium

Radiation

Microwaves, ultraviolet light, low-frequency electromagnetic fields, and sound

Particulate Matter

Fine dust, smoke from forest fires, burning stubbles and wood burning fires, asbestos, and cigarette smoke

important when assessing exposure to environmental contaminants to take as broad a perspective as possible to include all potential environmental factors.

Water Safety

Water is fundamental to all life on the planet. Uneven distribution of this resource around the globe means that some regions, such as Canada, have an abundance of fresh water, whereas other regions, such as the Middle East and northern Africa, suffer from a shortage. It is estimated that 500 million people in the world live in countries that are short of water and that, by 2025, this number will dramatically rise to 3 billion (Mitchell, 2001). Water use worldwide has risen sixfold between 1900 and 1995, more than double the population increase.

Internationally, the World Health Organization/United Nations Children's Fund [WHO/UNICEF] (2008) report that tremendous progress has been made in access to improved water supplies worldwide. Told as a "good news story," in relation to the more dismal reality of adequate sanitation facilities, the number of people without an improved drinking water source now numbers below one billion (WHO/UNICEF, 2008, Special focus on drinking water and sanitation, p. 58).

In countries such as Canada, the abundance of water has led to waste and increased pollution of this resource. Although water is the ultimate renewable resource, major problems now exist in that water sources are polluted with chemicals, fertilizers, heavy metals, hydrocarbons, and raw sewage (Robson & Schneider, 2001; UNEP, 1999; Wanke & Saunders, 1996). Industrial waste, runoff from large-scale farming operations, and the dumping of garbage in uncontrolled waste sites lead to continued pollution.

In nature, water is actually never "pure." As water flows, it gathers tiny pieces of everything it contacts, including minerals, earth, plants, fertilizers, and agricultural runoff. Even in what might seem like pristine locations, water in its natural state will likely require some type of treatment before it is safe to drink. However, you might be surprised to learn that the water you drink is a minor source of most pollutants; the largest percentage of our daily intake of pollutants is from food sources. Nonetheless, water is still the principle source of exposure to some microorganisms (CNA, 2005).

Drinking water in Canada comes either from surface water, such as lakes and rivers, or underground sources such as aquifers. Most Canadians get their drinking water from public water systems. Provincial and territorial governments set requirements for water quality for these public water sources. People living in rural and remote locations may get their drinking water from wells or from surface water sources on their own private property and are individually responsible for the safety of the drinking water (HC, 2008).

Aquifers, underground sources of water, are being drained more quickly than they are being replenished. Global warming has caused the atmosphere to retain more water in the form of vapor, which decreases the volume of water returned in the form of rain. An example of the overuse of subterranean water is the High Plains Aquifer that extends from South Dakota to Texas. The level of water has dropped by more than 40 meters as the population uses the water for irrigating land that was once barren. Solutions to this water depletion suggested by United States politicians and entrepreneurs are the bulk sale of water from Canada and the desalination of ocean water for human use. The short-term and long-term effects on the environment of either of these proposals are not known.

The need to provide a safe drinking water supply has been highlighted by outbreaks of *Escherichia coli* in the water supply at Walkerton, Ontario and *Cryptosporidium* species found in the water in North Battleford, Saskatchewan. The *E. coli* outbreak led to multiple gastrointestinal illnesses and, ultimately, to the deaths of nine people (Ahluwalia, 2000). Contamination of the water sources from manure from cattle farms in the area and the inadequate treatment of the water are suspected causes of this outbreak. The impact of these outbreaks has heightened public awareness and increased the need to examine and question water safety in the communities.

Cryptosporidium, although not a new organism, is becoming more prevalent. Animals and humans shed this protozoan parasite in their feces. The consumption of contaminated water or food, ingestion of recreational water, or contact with infected people can lead to infection. There are potentially life-threatening consequences for immunosuppressed people who become infected (Physicians for Social Responsibility [PSR], 2001b). Proper filtration, distillation, or reverse osmosis processes must be used to ensure that the organism has been removed from the water supply. *Giardia lamblia* is another parasite endemic to the ecosystem. *G. lamblia* causes gastrointestinal infections and can also produce life-threatening effects in an immunocompromised person. Contamination of water supplies with various microbial contaminants leads to multiple "boil water" alerts annually in all provinces.

In 2001, a government roundtable found that, although water quality is a serious problem throughout the country, there is particular concern regarding water supply to First Nations communities. A Health Canada report in 1995 signaled that 171 communities (one in five) had water systems that could negatively affect the health of the citizens (MacKinnon, 2001). Minimal improvements have occurred during the intervening years. As of 2001, there were no national regulations in Canada regarding water protection and safety, an indication that disasters can and will continue to occur. By the end of 2011, more than 130 First Nations communities across Canada were under a drinking water advisory (HC, 2011).

Air Pollution

Many regions of the world suffer from air pollution that leads to illness and death. In South America, about 4,000 premature deaths are estimated to occur annually in São Paulo and Rio de Janeiro as a result of severe air pollution (UNEP, 1999). The very young and the very old suffer a greater burden from air pollution than the people in the interim age ranges. The risk from air pollution for children increases because they breathe more rapidly and inhale more pollutants per pound of body weight than do adults. A wide range of negative effects from air pollution include impaired pulmonary function; reduced physical performance; multiple visits to physicians, emergency rooms, and hospitals; and premature death (HC, 1998; CNA, 2008a).

Air pollutants are generated from burning fossil fuels, such as oil, coal, gasoline, and diesel fuel, in vehicles and power generators. Industries, such as pulp and paper mills, oil refineries, and ore smelters, contribute to air pollution (CNA, 2008a). Oil, natural gas, and coal production has resulted in Alberta emitting 30% of the carbon dioxide, 26% of the nitrogen oxide, and 23% of the sulfur oxide emissions generated in Canada (Environment Canada [EC], 2000). Asthma is a respiratory disease that can be triggered by airborne contaminants. Air pollutants, such as ground-level ozone, sulfur dioxide, and particulate matter, are believed to be key factors in increased asthma rates (CNA, 2008a). Pope et al. (2002) analyzed the mortality statistics of participants in the Cancer Prevention Study II who resided in U.S. metropolitan areas where pollution data were available. They demonstrated that fine particulate air contamination is associated with cardiopulmonary and lung cancer mortality (Pope et al., 2002, p. 1137) and is a significant risk factor to population health.

An exponential increase in the incidence of asthma in children in Canada occurred in the 1990s. Rates of hospitalization for boys increased by 27% and for girls by 18% (HC, 1997). This raised annual hospital admissions of children to more than 60,000. According to Last et al. (1998), hospital admissions in Ontario for acute bronchitis, bronchiolitis, and pneumonia in children younger than 1 year of age "can be attributed to the summer pollutants, ozone and sulphates" (p. 21). According to the Canadian Lung Association, airborne contaminants including tobacco smoke and mold can cause or exacerbate asthma and other respiratory conditions; asthma now affects roughly 3 million Canadians (CNA, 2005).

Some authorities suggest that it would cost $6 billion to implement a program to decrease air pollution by developing cleaner vehicles and fuels in Canada (HC, 1998, p. 121). On the other hand, savings to the healthcare system are estimated to be $24 billion as a result of eliminating many of the negative health effects of air pollution. Improving ambient air quality in Canada alone could amount to $8 billion in healthcare savings over the next 20 years (Last et al., 1998). Last et al. (1998) suggest that the reduction of motor vehicle emissions would result in savings to the forest and agricultural sectors of the Canadian economy of between $11 billion and $30 billion.

Although chemically the same, ground-level ozone (found within 11 km of the earth's surface) and the "ozone layer" (found between 11 and 47 km above the earth in the stratosphere) need to be differentiated from each other. The ozone layer acts as a barrier against ultraviolet (UV) radiation (particularly UVB rays) from the sun (HC, 1998). As this layer is damaged or destroyed by chlorofluorocarbons, more radiation penetrates to earth. The result is an increase in skin cancer, particularly melanomas. There is also evidence that UVB exposure increases the risk for cataracts (Institute of Medicine, 1995).

Ground-level ozone, or smog, forms when nitrogen oxides and volatile organic compounds react in the presence of sunlight (HC, 1998). This reaction occurs on hot, still, summer days, and the resultant air pollution can lead to adverse cardiac and respiratory effects. Between 2003 and 2005, at least 40% of the Canadian population lived in areas with ozone levels higher than ambient ozone found at Canada-wide Standards goal (EC, 2007). Again, those most affected are the elderly and very young people. As the earth's average temperature rises, it is expected that more hot summer days with smog advisories or warnings will occur.

PCBs, dioxins, and other organic compounds can travel long distances through the air before being deposited on the land or in bodies of water. These toxins accumulate in the food chain, where they become a hazard to people who consume fish and wildlife as food, particularly when they are ingested faster than they can be excreted (HC, 1998). There is grave concern that seals and other Arctic animals are contaminated and pose a risk to Inuit communities that rely on these animals as a source of food.

Chemical Pollution

Humans are slowly coming to realize the effects of the huge quantities of manmade chemicals that have been discharged into the environment since the 1940s (Physicians for Social Responsibility,

2005). Excessive use of fertilizers, pesticides, and heavy metals such as arsenic, cadmium, lead, and mercury has polluted the land (UNEP, 1999). Local sources of contamination, such as sewage and waste disposal, and industrial discharge can be more readily identified. More diffuse contamination occurs through runoff from fields and lawns, motor vehicle emissions, and the long-distance contamination of acid rain (which develops from sulfur dioxide and nitrogen oxides from coal-fired power plants, smelters, and vehicular emissions). Once again, environmental contamination is an issue that disproportionately affects the health of children. Children, relative to their size, eat, drink, and breathe more than adults. Children are in closer contact with the environment through increased hand-to-mouth activity. Children absorb more chemicals through their skin and intestines than adults. Certain contaminants can have a major effect as children pass through critical developmental stages (Pronczuk, 2002). In addition, children and families living in poverty are likely to have increased exposure and less access to resources (i.e., nutrition and healthcare) to mitigate the negative effects of exposure to environmental contaminants (CNA, 2005).

Many of these chemical pollutants remain in the environment for long periods. They can be ingested and then accumulated in the tissues of humans if their excretion does not occur as quickly as their intake. Dioxins, furans, and PCBs build up in fatty tissue, whereas metals such as lead, mercury, and cadmium are stored in the liver, kidney, and bone. Mercury can be found in many lakes and rivers, where it converts to methyl mercury, a toxic substance that can affect the nervous systems of humans and animals (HC, 2007). An additional concern is long-term arsenic ingestion (through drinking water), which increases the risk for skin, bladder, lung, kidney, and other cancers (PSR, 2001a). The impact on human health of long-term low-level exposure to many chemical pollutants is unknown. Concerns focus on immune-system suppression, neurologic and behavioral changes, and the role that chemical toxins play in initiating cancer.

The term *pesticide* refers to a variety of chemicals that control weeds (herbicides), bacteria (disinfectants), fungi (fungicides), insects (insecticides), and rodents (rodenticides). Pesticides are widely used in agriculture and forestry to protect crops and forests. Large amounts of fertilizers and herbicides are used annually in urban and suburban environments in the care of lawns and golf courses. According to a review of the literature completed by the CNA, (2008d), a large body of research evidence has identified risks associated with pesticide use, particularly for children. The CNA (2008a, p. 21) document, "The Environment and Health," references the Toronto Health Department (2002, p. 1) statement that, "These substances [pesticides] are intended to be harmful to living organisms and because they are released into the environment, they pose an exposure and potential health risk to other organisms, including humans."

In Canada, more than 500 active ingredients have been registered for use as pesticides (HC, 1998). There is a growing movement within some municipalities across Canada to ban the use of herbicides because of the risk to human health. As of May 2008, there were 146 towns and cities with active pesticide ordinances, the largest of these being Toronto. A list of these communities can be found at http://www.flora.org/healthyottawa/BylawList.pdf

Of grave concern are the implications for the health of residents who live in the immediate vicinity of toxic waste sites or who now live in what was once a contaminated industrial site (Carruth et al., 1997). There are no biologic markers by which the level of exposure can be determined for many of the chemicals that are discharged into the environment. Further, the long-term impact of long-term exposure to some contaminants, such as malathion, is not known. Key concerns related to long-term exposure include the following:

- Those in lower socioeconomic conditions are often the people who live in areas closest to polluted sites.
- As knowledge of chemical pollutants grows, standards may change (i.e., norms or levels that were once considered safe may be now considered a health risk).

- Exposure to toxins may occur and may be undetected over extended periods of time.
- Exposure to contaminants may occur through multiple pathways (e.g., air, water, and soil) and enter the food chain in numerous ways, making detection more difficult.
- Action to curb exposure to contaminants has not kept pace with the society's abilities to detect contamination (CNA, 2000).

Inside Environments

The Ottawa Charter for Health Promotion [OCHP] (1986) credits adequate shelter as having a major effect on health. According to the report from the federal, provincial, and territorial governments, "Toward a Healthy Future: Second Report on the Health of Canadians," 1 in 5 Canadians who rent accommodations is living in substandard housing (HC, 1999). The people who most often live in these conditions are single-parent families, particularly ones in which parents are younger than 30 years of age; people with mental health problems; and senior citizens living alone. Of grave concern are the inadequate housing and crowded living conditions in which Aboriginal people live. This may be a major contributor to the fact that Aboriginal children suffer from much higher rates of respiratory and other infectious diseases than do non-Aboriginal children (HC, 1999).

HC estimates that Canadians spend up to 90% of their time indoors in their homes, work sites, and other buildings. In addition to outdoor contaminants, which can also be found indoors, inside air may contain tobacco smoke, formaldehyde, vapors from household products, carbon dioxide, and biologic agents, such as bacteria, fungi, molds, viruses, and mite byproducts (HC, 1998). The health of the residents may be adversely affected if the concentrations of any of these contaminants rise too high. The growing trend toward weatherizing homes and buildings in the interest of energy conservation may result in a lack of adequate air exchange because the ventilation systems were not designed for these well-insulated and sealed buildings. Therefore, the potential for contaminant build-up increases.

A principal contaminant in indoor environments is tobacco smoke, including sidestream smoke emitted from cigarettes, pipes, and cigars between puffs and mainstream smoke exhaled by smokers. In 2007, it was estimated that there were 18,560 deaths from lung cancer in Canada (Statistic Canada). In 2002, almost 80% of lung cancer–related deaths were due to smoking and in that same year, 252 non-smokers died from lung cancer (Rehm et al., 2006) due to environmental tobacco smoke (ETS). In addition, ETS is considered a significant cause of cardiovascular disease and death in non-smokers.

Canadian children are at an increased risk for health effects from ETS because they spend more time indoors than children in many other countries. As mentioned previously, children have smaller airways and breathe more rapidly than do adults, thus inhaling more pollutants per kilogram of body weight. There is a wide variation among provinces in the control and restriction of smoking in public areas. Restrictions against smoking range from being limited to designated smoking areas to a total ban on smoking on public premises. As the public becomes more aware and concerned with the health risks attributed to ETS, smoking bans are increasingly stringent. In 2008, the majority of the provinces and territories have legislated complete bans on smoking in public buildings.

Environmental Sensitivity

Environmental sensitivity (ES) has become an increasing problem in the industrialized era. Amongst other disabling characteristics, ES restricts the ability for a growing part of the population, particularly women, to participate in public life, such as through access to community services, education, homes of family and friends, and medical care (Gibson, 2010). As a rising disability, ES gives rise to detrimental symptoms from exposure to chemicals in ambient air, causing what can be referred to as multiple chemical sensitivity (MCS) and/or electro-magnetic fields, causing electromagnetic hypersensitivity (EH). Some of the most prevalent symptoms of ES are lethargy, difficulty concentrating, muscle aches, memory difficulties, and prolonged fatigue (Gibson & Vogel, 2009). The impact of developing ES may include social isolation (Chircop & Keddy, 2003), financial devastation, unemployment, and homelessness (Zwillenger, 1997).

As nurses, our understanding of this emerging problem is crucial not only for our support for those whose lives are affected, but also because it could guide the way we currently under-stand research and prevention of disease (Spencer & Schur, 2008). In addition, nurses can advo-cate for environmental issues by questioning the "influences of chemical industry on legislation, education, health care, research funding and the media" (Gibson, 2010, p. 13). Nurses could be informed by recalling examples such as the tobacco industry that discouraged research uncover-ing the hazards of smoking and funded research indicating it to be safe (Johnson, 2000). Further-more, nurses can lobby for a human rights approach, as promoted by Gibson (2010), by banning fragrant personal care products and cleaning supplies from public access, as they constitute the most common barriers for those whose lives are affected by ES.

Contaminated Social Environments

If consideration of environmental health risks is confined to the effects of pollution and hazards within the natural environment, a key component of the settings in which individuals and families live will be ignored. Impoverished neighborhoods with substandard housing, abject poverty, home-lessness, visible signs of people who are substance abusers and drug dealers, and violence and crime within the community are examples of contaminated social environments. The impact on the physi-cal, psychological, and emotional health of individuals living in such environments can be severe.

If the social environments in which people live are violent, degrading, and impoverished, there is a significant negative impact on the health of the residents. These negative effects are compounded by the toxic waste sites and heavy industry that are often near these communities. Healthcare professionals need to take into account the entire environmental context of the people and communities in which they are working.

SOCIO-POLITICAL ANALYSIS

Given what is known about current environmental risks and even dangers, it is challenging to understand how and why these issues continue to be unresolved. A socio-political analysis helps to explore issues in a way that asks difficult questions, such as whose needs are being served by the current state of affairs, and what knowledge counts as evidence in the discussion of conten-tious issues such as global warming.

It is hard not to notice that the interests of Canadian business that relies on the fossil fuel industry and the government are closely connected. The economic wellbeing of individuals and of a local, provincial, or, indeed, the national economy can be linked to environmental resources including logging, mining, and the oil and gas industries. Examples could be found at every level of government of the challenges to support economic development without risk to the environ-ment. The most recent and perhaps the most dramatic example of the national Conservative government in 2011 is turning away from the Kyoto Accord (Zuydam, 2011)—a lost opportunity for Canada to exhibit leadership on the world stage of environmental responsibility. Similarly, Canada's national governments have, for decades, failed to demonstrate a sustained and serious intention to address the deplorable environmental conditions in First Nations communities.

Throughout this chapter, the evidence cited points to politically, socially, and economically mar-ginalized Canadian citizens as being at the greatest risk for environmentally linked health challenges.

Children, those with chronic debilitating illness, and First Nations people residing in rural and remote communities are among those Canadians with the least political acumen and economic resources.

STRATEGIES TO OVERCOME BARRIERS

One of the greatest barriers to achieving environmental health has been the lack of public knowledge or education about the reality of increasing health risks connected to the environment. The more we know about and understand the links between the environment and human health, the more willing we are as a society to provide the economic support and the political will to make the changes that are needed.

One way to overcome this lack of knowledge in the public domain is for professional organizations to take a position on the issues and to make public their position statements. The CNA position statement titled, "Nurses and Environmental Health," states that "CNA expects that as nurses become more aware of environmental health issues, they will increasingly focus on reducing the environmental impact of the health setting in which they work and of their personal activities, and thus promote environmental sustainability" (CNA, 2009, p. 2). Of particular concern are the long-term health effects of contaminants on children, the chronically ill, and the elderly, especially those living in poverty in our communities, disproportionately members of First Nations communities. In a joint statement, the CNA and the Canadian Medical Association indicate that "environmental responsibility must be practiced at the individual level (in the workplace and in the home) and at the community level to achieve concrete results " (2009, p. 1). Through the revised "2008 Code of Ethics for Registered Nurses," the CNA (2008c) has made the position of the profession in Canada even stronger, by obligating nurses in "supporting environmental preservation and restoration and advocating for initiatives that reduce environmentally harmful practices in order to promote health and well-being" (p. 20) (Box 24.2).

In Canada, nurses and other healthcare professionals have the power to influence political decision making directly through lobbying members of parliament and indirectly through publishing position statements that exert pressure on politicians, governments, and health authorities. In taking this public stance, we must first recognize and address the impact that the waste from healthcare facilities has on the environment. In addition to addressing issues in the different areas of practice in their communities, individual nurses can also strive to increase their knowledge based on issues around their communities, bringing environmental issues to the forefront of their practice and personal lives. A total of 211 nurses completed the CNA (2008e) survey and although the sample was composed of a reasonably high proportion of nurses with graduate degrees, less than half had received any proper training in environmental health (EH). Although

---

BOX 24.2   Why Are Environmental Health Issues Important to Nurses?

Nurses in all settings should be well prepared to identify and assess potential environmental health issues related to workplaces, neighborhoods, houses, and schools.

Given that environmental health is a rapidly evolving field, nurses should know where to go to find current and credible scientific information.

Nurses are considered to be trusted sources of information regarding environmental health risks. As such, they are often in a position to translate information from other experts in fields such as toxicology and epidemiology.

Nurses are often in a position to identify environmental health issues because they may recognize patterns of symptoms in people who live or work in the same areas. Nurses should be prepared to investigate and act when they see such patterns.

From Canadian Nurses Association. (2005). *The ecosystem, the natural environment, and health and nursing: A summary of the issues*. Ottawa: Author (p. 5).

BOX 24.3   What Can Nurses Do about Environmental Health Issues?

Primary Prevention

- Counsel women of childbearing age about reducing their exposure to environmental hazards.
- Support the development of exposure standards for toxins and other contaminants.
- Advocate for safe air and water.
- Teach avoidance of ultraviolet exposure and use of sunscreen.
- Support programs for waste reduction and recycling as well as energy conservation in your community and workplace.

Secondary Prevention

- Assess homes, schools, worksites, and communities for environmental hazards.
- Screen children under 5 years of age for blood lead levels.

Tertiary Prevention

- Support cleanup of toxic waste sites and removal of other hazards.
- Refer homeowners to approved programs that eliminate contaminants, such as lead and asbestos.

Modified from Canadian Nurses Association. (2005). *The ecosystem, the natural environment, and health and nursing: A summary of the issues*. Ottawa: Author (p. 6).

the content on EH did not seem to be extensively available in either their undergraduate or graduate curricula, many of the participants were concerned that environmental hazards could affect the community in which they worked. In addition, these nurses utilized a range of teaching tools related to EH with their clients.

A study done by Tinker et al. (2010) concluded that public health nurses are well positioned to deliver environmental risk reduction, which is a program that assesses children's environmental health risks. We would argue that all nurses are in a position to raise awareness of environmental issues that affect the health and wellbeing of their clients (Box 24.3), and that continuing focus on EH education is crucial.

Nurses are well positioned to be leaders on related issues in EH. For example, members of the Registered Nurses' Association of Ontario (RNAO) campaigned alongside health and environmental groups for strong provincial regulation on the issue of pesticides. On Earth Day, 2009, a new law was legislated banning the cosmetic use of a comprehensive list of pesticides. Following this campaign, the RNAO (2009) published a statement, *Ontario nurses successfully campaign for comprehensive provincial pesticide ban,* an excellent demonstration of nurses' providing leadership in the political act of lobbying for needed changes to public health policy. This

BOX 24.4   Nursing Strategies for Reducing Waste

- Introducing recycling programs for hospital waste, 45% of which may be paper
- Supporting the purchase of reusable linens in hospital and clinic settings
- Lobbying and supporting suppliers willing to reduce packaging
- Ensuring that only material needing incineration goes to the medical incinerator by educating staff and making waste receptacles available and accessible
- Working with other members of hospital staff to purchase healthcare products that do not contain toxic substances such as mercury, so they do not end up in the waste stream.

Modified from Canadian Nurses Association. (2008). The role of nurses in greening the health system. Ottawa: Author (p. 6).

BOX 24.5 **Films Related to Environmental Concerns**

Peace Out (2011) (Canadian)
Avatar (2009)
Food Inc. (2009)
The 11th Hour (2007)
An Inconvenient Truth (2006)
A Crude Awakening: The Oil Crash (2006)
Erin Brockovich (2000)

successful campaign showcases nurses' visible leadership in shaping the healthcare system and influencing decisions that affect environmental health.

Nurses have the capacity to participate and to lead in the needed efforts to address environmental issues; the change in smoking practices in Canada over the past 20 years is another informative exemplar of overcoming what once seemed to be insurmountable barriers to change.

SUMMARY

Water safety, air purity or pollution, chemical spills and spread, the growing contamination of inside environments, and violent surroundings are serious environmental concerns across Canada, as is the relationship of the environment to the health of individuals, families, and populations whether in the home, community, or workplace. The information in this chapter represents a snippet of the volumes of literature available on the topic. Box 24.4 provides some strategies that nurses can use in reducing waste. Box 24.5 provides a list of films related to environmental concerns.

Add to your knowledge of this issue:	
Canadian Nurses Association	**www.cna-nurses.ca/cna**
Canadian Association of Physicians for the Environment	**www.cape.ca**
Environment Canada	**www.ec.gc.ca**
Canadian Council of Ministers of the Environment	**www.ccme.ca**
United Nations: Framework Convention on Climate Change	**www.unfccc.int**
Canadian Nurses for Health and the Environment	**www.cnhe-iise.ca**
First Nations Environment Network	**www.fnen.org**
International Council of Nurses	**www.icn.ch**
Canadian Health Networks	**www.canadian-health-network.ca**
Health Canada	**www.hc-sc.gc.ca**
World Health Organization	**www.who.int/peh**

Online

R E F L E C T I O N S *on the Chapter...*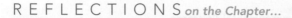

1 Cite-specific examples from courses in your nursing program that link health and environmental conditions.

2 Name three health issues related to environmental factors that have been in the news recently in your local region or in your province or territory. Were nurses evident in the discussions?

3 What evidence is there that global climate change will affect the health of individuals and communities across the globe?

4 What legislation has your provincial or territorial government or the federal government passed in the past year regarding pollution and contamination in the environment?

5 What types of medical waste might have an impact on the environment? What is the potential for contamination or pollution to occur from medical waste? Where and how might this contamination or pollution happen?

Want to know more? Visit the Point for additional helpful resources:

- Journal Articles
- Learning Objectives
- Nursing Professional Roles and Responsibilities
- Bonus chapters:
  - ○ Health and Nursing Policy: A Matter of Politics, Power and Professionalism
  - ○ The NP Movement: Recurring Issues
  - ○ When Difference Matters: The Politics of Privilege and Marginality

References

Ahluwalia, R. (2000, May). *Ontario's rural heartland in shock* [Television broadcast]. Toronto, ON: CBC TV News.

Berlinguer, G. (1999). Globalization and global health. *International Journal of Health Services, 29*(3), 579–595.

Brown, L., Flavin, C., & French, H. (2001). *State of the world 2001.* New York: W.W. Norton.

Canadian Nurses Association. (2000). *The environment is a determinant of health: Position statement.* Retrieved from http://www.cna-nurses.ca

———. (2005). *The ecosystem, the natural environment, and health and nursing: A summary of the issues.* Ottawa, ON: Author.

———. (2008a). *The environment and health: An introduction for nurses.* Ottawa, ON: Author.

———. (2008b). *The role of nurses in greening the health system.* Ottawa, ON: Author.

———. (2008c). *The code of ethics for registered nurses* (2008 centennial edition). Ottawa, ON: Author.

———. (2008d). *Nursing and environmental health.* Retrieved from www.cna-aiic.ca/CNA/issues/environment/default_e.aspx

———. (2008e). *Nurses and Environment Health: Survey Results.* Retrieved from http://www.cna-nurses.ca

———. (2009). *Nurses and environmental health: Position statement.* Retrieved from http://www.cna-nurses.ca

Canadian Nurses Association/Canadian Medical Association. (2009). *Environmentally responsible activity in the health sector. Joint CNA/CMA position statement.* Retrieved from http://www.cna-nurses.ca

Carruth, A.K., Gilbert, K., & Lewis, B. (1997). Environmental health hazards: The impact on a Southern community. *Public Health Nursing, 14*(5), 259–267.

Chaudhuri, N. (1998). Child health, poverty and the environment: The Canadian context. *Canadian Journal of Public Health, 89*(suppl 1), S26–S30.

Chircop, A., & Keddy, B. (2003). Women living with environmental illness. *Health Care for Women International, 24*(5), 371–383.

Clark, M.J. (1999). *Nursing in the community: Dimensions of community health nursing* (3rd ed.). Stamford, CT: Appleton & Lange.

Eigsti-Gerber, D., & McGuire, S.L. (1999). Teaching students about nursing and the environment. Part 1: Nursing role and basic curricula. *Journal of Community Health Nursing, 16*(2), 69–79.

Environment Canada. (2000). *Clean air.* Retrieved from www.ec.gc.ca/air/introduction_c.html

———. (2007). *Government of Canada five-year progress report: Canada-wide standards for particulate matter and ozone.* Retrieved from http://www.ec.gc.ca/cleanair-airpur/caol/pollution_issues/cws/s4_e.cfm

Fitzpatrick, M. (Reporter). (2011, December 13). *May accuses Harper of breaking law over Kyoto. CBC News, Politics.* Toronto, ON: Canadian Broadcasting Corporation. Retrieved from http://www.cbc.ca/news/politics/story/2011/12/13/pol-may-kyoto.html

Foley, D. (2001). *Fuelling the climate crisis: The continental energy plan.* Vancouver, BC: David Suzuki Foundation.

Gibson, P.R. (2010). Of the world but not in it: Barriers to community access and education for persons with environmental sensitivities. *Health Care for Women International, 31*(1), 3–16.

Gibson, P.R., & Vogel, V.M. (2009). Sickness related dysfunction in persons with self-reported multiple chemical sensitivity at four levels of severity. *Journal of Clinical Nursing, 18*(1), 72–81.

Health Canada. (1997). *Health and environment: Partners for life* (Cat. H49-112-1/1997E). Ottawa, ON: Minister of Public Works and Government Services.

———. (1998). *The health and environment handbook for health professionals* (Cat. H46-2/98-211E-2E). Ottawa, ON: Minister of Public Works and Government Services.

———. (1999). *Toward a healthy future: Second report on the health of Canadians* (Cat H39-468/1999E). Ottawa, ON: Minister of Public Works and Government Services.

———. (2007). *Mercury and health.* Retrieved from www.hc-sc.gc.ca/ewh-semt/pubs/contaminants/mercury

———. (2008). *Canadian drinking water guidelines.* Retrieved from www.hcsc.gc.ca/ewh-semt/water-eau/drink-potab/guide

———. (2011). *First Nations, Inuit and aboriginal health: Drinking water and wastewater.* Ottawa, ON: Author. Retrieved from http://www.hc-sc.gc.ca/fniah-spnia/promotion/public-publique/water-eau-eng.php

Hilfinger Messias, D.K. (2001). Globalization, nursing, and health for all. *Journal of Nursing Scholarship, 33*(1), 8–11.

Institute of Medicine Committee on Enhancing Environmental Health Content in Nursing Practice. (1995). *Nursing, health, & the environment.* Washington, DC: National Academy Press.

Intergovernmental Panel on Climate Change. (2007). *Climate change 2007: The physical science basis: Summary for policymakers.* Contribution of Working Group I to the Fourth Assessment Report of the Intergovernmental Panel on Climate Change. Cambridge, UK: Cambridge University Press.

Jefferson, J. (2006). *Energy efficiency opportunities in Ontario hospitals.* Toronto, ON: Ontario Hospital Association.

Johnson, D. (2011). *Thinking government: Public administration and politics in Canada.* Toronto, ON: University of Toronto Press.

Johnson, A. (2000). *Casualties of progress: Personal histories from the chemically sensitive.* Brunswick, ME: MCS Information Exchange.

Last, J., Trouton, K., & Pengally, D. (1998). Taking our breath away: The health effects of air pollution and climate change. Retrieved from http://www.davidsuzuki.org

MacKinnon, M. (2001, July 18). Vital to improve water quality on reserves, group says. *The Globe and Mail,* p. A5.

Malcolm, J., Liu, C., Miller, L., Allnutt, T., & Hansen, L. (2002). *Habitats at risk: Global warming and species loss in globally significant terrestrial ecosystems.* Gland, Switzerland: World Wide Fund for Nature.

McDevitt, J., & Wilbur, J. (2002). Locating sources of data. In N. Ervin (Ed.), *Advanced community health nursing practice* (pp. 109–148). Upper Saddle River, NJ: Prentice Hall.

McGuire, S.L., & Eigsti-Gerber, D. (1999). Teaching students about nursing and the environment. Part 2: Legislation and resources. *Journal of Community Health Nursing, 16*(2), 81–94.

Mikkonen, J., & Raphael, D. (2010). *Social determinants of health: The Canadian facts.* Toronto, ON: York University School of Health Policy and Management.

Mitchell, A. (2001, June 4). The world's "single biggest threat." *The Globe and Mail.*

Nickels, S., Furgal, C., Buell, M., Moquin, H., Shirley, J., & Carter, A. (2005). *Unikkaaqatigiit—Putting the human face on climate change: Perspectives from Inuit in Canada.* Ottawa, ON: Inuit Tapiriit Kanatami, Nasivvik Centre for Inuit Health and Changing Environments (Université Laval) & Ajunnginiq Centre (National Aboriginal Health Organization).

Nightingale, F. (1860). *Notes on nursing: What it is and what it is not.* (Reprinted London: J.B. Lippincott Company. 1992: Philadelphia).

Ottawa Charter for Health Promotion. (1986). *First international conference on health promotion.* Ottawa, ON. Retrieved from http://www.who.int/healthpromotion/conferences/previous/ottawa/en/

———. (2001a). *Arsenic: What health care providers should know* [Online]. Retrieved from http://www.envirohealthaction.org/upload_files/arsenicfs.pdf

———. (2001b). *Cryptosporidium: What health care providers should know* [Online]. Retrieved from http://www.envirohealthaction.org/upload_files/cryptofs.pdf

Pope, C.A., Burnett, R., Thun, M., et al. (2002). Lung cancer, cardiopulmonary mortality, and long-term exposure to fine particulate air pollution. *Journal of the American Medical Association, 287*(9), 1132–1141.

Pronczuk, J. (2002). Sentinel role of poisons centers in the protection of children's environmental health. *Journal of Toxicology - Clinical Toxicology, 40*(4):493–497. Retrived from http://informahealthcare.com/doi/pdf/10.1081/CLT-120006752

Registered Nurses' Association of Ontario (RNAO) (2009). *Nurses speak out about pesticides.* Retrieved Sept. 23 2012 from www.rnao.ca/search/content/pesticide ban

Rehm, J., Baliunas, D., Brochu, S., et al. (2006). *The costs of substance abuse in Canada 2002.* Ottawa, ON: Canadian Centre on Substance Abuse.

Robson, M., & Schneider, D. (2001). Environmental health issues in rural communities. *Environmental Health, 63*(10), 16–20.

Spencer, T. R., & Schur, P. M. (2008). The challenges of multiple chemical sensitivity. *Journal of Environmental Health, 70*(10), 24–27.

Tinker, E., Postma, J., & Butterfield, P. (2010). Barriers and facilitators in the delivery of environmental risk reduction by public health nurses in the home setting. *Public Health Nursing, 28*(1), 35–42.

United Nations Environment Programme. (1999). *Global environment outlook GEO-2000.* Retrieved from http://www.unep.org/geo2000

Wanke, M.I., & Saunders, D. (1996). Survey of local environmental health programs in Alberta. *Canadian Journal of Public Health, 87*(5), 345–350.

Wilkinson, C. (Producer) & Wilkinson, C. (Director). (2011). *Peace Out* [Motion picture]. Canada: IMDbPro.

World Health Organization. (2007). *Climate and health fact sheet.* Retrieved from www.who.int/media-center/factsheets/fs266/en/index/html

World Health Organization/United Nations Children's Fund. (2008). *Report on special focus on drinking water and sanitation.* Retrieved from www.who.int/water_sanitation-health/monitoring/jmp2008/en/index.html

Zwillinger, R. (l997). *The Dispossessed: Living with multiple chemical sensitivities.* Paulden, AZ: The Dispossessed Project.

Zuydam, S. (Reporter). (2011, December 12). *Canada pulls out of Kyoto protocol. CBC News, Politics.* Toronto, ON: Canadian Broadcasting Corporation. Retrieved from http://www.cbc.ca/news/politics/story/2011/12/12/pol-kent-kyoto-pullout.html

25 Interpersonal Violence and Abuse: Ending the Silence

Colleen Varcoe

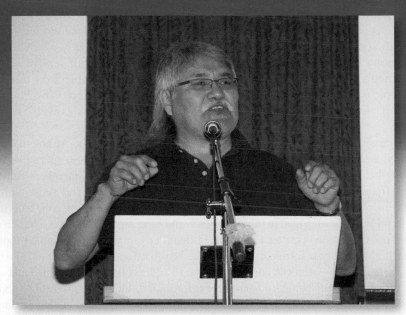

Paul Andrew of the Dene Nation shares with nurse educators the violations in residential schools that he and others experienced. The Truth and Reconciliation Commission established in 2008 to make the history of the Indian residential schools and its effects on generations of aboriginal people known to Canadians. (Used with permission. Photographer Anne-Mieke Cameron.)

Critical Questions

As a way of engaging with the ideas in this chapter, consider the following:

1. What do you think might be the prevalence of violence or abuse in your own community?

2. How do you think most people understand the causes of violence or abuse and who is held responsible based on that understanding?

3. What actions by professionals might silence the disclosure or reporting of experiences of violence or abuse?

4. Why might professionals be reluctant to address violence or abuse?

Chapter Objectives

After completing this chapter, you should be able to:

1. Understand the complex relationships among the many forms of violence and abuse.

2. Analyze political, legal, and ethical factors related to violence and abuse.

3. Relate the effects of violence and abuse to the health of individuals.

4. Evaluate the impact of violence and abuse on society, including the healthcare system.

5. Examine factors that contribute to the continued silencing of victims of violence and abuse.

6. Differentiate facilitators and barriers to resolution of various issues and generate strategies to address violence and abuse.

Interpersonal violence is a social problem of epidemic proportions around the world. Since the late 1970s, there has been a growing recognition that interpersonal violence and abuse have a significant impact on the health of individuals specifically and on Canadian society in general, including the healthcare system.

Violence involves exerting power over another person to control, disempower, or injure the other. As a social act, violence crosses legal, ethical, and healthcare boundaries with serious moral, sociocultural, political, and personal ramifications for society (Hoff, 1994). Violence is perpetrated against people of all ages, in every socioeconomic sector of society, and in all societies around the globe. However, violence is deeply gendered, and is perpetrated along various axes of power. Violence is enmeshed with sexism, racism, ableism, and homophobia. Women, young people, elderly people, people from racialized groups, and people with disabilities are often most vulnerable to violence. The long-term negative effects of violence have enormous implications for the victims as well as for all facets of society.

Discussion of violence is an everyday occurrence in the media. Although Canadian culture officially condemns violence, it is often glorified in film, television, sports, books, and music. The long-held myth that the family is a safe haven for all of its members has been dispelled through frequent accounts highlighting the magnitude of violence and abuse within that setting. There is increasing awareness of violence and abuse in the workplace, with bullying and specific acts of violence that may lead to injury or death and have significant mental health consequences. It is not possible in one chapter to present in-depth coverage of this complex topic. Rather, this chapter highlights some forms of violence, the health effects on individuals, and the role nurses and the nursing profession can and should take to address issues of violence and abuse. There is a vast array of multidisciplinary sources of information, including print, film, and audio, on the topic of violence. This chapter is meant to stimulate a rudimentary understanding of the topic, and readers are encouraged to expand their knowledge and understanding through the numerous other sources that are available. To begin, definitions of the multiple forms of violence and abuse are presented in Box 25.1.

THE MANY FORMS OF INTERPERSONAL VIOLENCE

Interpersonal violence encompasses much more than single physical acts of violence. First, such acts rarely occur without other forms of violation. Second, very harmful abuse can be perpetrated without any physical violence. Third, interpersonal violence and abuse usually occur as part of a pattern of relating. The word *violence* is derived from the Latin infinitive *violare,* to violate, rape, or injure. Violation of another person may result not only in visible physical harm, but also in emotional trauma that may be at least as harmful as physical battering and have more long-lasting effects. Within this chapter, the terms *violence* and *abuse* are used interchangeably, although abuse may not entail physical trauma.

- *Interpersonal violence* includes violence that occurs within relationships as well as that experienced from strangers and acquaintances. All types of violence are encompassed by this term, including violence against children, women, and elders; abuse of spouses or partners; violence within the context of dating; violence witnessed by children; and abuse and neglect of frail and vulnerable persons. Abuse may also be perpetrated by professionals. While violence associated with state violence (for example, war) is not the focus of this chapter, it is important to recognize that such violence is also interpersonal. Health professionals in Canada provide care to many people who have experienced such violence, including war veterans, refugees, and immigrants.

BOX 25.1   Forms of Violence and Abuse

Physical

Slapping, kicking, hitting with a fist, beating, choking, shoving
Using a weapon against another
Forcibly restraining, confining, or kidnapping another

Sexual

Forcing another to perform sexual acts, e.g., fellatio
Forcing another to have sexual intercourse

Psychological

Name calling, humiliating another, verbally degrading another
Harming property or pets
Creating an atmosphere of fear and terror
Using threats and coercion
Witnessing assault or abuse of another (parent, grandparent, sibling, friend, etc.)
Infantilization

Financial

Taking or withholding money
Extorting funds or property
Taking control of all expenditures
Forcing another to stop working and become dependent
Selling the home or possessions of elderly people without their consent

Social

Imposing (forced) isolation from friends and other family members
Monitoring all phone calls and connection with others

Physical Neglect

Failing to provide food, clothing, shelter, or medical care
Failing to supervise children or elders appropriately

- *Violence in relationships* of kinship, intimacy, dependency, or trust can take the form of physical assault, emotional abuse, intimidation, sexual assault, neglect, deprivation, and financial exploitation. Violence in relationships is commonly referred to as intimate partner violence (IPV).

The multiple definitions of violence and abuse influence how we view violence and where we place emphasis. Terms such as *family violence, domestic abuse, interpersonal violence,* and *violence in relationships* tend to downplay the gender relationships in violence and phrase the behavior in gender-neutral language. Holly Johnson, the primary researcher focused on violence at Statistics Canada (SC), noted that "Men's and boys' experiences of violence are different from women's and girls' in important ways. While men are more likely to be injured by strangers in a public or social venue, women are in greater danger of experiencing violence from intimate partners in their own homes. Women are also at greater risk of sexual violence" (Johnson, 2006, p. 1). According to the 2004 Canadian General Social Survey (GSS), the most recent Canadian population survey as of 2011, in the years between 1995 and 2004, males perpetrated 86% of one-time incidents, 94% of repeat (two to four) incidents, and 97% of chronic incidents of spousal violence

(SC, 2006). In Canada and globally, most perpetrators of violence in families are heterosexual males, and the victims of the most violent crimes are women and children (Bunge & Locke, 2000; Johnson, 2006; SC, 2006; World Health Organization [WHO], 2002). Terms such as *family violence* locate abuse within the family, and draw attention away from society's influence and effects. Nurses must be aware of how the terminology used affects the perceptions of professionals and society at large. Using language that downplays gender relationships and societal influences emphasizes the responsibility of individuals and victims over the responsibility of society.

HISTORICAL PERSPECTIVES ON VIOLENCE AND ABUSE

The abuse of children and of female partners has deep historical roots. Even today, abuse is condoned to varying extents in all societies. Throughout history, children have been sacrificed to appease the gods, killed if they suffered handicapping conditions, and beaten and tortured to "rid them of demons" or to educate them (Humphreys & Ramsey, 1993). It was only in 1962 that Dr. Henry Kempe coined the term *battered child syndrome* (Helfer & Kempe, 1968), which was the impetus for educational campaigns and increased efforts in the United States and Canada to protect children from violence and abuse.

Humphreys and Ramsey (1993) noted that it was the interaction of several factors that focused societal attention and helped raise public concern regarding child abuse. They suggested that the public was affected by the violence in Southeast Asia, namely the United States/Vietnamese conflict, and the rising homicide rates in the United States. Other factors that heightened public awareness of violence were the women's movement, of which the "battered women's movement" was a component (Morrow, 2007), and the interest demonstrated by social scientists studying the phenomenon. This combination of influences led to multiple studies on violence and abuse, with resultant books and articles on the topic. Social agencies were formed, the Society for the Prevention of Child Abuse and Neglect was developed, and laws mandating the prevention of the abuse and neglect of children were updated. In Canada, child abuse and exploitation are prohibited by the Criminal Code (Department of Justice Canada [DJC], 2007a), although policies are inherently contradictory (Varcoe & Einboden, 2010). Most provinces and territories have legislation that makes the reporting of child abuse by the public, including health professionals, mandatory. "Child Welfare in Canada 2000" (Human Resources and Child Welfare Canada [HRCWC], 2000) outlines the roles and responsibilities of provincial and territorial child welfare authorities in the provision of child protection and preventive and support services. If you are working with children, you should review the specific requirements for the jurisdiction in which you are working.

Equally, the abuse of female partners has deep historical roots. Within Christianity, the Bible provides "the earliest prescription for physical punishment of wives" (Campbell & Fishwick, 1993, p. 73). According to these authors, documentation of wife beating can be found throughout European literature—women accused of adultery could be killed with impunity, and instructions for "correcting" wives by beating were available. While violence against women remains a significant problem around the world, the World Health Organization's (WHO's) "World Report on Violence and Health" (2002) and the subsequent WHO multicountry study on women's health and domestic violence (García-Moreno et al., 2005) found that rates varied considerably among different countries, and describes violence against women as both a manifestation and cause of gender inequity, emphasizing the importance of economic inequity. The WHO Summary Report (2005) noted that risk factors for violence against women relating to the immediate social context "included the degree of economic inequality between men and women, levels of female mobility and autonomy, attitudes toward gender roles and violence against women, the extent to which extended family, neighbours, and friends intervene in domestic violence incidents, levels of male–male aggression and crime, and some measure of social capital" (p. 4). While forms of violence against women may have culturally specific features, such as "dowry deaths" in India, the use of wood axes to kill women in Canada, or the stoning of women in some countries, it is important to remember that these are manifestations of gender inequality, not evidence of a cultural propensity to violence.

The prevalence of elder abuse only began to be recognized in the 1970s with initial efforts to "identify the kind and extent of abuse and neglect of seniors" (MacLean & Williams, 1995, p. xi). The Manitoba Association on Gerontology was the first provincial association to begin addressing this subject by developing guidelines to identify elder abuse and protocols for practice (Interdepartmental Working Group on Elder Abuse and Manitoba Seniors Directorate [IWGEAMSD], 1993). In Canada, Elizabeth Podnieks, a nurse, provided early leadership in the study of elder abuse (Podnieks, 1985; Podnieks & Baillie, 1995; Podnieks et al., 1990; Podnieks, 2008). The national prevalence study that she undertook emphasized the scope of elder abuse in Canada and laid the groundwork for further research and intervention efforts.

Increasingly, violence and abuse are seen from an intersectional perspective that moves beyond a gender-only analysis to take into account how class, racialization, colonization, heterosexism, homophobia, and other forms of inequity shape the extent and impact of violence and have particular effects for groups such as Aboriginal women, immigrant and refugee women, women of color, people with disabilities, gay men, and lesbians. Hankivsky and Varcoe (2007) argue that an intersectional perspective:

- shifts from individual to social explanations of violence.
- shifts away from assigning blame and responsibility to victims of violence.
- turns attention to structural inequalities as causing and perpetuating violence.
- focuses on the importance of social policy in reducing and ending violence.

An intersectional perspective on violence is used throughout the remainder of this chapter.

STATISTICS IN THE CANADIAN CONTEXT

Multiple factors contribute to the underreporting of violence and abuse. Widespread ideologies about the causes of violence ("don't some women just ask for it?") and personal responsibility ("why doesn't she just leave?") contribute to misunderstandings and silencing. Shame on the part of the victim and the perpetrator, dependency of the victim on the perpetrator, ignorance of resources, fear of repercussions, and an inability to seek help because of forced restraint all contribute to a code of silence. Judgmental, blameful, incredulous, and other unhelpful or inappropriate responses by potential helpers, including friends, family, and professionals, further such silencing (e.g., Cooper et al., 2004; Lempert, 1997; Tower, 2007; Wilson et al., 2007). For women living in rural and remote areas, distance and lack of resources hinder attempts to escape abusive relationships (Biesenthal et al., 1997; Riddell et al., 2009), factors that are compounded for rural Aboriginal women by racialized discriminatory policies and practices (Varcoe & Dick, 2008). This remoteness helps conceal the true number of incidents of violence. These factors compound the difficulties for young people, elderly people, people with disabilities, and immigrants and other women who may not know where to seek help, may not have the physical means to do so, and may fear and encounter judgment and other inappropriate responses.

The study of violence is hampered by the same factors that lead to underreporting and by the way violence is measured and data collected. To date, the most comprehensive national study of violence against women remains the 1993 Violence Against Women (VAWS) study, conducted by SC and analyzed by numerous researchers (e.g., Johnson, 1996; Kaukinen, 2002). The study used a large random sample and made special efforts to ensure safety so that a range of women could respond. Findings from this study indicated that 29% of women had experienced at least one episode of violence and that two thirds of these women reported that it had happened more than once. Since that time, SC primarily has relied upon modules within the Canadian GSS to obtain data on violence (Johnson, 2006). This data is collected within a more general survey, and does not employ the same safeguards. Johnson notes that because the VAWS was a dedicated survey it focused exclusively on matters relating to violence against women and employed only female interviewers. The 1999 and 2004 GSSs, on the other hand, are general victimization surveys with a special module of questions based on the VAWS related to spousal violence. The GSS employs both male and female interviewers, although respondents are offered the opportunity to switch to an interviewer of the other sex if they are uncomfortable responding to sensitive questions during the interview. As a result of these methodological differences, comparisons between the two surveys must be made with caution (Clark & Dumont, 2003). Seven percent of women who were living in a common-law or marital relationship reported to the 2004 GSS that they had been physically or sexually assaulted by a spousal partner at least once during the previous 5 years, which is a small but statistically significant drop from 8% in 1999, and a decline from the 12% reported in the 1993 VAWS.

Violence Against Women

Criticisms regarding the use of the terms *spousal abuse, conjugal violence, partner violence,* and *domestic abuse* center on the implication that the abuse that women direct against male partners is equal in nature and degree to that committed by men against female partners (Campbell & Fishwick, 1993). There remains a consensus in the statistics on violence and abuse that women continue to suffer the most severe, repetitive, protracted forms of abuse, often resulting in injury and requiring medical attention (Bunge & Locke, 2000; Dobash & Dobash, 1979; SC, 2006). There is also concurrence in the research that female-to-male violence results primarily from acts of self-defense (DeKerseredy & Kelly, 1993). This is consistent with the fact that in Canada men reported far greater incidents of hitting, kicking, biting, and having objects thrown at them than did women (Bunge & Locke, 2000; Johnson, 2006). The concerns regarding the impact of terminology in focusing attention away from the reality of who constitutes the majority of abusers must be kept at the forefront while reading the following statistics.

Findings of the 2004 GSS suggest that, within the previous 5 years, 7% of people who were married or in common-law relationships experienced some form of violence from their intimate partners, with the rates for women and men being similar. However, both the report "Family Violence in Canada: A Statistical Profile 2000" and the more recent "Family Violence in Canada: A Statistical Profile 2006" continue to emphasize that the most severe and consistent forms of violence were reported by women. In general, women are more frequently subjected to severe forms of violence from men than men are from women. For example, women continue to be about four times more likely to be victims of spousal homicide than men. SC reported that in 2007 there were 51 women and 13 men killed by a current or former spouse (Li, 2007).

In 2004, twice as many women than men were beaten by their partners; four times as many were choked; and twice as many female as male victims of spousal assault reported chronic, ongoing assaults (10 or more). In 2000, women made up the vast majority of victims of sexual assault (86%) and other types of sexual offences (78%) (SC, 2001). While 23% of women who report being sexually assaulted are assaulted by strangers (Matas, 2001), based on anonymous surveys, it has been estimated that as many as 90% of sexual assaults are never reported.

Violence in Gay and Lesbian Relationships

Until recent decades, there have been relatively few studies of violence in gay and lesbian relationships. The 2004 GSS was the first to ask Canadians to identify their sexual orientation. In the 2004 GSS gay, lesbian, and bisexual people reported experiencing higher rates of violent victimization including sexual assault, robbery, and physical assault, both by family members and strangers, than did their heterosexual counterparts. Ristock (2001) conducted a multisite qualitative study of violence experienced in lesbian relationships. Service providers (counselors, shelter workers, and social workers) who participated in focus groups noted that basing their efforts on heterosexual dynamics limited their practice. Ristock highlighted that some concerns were raised—chief among them that drawing attention to violence in lesbian relationships will detract from feminist efforts to raise awareness that violence perpetrated by men continues to be a significant social issue.

Although the focus on gender-based violence is challenged by the reporting of same-sex violence, these reports emphasize the need for the further examination of power and control as key factors in violence and abuse. Key questions that may be asked are, "where is power held within a society?" and "what is the relationship between gender and power?" Of importance in this discussion is the relationship to the social context in which this violence occurs. Victims of same-sex violence may fear being stigmatized as gay or lesbian and may expect their complaints to be trivialized (Duffy & Momirov, 2000). In a society that remains largely homophobic, the dynamics of violence within same-sex relationships are even more complex than those of opposite-sex relationships. This complexity will continue to contribute to the silencing of the issues in violent and abusive same-sex relationships.

Abuse and Neglect of Older Canadians

Elder abuse and neglect encompasses IPV that continues into older adulthood and forms of abuse and neglect that arise as persons become more vulnerable with age. As with any form of IPV, IPV in older adults is gendered—that is, older women are at higher risk than men. One of the leading studies on the abuse and neglect of older Canadians found that 4% of respondents reported financial, material, and verbal abuse by family members and other people (Podnieks et al., 1990). Ten years later, 7% of older adults in the GSS reported experiencing emotional abuse in the form of name calling, being put down, being isolated from friends and family, or being taken advantage of financially by a spouse, caregiver, or child (Bunge & Locke, 2000). One must keep in mind that older people may be reluctant or afraid to report abuse by family members for various reasons, among them dependency, feelings of shame, and fear of retaliation.

Elder abuse and neglect includes violence in the home, violence in institutions, and self-neglect (McDonald & Collins, 2000). Older adults who become frail and require medical or other health-related services may experience abuse. In this context, abuse of older adults may involve failing to facilitate their access to medical or health services, failing to provide medical attention due to age, or conducting a procedure or providing treatment without the informed consent of the patient or their recognized substitute. Although age can increase vulnerability, it is important to note that other factors such as economic dependence; disabilities, such as developmental, mental, and physical; and rural isolation also increase vulnerability to violence, intersecting with age and gender. Walsh et al. (2011) found that increased vulnerability to elder abuse was related to oppression experienced as a consequence of ageism, sexism, ableism/disability, racism, heterosexism/homophobia, classism, and various intersecting types of oppression. Similarly, Brozowski and Hall (2010) found that women, Aboriginal Canadians, and elders who are divorced and living in urban areas with low income experienced higher levels of physical and sexual abuse. Importantly, as elder care is increasingly shifted to family care providers, nurses must consider how their expectations for family caregiving might contribute to conditions that give rise to abuse.

Research is increasingly focused on violence and abuse of elderly people living in institutions (e.g., Conner et al., 2011; Post et al., 2010; Zhenmei et al., 2011). Abuse of the elderly in institutional settings includes overt acts of physical abuse such as extensive use of restraints as well as hitting, pinching, and shoving, and more covert abuses such as limiting freedom and choice, providing inadequate nutrition, and isolating people. Those with responsibility for the care of the residents—the people who were in power—are commonly the abusers.

In police-reported statistics of elder abuse, most offenders are strangers and people outside the family. According to statistics from the "Incident-based Uniform Crime Reporting Survey," older Canadians were 67% more likely to be abused by strangers than by family members (Bunge & Locke, 2000). Although the numbers are relatively small, people who deliberately target elderly people in home invasions and fraud figure prominently in the media. The most recent statistics available are based on police reports (SC, 2007).

Violence Against Children and Youth

Child maltreatment is an all-encompassing term that includes the physical, sexual, and emotional abuse and neglect of children. Although child maltreatment is recognized as a significant problem in Canada, no data set consolidates all of the provincial statistics to present a comprehensive national picture. Data on cases of child maltreatment are based on child welfare caseloads, police files on assault and homicide, and hospitalizations for violence-related injuries (Bunge & Locke, 2000). Child welfare is a provincial responsibility, and, although each province has legislation defining child abuse and neglect, a lack of common definitions across jurisdictions precludes the formation of a single national data set.

Understandings of child abuse often focus on the problem as though it occurs in isolation from other forms of abuse and wider social conditions, and often focus on severe forms of physical abuse or more sensational incidents of sexual abuse, rather than on the more common forms of child maltreatment—neglect and emotional abuse. It is important to note that child abuse often overlaps with IPV against women with estimates that children are abused in up to 70% of families in which women are abused (Folsom et al., 2003). It is also important to note that perceptions of what constitutes abuse shift over time and are shaped by changing class and social attitudes. For example, in many Canadian jurisdictions, children who witness violence (usually against their mothers) are considered to be abused, and in such cases fear of child apprehension by the state may be a barrier to women seeking help in relation to abuse. Finally, it is critical to note that there is a high rate of unsubstantiated reports of child abuse.

Estimates of child abuse are difficult to make because they largely rely on *reported* cases. Based on data from child welfare authorities, the "Canadian Incidence Study of Reported Child Abuse and Neglect" estimated that there were 135,573 child maltreatment investigations in Canada in 1998. This was a rate of 21.52 investigations of child maltreatment per 1,000 children. Forty-five percent of these investigations were substantiated; 22% remained suspected; and 33% were found to be unsubstantiated (Public Health Agency of Canada, 2001). The greatest proportion of both reported and substantiated child abuse cases were of neglect. This report suggests that insufficient attention has been paid to neglect in comparison with the attention to risk assessment and urgent intervention for severe physical abuse and in comparison to sexual abuse, possibly in part because it is more sensational. Trocmé et al. (2003) argue that because 96% of substantiated cases did not involve severe physical harm, assessment and investigation priorities need to be revised and include consideration of long-term service needs. Importantly, socioeconomic status has been consistently shown to be related to parenting effectiveness (Wekerle et al., 2009), also suggesting that assessment for longer-term, broader social support is required.

Although there are mandatory reporting laws for child abuse, it is accepted that official accounts of child maltreatment underestimate the prevalence because of the failure to report by perpetrators and victims, by community members who observe abuse, and by professionals who fail to recognize the maltreatment (MacMillan et al., 1997). It is thought that as many as 90% of cases are not reported to child welfare authorities (MacMillan et al., 1997). An issue is why, with mandatory reporting laws for child abuse and neglect, underreporting persists. A question for professionals and for society is why and how this silence regarding a significant social and health problem continues.

Children and youth represented 60% of sexual assault victims and 20% of physical assault victims reported in Canada in 1999 (Bunge & Locke, 2000). Acquaintances were the primary abusers (52%), with the remaining perpetrators being family members (24%) and strangers (19%). Girls were victimized more often than boys in 80% of sexual assault cases and 53% of physical assault cases.

An additional concern is the incidence of violence toward children and youth, perpetrated by their peers. In a compelling account of prejudice in public schools, Adrienne Dessel (2010) relates that prejudicial attitudes contribute to problematic inter-group relations and bullying among children and youth. Of particular note is the bullying of children who are seen as falling outside of a typical gender presentation by their peers and are subsequently labeled as gay, lesbian, bisexual, transgendered, or queer (lgbtq). Whether or not these children actually identify as nonheterosexual, the harassment and bullying of youth in these circumstances leads to significant distress and in some cases to youth suicide (Savage & Miller, 2011). Media attention has been focused on this issue through the internet "It get's better campaign," which has drawn participation from across North America and abroad with more than 10,000 video postings on YouTube to the project since it's 2010 inception. Closer to home, in 2007, two Nova Scotia high school students began the Pink Shirt Day campaign in response to the bullying of a grade 9 student labeled homosexual and threatened with violence for wearing a pink polo shirt to school. This innovative strategy has spread across the country as an annual campaign to combat bullying in schools. Check out the Pink Shirt Day Web site to find out about the annual day to stand up against bullying in your province.

Violence in Aboriginal Communities

Violence in Aboriginal communities must be understood in the context of historical and ongoing colonization of Aboriginal people in Canada. Aboriginal people in Canada have been systematically stripped of their lands, ways of living, culture, language, and freedom, with extensive effects on their health and well-being. These colonizing practices and the system of confining Aboriginal people to reserves and requiring children to attend residential school has had extensive long-term effects (Adelson, 2005; Smith et al., 2005). Aboriginal people face ongoing discrimination and racialization, including in their experiences of health care (Bourassa et al., 2004; Browne, 2007; Fiske & Browne, 2006). Aboriginal women have been particularly disadvantaged through gender-biased policies and face disproportionate socioeconomic burdens—such as poverty and isolation—that magnify the difficulties they face in dealing with violence (Dion Stout, 1998; MacMillan et al., 1996).

High rates of violence experienced by Aboriginal people generally, and women and children particularly, and social responses to their experiences of violence are shaped by these colonizing processes (Brownridge, 2003; SC, 2006). According to SC, 24% of Aboriginal women experienced spousal abuse in the 5 years preceding the 2004 GSS, compared with 7% of women in the general population. Aboriginal women in Canada are eight times more likely than non-Aboriginal women to be killed by their partners and experience more severe IPV than the rest of the population (SC, 2006). Aboriginal children are much more likely to be investigated for maltreatment, and investigations are more likely to be substantiated, more likely to be kept open for ongoing services, and more likely to result in children being placed in out-of-home care (Blackstock et al., 2004).

While all victims of violence face possible judgment, disbelief, and discrimination, Aboriginal people in particular can anticipate such responses that operate as barriers to help. In one community survey, 63% of respondents reported they had experienced violence and abuse, whereas 76% were aware that family members had been abused (Thomlinson et al., 2000). However, only 37% disclosed that violence to people in authority. Fear of repercussions and a lack of trust that reporting would introduce a change contributed to this lack of reporting.

According to the Report of the Royal Commission on Aboriginal Peoples (1996), although it is impossible to ascertain the full extent of violence in Aboriginal communities, the topic is distinctive from other communities in that "[violence] has invaded whole communities and cannot be considered a problem of a particular couple or an individual household" (p. 56). The interrelationship of poverty and social and economic marginalization of many Aboriginal communities is believed to contribute to an increase in violence and abuse (Hamby, 2000). Without efforts that will substantially change conditions in the community, attempts to address violence will continue to experience only minor success.

Dating Violence

As they do in other forms of violence, women suffer more severe, pervasive, and systematic victimization in dating relationships (Canadian Public Health Association [CPHA], 1994) than do men. The "Department of Justice Canada's Fact Sheet" (2007b) on dating violence summarizes the few available studies and concludes that although it is difficult to know the prevalence with any accuracy, violence in dating relationships is common. According to a survey of college and university students, 45% of women had been sexually assaulted while in a dating relationship, 79% had been psychologically abused, and 35% had been physically abused (DeKerseredy & Kelly, 1993). DeKerseredy and Kelly caution that although this survey pointed to high percentages of dating violence, these statistics should be regarded as underestimates for reasons similar to those of other forms of violence and abuse.

Violence in the Workplace

Violence in the workplace, including sexual harassment, is also deeply gendered (Hinch & DeKeseredy, 1994). According to Mireille Kingma, nurse consultant with the International Council of Nurses, "72% of nurses do not feel safe from assault in their workplace," and "97% of nurse respondents in a British survey knew a nurse who had been physically assaulted in the past year and up to 95% reported having been bullied at work" (International Council of Nurses [ICN], 1999). In the United States, Carroll and Morin (1998) reported that one third of nurses working in general areas were affected by workplace violence. In Sweden, Arnetz et al. (1998) found that the incidence of violence toward practical nurses was 31 incidents per 100 person years. Poster (1996) found that 75% of 999 psychiatric nursing staff in Canada, the United States, the United Kingdom, and South Africa reported being assaulted at least once during their careers.

In Canada, the CPHA (1994) concluded that up to 70% of nurses have been abused or threatened on the job, including being hit, kicked, verbally abused, and sexually harassed. A survey of hospital nurses in British Columbia and Alberta found that 46% of those surveyed had experienced one or more types of violence in the last five shifts worked, including emotional abuse 38%, threat of assault 19%, physical assault 18%, verbal sexual harassment 7.6%, and sexual assault 0.6% (Duncan et al., 2001). Such abuse has profound health and social effects (Chapman et al., 2009; O'Donnell et al., 2010; MacIntosh et al., 2010).

One of the issues that is relevant to the safety of nurses and that ultimately affects the recruitment and retention of nurses in the workplace is the continued lack of reporting and tolerance of abuse against nurses. Of the 5,000 nurses who responded to a survey by the Manitoba Association of Registered Nurses (1989), between one fourth and one third noted that they chose to ignore abusive behavior directed toward them in the workplace. Factors affecting this decision are relevant to analysis of this issue. More recently, Duncan et al. (2001) found that 70% of those who had experienced violence indicated they had not reported it.

UNDERSTANDING VIOLENCE: THEORETICAL PERSPECTIVES

Since the 1970s, a number of theoretical approaches have been proposed in the effort to understand factors related to the violence and abuse of people, mainly women and children (Campbell & Fishwick, 1993; Duffy & Momirov, 2000; Gelles, 1980; Hankivsky & Varcoe, 2007). Gelles classified three different types of models: The psychiatric or intraindividual model, the social–psychological model, and the sociologic model. The focus of assessments and interventions varies depending on the type of model to which one subscribes: Individuals, individuals in context, or society at large. Beliefs and myths regarding violence and abuse that arise from the underlying theoretical framework will affect how one chooses to interact with individuals who are experiencing abusive situations.

From Inside the Individual

Intraindividual explanations tend to pathologize abusive men as psychopaths and female victims as masochists. Innes et al. (1991) noted that studies focusing on the mental health of men and women in abusive relationships demonstrated a bias against women by blaming the victims. Campbell and Fishwick (1993) contend that vestiges of the masochism myth remain today when authors suggest that a woman provoked a man to batter her. As early as 1979, Walker, (1979) stated that by blaming the victims, men are ultimately excused of their abusive behaviors. Innes, et al. (1991) further noted that men rarely demonstrate the same violent actions outside the home but confine their abuse to where they will avoid castigation, thus pointing to the importance of the social environment.

Environment and Interaction

The social–psychological model focuses on the interaction of the environment and the individual and the family. In child abuse cases, Helfer and Kempe hypothesized that an interaction occurs between the child, the caretaker, and the circumstance that predisposes toward violence (Helfer & Kempe, 1968). Social learning theory (Bandura, 1969) is the basis for the suggestion that growing up in violent homes predisposes children toward violent behavior (Duffy & Momirov, 2000). This model has been used to explain the intergenerational transmission of violence in which the members of each generation of a family continues the violent and abusive behaviors that were perpetrated against them or that they observed against others in the family; however, the evidence for this theory is questionable (Ozturk Ertem et al., 2000).

Tolerance of Violence

Sociologic models contend that violence and abuse occur in environments that tolerate, and even foster, violent actions. Garbarino's ecologic model of child abuse stresses the effect of the continued support of force in the care of children and multiple factors that affect the family (Garbarino, 1977; Garbarino, 1995; Garbarino & Kostelny, 1992; Garbarino & Sherman, 1980). A key component of this model is the incorporation of societal beliefs and values along with other factors that affect the family, such as housing, poverty, social supports, and reactions of others in the family and community.

Feminist Perspective

Feminist analysis emphasizes the role of patriarchal culture in legitimizing male violence against both women and children (Duffy & Momirov, 2000). The power and control that men hold in the corporate world, in government, in religious institutions, and in society as a whole facilitate male use of power and control in the home (Wiehe, 1998). Violence and abuse ensure continued control over women and children. Feminist analysis has contributed to the exploration of violence through examination of how race, culture, disability, social class, age, and sexual orientation affect the experiences that women of all ages have in society. Duffy and Momirov (2000) suggest that inclusion of violence in lesbian relationships in this dialogue has forced feminists to focus more attention on the issues of power and control rather than remaining concentrated on gender-based relationships.

Intersectional Analysis

As outlined at the beginning of this chapter, an intersectional analysis (which is a sociological model) explicitly examines how multiple forms of oppression and privilege operate simultaneously to shape experiences of violence (Crenshaw, 1994; Mosher, 1998; Hankivsky & Varcoe, 2007). This perspective overlaps with feminist perspectives, which often treat gender as the most salient aspect of social location. However, while gender is important, we are all shaped by the privileging and marginalizing processes of class, racialization, sexual orientation, ability, and so on. Taking larger societal variables, including historical and cultural perspectives, into account helps explain why certain groups of women (e.g., Aboriginal women, rural women, immigrant women, women of color, women living with disabilities, and women living in poverty) face more violence and more barriers to social support in relation to violence. Prejudice, economic marginalization, and social powerlessness are key factors in the lives of both the abused and the abusers.

IMPACT ON HEALTH AND THE HEALTHCARE SYSTEM

Violence and abuse present formidable costs to the health of individuals and families and to society. The short- and long-term effects of violence on health are well established. IPV against women is associated with *direct effects* of physical injuries such as bruises and fractures (Muellman et al., 1996); *chronic physical health problems,* such as chronic pain, arthritis, frequent headaches and migraines, visual problems, unexplained dizziness and fainting, sexually transmitted infections, unwanted pregnancies, gynecological symptoms, hypertension, viral infections such as the flu, peptic ulcers, and functional or irritable bowel disease (Campbell & Lewandowski, 1997; Carbone-López et al., 2006; Hill et al., 2009; Leserman & Drossman, 2007; Kendall-Tackett et al., 2003; Wuest et al., 2007); and *mental health problems,* including clinical depression, acute and chronic symptoms of anxiety, serious sleep disturbances, symptoms consistent with post-traumatic stress syndrome (PTSD), substance use and dependence, and thoughts of suicide (Campbell, 2002; Cascardi et al., 1999; Fischbach & Herbert, 1997; Mechanic et al., 2008; Sleutel, 1998; Wiehe, 1998). These health effects lead to significant suffering for women and incur significant interference with their lives. For example, various sources estimate that abused women suffer losses of up to $7 million annually in wages and productivity (Duffy & Momirov, 2000).

Violence also incurs expenditures for the state, including the Canadian healthcare system, when victims seek medical care. Financial costs to police, child welfare and victim counseling services, the court system, social services, shelters, and foster-home care as well as costs incurred for imprisoning offenders, for second-stage housing, and the incalculable costs in human suffering contribute to the impact of violence and abuse on individuals and society. Greaves, Hankivsky, and Kingston-Riechers (1995) used the Canadian Violence Against Women study to calculate the proportion of some costs attributable to violence in three forms of violence—sexual assault, violence in intimate partnerships, and incest and child sexual assault—and estimated $4.2 billion spent in four policy areas—health and medicine, criminal justice, social services and education, and labor and employment. In 1996, Kerr and McLean estimated that the health costs in British Columbia were at least $385 million annually. Estimates suggest that more than 100,000 inpatient hospital days can be attributed to violence (CPHA, 1994). With hospital bed costs ranging from $400 to $800 a day, this would result in expenditures between $40 and $80 million annually in Canada as a result of violence. More recently it was estimated that the partial excess costs attributable to violence incur a national annual cost of $6.9 billion just for women aged 19 to 65 who have left abusive partners (Varcoe et al., in press).

Child maltreatment can lead to severe, long-term emotional and academic problems. Abused children have difficulty concentrating, have little anger control, may suffer from eating disorders, and are at high risk for dropping out of school (Wiehe, 1998). Koniak-Griffin and Lesser (1996) found that child maltreatment was a significant predictor of self-injurious behavior and attempted suicide. In Canada from 1997 to 1998, childhood admissions for acknowledged cases of assault and other maltreatment such as battering, rape, fighting, strangulation, firearms, and stabbings were 2,359 per 100,000 population (Bunge & Locke, 2000). A total of 38 in every 100,000 children under the age of 1 year were admitted to a hospital as a result of child abuse. Considering that many more cases of abuse are never reported or go unrecognized, these are significant numbers. The cost to the healthcare system and in lost human potential and suffering because of the maltreatment of children and youth is incalculable.

As noted previously, there is a growing awareness that even if they themselves are not abused, children who live in a home where mothers are battered and where violence between parents occurs may experience PTSD (Humphreys, 1993; Lehmann, 2000). Behavioral responses of these children include truancy, disturbed sleep patterns, decreased school performance, lack of positive peer relations, increased worry for their mothers, and fear. Children who are exposed to violence and abuse learn that violence is the way to settle problems and achieve their own ends (Beauchesne et al., 1997). Pynoos and Nader (1990) examined four main types of symptoms experienced by children who have observed violent and abusive incidents: PTSD, grief reactions, separation anxiety symptoms, and exacerbation or renewal of previous symptoms. They found that exposure to violence may have long-term detrimental effects on a child's cognitive development.

ISSUES FOR NURSES AND THE NURSING PROFESSION

Nursing associations at all levels, provincially, nationally, and internationally, advocate that nurses take an active role in addressing problems of violence by increasing their knowledge of issues associated with violence and abuse (e.g., Registered Nurses Association of Ontario [RNAO], 2009).

Many nursing associations advocate zero tolerance for interpersonal violence and violence in the workplace. How should nurses enhance their nursing practice?

Language

The use of gender-neutral language in discussing all types of interpersonal violence erroneously creates the impression that violence and abuse are committed equally by men and women in society. A careful examination of the statistics on the types and circumstances surrounding any violence and abuse provides a more comprehensive picture of what actually is occurring. Nurses, as professionals and as members of society, have a role to play in recognizing that the use of a particular language can obscure and slant perceptions of what really is happening in violent and abusive relationships. Further, language that labels (e.g., "battered women") reduces the person to their experience of violence. Hence, it is important to use language that acknowledges the person, not just the problem (e.g., "women who have been battered").

Lack of Understanding

A second issue arises from a lack of understanding about the pervasiveness of violence. Multiple myths about violence and abuse affect how healthcare professionals respond to and treat people involved in violent situations. One myth that continues to pervade society is that it is mainly people living in poverty who act violently toward others. Healthcare providers, then, do not consider that professionals and people from upper socioeconomic brackets could be victims or perpetrators of violence within their families. The effect of holding onto this perception is that poor people may be stereotyped as violent and the effects minimized as being part of the culture, whereas others receive little intervention because "[violence] cannot possibly be happening in that home." A related myth is the idea that people from certain racialized groups are inherently more violent. It is critical for nurses to recognize that it is mistaken to use population statistics, such as higher rates of violence experienced by Aboriginal women, to predict individual behaviors such as anticipating violence when caring for a particular Aboriginal person. For example, in one Canadian study, nurses acting on stereotypes and inappropriate application of population statistics tended to anticipate IPV among poor and racialized people and to anticipate child abuse in Aboriginal families (Varcoe, 2001).

Other Issues

Other issues that require analysis include the following:

- The persistent underreporting of child abuse cases
- The need for prevention and recognition of abuse of elders who live in their own homes or the homes of family members, not in institutions, especially as more families are expected to provide care
- The need for comprehensive approaches to interpersonal violence within healthcare settings
- The ongoing lack of reporting of violence against nurses in the workplace.

BARRIERS TO RESOLUTION

The pervasiveness of abuse and violence through all ages, classes, cultures, and ethnicities and across genders and national and international political boundaries underlies and hampers efforts to address the issues surrounding the topic. This pervasiveness means that victims of violence, as well as the perpetrators, exist in all sectors of society, including the healthcare professions. The strong need to deny abuse, to keep silent, pervades society. This social and political reality counters efforts for change. The silence that has permitted and even encouraged violence and abuse is complex, not easily understood, and universal.

A key factor that reinforces the silencing of abuse is a societal belief in the sanctity of the family: What occurs within the walls of the home is private. A belief that parents and spouses are permitted to control what goes on in the family and to discipline family members is another component. Power differences based on age, gender, ability, ethnicity, class, geography, citizenship, language, and sexual orientation that underlie society, as noted previously in the chapter, affect relationships at all levels. The perpetrators of abuse may be in positions of power in government, justice, and throughout the rest of society. Secrecy permits them to continue to abuse. Power in relationships such as nurse–patient interactions contributes to the opportunity for abuse to occur; there is sometimes little recognition given to the type and amount of power that health professionals hold over their patients. Indeed, failure to recognize and counter barriers to social support, such as using interpreters for those who cannot adequately communicate in the dominant language, recognizing the dynamics of economic dependence, and countering racial stereotypes, can directly contribute to the continuation of abuse.

Another element may be the helplessness that professionals may feel regarding their inability to understand the dynamics of violence and to intervene. It is easier not to ask questions about violence than to ask questions that might reveal an abusive relationship and not know how to interact and intervene. Professionals may subvert their assessments by the manner in which they ask questions regarding violence. Those who choose to speak out may be silenced by coworkers and others who wish to have the abuse and violence remain secret. The complex interactions that yield this ongoing silencing suggest that there may be no easy solutions.

STRATEGIES FOR RESOLUTION

No one professional can successfully work toward ending the silence about abuse and violence in isolation from others. Developing partnerships across disciplines and with victims of violence requires concerted effort to build confidence and trust. Although this is a time-consuming process, effective intervention programs can develop out of such alliances. Interdisciplinary courses are an important component.

Interdisciplinary Education and Intervention

Interdisciplinary education programs and intervention protocols for health and social service professionals remain underdeveloped. This issue is particularly relevant to nurses because they are in key positions to advocate for patients, to educate others, to promote healthy relationships, to identify abuse and violence, and to intervene. To act, nurses must be knowledgeable about the dynamics of abuse; they must understand the extent to which those with whom they work share that knowledge; and they must understand the roles the nursing profession has in addressing violence and abuse.

Victims of violence consistently reported that healthcare providers are judgmental, uncaring, and often the least helpful category of professionals to whom they have gone for assistance (American Academy of Nurses Expert Panel on Violence [AANEPV], 1993; Bacchus et al., 2003; Gerbert et al., 1999; McCloskey & Grigsby, 2005; Tower, 2007). Globally, nursing associations condemn violence of all forms. Yet, despite this convergence of opinion and the consensus that everyone has the right to a life free of violence and abuse, the development of interdisciplinary curricula has been slow. This suggests that political action is necessary.

Political Action

The societal and cultural issues underlying the reticence to deal with issues involving violence and abuse are key factors affecting the procrastination in developing joint curricula. The approach of healthcare professionals to focus on the short-term treatment of the signs and symptoms of violence places the onus on the individual to correct the problem and does not demand change within society. Compartmentalization and a focus on the physical effects of violence and abuse also, then, do not require that professionals accept responsibility to address the broader implications of abuse and violence.

Continued joint efforts of professional associations at the national and provincial levels are needed for developing interdisciplinary curricula on abuse and violence. As with all other issues, there must be individuals within the various organizations who will advocate for these education programs. The efforts to lobby faculties of nursing, medicine, dentistry, physiotherapy, and occupational therapy must be undertaken by those who recognize and believe in the need to address this issue. An example of an organization that could be used in this lobby in western Canada is

RESOLVE (Research and Education for Solutions to Violence and Abuse), an interdisciplinary community and academic organization working across Manitoba, Saskatchewan, and Alberta toward ending abuse and violence (http://www.umanitoba.ca/resolve). Joint research and education organizations exist in other regions of the country and the involvement of professionals from multiple disciplines working with community members strengthens the efforts and potentiates success. Importantly, the Nursing Network On Violence Against Women International is an organization that brings together women, nurses, and researchers from around the world. The commitment of time and energy to establish working relationships with members of other disciplines can facilitate efforts to address this issue.

SUMMARY

The enormity and pervasiveness of violence and abuse across society are emphasized and validated by the thousands of books and articles on the topic. The financial and human costs of violence are incalculable but extensive, affecting intimate relationships and all segments of society, particularly the people who are most vulnerable: Elderly people, disabled people, Aboriginal people, immigrant people and those from racialized minorities, and children. Violence in the workplace affects nurses and other health professionals.

Nurses are in strategic positions to address issues of violence and abuse because they are among the most trusted professionals, are accessible to the public, and are often the first professionals met by those seeking health care.

Nurses, therefore, must become knowledgeable about violence and abuse, develop the skills to assess and intervene in cases of violence and abuse, and work in interdisciplinary teams to provide comprehensive care. To do any less is a disservice to patients and the profession.

Add to your knowledge of this issue: *Online*

Canadian Network for the Prevention of Elder Abuse	**http://www.cnpea.ca**
Canadian Women's Foundation Violence Prevention Fund	**http://www.cdnwomen.org**
Center for Research on Violence Against Women and Children	**http://www.crvawc.ca**
Family and Intimate Partner Violence Prevention Team	**www.cdc.gov**
Family Violence in Canada	**www.statcan.ca**
National Clearinghouse on Family Violence	**www.hc-sc.gc.ca**
National Council Against Domestic Violence	**www.ncadv.org**
National Council on Child Abuse and Family Violence	**www.nccafv.org**
Nursing Network On Violence Against Women International	**http://www.nnvawi.org**
Seniors Canada—Elder Abuse	**http://www.seniors.gc.ca**

R E F L E C T I O N S *on the Chapter...*

1 What images do you have when you hear the terms *family violence, woman abuse,* and *abuse of the elderly*? Who are the main characters in your images and what are they doing?

2 Compile a list of accounts from newspapers, television, and radio from the past week that dealt with violence and abuse. How do these reports counter or reinforce harmful stereotypes? What impact would these incidents have on the health of the population? Were health issues addressed in these accounts?

3 If you have had a patient divulge that she or he had been abused, what steps did you take to assist this person? What steps might you take having read this chapter? What resources could you draw on to guide your actions?

4 What attitudes have you heard expressed that would provide a caring atmosphere for any person (patient or nurse) who divulges abuse? What attitudes would hinder or suppress disclosing this type of information?

5 On which of the many facets of violence and abuse would you choose to focus your attention if you were asked to undertake a project of prevention? Where would you begin your efforts?

6 What resources are available in your work environment that would help you care for and deal with the emotional impact of working with victims of violence?

Want to know more? Visit the Point for additional helpful resources:

- Journal Articles
- Learning Objectives
- Nursing Professional Roles and Responsibilities
- Bonus chapters:
  - Health and Nursing Policy: A Matter of Politics, Power and Professionalism
  - The NP Movement: Recurring Issues
  - When Difference Matters: The Politics of Privilege and Marginality

References

Adelson, N. (2005). The embodiment of inequity: Health disparities in Aboriginal Canada. *Canadian Journal of Public Health, 96*(Suppl. 2), S45–S61.

American Academy of Nurses Expert Panel on Violence. (1993). Violence as a nursing priority: Policy implications. *Nursing Outlook, 41*(2), 83–92.

Arnetz, J.E., Arnetz, B.B., & Soderman, E. (1998). Violence toward health care workers: Prevalence and incidence at a large regional hospital in Sweden. *AAOHN, 46*(3), 107–114.

Bacchus, L., Mezey, G., & Bewley, S. (2003). Experiences of seeking help from health professionals in a sample of women who experienced domestic violence. *Health & Social Care in the Community, 11*(1), 10–18.

Bandura, A. (1969). Social-learning theory of identificatory processes. In D.A. Goslin (Ed.), *Handbook of socialization theory and research* (pp. 213–262). Chicago, IL: Rand McNally.

Beauchesne, M., Kelley, B.R., Lawrence, P.R., & Farquharson, P.E. (1997). Violence prevention: A community approach. *Journal of Pediatric Health Care, 11*, 179–188.

Biesenthal, L., Sproule, L.D., & Plocica, Z. (1997). *Violence against women in rural communities in Canada: Research project backgrounder.* Ottawa, ON: Research and Statistics Division, Department of Justice, Canada.

Blackstock, C., Trocmé, N., & Bennett, M. (2004). Child maltreatment investigations among Aboriginal and non-Aboriginal Families in Canada. *Violence Against Women, 10*(8), 901–916.

Bourassa, C., McKay-McNabb, K., & Hampton, M.R. (2004). Racism, sexism, and colonialism: The impact on the health of Aboriginal women in Canada. *Canadian Woman Studies, 24*(1), 23–29.

Browne, A.J. (2007). Clinical encounters between nurses and First Nations women in a Western Canadian hospital. *Social Science & Medicine, 64*(10), 2165–2176.

Brownridge, D. (2003). Male partner violence against Aboriginal women in Canada: An empirical analysis. *Journal of Interpersonal Violence, 18*(1), 65–83.

Brozowski, K., & Hall, D.R. (2010). Aging and risk: Physical and sexual abuse of Elders in Canada. *Journal of Interpersonal Violence, 25*, 1183–1199.

Bullied student tickled pink by schoolmates' T-shirt campaign. Wednesday, September 19, 2007 CBC News http://www.cbc.ca/news/canada/nova-scotia/story/2007/09/18/pink-tshirts-students.html

Bunge, V.P., & Locke, D. (2000). *Family violence in Canada: A statistical profile.* Ottawa, ON: Minister of Industry. Retrieved from http://www.statcan.ca (Catalogue 85-224-XIE Canadian Centre for Justice Statistics).

Campbell, J.C., & Fishwick, N. (1993). Abuse of female partners. In J. Campbell & J. Humphreys (Eds.), *Nursing care of survivors of family violence* (pp. 68–106). St. Louis, MO: Mosby.

Campbell, J.C., & Lewandowski, L. (1997). Mental and physical health effects of intimate partner violence on women and children. *Psychiatric Clinics of North America, 20*(2), 353–374.

Campbell, J.C. (2002). Health consequences of intimate partner violence. *The Lancet, 359*, 1331–1336.

Canadian Public Health Association. (1994). *Violence in society: A public health perspective* (Issue Paper). Ottawa, ON: Author.

Carbone-López, K., Kruttschnitt, C., & MacMillan, R. (2006). Patterns of intimate partner violence and their associations with physical health, psychological distress, and substance use. *Public Health Reports, 121*(4), 382–392.

Carroll, V., & Morin, K.H. (1998). Workplace violence affects one-third of nurses: Survey of nurses in seven SNA's reveals staff nurses most at risk. *American Nurses, 30*(5), 15.

Cascardi, M., O'Leary, D.K., & Schlee, K.A. (1999). Co-occurrence and correlates of posttraumatic stress disorder and major depression in physically abused women. *Journal of Family Violence, 14*(3), 227–249.

Chapman, R., Perry, L., Styles, I., & Combs, S. (2009). Consequences of workplace violence directed at nurses. *British Journal of Nursing (BJN), 18*, 1256–1261.

Clark, J., & DuMont, J. (2003). Intimate partner violence and health: A critique of Canadian prevalence studies. *Canadian Journal of Public Health, 94*(1), 52–58.

Conner, T., Prokhorov, A., Page, C., Fang, Y., Xiao, Y., & Post, L.A. (2011). Impairment and abuse of elderly by staff in long-term care in Michigan: Evidence from structural equation modeling. *Journal of Interpersonal Violence, 26*, 21–33.

Cooper, H., Moore, L., Gruskin, S., & Krieger, N. (2004). Characterizing perceived police violence: Implications for public health. *American Journal of Public Health, 94*(7), 1109–1118.

Crenshaw, K.W. (1994). Mapping the margins: Intersectionality, identity politics, and violence against women of color. In M.A. Fineman & R. Mykitiuk (Eds.), *The public nature of private violence* (pp. 93–118). New York: Routledge.

DeKerseredy, W.S., & Kelly, K. (1993). The incidence and prevalence of woman abuse in Canadian university and college dating relationships. *Canadian Journal of Sociology, 18*(2), 137–159.

Department of Justice Canada. (2007a). Child abuse fact sheet. *Journal.* Retrieved from http://www.justice.gc.ca/en/ps/fm/childafs.html

———. (2007b). Dating violence: A fact sheet from the Department of Justice Canada. *Journal.* Retrieved from http://www.justice.gc.ca/en/ps/fm/datingfs.html#head2

Dessel, A. (2010). Prejudice in schools: Promotion of an inclusive culture and climate. *Education and Urban Society, 42*, 407–429.

Dion Stout, M. (1998). *Aboriginal Canada: Women and health—A Canadian perspective.* Retrieved April 29, 1998 from http://www.hc-sc.gc.ca/hl-vs/alt_formats/hpb-dgps/pdf/indigen_e.pdf.

Dobash, R.E., & Dobash, R.P. (1979). *Violence against wives.* New York: Free Press.

Duffy, A., & Momirov, J. (2000). Family violence: Issues and advances at the end of the twentieth century. In N. Mandell & A. Duffy (Eds.), *Canadian families: Diversity, conflict, and change* (pp. 290–322). Toronto, ON: Harcourt Canada.

Duncan, S., Hyndman, K., Estabrooks, C., et al. (2001). Nurses' experience of violence in Alberta and British Columbia hospitals. *Canadian Journal of Nursing Research, 32*(4), 57–78.

Fischbach, R., & Herbert, B. (1997). Domestic violence and mental health: Correlates and conundrums within and across cultures. *Social Science & Medicine, 45*(8), 1161–1176.

Fiske, J.A., & Browne, A. (2006). Aboriginal citizen, discredited medical subject: Paradoxical constructions of Aboriginal women's subjectivity in Canadian health care policies. *Policy Sciences, 39*(1), 91–111.

Folsom, W., Christensen, M., Avery, L., & Moore, C. (2003). The co-occurrence of child abuse and domestic violence. *Child and Adolescent Social Work Journal, 20*(5), 375–387.

Garbarino, J., & Kostelny, K. (1992). Child maltreatment as a community problem. *Child Abuse and Neglect, 16*, 455–464.

Garbarino, J., & Sherman, D. (1980). High-risk neighborhoods and high-risk families: The human ecology of child maltreatment. *Child Development, 51*, 188–198.

Garbarino, J. (1977). The human ecology of child maltreatment: A conceptual model for research. *Journal of Marriage and the Family, 39*, 721–735.

———. (1995). Growing up in a socially toxic environment: Life for children and families in the 1990s. In G.B. Melton (Ed.), *The individual, the family, and social good: Personal fulfillment in times of change* (Vol. 42, pp. 1–20). Lincoln: University of Nebraska Press.

García-Moreno, C., Jansen, H.A.F.M., Ellsberg, M., Heise, L., & Watts, C. (2005). *WHO multi-country study on women's health and domestic violence against women: Initial results on prevalence, health outcomes and women's responses.* Geneva: World Health Organization.

Gelles, R.J. (1980). Violence in the family: A review of research in the seventies. *Journal of Marriage and the Family, 42*, 873–885.

Gerbert, B., Abercrombie, P., Caspers, N., Love, C., & Bronstone, A. (1999). How health care providers help battered women: The survivor's perspective. *Women & Health, 29*(3), 115–135.

Greaves, L., Hankivsky, O., & Kingston-Riechers, J. (1995). *Selected estimates of the costs of violence against women.* London, ON: Centre for Research on Violence against Women and Children.

Hamby, S.L. (2000). The importance of community in a feminist analysis of domestic violence among American Indians. *American Journal of Community Psychology, 28*(5), 649–669.

Hankivsky, O., & Varcoe, C. (2007). From global to local and over the rainbow: Violence against women. In M. Morrow, O. Hankivsky, & C. Varcoe (Eds.), *Women's health in Canada: Critical perspectives on theory and policy* (pp. 478–507). Toronto, ON: University of Toronto.

Helfer, R., & Kempe, C.H. (1968). *The battered child.* Chicago, IL: University of Chicago Press.

Hill, T.D., Schroeder, R.D., Bradley, C., Kaplan, L.M., & Angel, R.J. (2009). The long-term health consequences of relationship violence in adulthood: An examination of low-income women from Boston, Chicago, and San Antonio. *American Journal of Public Health, 99*(9), 1645–1650.

Hinch, R., & DeKeseredy, W.S. (1994). Corporate violence and women's health at home and in the work place. In B.S. Bolaria & H.D. Dickinson (Eds.), *Sociology of health care in Canada* (pp. 326–344). Toronto, ON: Harcourt Brace Jovanovich.

Hoff, L.A. (1994). *Violence issues: An interdisciplinary curriculum guide for health professionals* (H72-21/129-1995E). Ottawa, ON: Mental Health Division Health Canada.

Human Resources and Child Welfare Canada. (2000). *Child Welfare in Canada.* Retrieved from http://www.hrsdc.gc.ca/en/cs/sp/sdc/socpol/publications/reports/2000-000033/page00.shtml.

Humphreys, J. (1993). Children of battered women. In J. Campbell & J. Humphreys (Eds.), *Nursing care of survivors of family violence* (pp. 107–131). St. Louis, MO: Mosby.

Humphreys, J., & Ramsey, A.M. (1993). Child abuse. In J. Campbell & J. Humphreys (Eds.), *Nursing care of survivors of family violence* (pp. 36–67). St. Louis, MO: Mosby.

Innes, J.E., Ratner, P.A., Finlayson, P.F., Bray, D., & Giovanneti, P.B. (1991). *Models and strategies of delivering community health services related to woman abuse.* Edmonton: University of Alberta.

Interdepartmental Working Group on Elder Abuse and Manitoba Seniors Directorate. (1993). *Abuse of the elderly: A guide for the development of protocols.* Winnipeg, MB: Government of Manitoba.

International Council of Nurses. (1999). *Increasing violence in the workplace is a threat to nursing and the delivery of health care* . Retrieved from http://www.icn.ch

It Gets Better Project www.itgetsbetter.org accessed August 1, 2011.

Johnson, H. (1996). *Dangerous domains: Violence against women in Canada.* Scarborough, ON: International Thomson Publishing.

———. H. (2006). *Measuring violence against women: Statistical trends.* Ottawa, ON: Statistics Canada.

Kaukinen, C. (2002). The help-seeking of women violent crime victims: Findings from the Canadian violence against women survey. *International Journal of Sociology and Social Policy, 22*(7/8), 5–44.

Kendall-Tackett, K., Marshall, R., & Ness, K. (2003). Chronic pain syndromes and violence against women. *Women & Therapy, 26,* 45–56.

Kerr, R., & McLean, J. (1996). *Paying for violence: Some of the costs of violence against women in BC.* Victoria, BC: Ministry of Women's Equality.

Koniak-Griffin, D., & Lesser, J. (1996). The impact of childhood maltreatment on young mothers' violent behavior toward themselves and others. *Journal of Pediatric Nursing, 11*(5), 300–308.

Lehmann, P. (2000). Posttraumatic stress disorder (PTSD) and child witnesses to mother-assault: A summary and review. *Children and Youth Services Review, 22*(3/4), 275–396.

Lempert, L.B. (1997). The other side of help: Negative effects in the help-seeking processes of abused women. *Qualitative Sociology, 20*(2), 289–309.

Leserman, J., & Drossman, D.A. (2007). Relationship of abuse history to functional gastrointestinal disorders and symptoms. *Trauma, Violence & Abuse, 8*(3), 331–343.

Li, G. (2007). *Homicide in Canada,* 2007 from http://www.statcan.gc.ca/pub/85-002-x/2008009/article/10671-eng.htm#a8

MacIntosh, J., Wuest, J., Gray, M.M., & Cronkhite, M. (2010). Workplace bullying in health care affects the meaning of work. *Qualitative Health Research, 20,* 1128–1141.

MacLean, M.J., & Williams, R.M. (1995). Introduction. In M.J. MacLean (Ed.), *Abuse & neglect of older Canadians: Strategies for change* (pp. ix–xii). Toronto, ON: Canadian Association on Gerontology and Thompson Educational Publishing.

MacMillan, H.L., Fleming, J.E., Trocmé, N., et al. (1997). Prevalence of child physical and sexual abuse in the community. *Journal of the American Medical Association, 278*(2), 131–135.

MacMillan, H.L., MacMillan, A.B., Offord, D.R., et al. (1996). Aboriginal health. *Canadian Medical Association Journal, 155*(11), 1569–1578.

Manitoba Association of Registered Nurses. (1989). *Nurse abuse report.* Winnipeg, MB: Author.

Matas, R. (2001). "He said if I ever told anyone, he will kill me when he gets out." *Globe and Mail,* A9–A10.

McCloskey, K., & Grigsby, N. (2005). The ubiquitous clinical problem of adult intimate partner violence: The need for routine assessment. *Professional Psychology: Research and Practice, 36*(3), 264–275.

McDonald, L., & Collins, A. (2000). *Abuse and neglect of older adults: A discussion paper.* Ottawa, ON: Health Canada.

Mechanic, M., Weaver, T., & Resick, P. (2008). Mental health consequences of intimate partner abuse: A multidimensional assessment of four different forms of abuse. *Violence Against Women, 14,* 634–654.

Morrow, M. (2007). Our bodies, ourselves in context: Reflections on the women's health movement in Canada. In M. Morrow, O. Hankivsky, & C. Varcoe (Eds.), *Women's health in Canada: Critical perspectives on theory and policy* (pp. 33–63). Toronto, ON: University of Toronto.

Mosher, J.E. (1998). Caught in tangled webs of care: Women abused in intimate relationships. In C.T. Baines, P.M. Evans, & S.M. Neysmith (Eds.), *Women's caring: Feminist perspectives on social welfare* (2nd ed., pp. 139–159). Toronto, ON: Oxford University Press.

Muellman, R.L., Lenaghan, P.A., & Pakieser, R.A. (1996). Battered women: Injury locations and types. *Annals of Emergency Medicine, 28*(5), 468–492.

O'Donnell, S., MacIntosh, J., & Wuest, J. (2010). A theoretical understanding of sickness absence among women who have experienced workplace bullying. *Qualitative Health Research, 20,* 439–452.

Ozturk Ertem, I., Leventhal, J.M., & Dobbs, S. (2000). Intergenerational continuity of child physical abuse: How good is the evidence? *Lancet, 356*(9232), 814.

Podnieks, E. (1985). Elder abuse: It's time we did something about it. *Canadian Nurse, 81*(11), 36–39.

———. (2008). Elder abuse: The Canadian experience. *Journal of Elder Abuse & Neglect, 20,* 126–150.

Podnieks, E., & Baillie, E. (1995). Education as the key to the prevention of elder abuse and neglect. In M.J. MacLean (Ed.), *Abuse & neglect of older Canadians: Strategies for change* (pp. 81–93). Toronto, ON: Canadian Association on Gerontology and Thompson Educational Publishing.

Podnieks, E., Pillemer, K., Nicholson, J.P., Shillington, T., & Frizzel, A. (1990). *National survey on abuse of the elderly in Canada.* Toronto, ON: Ryerson Polytechnical Institute.

Post, L., Page, C., Conner, T., Prokhorov, A., Fang, Y., & Biroscak, B.J. (2010). Elder abuse in long-term care: Types, patterns, and risk factors. *Research on Aging, 32,* 323–348.

Poster, E. (1996). A multi-national study of psychiatric nursing staffs' beliefs and concerns about work safety and patient assault. *Archives of Psychiatric Nursing 10*(6), 365–373.

Public Health Agency of Canada (2001). Canadian incidence study of reported child abuse and neglect: Selected results. Retrieved from www.publichealth.gc.ca. Retrieved October 12, 2012.

Pynoos, R.S., & Nader, K. (1990). Children's exposure to violence and traumatic death. *Psychiatric Annals, 20*(6), 334–344.

Registered Nurses Association of Ontario (2009). *Preventing and Managing Violence in the Workplace* Available from http://www.rnao.org/Storage/61/5519_RNAO_Violence_in_work_WEB_2.pdf

Report of the Royal Commission on Aboriginal Peoples. (1996). *For seven generations* (Vol. 3). Ottawa, ON: Libraxus.

Riddell, T., Ford-Gilboe, M., & Leipert, B. (2009). Strategies used by rural women to stop, avoid, or escape from intimate partner violence. *Health Care for Women International, 30,* 134–159.

Ristock, J.L. (2001). Decentering heterosexuality: Responses of feminist counselors to abuse in lesbian relationships. *Women & Therapy, 23*(3), 59–72.

Savage, D., & Miller, T. (2011). *It gets better: Coming out, overcoming bullying and creating a life worth living.* New York: Dutton

Sleutel, M.R. (1998). Women's experiences of abuse: A review of qualitative research. *Issues in Mental Health Nursing, 19,* 525–539.

Smith, D., Varcoe, C., & Edwards, N. (2005). Turning around the intergenerational impact of residential school on Aboriginal people: Implications for health policy and practice. *Canadian Journal of Nursing Research, 37*(4), 39–60.

Statistics Canada. (1997). *Graphical overview of crime and the administration of criminal justice in Canada, 1997 (Catalogue No. 85F0018XIE).* Ottawa, ON: Minister of Industry.

———. (2005). Statistics Canada—The Daily. *Homicides.* Retrieved from http://www.statcan.ca/Daily/English/051006/d051006b.htm.

———. (2006). *Family violence in Canada: A statistical profile 2006.* Ottawa, ON: Canadian Centre for Justice Statistics.

———. (2007). *Family violence in Canada,* from ≤http://www.statcan.ca/english/freepub/85-224-XIE/85-224-XIE2007000.pdf≥

Thomlinson, E.B., Erickson, N., & Cook, M. (2000). Could this be your community? In J. Proulx & S. Perrault (Eds.), *No place for violence: Canadian aboriginal alternatives* (Vol. 1, pp. 22–38). Halifax: Fernwood Publishing and RESOLVE (Research and Education for Solutions to Violence and Abuse).

Tower, M. (2007). Intimate partner violence and the health care response: A postmodern critique. *Health Care for Women International, 28*(5), 438–452.

Trocme, N., MacMillan, H., Fallon, B., & De Marco, R. (2003). Nature and severity of physical harm caused by child abuse and neglect: Results from the Canadian incidents study. *Canadian Medical Association Journal, 169*(9), 911–915.

Varcoe, C. (2001). Abuse obscured: An ethnographic account of emergency nursing in relation to violence against women. *CJNR, 32*(4), 95–115.

Varcoe, C., & Dick, S. (2008). Intersecting risks of violence and HIV for rural and Aboriginal women in a neocolonial Canadian context. *Journal of Aboriginal Health, 4,* 42–52.

Varcoe, C., & Einboden, R. (2010). Family violence and ethics. In J. Humphreys & J. C. Campbell (Eds.), *Family violence and nursing practice* (2nd ed., pp. 381–410). New York: Springer.

Varcoe, C., Hankivsky, O., Ford Gilboe, M., Wuest, J., Wilk, P., Hammerton, J., & Campbell, J. (2011). Attributing selected costs to intimate partner violence in a sample of women who have left abusive partners: A social determinants of health approach. *Canadian Public Policy, 37*(3), 359–380.

Walker, L.E. (1979). *The battered woman.* New York: Harper & Row.

Walsh, C.A., Olson, J.L., Ploeg, J., Lohfeld, L., & MacMillan, H.L. (2011). Elder abuse and oppression: Voices of marginalized elders. *Journal of Elder Abuse & Neglect, 23*, 17–42.

Wekerle, C., Leung, E., Wall, A., MacMillan, H., Boyle, M., Trocme, N., & Waechter, R. (2009). The contribution of childhood emotional abuse to teen dating violence among child protective serves-involved youth. *Child Abuse and Neglect, 33*, 45–58.

Wiehe, V.R. (1998). *Understanding family violence: Treating and preventing partner, child, sibling, and elder abuse.* Thousand Oaks, CA: Sage.

Wilson, K.S., Silberberg, M.R., Brown, A.J., & Yaggy, S.D. (2007). Health needs and barriers to healthcare of women who have experienced intimate partner violence. *Journal of Women's Health (15409996), 16*(10), 1485–1498.

World Health Organization. (2002). *World report on violence and health.* Geneva: World Health Organization.

———. (2005). *WHO multi-country study on women's health and domestic violence against women: Summary report of initial results on prevalence, health outcomes and women's responses.* Geneva: World Health Organization.

Wuest, J., Merritt-Gray, M., Lent, B., Varcoe, C., Connors, A.J., & Ford-Gilboe, M. (2007). Patterns of medication use among women survivors of intimate partner violence. *Canadian Journal of Public Health, 98*(6), 460–464.

Zhenmei, Z., Schiamberg, L.B., Oehmke, J., et al. (2011). Neglect of older adults in Michigan nursing homes. *Journal of Elder Abuse & Neglect, 23*, 58–74.

26 Looking Back, Moving Forward: The Promise of Nursing in the 21st Century

Susan M. Duncan

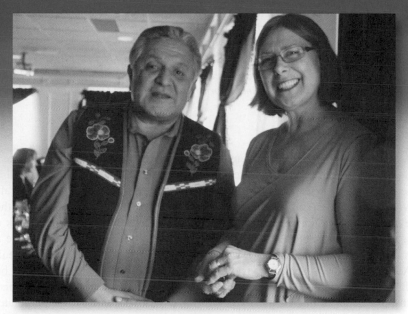

Pertice Moffit of Aurora College NWT and the Honorable George Tuccaro, Commissioner of the North West Territories meet with nurse educators visiting Yellowknife. (Used with permission. Photographer Anne-Mieke Cameron.)

Critical Questions

As a way of engaging with these ideas in this chapter, consider the following:

1. How do you envision your career unfolding with respect to change and transformation in nursing roles over the next several decades to 2035? to 2050?

2. As a nurse in the 21st century, how should you be thinking about your nursing education? What competencies must you have, and how will your experiences prepare you to practice in the knowledge economy of the 21st century?

3. How might student nurses seek educational experiences in a global context and what perspectives and values might inform these experiences?

4. How will you use power in transforming nursing, health, and public policy?

Chapter Objectives

After completing the chapter, you will be able to:

1. Reflect on future nursing practice scenarios and competencies required of nurses as knowledge workers.

2. Discuss and consider implications of landmark policy documents that inform the future of Canadian nursing in global contexts.

(continued on page 452)

3. Consider how nursing education is and must continue to be visionary and provide leadership for systems transformation.

4. Envision the future realities of Canadian nursing through the lenses of politics, history, society, power, and economics.

The key question that dominated the 20th century was: "What do nurses do?" In the 21st century, the key questions will become: "What do nurses know?" and "How do they use that knowledge to benefit people?"

—(Hildegard Peplau, renowned world nurse leader and visionary upon her acceptance of nursing's highest honor—the Christiane Reimann prize at the 1997 ICN Quadrennial Congress.)

How will nursing continue to make a difference to worldwide health? The answer to this question is that global needs for nurses and nursing care in the 21st century will be intense and can be met only if nurses are able to transform roles and influence nursing, health, and public policy. Premises underlying the final chapter of this textbook are consistent with those developed in previous chapters: Nursing practice in the mid- to late 21st century will look different from today, and nurses must engage politically to shape their new reality. And, there are significant power issues that nurses must address in order to maximize their influence on health.

An emerging transformative vision of nursing is described in this chapter, building on the foundation of previous chapters. Historical, socioeconomic, and critical-feminist perspectives inform this vision. In this chapter, you will have the opportunity to contemplate the future of Canadian nursing in the mid-21st century through these perspectives, as they inspire possibilities for nurses to build a healthy society. This new millennium, characterized by a knowledge economy and rapid technological change, will engage nurses as knowledge workers in the promotion of health and delivery of nursing care. In this context of the future, nurses must continue to be bold in their vision, and informed by what people throughout the world need to attain health. In this inspiring future nurses acknowledge the challenge of persistent issues and tensions as well as the promise of nursing in the 21st century.

This chapter begins with a discussion of the promise of nursing in the 21st century. The balance of the chapter is organized around key issues in nursing practice and education analyzed according to historical, socioeconomic, and critical-feminist lenses on the future. Threaded through these sections are the themes of persistence and tension—persistence of nurses in advancing a vision of nursing to meet societal health needs and the tension resulting from nurses' capacity for power and constraints on attaining and using that power.

THE PROMISE OF NURSING IN THE 21ST CENTURY

While we accept that nursing practice and education in the mid-21st century will be markedly different from today, we are challenged to identify how nurses can lead transformations in nursing knowledge and health systems. Undeniably, the future holds that nurses will lead and influence change in ways that we may not yet contemplate. As this chapter goes to press, there are policy papers and positions that can help us envision the changes in nursing practice, education, research, and healthcare systems that are needed now to position us on this course of change toward the ultimate of goal of health equity (Reutter & Kushner, 2010). Health equity can only be achieved if the systemic conditions of health disparities are confronted and changed (Sachs, 2011). The positions and policy papers described in this chapter span international, national, and local contexts and bring a global perspective on the issues pertaining to health and health equity. A discussion of international policy directions including the United Nations (UN), World Health Organization (WHO), and the International Council of Nurses (ICN) provides context for nursing education and practice in Canada. The context and perspective on the future of Canadian nursing as articulated by national nursing organizations including the Canadian Nurses Association (CNA) and the Canadian Association of Schools of Nursing (CASN) is also discussed.

This chapter emphasizes nursing education as the sector that can inspire and lead change (Duncan et al., 2012; Hewlett et al., 2009; IOM, 2010). There is strong consensus among nursing and health professional educators worldwide that changes in nursing education are needed to prepare practitioners with competencies to practice in a new reality (Canadian Association of Schools of Nursing [CASN], 2010; IOM, 2010; Frenk et al., 2010). As identified in the report of a Global Commission (Frenk et al., 2010), "all health professionals in all countries should be educated to mobilize knowledge and to engage in critical reasoning and ethical conduct so that they are competent to participate in patient and population-centered health systems as members of locally responsive and globally connected teams" (p. 1924). This vision for change also requires that nurses and others acquire global citizenship competencies based on understanding the day-to-day interrelationships between local and global community experiences and contexts (Mill et al., 2010). Achieving these competencies will depend on a system of nursing education that inspires vision and innovation. Most important, this transformation depends on faculty, students, and practitioners with diverse and critical ways of viewing the world and health challenges. This vision of nursing education fits well with emerging views of nursing practice within the healthcare system and global health policy perspectives (National Expert Commission, 2012).

Nursing and Healthcare Policy Perspectives on the Future

Primary healthcare (PHC) is the overarching philosophy to guide healthcare policy transformation; its principles and values have been affirmed and reaffirmed for over 3 decades (World Health Organization [WHO], 1978). Viewed as the way of achieving the Millennium Development Goals (MGDs) (see the link to United Nations Millennium Development Goals listed in online resources at the end of the chapter) and health equity on a global scale, PHC requires commitment and tenacity in moving forward. The WHO (2008, 2009, 2010) and the International Council of Nurses [ICN] (2012) have affirmed the central role of nurses in reforming systems and influencing public policy so PHC can be realized. Such leadership requires that nurses understand PHC as a philosophy extending beyond their work in the healthcare system, to the achievement of social justice and global health equity.

Twenty-first century reforms central to the PHC agenda include:

- Correcting inequities by moving to universal health coverage;
- Reforming service delivery to make health systems people-centered;
- Reforming leadership to make health authorities more reliable;
- Reforming public policy to promote and protect the health of communities (2008, p. xvi).

In considering these reforms, you may draw on the foundational perspectives presented in the chapters of this textbook in affirming how and why nursing knowledge and leadership is central to their achievement.

As this textbook is published, the world is but 2 years from the target goal of achieving the MDGs, scheduled for 2015. We can anticipate gains in key areas of the MDGs where nurses and nursing make a significant difference: Maternal and child health, prevention and treatment of

BOX 26.1   World Health Organization Key Results Areas for Nurses and Midwives

- *KRA1*—Strengthening of health systems and service: *Nursing and midwifery services-led models form the basis of PHC reforms, especially in the areas of universal coverage and leadership for health.*
- *KRA2*—Nursing and midwifery policy and practice: *Nurses and midwives play a proactive part in ensuring that the health policies plans and decisions affecting their professions are country specific and in keeping with the principles of inclusive leadership, effective governance, and regulated practice.*
- *KRA3*—Education, training, and career development: *Institutional capacity enhanced for the intake and production of suitably skilled practitioners to provide comprehensive people-centered services.*
- *KRA4*—Nursing and midwifery workforce management: *Policy-makers create an enabling environment for the nursing and midwifery workforce to meet changing health needs.*
- *KRA5*—Partnership for nursing and midwifery services: *Active systematic collaboration is encouraged among nursing and midwifery organizations and with community-based organizations, health professional groups, and governments.*

communicable and noncommunicable disease, elimination of poverty and hunger, and advocacy for safe water supplies and other areas of environmental sustainability through global partnerships. At this juncture, nursing must critically appraise its contributions to the MDGs. The profession must also position itself to address ongoing and emerging population health challenges and shape the definition of 21st century goals.

WHO (2010) has laid out the new strategic directions for nursing and midwifery services (2011–2015). The foundational premise of these directions is that nurses and midwives must be proactive by leading in areas of health policy, systematic collaboration, and governance (p. 5). Leadership required to transform health systems "from the bedside to the boardroom" will see nurses engaged as full partners in systems transformation and change at local, organizational, national, and international levels (IOM, 5–1). To these ends, WHO identifies five *Key Results Areas* (KRAs) for nurses and midwives to 2015.

In Box 26.1, we see that the KRAs have implications for nursing education and practice as nurses are expected to play a central role in developing new service delivery models and to provide inclusive leadership for the changes, as well as provide highly skilled people-centered services. Nurses must have the political acumen to preserve universal healthcare where it exists in Canada and work with colleagues around the world to reform existing systems. For example, nurses must oppose for-profit user-pay models that stand in contradiction to PHC values and social justice. This will be a tall order in some political arenas, but one that nurses can and must rise to.

A perspective on the future is required to project trends and anticipate how nursing can stay ahead of the curve of change in meeting health needs and proactively influence health policy. Projections range from anticipating how global economics will influence determinants of health to local adaptations of emerging technologies, and understanding social demographics. Nursing associations must scan the environment in areas outside of the health sector including technology, finance, business, and the environment in order to position nursing on the forefront of health and public policy agendas. Nurses have a key role in bringing critical observations about emerging trends to the attention of policy makers, and nurses themselves will become policy makers in areas of health and determinants of health.

Nurses and others must also challenge dominant bio-medical paradigms when knowledge and system development may privilege advances that are accessible to only a few people. Investment in privileged technologies may preclude the development of nonmedical technologies necessary for the achievement of PHC. This is not to say that bio-medical advances are not important facets of PHC, but rather that they must be balanced with other programs and models in the realm of addressing the social determinants of health. There is also evidence to suggest that technological innovations are potentially the most significant drivers of healthcare costs therefore requiring judicious review and decision making with respect to the use of resources (Canadian Institute for Health Information [CIHI], 2011a).

For example, future projections often focus on emerging medically focused technologies such as genomics and robotics as indicators of progress and innovation in the treatment of disease. Although such scientific advancements are valued, nurses and others must also advocate for the development of other technologies and programs that will impact PHC and health equity on a wider scale such as green technologies that reduce environmental toxins, development of water sanitation and sources, and vaccine development for widespread diseases such as malaria (Edwards & Riley, 2006).

Emerging communication and information technologies pose significant professional and ethical issues for nurses that require vigilance in identifying and creating policies for maintaining patient privacy and confidentiality, nurses' professionalism, and the quality of information provided to patients (Aylott, 2011; Mostaghimi & Crotty, 2011). These issues are likely to become more complex as technology evolves, requiring more sophisticated scrutiny and moral leadership within the nursing profession. A current example is the issue of boundaries when nurses share information about their personal and professional lives on social media networks such as Facebook with no control over the boundaries of where and how that information is further communicated, potentially resulting in breaches of professional conduct and inadvertent disclosures of confidential patient information (Aylott, 2011). Further, nurses must be critical consumers of sources of health information such as the use of apps and other electronic sources of health information in order to assist the public to access best sources for health promotion and to participate in public discourses of health issues, and to support professional nursing practice (Golterman & Banasiak, 2011; Regenberg, 2010). Furthermore, nurses and others must advocate for equity in public access to information through internet connections such as broadband to ensure that those living outside of urban centers or those who cannot afford state-of-science technology are not disadvantaged (Smith, 2012).

Nurses must also ask critical questions about widely held assumptions, for instance, that an aging demographic results in increased healthcare delivery costs. Emerging data suggests a more informed view based on a healthier senior population and a reformed system of care and advocacy will make the difference (CIHI, 2011b). Nurses are positioned to be key reformers of long-term and home care by introducing and leading not-for-profit organizations that emulate best practices in the most cost-effective delivery of care for seniors and those who have chronic illnesses, and supporting exemplary practices such as fall prevention programs.

The Promise of Nursing Education—Taking Center Stage

A vision of promise was developed by a Global Independent Commission (2010) on the Education of Health Professionals for the 21st century. The findings of the Commission invite reflections on nursing's future as collaborators with a diverse stakeholder group and public. In the article "Health professionals for a new century: transforming education to strengthen health systems in an interdependent world," authors Frenk et al. (2010) depict sweeping reforms in education based on the development of global and local academic systems in which universities collaborate with practice agencies and nongovernmental agencies toward the goal of transformative and interdependent professional education for global equity in health. This is an exciting vision for students to contemplate, as many are eager to engage in international experiences and develop competencies in global citizenship.

There are opportunities to work across borders with others in health, education, and nongovernmental organizations in mutually promising areas of development and research. Students working together with their colleagues in other countries can ask critical questions about relationships between local and global health and engage in collective action to improve health and advocate for conditions for health and education. These outcomes can only be achieved if we develop and link networks of health systems and academic systems that would provide opportunities for students to develop competencies required for practitioners and researchers to make a difference to global health in the 21st century (Frenk et al., 2010).

It is timely for you to reflect on how your nursing education program is preparing you for the future. Nurse educators agree on how basic competencies of nurses at graduation are shifting. Referring to the competency frameworks presented in Table 26.1, we can see how important it is that nurses are able to lead diverse teams, collaborate across multiple types of agencies, and develop new systems of care to meet existing and new population health challenges. Most schools of nursing have made significant shifts in nursing curricula so that students have a range of community experiences in health and nonhealth agencies and develop a broad view of health. Making these shifts can be difficult when the future-oriented practice experiences necessary to prepare nurses with the competencies required for PHC do not yet exist.

Projections over the past decade or more indicate that most healthcare will be delivered in community settings outside of institutions; however, this has not yet materialized. Recent statistics on nurses' place of work show an increase in the proportion of RNs employed in the community health sector up slightly from 13.5% in 2005 to 14.2% in 2009, and we can be sure that this will continue to rise (CIHI, 2010). The projected reality of PHC reform is that most nurses will practice in a community sector including public health and there is growing concern about how we are preparing students for this reality (Public Health Agency of Canada [PHAC], 2008; Underwood et al., 2009).

In light of the competencies required of nurses, we can project continuous changes in nursing education both in terms of the content as well as the process of delivery. CASN (2010), in its landmark document titled *Nursing Workforce Education for the 21st Century,* discussed the need for increasingly diverse student practice opportunities to allow students to develop competencies identified in Table 26.1. Along with the need to expand student experiences, CASN also identified the need to expand graduate education for nurses to prepare educators and researchers needed to sustain nursing education now and in the future. A pressing challenge in nurse education is the looming faculty shortage: "Who will teach the nurses of the future?" (Bartfay & Howse, 2007, p. 24; CASN, 2010; NECBC, 2010). An equally critical question is: Who will do the research to develop the body of knowledge required of nurses? Graduate education for nurses is a growing priority in meeting these challenges.

If this vision of promise is sustained, nursing education will be transformed in concert with innovations in nursing, health systems, and society. An exciting future is emerging where nurses work as full partners in health promotion, social advocacy, and primary care to fulfill a social mission toward greater equity in health. In future, nurses will continue to be prepared for entry-level practice at the baccalaureate level, graduating with the generalist skills required to lead systems change and collaborate with a myriad of partners including community members, nongovernmental organizations, and those working in other sectors such as finance and urban planning. This requires nurses to develop competencies for diverse forms of collaboration with teams and organizations. As interprofessional competencies are developed, nurses and others must develop strong identities rooted in their respective disciplines. Nursing practice of the 21st century must be embedded in the unique body of knowledge that it brings to PHC.

Today's nursing education must prepare nurses for future-oriented competencies and inspire systemwide innovation. In many ways, this has been happening through the offering of courses such as Nursing Leadership and Societal Health (Collaboration for Academic Education in Nursing [CAEN], 2010), where students conceive of innovative projects and delivery models that may not yet exist within nursing practice roles. Box 26.2 contains examples of baccalaureate nursing students' health promotion initiatives as illustrations of how they are developing 21st century competencies in nursing practice courses that provide them with opportunities to work with communities to address determinants of health.

Although in the past nursing education was seen as somehow distinct from practice, the emerging and dominant perspective on nursing education is one of a continuous and reflexive

Table 26.1   Educating Health Professionals in the 21st Century: Organizational Perspectives on Basic Education Requirements and Competencies

ORGANIZATION/POLICY DOCUMENT	POLICY PERSPECTIVE: NURSING AND HEALTH PROFESSIONAL EDUCATION
Canadian Association of Schools of Nursing Workforce Development in the 21st Century (2010)	Emerging educational requirements: • Public and population health competencies • Inter-professional and team-based practice • Elder care • Highly specialized critical care and home care • Cultural competence and service provision to underserved groups • Evidence informed practice and knowledge translation • Delegation and supervision of assistive personnel • Use of informatics and electronic information systems
Institute of Medicine— Committee on the Robert Wood Johnson Foundation Initiative on the Future of Nursing: Education [IMCRWJFIFNE] (2010)	The "new basics in nursing education": • Collaboration within the profession and across other health professions • Communication • Systems thinking (p. x) • Care of the older adult • Fostering diversity in care (p. 10) Nursing pedagogy linked to the dissemination of knowledge (p. 9)
WHO Global Standards for the Initial Education of Nurses and Midwives (2009)	Program graduate attributes: • Use of evidence in practice • Cultural competence • The ability to practice in the healthcare systems of their respective countries and meet population needs • Critical and analytical thinking • The ability to manage resources and practice safely and effectively • The ability to be effective client advocates and professional partners with other disciplines in health-care delivery • Community service orientation • Leadership ability and continual professional development
Global Commission on the Education of Health Professionals in the 21st Century (2010)	A transformative use of competencies that would engage professionals across traditional boundaries in achieving teamwork necessary for health system transformation • Transformational teamwork that includes nonprofessional workers may be most important for health systems globally All health professionals should be educated to: • Mobilize knowledge • Engage in critical reasoning and ethical conduct • Participate in patient- and population-centered health systems • Act as members of locally responsive and globally connected teams
Canadian Inter-professional Health Collaborative: A National Inter-professional Competency Framework (2010)	National Framework—Competency Domains: • Role clarification • Inter-professional conflict resolution • Team functioning • Collaborative leadership
Public Health Agency of Canada Core Competencies for Public Health In Canada (2008)	Core Competencies for Public Health in Canada: • Public health sciences—core knowledge of population health, • Assessment and analysis: evidence-based decisions • Policy and program planning, implementation and evaluation • Partnerships, collaboration and advocacy • Diversity and inclusiveness • Leadership

BOX 26.2   Baccalaureate Student Health Promotion Initiatives

- Contributing a nursing perspective on homelessness and affordable housing through participation in a coalition of nongovernmental organizations working to advance societal understanding of the determinants of health;
- Collaborating with teams of practical nurses and healthcare attendants to identify leadership and support initiatives in long-term care;
- Working with an international community to advance mutual interests in learning about community health needs and global citizenship competencies;
- Working to engage street involved individuals in health promotion initiatives and engage their voices in planning;
- Collaborating with students in journalism to make the public aware of research findings in the areas of best practices in end-of-life care and access to reproductive healthcare for youth in rural communities;
- Working with First Nations organizations to plan accessible and culturally safe services for people with diabetes;
- Engaging youth in schools to advocate for socially responsible marketing of products.

relationship with society and practice. This is indeed good news as we have long known that education and practice must be reciprocal and the sectors must work synergistically (in relationship). It is time for nursing education to take centre stage.

PERSISTENCE AND TENSION: THEMES IN NURSING'S TRANSFORMATION

By now, you will likely be convinced that your future in nursing presents exciting opportunities to lead change and transform health systems in order to make a difference to health on a global level. You may ask: Why does nursing have this remarkable future and opportunity? And you may question: What are the challenges ahead? How can nursing's power to make a critical difference in health be assured? Answers to these important questions are found, in part, by viewing nursing's place as a profession through the lenses of history, social, and economic contexts, a critical-feminist examination of nursing's power and influence. It is to these analytical lenses that we now turn.

Historical Analysis

Nursing education organizations such as CASN, CASN's counterparts in other countries, and nursing education leaders continue a historic tradition of recognizing nursing as a knowledge-based profession and discipline. Their ideal is an academic education for nurses at the level of the baccalaureate degree as required preparation for professional practice. Through the years, this ideal has been continuously challenged, and never more acutely than at times of a shortage of nurses, such as the present. Nursing education leaders have fought for the education of registered nurses in Canada and worldwide. Although the baccalaureate requirement has been achieved in most Canadian jurisdictions including Quebec as of 2011, nurses must be ever vigilant so that this standard will not be eroded in favor of more practical and less academic preparation.

Canadian nursing history scholars have researched the tenacity of nursing education leaders to achieve nursing's place in universities since early 20th century, and their research shows that nursing has a legacy of visionary leadership. The vision and courage of leaders such as Ethel Johns, Kathleen Russell, and Bertha Harmour are sources of inspiration, and historical accounts of their achievements are well worth reading (Paul & Ross-Kerr, 2011; Street, 1973). These leaders maintained that the complexity of nursing necessitated an educational system outside of the oppression of hospital apprenticeship. In the face of scant support, resources, or acknowledgment, these leaders were able to position nursing within the university.

A historical account from the biography of Ethel Johns, one of Canada's most celebrated nurse leaders, is an exemplar. Speaking to a mass meeting of the student body and graduate staff as well as the members of the Training School Committee at UBC in 1919, her words compelled the need for a nurse's education to be both broad and deep:

> Now where do we come in? Is there a phase of life where we do not come in? There is no avocation, not even medicine itself which transcends ours in its intimate association with life. Do you think any preparation too broad and deep as this? . . . Now what are we nurses going to do about it? (Street, 1973, p. 123–124)

A full account of this "cradle to the grave speech" can be found in Margaret Street's (1973) biography of Johns titled *Watchfires on the Mountain*. This biography is a moving historical reference that sheds light on how and why nurses' persistence in actualizing nursing's progress as a profession sets us up to continue to succeed in the arena of the 21st century.

Despite the insistence and tenacity of nurse leaders throughout the late 19th and early 20th centuries, nurses and nursing continue to be plagued by challenges to their education. Some in various positions of power fail to acknowledge the knowledge and skill required to nurse, insisting on a vocational or practical educational preparation. Remarkably, as early as 1932, Dr. George Weir (1932) undertook an in-depth examination of nursing education and concluded that nursing is no more practical in nature than law, medicine, or teaching and he further recommended that nursing must be recognized as a profession requiring a university education as essential preparation.

Despite ongoing challenges, the Canadian Nurses Association at its Biennium in 1982 affirmed the baccalaureate as the essential preparation for the practice of nursing, and since then every Canadian province has made strides toward the goal by increasing access to this level of education in universities and through collaborative partnerships between postsecondary educational institutions. WHO (2009) calls for every country to require the baccalaureate for entry level nursing, a considerable challenge for countries with far fewer resources than Canada. As a nursing student of the 21st century, you can celebrate this legacy of past and ongoing achievements in nursing education and the quality of your nursing education today. It is important to recognize that these achievements have been hard won and must be continuously affirmed and strengthened through progressive policy and political action, and to extend the learning and privileges of Canada to others in the world. In this age of knowledge, nursing knowledge and nurses as knowledge workers are needed more than ever. Thus, nurses must be ever vigilant to the lessons and challenges of the past in advocating and extending nursing standards and quality of nursing education.

Socio-Economic Analysis

Nursing education standards and competencies must always be viewed within the context of their service to society. Achievement of the UN MDGs will require nurses and others to challenge social and economic contexts that are contradictory to the values of social justice and equity in health, requiring nurses to have competencies in leadership, change, and politics. We can anticipate that global resources will dwindle as the world is challenged by climate change and a shifting world economy. It is in this context that nurses must understand health challenges and how to transform systems for greater equity in health.

The ICN (2010) asserts that:

Strong health systems with effective nursing workforces bring economic benefits to people and the society. Continuing to compile and disseminate the evidence of this is critical. Nurses also need to protect the public interest by ensuring the most efficient and equitable use of available health resources." *(p. 10)*

Nurses and others must understand that the values of PHC are not compatible with all political and economic ideologies including that of neoliberalism, which is growing in influence in the 21st century (Duncan & Reutter, 2006; Labonte, 2009). New awareness and strategies are needed to engage a wider public in confronting discrepant values that prohibit moving forward in health equity.

The Union Nations [UN] (2010) has an action plan to meet the MDGs by 2015. The plan includes strategies and policies aimed at supporting country-led development; fostering inclusive pro-poor economic growth; increasing investments in education, health, water, sanitation, and infrastructure; and expanding opportunities for women and girls in economic and political empowerment (p. vi). One can see that these policies will surely be in contradiction to some political approaches such as neoliberalism (Labonte, 2009), yet the goals of health equity and PHC will not be met without countries' reform of macro-level public policy. Nurses must therefore play a role in public policy reform through collaboration with other sectors in society and by inspiring public participation in healthy public policy.

We can turn to a contemporary example of how nurses have worked together through their organizations to reform healthcare practices in the interests of health equity for those most vulnerable. This example points to the importance of a unified voice for nurses in influencing policy based on social justice values. Working with the Registered Nurses Association of British Columbia, which confirmed that supervision of injections is within the scope of registered nursing practice in order to prevent illness and promote health, the nurses of the Dr. Peter Centre introduced supervised injection into a comprehensive day program based on the principles of harm reduction (Wood et al., 2003). Based on the values and conceptual framework described in the CNA policy document on harm reduction (Canadian Nurses Association, 2011a, 2011b; [CNA], 2011), nurses collaborated with other individuals and organizations including the professional association and the union to support the introduction of a supervised injection facility known as "Insite" for people who experience addictions, mental illness, and poverty in the Downtown Eastside of the city of Vancouver (Gold, 2003; Pauly et al., 2007; Lightfoot et al., 2009). Nurses' role as advocates on behalf of supervised injection has been highly visible to the public in, for example, the film *Fix: The Story of an Addicted City* (Carson & Wild, 2002) and a press conference organized by BCNU and the Portland Hotel Society. Recently, when challenged by the federal government's move to force the closure of the program, the professional associations (CNA, Registered Nurses Association of Ontario, Association of Registered Nurses of British Columbia) and the union (British Columbia Nurses Union [BCNU]) each acted as interveners in support of Insite at the Supreme Court of Canada. The court ruled in favor of maintaining the program. Nurse Irene Goldstone worked for many years to support the role nurses play in providing care for this marginalized population and has written about nurses' role in advocacy on behalf of Insite in the form of a blog post to the Association of Registered Nurses of British Columbia Web site (see online resources at the end of the chapter). Her writing is a powerful example of how the coalescence of nursing advocacy, multisectoral collaboration (Small et al., 2006) and the power of the Canadian Charter of Rights and Freedoms (1982) and the Canadian legal process made a difference for those who are among the most marginalized in society.

Critical-feminist Analysis: Nursing's Power and Influence

Nursing power is paradoxical: Although nurses have an immense capacity for power due to their numbers, knowledge, and position in society, there are forces that limit this potential. This power paradox has been persistent in nursing and at a time when immense progress is possible, nurses must understand what this tension means and how it can be resolved. As presented in previous chapters, a critical-feminist lens is one that exposes power differentials in relationships and analyzes issues of gender related to nursing's status and power as a profession in the 21st century.

A contemporary example is the absence of nurses and leadership for nursing in the WHO organization. As discussed previously in this chapter, the *WHO Strategic Directions for Strengthening Nursing and Midwifery Services, 2011–2015,* clearly states that despite the centrality of nurses across healthcare settings, they are frequently excluded from health policy deliberations (Bryant, 2011; WHO, 2010). Yet, this absence of nurses in health policy exists in the organizational culture of WHO itself. In the face of this contradiction to WHO's own policy direction to strengthen nursing, ICN at its Congress in May 2011 took political action to table a resolution to the 64th World Health Assembly that included the following request of the Director General of WHO:

> To strengthen WHO's capacity for development and implementation of effective nursing and midwifery policies and programmes through continued investment and appointment of professional nurses and midwives to specialist posts in the Secretariat both at headquarters and in the regions" (p. 3).

Clearly this action is essential if WHO's own strategic directions to strengthen nursing and midwifery are to be realized. The nursing profession must continue to push back against this and other contradictions in nursing power. The outcomes of this action must be the reinstatement of a Senior Nurse Advisor at the highest levels of WHO leadership, and there must be a significant increase in numbers of nurses and midwives throughout the organization. Other tensions in the expression of nursing's power are found in the persistent challenge to nursing as a knowledge-based profession, along with the emergence of care delivery models that are contrary to the evidence of what should be in place for the delivery of quality nursing care. For example, while nursing as a profession and discipline is positioned to influence health and systems globally, two levels of entry into the practice of nursing continue to exist in many countries including Canada. The persistence of both practical and baccalaureate forms of nursing education must be questioned as we recognize the depth and breadth of education required to prepare nurses with competencies required for the 21st century. Another tension exists in the call for interprofessional practice and education. In many settings, we continue to see the dominance of physicians in systems of care, which stands in contradiction to models and competencies required for PHC and collaborative models.

A critical-feminist analysis helps us to understand these tensions in relationships and power in nursing. Feminist values place the mostly female nursing profession as equal to, rather than in subservience to, the medical profession. These values are in tension with the continuous calling into question of nursing education. When nurses argue that a 1- or 2-year practical or vocational level of education is inadequate to prepare practitioners for the complexity of care required, they are also criticized for oppressing another primarily female group of health providers, prepared as practical nurses. At the same time, one can see that nursing as a female gendered profession experiences ongoing oppression within a patriarchal society that continuously challenges the foundational premise of nurses as knowledge workers.

This tension that originates in the persistence of two levels of nursing and nurses remains unresolved (Gebbie, 2009). These examples provoke critical questions about how nurses relate to others: How should nurses and nursing students be practicing with other professionals to develop a system of collaborative practice and avoid the dominance of one profession? How should nurses value and support LPNs as colleagues, while simultaneously questioning the adequacy of a practical education and the potential for collaboration? How can nurses acknowledge their own power over unregulated health workers while developing collaborative relationships and

BOX 26.3   Projection

Scenario: The year is 2030—you are an RN working in a home care program developed within the philosophy of PHC. Anticipate the needs of the population you serve and the nature of your practice: What health challenges are present? What services do you provide and where does the population access nursing services? Who do you work with? How have nurses played a role in developing and managing the system of home care? What are the dominant social determinants of health? How are you engaged in PHC as well as primary care?

Your Task: As a member of the school of nursing advisory committee, your task is to identify the nursing practice competencies you require and to make recommendations for the education of new nurses. You are also asked for your ideas on how to best develop systems of home care in countries with fewer resources than Canada.

Consider: The competencies required of nurses in the delivery of home care within the broad scope of PHC, for instance those required to engage the community in wider discussions of priority health issues and services, and public policy shifts necessary to address the determinants of health.

supporting those workers who are close to their communities in understanding health needs and solutions? These are critical questions for nurses and nursing in their quest to both maximize power and influence and share power with others.

S U M M A R Y

Nursing stands poised on a future inspired by a transformative vision of practice and education in the 21st century. Nurses can create the future they want by anticipating the needs of populations (Box 26.3). This vision requires that nursing continue its tradition of values and commitment to quality and breadth in health and education. Nursing must affirm a commitment to PHC values and social justice. The future of nursing demands that nurses engage with communities in local and global contexts to implement PHC. Nurses will also work with others outside of the health sector and bring the nursing and PHC lens to bear on policies related to the determinants of health and social justice. As we have discussed in this chapter, nurses must develop competencies for this level of collaboration, political influence, and leadership. These competencies define the nature of nursing practice in the 21st century. There will continue to be challenges to nursing's influence to achieve health equity and PHC goals. We gain inspiration from understanding nursing's history of leadership and influence and from our will to confront the consistent contradictions in the collective power of nursing as forces that may detract from the collective will toward health equity, PHC, and the MDGs. We can also be inspired by our colleagues in countries with fewer resources who continue to make strides in their ability to influence healthcare, and we can join with them in our efforts to connect the local with the global momentum for change (Duncan & Whyte, 2010).

The focus of nursing research and scholarship must be to develop a body of knowledge to prepare nurses to engage with other disciplines and with communities to influence change in policy and political arenas. This will require new methodologies to focus on curricular issues and innovations in preparing nurses for competencies discussed in this chapter. The nursing profession will be able to track its record of action and influence relative to the goals identified in the WHO Strategic Directions for Nursing and Midwifery by 2015, and its record of populating the WHO with nurses who can influence policy in the organization.

The focus of this chapter on the future and transformative change required for health in the 21st century has drawn on contemporary policy documents with implications for health equity, PHC, and the MDGs. It is indeed a most exciting time as nursing students and nurses can consider how their local community health issues and programs are connected to others worldwide and value the interconnectedness of health. Within this web of interconnectedness, there are boundless opportunities and challenges to make a difference to health at home and worldwide.

Add to your knowledge of this issue:	
ARNBC Getting to Insite Blog	**www.arnbc.ca**
Canadian Association of Schools of Nursing	**www.casn.ca**
Canadian Nurses Association	**www.cna.ca**
Canadian Inter-professional Health Collaborative	**www.cihc.ca**
Commission on the Education of Health Professionals for a New Century	**http://www.healthprofessionals21.org**
International Council of Nurses	**www.icn.org**
Public Health Agency of Canada Core Competencies	**http://www.phac-aspc.gc.ca**
Millennium Project—Global Futures Studies and Research	**www.millennium-project.org**
United Nations Millennium Development Goals	**http://www.un.org**
World Health Organization Primary Health Care Now More Than Ever	**http://www.who.int**

Online

R E F L E C T I O N S *on the Chapter...*

1 Visualize a preferred future for the role of the registered nurse in PHC in 2030? What new roles for nurses do you envision? How will the setting of nursing practice change? What is most exciting about this future?

2 Think about how you can focus your educational experiences to prepare you for the competencies identified in the policy documents presented in this chapter. Identify recommendations that you as a nursing student might make for nursing programs to ensure that students are prepared with competencies required for practice in this century.

3 Reflect on how your view of your future nursing career changed in the past year. What trends or insights are most important to how you view your career pathway?

4 Consider how you will stay on top of future trends and changes in order to position your career as a nurse. In particular, consider the roles of nursing associations in environmental scanning.

Want to know more? Visit thePoint for additional helpful resources:

* Journal Articles
* Learning Objectives
* Nursing Professional Roles and Responsibilities
* Bonus chapters:
  ◦ Health and Nursing Policy: A Matter of Politics, Power and Professionalism
  ◦ The NP Movement: Recurring Issues
  ◦ When Difference Matters: The Politics of Privilege and Marginality

References

Aylott, M. (2011). Blurring the boundaries: Technology and the nurse-patient relationship. *British Journal of Nursing, 20*(13), 810–816.

Bartfay, W.J., & Howse, E. (2007). Who will teach the nurses of the future? *The Canadian Nurse, 103*(7), 24–27.

Bryant, R. (2011). Nursing and health policy perspectives. *International Nursing Review, 58*(2), 148.

Canadian Association of Schools of Nursing (CASN). (2010). *The case for healthier Canadians: Nursing workforce education for the 21st century.* Ottawa: CASN.

Canadian Association of Schools of Nursing Standing Committee on Public Health/Community Health Nursing. (2010). *Guidelines for quality community health nursing clinical placements for baccalaureate students.* Ottawa: CASN.

Canadian Institute for Health Information (CIHI). (2011a). *Health care cost drivers: The facts.* Ottawa: Author.

———. (2011b). *Health care in Canada, 2011—A focus on seniors and aging.* Ottawa: Author.

Canadian Nurses Association & Canadian Association of Schools of Nursing. (2011). *Registered nurses education in Canada statistics 2009–2010.* Ottawa: Authors.

Canadian Nurses Association (CNA). (2011a). Nurses praise Insite ruling. *Canadian Nurse, 107*(9), 16.

———. (2011b). Harm reduction and currently illegal drugs: Implications for nursing policy, practice, education and research. Discussion paper. Available: http://www.cna-aiic.ca/CNA/documents/pdf/publications/Harm_Reduction_2011_e.pdf.

Carson, B., & Wild, N. (Producers). (2002). *Fix: the story of an addicted city.* Canada: Canada Wild Productions.

Charter of Rights and Freedoms—Part 1 of the Constitution Act, Department of Justice Canada, (1982). Available: http://laws-lois.justice.gc.ca/eng/charter/page-1.html

Collaboration for Academic Education in Nursing (CAEN). (2010). *Unpublished curriculum guide.* Victoria: Author.

Duncan, S.M., & Reutter, L. (2006). A critical policy analysis of an emerging agenda for home care in one Canadian province. *Health and Social Care in the Community, 14*(3), 242–253.

Duncan, S.M., & Whyte, N. (2010). Global leadership priorities for Canadian nursing: A perspective on the ICN 24th Quadrennial Congress, Durban, South Africa. *Canadian Journal of Nursing Leadership, 23*(1), 16–21.

Duncan, S.M., Thorne, S., VanNeste-Kenny, J., & Tate, B. (2012). Policy analysis and advocacy in nursing education: The Nursing Education Council of British Columbia Framework. *Nurse Education Today, 32*, 432–437.

Edwards, N.C., & Riley, B. (2006). Can we develop wait lists for public health issues? *Canadian Medical Association Journal, 174*(6), 747–749.

Frenk, J., Chen, L., Buhtta, Z.A., et al. (2010). Health professionals for a new century: transforming education to strengthen health systems in an interdependent world. *The Lancet, 376*, 1923–1958.

Gebbie, K. (2009). 20th century reports on nursing education: What difference did they make? *Nursing Outlook, 57*(2), 84–92.

Gold, F. (2003). Advocacy and activism: Supervised injection facilities. *Canadian Nurse, 99*(2), 14–18.

Goldstone, I. (2011, November 9). What did it take to get Insite? [Web log post]. Retrieved from: http://www.arnbc.ca/blog/what-did-it-take-to-get-insite/.

Golterman, L., & Banasiak, N.C. (2011). Evaluating web sites: Reliable child health resources for parents. *Pediatric Nursing, 37*(2), 81–83.

Hewlett, P.O., Bleich, M., Cox, M.F., & Hoover, K.W. (2009). Changing times: The role of academe in health reform. *Journal of Professional Nursing, 25*(6), 322–328.

Institute of Medicine Committee: on the Robert Wood Johnson Foundation Initiative on the Future of Nursing Education. (2010). Washington D.C: The National Academies Press.

International Council of Nurses. (2010). *The nursing community, macroeconomic and public finance policies: Towards a better understanding.* Geneva: Author. http://www.icn.ch/images/stories/documents/publications/free_publications/Nursing_macroeconmic_public_finance_policies_FINAL_with_covers.pdf

Labonte, R. (2009). The global financial crisis and health: Scaling up our effort. *Canadian Journal of Public Health, 100*(3), 173–175.

Lightfoot, B., Panessa, C., Hayden, S., Thumath, M., Goldstone, I., & Pauly, B. (2009). Gaining Insite: Harm reduction in nursing practice. *Canadian Nurse, 105*(4), 16–22.

Mill, J., Astle, B.J., Ogilvie, L., & Gastaldo, D. (2010). Linking global citizenship, undergraduate nursing education, and professional nursing: Curricular innovation in the 21st century. *Advances in Nursing Science, 33*(3), E1–E11.

Mostaghimi, A., & Crotty, B.H. (2011). Professionalism in the digital age. *Annals of Internal medicine, 154*(8), 560–562.

National Expert Commission. (2012). *A nursing call to action. The health of our nation, the future of our health system.* Ottawa: Canadian Nurses Association. http://www.cna-aicc.ca/expert commission/

Nursing Education Council of British Columbia (NECBC). (2010). A policy framework for nursing education in BC. Unpublished document. Available: http://www.bcahc.ca

Paul, P., & Ross-Kerr, J.C. (2011). The origins and development of nursing education in Canada. In J.C. Ross-Kerr & M. Wood (Eds.), *Canadian nursing: Issues and perspectives* (5th ed., pp. 327–358). Toronto, ON: Elsevier.

Pauly, B., Goldstone, I., McCall, J., Gold, F., & Payne, S. (2007). The ethical, legal and social context of harm reduction. *Canadian Nurse, 103*(8), 19–23.

Public Health Agency of Canada. (2008). *Core competencies for public health in Canada.* Ottawa: Author.

Regenberg, A.C. (2010). Tweeting science and ethics. Social media as a tool for constructive social engagement. *American Journal of Bioethics, 10*(5), 30–31.

Reutter, L., & Kushner, K.E. (2010). "Health equity through action on the social determinants of health": Taking up the challenge in nursing. *Nursing Inquiry, 17*(3), 269–280.

Sachs, J. (2011). *The price of civilization: Economics and ethics after the fall.* Toronto, ON: Random House of Canada.

Small, D., Peters, H., & Tyndall, M.W. (2006). The establishment of North America's state sanctioned supervised injection facility: A case study in culture change. *International Journal of Drug Policy, 17*(2), 73–82.

Smith, R. (2012). The last word: Broadband access equals better connections. *Canadian Nurse, 108*(8), 44.

Street, M. (1973). *Watch-fires on the mountains: The life and writings of Ethel Johns.* Toronto, ON: University of Toronto Press.

Underwood, J.M., Mowat, D.L., Meagher-Stewart, D.M., et al. (2009). Building community and public health capacity: A synthesis report of the National Community Health Nursing Study. *Canadian Journal of Public Health, 100*(5), 11–21.

United Nations. (2010). What will it take to meet the MDGs? http://content.undp.org/go/cms-service/stream/asset/;jsessionid=aMgXw9lbMbH4?asset_id=2620072

Weir, G.M. (1932). *Survey of nursing education in Canada.* Toronto, ON: University of Toronto Press.

World Health Organization (WHO). (1978). *Primary health care: Report on the international conference on primary health care.* Alma Ata, Kazakstan: Author.

———. (2008). *Primary health care: Now more than ever.* Geneva: Author.

————. (2009). *Global standards for the initial education of professional nurses and midwives.* Geneva: Author.

————. (2010). *Strategic directions for strengthening nursing and midwifery service 2011–2015.* Geneva: Author. Available at: http:www.who.int.hrh/resources/nmsd/en/index.html

————. Strengthening nursing and midwifery. *Sixty-fourth World health assembly resolution.* (May 24, 2011). Agenda item 13.4. http://apps.who.int/gb/ebwha/pdf_files/WHA64/A64_R7-en.pdf

Wood, A., Zettel, P., & Stewart, W. (2003). The Dr. Peter Centre: Harm reduction nursing. *Canadian Nurse, 99*(5), 20–24.

Index

Note: Page number followed by b, f, and t indicates boxed text, figure, and table respectively.